MOVEMENT DISORDERS IN CHILDHOOD

SECOND EDITION

ELSEVIER *science &* *technology books*

ELSEVIER

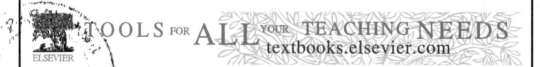
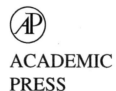

ACADEMIC PRESS

MOVEMENT DISORDERS IN CHILDHOOD

SECOND EDITION

HARVEY S. SINGER
Department of Neurology, Johns Hopkins Hospital, Baltimore, MD, USA

JONATHAN W. MINK
Division of Child Neurology, University of Rochester Medical Center, Rochester, NY, USA

DONALD L. GILBERT
Division of Neurology, Cincinnati Children's Hospital Medical Center, Cincinnati, OH, USA

JOSEPH JANKOVIC
Department of Neurology, Baylor College of Medicine, Houston, TX, USA

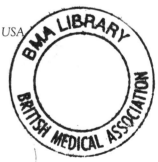

AMSTERDAM • BOSTON • HEIDELBERG • LONDON
NEW YORK • OXFORD • PARIS • SAN DIEGO
SAN FRANCISCO • SINGAPORE • SYDNEY • TOKYO
Academic Press is an imprint of Elsevier

ELSEVIER

Academic Press is an imprint of Elsevier
125, London Wall, EC2Y 5AS
525 B Street, Suite 1800, San Diego, CA 92101-4495, USA
225 Wyman Street, Waltham, MA 02451, USA
The Boulevard, Langford Lane, Kidlington, Oxford OX5 1GB, UK

ISBN: 978-0-12-411573-6

British Library Cataloguing-in-Publication Data
A catalogue record for this book is available from the British Library

Library of Congress Cataloging-in-Publication Data
A catalog record for this book is available from the Library of Congress

For information on all Academic Press publications
visit our website at http://store.elsevier.com/

Typeset by MPS Limited, Chennai, India
www.adi-mps.com

Printed and bound in the United States of America

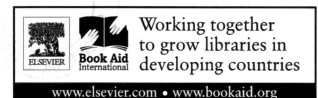

Publisher: Mica Haley
Acquisition Editor: Melanie Tucker
Editorial Project Manager: Kristi Anderson
Production Project Manager: Caroline Johnson
Designer: Victoria Pearson

Contents

V

SELECTED SECONDARY MOVEMENT DISORDERS

Preface

Movement disorders are an expanding area of specialization within the field of child neurology. Clinics devoted to pediatric movement disorders are rapidly appearing in the United States and in developed countries throughout the world. The number of fellowship training positions and child neurology residents entering the field continues to grow, although not sufficient to satisfy the growing need for pediatric movement disorder experts. National and international societies are devoting major segments of their conferences, or even entire meetings, to issues pertaining to movement disorders in children. We are also pleased to note increasing collaborations, among pediatric and adult neurologists and basic scientists, with the common goal to better understanding the etiology, mechanism, and treatment of conditions discussed in this book.

It is likely that multiple factors have contributed to the expansion of interest in the field of pediatric movement disorders. Researchers are providing new insights into the development and maintenance of motor control, volitional, and habitual behaviors. Advances have been made in identifying the underlying pathophysiologic mechanisms in several hyper- and hypokinetic movement disorders, especially regarding the circuitry interconnecting the cerebral cortex, basal ganglia, cerebellum, and brainstem. Recognizing that these same circuits are also involved in cognition and emotion, the interest and number of multi-faceted, multi-disciplinary research protocols has expanded. Progress in the areas of molecular and clinical genetics, developmental and metabolic disorders, and immunologic disorders, such as autoimmune encephalitis, has provided investigators with exciting methodologies with which to diagnose and better understand underlying disease processes. Lastly, there is the ever present awareness and desire to improve care and to develop new and improved therapies for children affected with movement disorders.

Our decision to write the first edition of this book was based on a perceived need for a high-quality, comprehensive text devoted to movement disorders in children. In order to develop this useful resource, several working guidelines were established. First and foremost, each chapter was to be written by a neurologist with a strong clinical and scientific background and expertise in the field of childhood movement disorders. Second, the number of authors would be limited, in order to maintain an active dialogue and comprehensive review of each chapter. Lastly, recognizing the educational limitations of written descriptions of abnormal movements, the inclusion of videos was a requirement. These same guidelines, successfully implemented in the first book, were again used in this second edition.

In the six years since publication of the first edition, our understanding of processes responsible for typical motor development and those underlying pathologic disorders has grown dramatically. Advances in basic and translational neuroscience, expanded clinical characterizations, availability of new diagnostic tests, and the discovery of new therapies has required a substantial revision of each chapter. However, based on the positive feedback from the initial edition, the basic format of the book was maintained. We have also added four new chapters reflecting expanded information on motor assessments, hereditary spastic paraplegias, movement disorders in auto-immune diseases, and motor disorders in neuropsychiatric conditions. We have once again attempted to provide a resource that provides a fundamental background of neuronal circuitry, a guide to efficient patient evaluation, and a comprehensive review of disorders. We hope that this information is of interest and value to readers at all levels of experience. In closing, we look forward with great anticipation to future clinical and scientific advances in the area of 'movement disorders in childhood.'

Fall 2015

Harvey S. Singer MD,
Jonathan W. Mink MD, PhD,
Donald L. Gilbert MD, MS and
Joseph Jankovic MD

Acknowledgment

The authors would like to thank the staff at Elsevier for their assistance and flexibility. In particular, we acknowledge the efforts of Melanie Tucker, Kristi Anderson and Caroline Johnson.

OVERVIEW

1

Basal Ganglia Anatomy, Biochemistry, and Physiology

Harvey S. Singer[1], Jonathan W. Mink[2],
Donald L. Gilbert[3] and Joseph Jankovic[4]

[1]Department of Neurology, Johns Hopkins Hospital, Baltimore, MD, USA;
[2]Division of Child Neurology, University of Rochester Medical Center,
Rochester, NY, USA; [3]Division of Neurology, Cincinnati Children's Hospital
Medical Center, Cincinnati, OH, USA; [4]Department of Neurology, Baylor
College of Medicine, Houston, TX, USA

Movement Disorders in Childhood, Second Edition.
DOI: http://dx.doi.org/10.1016/B978-0-12-411573-6.00001-2

3

INTRODUCTION

The basal ganglia are large subcortical structures comprising several interconnected nuclei in the forebrain, diencephalon, and midbrain. Historically, the basal ganglia have been viewed as a component of the motor system. However, there is now substantial evidence that the basal ganglia interact with all of frontal cortex and with the limbic system. Thus, the basal ganglia likely have a role in cognitive and emotional function in addition to their role in motor control.[1] Indeed, diseases of the basal ganglia often cause a combination of movement, affective, and cognitive disorders. The motor circuits of the basal ganglia are better understood than the other circuits, but because of similar organization of the circuitry, conceptual understanding of basal ganglia motor function can provide a useful framework for understanding cognitive and affective function too.

CIRCUITS AND NEUROTRANSMITTERS IN THE BASAL GANGLIA

The basal ganglia include the striatum (caudate, putamen, and nucleus accumbens), the subthalamic nucleus (STN), the globus pallidus (internal segment (GPi), external segment (GPe), and ventral pallidum (VP)), and the substantia nigra (pars compacta (SNpc) and pars reticulata (SNpr)) (Figure 1.1). The striatum and STN receive the majority of their inputs from outside of the basal ganglia. Most of those inputs come from cerebral cortex, but thalamic nuclei also provide strong inputs to striatum. The bulk of the outputs from the basal ganglia arise from the GPi, VP, and SNpr. These outputs are inhibitory to the pedunculopontine area in the brainstem and to thalamic nuclei that in turn project to frontal lobe.

The striatum receives the bulk of extrinsic input to the basal ganglia. The striatum receives excitatory input from virtually all of cerebral cortex.[2] In addition, the ventral striatum (nucleus accumbens and rostroventral extensions of caudate and putamen) receives inputs from hippocampus and amygdala.[3] The cortical input uses glutamate as its neurotransmitter and terminates largely on the heads of the dendritic spines of medium spiny neurons.[4] The projection from the cerebral cortex to striatum has a roughly topographic organization that provides the basis for an organization of functionally different circuits in the basal ganglia.[5,6] Although the topography implies a certain degree of parallel organization, there is also evidence for convergence and divergence in the corticostriatal projection. The large dendritic fields of medium spiny neurons[7] allow them to receive input from adjacent projections, which arise from different areas of cortex. Inputs to striatum from several functionally related cortical areas overlap and a single cortical area projects divergently to multiple striatal zones.[8,9] Thus, there is a multiple convergent and divergent organization within a broader framework of functionally different parallel circuits. This organization provides an anatomical framework for the integration and transformation of cortical information in the striatum.

Cell types in the Basal Ganglia

Medium spiny striatal neurons make up 90–95% of the striatal neuron population. They project outside of the striatum and receive a number of inputs in addition to the important

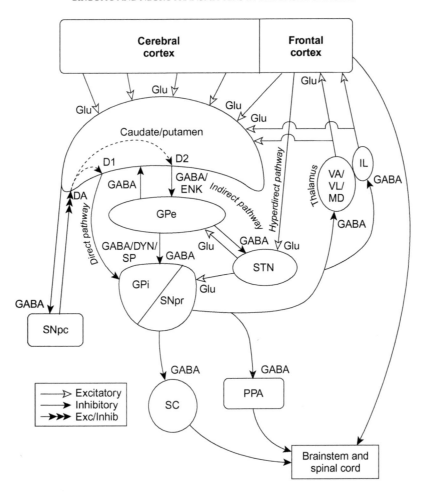

FIGURE 1.1 Simplified schematic diagram of basal ganglia-thalamocortical circuitry. Excitatory connections are indicated by open arrows and inhibitory connections by filled arrows. The modulatory dopamine projection is indicated by a three-headed arrow. dyn, dynorphin; enk, enkephalin; GABA, gamma-amino-butyric acid; glu, glutamate; GPe, globus pallidus pars externa; GPi, globus pallidus pars interna; IL, intralaminar thalamic nuclei; MD, mediodorsal nucleus; PPA, pedunculopontine area; SC, superior colliculus; SNpc, substantia nigra pars compacta; SNpr, substantia nigra pars reticulata; SP, substance P; STN, subthalamic nucleus; VA, ventral anterior nucleus; VL, ventral lateral nucleus.

cortical input, including (1) excitatory glutamatergic inputs from thalamus; (2) cholinergic input from striatal interneurons; (3) gamma-amino-butyric acid (GABA), substance P, and enkephalin input from adjacent medium spiny striatal neurons; (4) GABA input from fast-spiking interneurons; (5) a large input from dopamine-containing neurons in the SNpc; (6) a more sparse input from the serotonin-containing neurons in the dorsal and median raphe nuclei.

The fast-spiking GABAergic striatal interneurons make up only 2–4% of the striatal neuron population, but they exert powerful inhibition on medium spiny neurons. Like medium spiny neurons, they receive excitatory inputs from cerebral cortex. They appear to play an important role in limiting the activity of medium spiny neurons and in focusing the spatial pattern of their activation.[10] Abnormalities in the number or function of these neurons have been linked to the pathobiology of involuntary movements.[11–13]

Dopamine

The dopamine input to the striatum terminates largely on the shafts of the dendritic spines of medium spiny neurons where it is in a position to modulate transmission from the cerebral cortex to the striatum.[14] The action of dopamine on striatal neurons depends on the type of dopamine receptor involved. Five types of G protein-coupled dopamine receptors have been described (D1 … D5).[15] These have been grouped into two families based on their linkage to adenyl cyclase activity and response to agonists. The D1 family includes D1 and D5 receptors and the D2 family includes D2, D3, and D4 receptors. The conventional view has been that dopamine acts at D1 receptors to facilitate the activity of postsynaptic neurons and at D2 receptors to inhibit postsynaptic neurons.[16] Indeed, this is a fundamental concept for currently popular models of basal ganglia pathophysiology.[17,18] However, the physiologic effect of dopamine on striatal neurons is more complex. While activation of dopamine D1 receptors potentiates the effect of cortical input to striatal neurons in some states, it reduces the efficacy of cortical input in others.[19] Activation of D2 receptors more consistently decreases the effect of cortical input to striatal neuron.[20] Dopamine contributes to focusing the spatial and temporal patterns of striatal activity.

In addition to short-term facilitation or inhibition of striatal activity, there is evidence that dopamine can modulate corticostriatal transmission by mechanisms of long-term depression (LTD) and long-term potentiation (LTP). Through these mechanisms, dopamine strengthens or weakens the efficacy of corticostriatal synapses and can thus mediate reinforcement of specific discharge patterns. LTP and LTD are thought to be fundamental to many neural mechanisms of learning and may underlie the hypothesized role of the basal ganglia in habit learning.[21] SNpc dopamine neurons fire in relation to behaviorally significant events and reward.[22] These signals are likely to modify the responses of striatal neurons to inputs that occur in conjunction with the dopamine signal resulting in the reinforcement of motor and other behavior patterns. Striatal lesions or focal striatal dopamine depletion impairs the learning of new movement sequences,[23] supporting a role for the basal ganglia in certain types of procedural learning.

GABA

Medium spiny striatal neurons contain the inhibitory neurotransmitter GABA and co-localized peptide neurotransmitters.[24,25] Based on the type of neurotransmitters and the predominant type of dopamine receptor they contain, the medium spiny neurons can be divided into two populations. One population contains GABA, dynorphin, and substance P and primarily expresses D1 dopamine receptors. These neurons project to the basal ganglia output nuclei, GPi, and SNpr. The second population contains GABA and enkephalin and primarily expresses D2 dopamine receptors. These neurons project to the external segment of the globus pallidus (GPe).[17]

Acetylcholine

Although there are no apparent regional differences in the striatum based on cell type, an intricate internal organization has been revealed with special stains. When the striatum is stained for acetylcholinesterase (AChE), there is a patchy distribution of lightly staining regions within more heavily stained regions.[26] The AChE-poor patches have been called *striosomes* and the AChE-rich areas have been called the extrastriosomal *matrix*. The matrix forms the bulk of the striatal volume and receives input from most areas of cerebral cortex. Within the matrix are clusters of neurons with similar inputs that have been termed *matrisomes*. The bulk of the output from cells in the matrix is to both segments of the GP, VP, and to SNpr. The striosomes receive input from prefrontal cortex and send output to SNpc.[27] Immunohistochemical techniques have demonstrated that many substances such as substance P, dynorphin, and enkephalin have a patchy distribution that may be partly or wholly in register with the striosomes. The striosome-matrix organization suggests a level of functional segregation within the striatum. The clinical significance of this organization is not well understood.

SUBTHALAMIC NUCLEUS (STN)

The STN receives an excitatory, glutamatergic input from many areas of frontal lobes with especially large inputs from motor areas of cortex.[28] The STN also receives an inhibitory GABA input from GPe. The output from the STN is glutamatergic and excitatory to the basal ganglia output nuclei, GPi, VP, and SNpr. STN also sends an excitatory projection back to GPe. There is a somatotopic organization in STN[29] and a relative topographic separation of "motor" and "cognitive" inputs to STN.

OUTPUT NUCLEI: GLOBUS PALLIDUS INTERNA (GPi) AND SUBSTANTIA NIGRA PARS RETICULATA (SNpr)

The primary basal ganglia output arises from GPi, a GPi-like component of VP, and SNpr. As described above, GPi and SNpr receive excitatory input from STN and inhibitory input from striatum. They also receive an inhibitory input from GPe. The dendritic fields of GPi, VP, and SNpr neurons span up to 1 mm diameter and thus have the potential to integrate a large number of converging inputs.[30] The output from GPi, VP, and SNpr is inhibitory and uses GABA as its neurotransmitter. The primary output is directed to thalamic nuclei that project to the frontal lobes: the ventrolateral, ventroanterior, and mediodorsal nuclei. The thalamic targets of GPi, VP, and SNpr project, in turn, to frontal lobe, with the strongest output going to motor areas. Collaterals of the axons projecting to thalamus project to an area at the junction of the midbrain and pons in the region of the pedunculopontine nucleus.[31] Other output neurons (20%) project to intralaminar nuclei of the thalamus, to the lateral habenula, or to the superior colliculus.[32]

The basal ganglia motor output has a somatotopic organization such that the body below the neck is largely represented in GPi and the head and eyes are largely represented in SNpr.

The separate representation of different body parts is maintained throughout the basal ganglia. Within the representation of an individual body part, it also appears that there is segregation of outputs to different motor areas of cortex and that an individual GPi neuron sends output via thalamus to just one area of cortex.[33] Thus, GPi neurons that project via thalamus to motor cortex are adjacent to, but separate from, those that project to premotor cortex or supplementary motor area. GPi neurons that project via thalamus to prefrontal cortex are also separate from those projecting to motor areas and from VP neurons projecting via thalamus to orbitofrontal cortex. The anatomic segregation of basal ganglia-thalamocortical outputs suggests functional segregation at the output level, but other anatomic evidence suggests interactions between circuits within the basal ganglia.[5,34]

GLOBUS PALLIDUS EXTERNA (GPe)

The GPe and the GPe-like part of VP may be viewed as intrinsic nuclei of the basal ganglia. Like GPi and SNpr, GPe receives an inhibitory projection from the striatum and an excitatory one from STN. Unlike GPi, the striatal projection to GPe contains GABA and enkephalin but not substance P.[17] The output of GPe is quite different from the output of GPi. The output from GPe is GABAergic and inhibitory and the majority of the output projects to STN. The connections from striatum to GPe, from GPe to STN, and from STN to GPi form the "indirect" striatopallidal pathway to GPi[35] (Figure 1.1). In addition, there is a monosynaptic GABAergic inhibitory output from GPe directly to GPi and to SNpr and a GABAergic projection back to striatum.[36] Thus, GPe neurons are in a position to provide feedback inhibition to neurons in striatum and STN and feedforward inhibition to neurons in GPi and SNpr. This circuitry suggests that GPe may act to oppose, limit, or focus the effect of the striatal and STN projections to GPi and SNpr as well as focus activity in these output nuclei.

Dopamine input to the striatum arises from SNpc and the ventral tegmental area (VTA). SNpc projects to most of the striatum; VTA projects to the ventral striatum. The SNpc and VTA are made up of large dopamine-containing cells. SNpc receives input from the striatum, specifically from the striosomes. This input is GABAergic and inhibitory. The SNpc and VTA dopamine neurons project to caudate and putamen in a topographic manner,[34] but with overlap. The nigral dopamine neurons receive inputs from one striatal circuit and project back to the same and to adjacent circuits. Thus, they appear to be in a position to modulate activity across functionally different circuits.

INHIBITING AND DISINHIBITING MOTOR PATTERNS

Although the basal ganglia intrinsic circuitry is complex, the overall picture is of two primary pathways through the basal ganglia from cerebral cortex with the output directed via thalamus at the frontal lobes. These pathways consist of two disynaptic pathways from cortex to the basal ganglia output (Figure 1.2). In addition, there are several multisynaptic pathways involving GPe. The two disynaptic pathways are from cortex through (1) striatum (the *direct pathway*) and (2) STN (the *hyperdirect pathway*) to the basal ganglia outputs. These

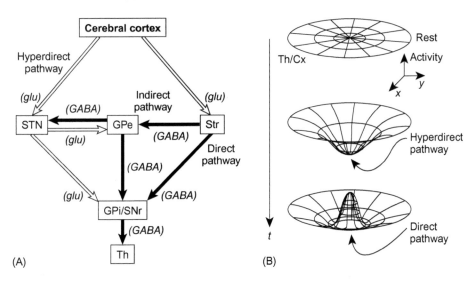

FIGURE 1.2 (A) Schematic diagram of the hyperdirect cortico-subthalamo-pallidal, direct cortico-striatopalli-dal, and indirect cortico-striato-GPe-subthalamo-GPi pathways. White and black arrows represent excitatory glu-tamatergic (glu) and inhibitory GABAergic (GABA) projections, respectively. GPe, external segment of the globus pallidus; GPi, internal segment of the globus pallidus; SNr, substantia nigra pars reticulata; STN, subthalamic nucleus; Str, striatum; Th, thalamus. (B) A schematic diagram explaining the activity change over time (*t*) in the thalamocortical projection (Th/Cx) following the sequential inputs through the hyperdirect cortico-subthalamo-pallidal (*middle*) and direct cortico-striatopallidal (*bottom*) pathways. *Modified from Ref. [37].*

pathways have important anatomical and functional differences. First, the cortical input to STN comes only from frontal lobe whereas the input to striatum arises from virtually all areas of cerebral cortex. Second, the output from STN is excitatory, whereas the output from striatum is inhibitory. Third, the excitatory route through STN is faster than the inhibitory route through striatum.[37] Finally, the STN projection to GPi is divergent and the striatal projection is more focused.[38] Thus, the two disynaptic pathways from cerebral cortex to the basal ganglia output nuclei, GPi and SNpr, provide fast, widespread, divergent excitation through STN and slower, focused, inhibition through striatum. This organization provides an anatomical basis for focused inhibition and surround excitation of neurons in GPi and SNpr (Figure 1.3). Because the output of GPi and SNpr is inhibitory, this results in focused facilitation and surround inhibition of basal ganglia-thalamocortical targets. The tonically active inhibitory output of the basal ganglia acts as a "brake" on motor pattern generators (MPGs) in the cerebral cortex (via thalamus) and brainstem. When a movement is initiated by a particular MPG, basal ganglia output neurons projecting to competing MPGs increase their firing rate, thereby increasing inhibition and applying a "brake" on those generators. Other basal ganglia output neurons projecting to the generators involved in the desired movement decrease their discharge, thereby removing tonic inhibition and releasing the "brake" from the desired motor patterns. Thus, the intended movement is enabled and competing movements are prevented from interfering with the desired one.[28,39]

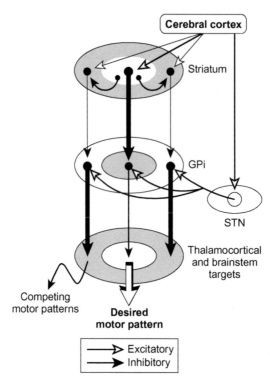

FIGURE 1.3 Schematic of normal functional organization of the basal ganglia output. Excitatory projections are indicated with open arrows; inhibitory projections are indicated with filled arrows. Relative magnitude of activity is represented by line thickness. *Modified from Ref. [40].*

IMPLICATIONS FOR DISEASE: FOCAL LESIONS AND ABNORMAL MOVEMENTS

This scheme provides a framework for understanding both the pathophysiology of Parkinsonism[28,41] and involuntary movement.[28,39] Different involuntary movements such as Parkinsonism, chorea, dystonia, or tics result from different abnormalities in the basal ganglia circuits. Loss of dopamine input to the striatum results in a loss of normal pauses of GPi discharge during voluntary movement. Hence, there is excessive inhibition of MPGs and ultimately bradykinesia.[41] Furthermore, loss of dopamine results in abnormal synchrony of GPi neuronal discharge and loss of the normal spatial and temporal focus of GPi activity.[41–43] Broad lesions of GPi or SNpr disinhibit both desired and unwanted motor patterns leading to inappropriate activation of competing motor patterns, but normal generation of the wanted movement. Thus, lesions of GPi cause cocontraction of multiple muscle groups and difficulty turning off unwanted motor patterns, similar to what is seen in dystonia, but do not affect movement initiation.[44] Lesions of SNpr cause unwanted saccadic eye movements that interfere with the ability to maintain visual fixation, but do not impair the initiation of voluntary saccades.[45] Lesions of putamen may cause dystonia due to the loss of focused inhibition in GPi.[39] Lesions of STN produce continuous involuntary movements of the contralateral limbs (hemiballism or hemichorea).[39] Despite the involuntary movements, voluntary movements can still be performed. Although structural lesions of putamen, GPi,

SNpr, or STN produce certain types of unwanted movements or behaviors, they do not produce tics. Tics are more likely to arise from abnormal activity patterns in the striatum.[12,39]

Although the focus of this discussion of basal ganglia circuits has been on motor control and movement disorders, it is likely that the fundamental principles of function in the somatomotor, oculomotor, limbic, and cognitive basal ganglia circuits are similar. If the basic scheme of facilitation and inhibition of competing movements is extended to encompass more complex behaviors and thoughts, many features of basal ganglia disorders can be explained as a failure to facilitate wanted behaviors and simultaneously inhibit unwanted behaviors due to abnormal basal ganglia output patterns. Indeed, many movement disorders are accompanied by cognitive and affective symptoms.[46–48]

References

1. Baez-Mendoza R, Schultz W. The role of the striatum in social behavior. *Front Neurosci*. 2013;7:233.
2. Kemp JM, Powell TPS. The corticostriate projection in the monkey. *Brain*. 1970;93:525–546.
3. Fudge J, Kunishio K, Walsh C, Richard D, Haber S. Amygdaloid projections to ventromedial striatal subterritories in the primate. *Neuroscience*. 2002;110:257–275.
4. Cherubini E, Herrling PL, Lanfumey L, Stanzione P. Excitatory amino acids in synaptic excitation of rat striatal neurones in vitro. *J Physiol*. 1988;400:677–690.
5. Kelly R, Strick PL. Macro-architecture of basal ganglia loops with the cerebral cortex: use of rabies virus to reveal multisynaptic circuits. *Prog Brain Res*. 2004;143:449–459.
6. Alexander GE, DeLong MR, Strick PL. Parallel organization of functionally segregated circuits linking basal ganglia and cortex. *Ann Rev Neurosci*. 1986;9:357–381.
7. Wilson CJ, Groves PM. Fine structure and synaptic connections of the common spiny neuron of the rat neostriatum: a study employing intracellular injection of horseradish peroxidase. *J Comp Neurol*. 1980;194:599–614.
8. Selemon LD, Goldman-Rakic PS. Longitudinal topography and interdigitation of corticostriatal projections in the rhesus monkey. *J Neurosci*. 1985;5:776–794.
9. Flaherty AW, Graybiel AM. Corticostriatal transformations in the primate somatosensory system. Projections from physiologically mapped body-part representations. *J Neurophysiol*. 1991;66(4):1249–1263.
10. Mallet N, Le Moine C, Charpier S, Gonon F. Feedforward inhibition of projection neurons by fast-spiking GABA interneurons in the rat striatum in vivo. *J Neurosci*. 2005;25(15):3857–3869.
11. Kataoka Y, Kalanithi PS, Grantz H, et al. Decreased number of parvalbumin and cholinergic interneurons in the striatum of individuals with Tourette syndrome. *J Comp Neurol*. 2010;518(3):277–291.
12. McCairn KW, Bronfeld M, Belelovsky K, Bar-Gad I. The neurophysiological correlates of motor tics following focal striatal disinhibition. *Brain*. 2009;132(Pt 8):2125–2138.
13. Gittis AH, Leventhal DK, Fensterheim BA, Pettibone JR, Berke JD, Kreitzer AC. Selective inhibition of striatal fast-spiking interneurons causes dyskinesias. *J Neurosci*. 2011;31(44):15727–15731.
14. Bouyer JJ, Park DH, Joh TH, Pickel VM. Chemical and structural analysis of the relation between cortical inputs and tyrosine hydroxylase-containing terminals in rat neostriatum. *Brain Res*. 1984;302:267–275.
15. Sibley DR, Monsma FJ. Molecular biology of dopamine receptors. *Trends Pharm Sci*. 1992;13:61–69.
16. Gerfen CR, Engber TM, Mahan LC, et al. D_1 and D_2 dopamine receptor-regulated gene expression of striatonigral and striatopallidal neurons. *Science*. 1990;250:1429–1432.
17. Albin RL, Young AB, Penney JB. The functional anatomy of basal ganglia disorders. *Trends Neurosci*. 1989;12:366–375.
18. DeLong MR. Primate models of movement disorders of basal ganglia origin. *Trends Neurosci*. 1990;13:281–285.
19. Hernandez-Lopez S, Bargas J, Surmeier DJ, Reyes A, Galarraga E. D1 receptor activation enhances evoked discharge in neostriatal medium spiny neurons by modulating an L-type Ca2+ conductance. *J Neurosci*. 1997;17(9):3334–3342.
20. Nicola S, Surmeier J, Malenka R. Dopaminergic modulation of neuronal excitability in the striatum and nucleus accumbens. *Ann Rev Neurosci*. 2000;23:185–215.
21. Jog M, Kubota Y, Connolly C, Hillegaart V, Graybiel A. Building neural representations of habits. *Science*. 1999;286:1745–1749.

22. Schultz W, Romo R, Ljungberg T, Mirenowicz J, Hollerman JR, Dickinson A. Reward-related signals carried by dopamine neurons. In: Houk JC, Davis JL, Beiser DG, eds. *Models of Information Processing in the Basal Ganglia*. Cambridge, MA: MIT Press; 1995:233–249.

23. Matsumoto N, Hanakawa T, Maki S, Graybiel AM, Kimura M. Role of nigrostriatal dopamine system in learning to perform sequential motor tasks in a predictive manner. *J Neurophysiol*. 1999;82:978–998.

24. Kreitzer AC. Physiology and pharmacology of striatal neurons. *Ann Rev Neurosci*. 2009;32:127–147.

25. Penny GR, Afsharpour S, Kitai ST. The glutamate decarboxylase-, leucine enkephalin-, methionine enkephalin- and substance P-immunoreactive neurons in the neostriatum of the rat and cat: evidence for partial population overlap. *Neuroscience*. 1986;17:1011–1045.

26. Graybiel AM, Aosaki T, Flaherty AW, Kimura M. The basal ganglia and adaptive motor control. *Science*. 1994;265:1826–1831.

27. Gerfen CR. The neostriatal mosaic: multiple levels of compartmental organization in the basal ganglia. *Ann Rev Neurosci*. 1992;15:285–320.

28. Mink JW. The basal ganglia: focused selection and inhibition of competing motor programs. *Prog Neurobiol*. 1996;50:381–425.

29. Nambu A, Takada M, Inase M, Tokuno H. Dual somatotopical representations in the primate subthalamic nucleus: evidence for ordered but reversed body-map transformations from the primary motor cortex and the supplementary motor area. *J Neurosci*. 1996;16(8):2671–2683.

30. Percheron G, Yelnik J, Francois C. A Golgi analysis of the primate globus pallidus. III. Spatial organization of the striato-pallidal complex. *J Comp Neurol*. 1984;227:214–227.

31. Parent A. Extrinsic connections of the basal ganglia. *Trends Neurosci*. 1990;13(7):254–258.

32. Francois C, Percheron G, Yelnik J, Tande D. A topographic study of the course of nigral axons and of the distribution of pallidal axonal endings in the centre median-parafascicular complex of macaques. *Brain Res*. 1988;473:181–186.

33. Hoover JE, Strick PL. Multiple output channels in the basal ganglia. *Science*. 1993;259:819–821.

34. Haber SN, Fudge JL, McFarland NR. Striatonigrostriatal pathways in primates form an ascending spiral from the shell to the dorsolateral striatum. *J Neurosci*. 2000;20:2369–2382.

35. Alexander GE, Crutcher MD. Functional architecture of basal ganglia circuits: neural substrates of parallel processing. *Trends Neurosci*. 1990;13(7):266–271.

36. Bolam JP, Hanley JJ, Booth PA, Bevan MD. Synaptic organisation of the basal ganglia. *J Anat*. 2000;196:527–542.

37. Nambu A, Tokuno H, Hamada I, et al. Excitatory cortical inputs to pallidal neurons via the subthalamic nucleus in the monkey. *J Neurophysiol*. 2000;84:289–300.

38. Parent A, Hazrati L-N. Anatomical aspects of information processing in primate basal ganglia. *Trends Neurosci*. 1993;16(3):111–116.

39. Mink J. The basal ganglia and involuntary movements: impaired inhibition of competing motor patterns. *Arch Neurol*. 2003;60:1365–1368.

40. Mink JW. Basal ganglia dysfunction in Tourette's syndrome: a new hypothesis. *Pediatr Neurol*. 2001;25:190–198.

41. Boraud T, Bezard E, Bioulac B, Gross CE. From single extracellular unit recording in experimental and human Parkinsonism to the development of a functional concept of the role played by the basal ganglia in motor control. *Prog Neurobiol*. 2002;66:265–283.

42. Raz A, Vaadia E, Bergman H. Firing patterns and correlations of spontaneous discharge of pallidal neurons in the normal and the tremulous 1-methyl-4-phenyl-1,2,3,6-tetrahydropyridine vervet model of Parkinsonism. *J Neurosci*. 2000;20:8559–8571.

43. Tremblay L, Filion M, Bedard PJ. Responses of pallidal neurons to striatal stimulation in monkeys with MPTP-induce Parkinsonism. *Brain Res*. 1989;498:17–33.

44. Mink JW, Thach WT. Basal ganglia motor control. III. Pallidal ablation: normal reaction time, muscle cocontraction, and slow movement. *J Neurophysiol*. 1991;65:330–351.

45. Hikosaka O, Wurtz RH. Modification of saccadic eye movements by GABA-related substances. II. Effects of muscimol in monkey substantia nigra pars reticulata. *J Neurophysiol*. 1985;53(1):292–308.

46. Asmus F, Gasser T. Dystonia-plus syndromes. *Eur J Neurol*. 2010;17(suppl 1):37–45.

47. Poletti M, De Rosa A, Bonuccelli U. Affective symptoms and cognitive functions in Parkinson's disease. *J Neurol Sci*. 2012;317(1–2):97–102.

48. Ross CA, Aylward EH, Wild EJ, et al. Huntington disease: natural history, biomarkers and prospects for therapeutics. *Nat Rev Neurol*. 2014;10(4):204–216.

Cerebellar Anatomy, Biochemistry, Physiology, and Plasticity

Harvey S. Singer[1], Jonathan W. Mink[2],
Donald L. Gilbert[3] and Joseph Jankovic[4]

[1]Department of Neurology, Johns Hopkins Hospital, Baltimore, MD, USA;
[2]Division of Child Neurology, University of Rochester Medical Center,
Rochester, NY, USA; [3]Division of Neurology, Cincinnati Children's Hospital
Medical Center, Cincinnati, OH, USA; [4]Department of Neurology, Baylor
College of Medicine, Houston, TX, USA

OUTLINE

Movement Disorders in Childhood, Second Edition.
DOI: http://dx.doi.org/10.1016/B978-0-12-411573-6.00002-4

13

INTRODUCTION

The objective of this chapter is to provide an overview of the basic anatomic and functional organization of the cerebellum and its inflow and outflow pathways. Structures, pathways, circuits, and receptor systems are emphasized with regard to their relevance to diagnosis and management in children. This information provides a context for understanding the development of motor control in healthy children as well as the failure to develop it, or loss of it, in conditions such as the ataxias. Topics of anatomy of more limited relevance to children, such as the circulatory system, are omitted.

A number of challenges make diagnosis of cerebellar disorders and diseases more difficult in pediatrics. First, in children, symptoms of cerebellar dysfunction emerge in the context of a developing motor system. The child is developing motor control of eye movements, muscles of speech, axial truncal muscles, and distal muscles. Clinical experience with the range of trajectories of typical development in healthy children is often vital for detecting pathology. Second, movement disorders in children are usually mixed. For example, diseases named for their ataxia may have prominent dystonia, and complicated spastic paraplegias may involve cerebellum and basal ganglia. Third, in the presence of epilepsy, cognitive dysfunction, or behavior problems, medications may be prescribed that precipitate, exacerbate, or cause cerebellar dysfunction. These issues are addressed more specifically in the chapters on the relevant disease phenomenologies.

This chapter provides a clinically relevant overview. For more comprehensive descriptions, readers are referred to a number of excellent reviews.[1–7]

OVERVIEW OF CEREBELLAR STRUCTURE, FUNCTION, AND SYMPTOMS

Our present understanding of cerebellar function and disease has evolved over the last 100 years through painstaking clinical and pathologic observation and gross ablational studies in animals.[8,9] More recently, insights from imaging studies[10] have been augmented through experiments utilizing virus transneuronal tracers to identify cerebellar projections and loops to motor and nonmotor cerebral and basal ganglia nodes.[4] Understanding the roles of specific cell types, synapses, and calcium, flux in motor control and neuroplasticity has expanded due to electrophysiological recording and targeted mutations in transgenic mice.[2,3] Increasingly, it has become possible to test and validate some of these relationships noninvasively in healthy (primarily adult) humans stimulating cerebellum using transcranial magnetic stimulation (TMS; single pulse, paired pulse, or repetitive) and transcranial direct current stimulation (tDCS; anodal or cathodal).[11] Collectively, these techniques will continue to advance our understanding of motor and nonmotor functions of the cerebellum and improve our therapeutics for diseases of the cerebellum.

Of particular recent interest is testing of models to understand the basic operations by which the cerebellum integrates sensory information to produce adaptive, controlled movements. Models account for the necessary time interval between motor activities and the sensory feedback of those motor activities and posit a need to "estimate" future motor positions in order to perform fast and accurate movements. Trial and error in motor learning may involve climbing fiber inputs carrying error signals to specific Purkinje neurons. Motor learning may also generate internal models in the cerebellum which would allow for subsequent movements to be assembled and performed without conscious control of specific movement of elements.[7]

MACROSCOPIC TO MICROSCOPIC CEREBELLAR STRUCTURE

The cerebellum contains more than half of all neurons in the central nervous system.[12] Its organization is hierarchic and has been considered to be highly regular. Some recent evidence has emerged that the mammalian cerebellar cortex's cytoarchitecture contains microcircuits with differing properties, underlying functional variations in information processing.[13] This section presents a simplified, hierarchical model of cerebellar anatomy, circuits, and neurotransmission as a basis for understanding the cerebellum's role in development of motor and behavioral control as well as symptoms of and treatments for cerebellar diseases.

Cerebellar Structural "Threes"

Heuristically, *three* is a helpful mnemonic for remembering cerebellar anatomy. The cerebellum has three major anatomic components that may be affected by focal pathologic processes; three major functional regions that correspond moderately to these components and subserve somewhat distinct functions; three sets of paired peduncles that carry information into and out of the cerebellum via the pons; three cortical cell layers that interconnect via predominantly glutamatergic and GABAergic signals; and three deep cerebellar output nuclei that transmit cerebellar signal out to the cerebrum.

The Three Anatomic Regions—Structures and Afferent Connections

The cerebellum has surface gray matter, medullary white matter, and deep gray matter nuclei. Analogous to cerebral gyri and sulci, folia make up the surface of the cerebellum. Beneath the folia, the myelin develops during childhood and is susceptible to a wide variety of diseases affecting white matter. Innermost are the deep cerebellar nuclei.

The clefts between folia run transversely, demarcating the three main anatomic regions, the flocculonodular, anterior, and posterior lobes, as shown in Figure 2.1 and described in Table 2.1.

The Three Cerebellar Functional Regions Connect to Three Deep Cerebellar Nuclei

At a gross structural level, it can be helpful to think about the motor control and signs of cerebellar disease in terms of the three functional divisions of the cerebellum: (1) the *vestibulocerebellum*, in the flocculonodular lobe, involved in axial control and balance and positional reflexes; (2) the *spinocerebellum*, in the vermis and medial portion of the cerebellar hemispheres, involved in ongoing maintenance of tone, execution, and control of axial and

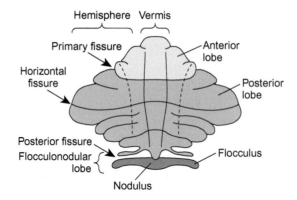

FIGURE 2.1   Schematic of the three lobes of the cerebellum (anterior, posterior, and flocculonodular) and three anatomic regions (hemispheres, vermis, and nodulus). *From Ref. [14].*

TABLE 2.1   Lobes and Pathways in the Cerebellum

Anatomic region	Structures	Input
Flocculonodular lobe	Flocculus—two small appendages inferiorly located	Vestibular
	Nodulus—inferior vermis	
Anterior lobes	A smaller region of the cerebellar hemispheres and vermis anterior to the primary cerebellar fissure	Spinal cord—spinocerebellar pathways
Posterior lobes	Largest, most lateral, and phylogenetically latest region of cerebellar hemispheres	Cerebrocortical, via pons

proximal (vermis) and distal movements; and (3) the *cerebrocerebellum*, in the lateral part of the hemisphere, involved in initiation, motor planning, and timing of coordinated movements. Functional anatomy of the cerebellum and associated, localizing signs of cerebellar diseases are presented in Table 2.2.

The vestibulocerebellum, spinocerebellum, and cerebrocerebellum subserve basic functions of execution and integration of information about balance, body position and movement, and motor planning and timing. Output from these regions goes to the deep cerebellar nuclei.

The deep cerebellar nuclei, arranged medially to laterally, are the fastigial, interposed, and dentate nuclei. The interposed nucleus consists of the globose (medial) and emboliform (lateral) nuclei. Anatomy, output nuclei, and function of these regions are described in Table 2.3.

The Three Cerebellar Peduncles

Three paired sets of peduncles carry fibers to and from the cerebellum. The cerebellum has a direct connection to the spinal cord. Cerebellar connections with the spinal cord and body (spinocerebellar) are ipsilateral. Cerebellar connections with the cerebrum (cerebrocerebellar, via dentate-rubral-thalamic tract) are contralateral. That is, motor control of the right side of

TABLE 2.2   Functional Anatomy of the Cerebellum

EYE MOVEMENTS

Anatomy	Vestibulocerebellum
	Vestibular system afferents to the cerebellar flocculus, paraflocculus, dorsal vermis
Function	Integration of both position and velocity information so that the eyes remain on target
Signs	*Nystagmus*—oscillatory, rhythmical movements of the eyes
	Impairment with maintaining gaze
	Difficulties with smooth visual pursuit
	Undershooting (hypometria) or overshooting (hypermetria) of saccades

---

SPEECH

Anatomy	Spinocerebellum—vermis
	Cerebrocerebellum
	Sensory afferents from face
	Corticocerebellar pathway afferents, via pons
Function	Ongoing monitoring, control of facial muscles
Signs	Dysarthria, imprecise production of consonant sounds
	Dysrhythmia of speech production
	Poor regulation of prosody. Slow, irregularly emphasized, i.e., *scanning*, speech

---

TRUNK MOVEMENTS

Anatomy	Vestibulocerebellum
	Spinocerebellum
	Sensory, vestibular, and proprioceptive afferents
Function	Integration of head and body position information to stabilize trunk and head
Signs	Unsteadiness while standing or sitting, compensatory actions such as use of visual input or stabilization with hands
	Titubation—Characteristic bobbing of the head and trunk

LIMB MOVEMENTS

Anatomy	Spinocerebellum
	Cerebrocerebellum
	Sensory and proprioceptive afferents to spinocerebellum
	Corticocerebellar pathway afferents via pons
Function	Integration of input from above—cortical motor areas—about intended commands allows for control of muscle tone in the execution of ongoing movement
	The spinocerebellum monitors and regulates ongoing muscle activity to compensate for small changes in load during activity and to dampen physiological oscillation
	. The cerebrocerebellar pathway input contains information about intended movement

(Continued)

TABLE 2.2   (Continued)

Signs	Hypotonia—diminished resistance to passive limb displacement
	Rebound—delay in response to rapid imposed movements and overshoot
	Pendular reflexes
	Imprecise targeting of rapid distal limb movements
	Delays in initiating movement
	Intention tremor—tremor at the end of movement seen on finger-to-nose and heel-to-shin testing
	Dysynergia/asynergia—decomposition of normal, coordinated execution of movement—errors in the relative timing of components of complex multijoint movements
	Difficulties with spatial coordination of hand and fine fractionated finger movements
	Dysdiadochokinesia—errors in rate and regularity of movements, including alternating movements.

GAIT

Anatomy	Vestibulocerebellum
	Spinocerebellum
	Cerebrocerebellum
Function	Maintenance of balance, posture, tone, ongoing monitoring of gait execution
Symptoms	Broad based, staggering gait

TABLE 2.3   Summary of Cerebellar Structure and Function

Functional	Anatomic	Output nuclei	Function
Vestibulocerebellum	Flocculonodular	Vestibular nuclei (medulla, not cerebellum)	Balance, vestibular reflex, axial control
Spinocerebellum	Vermis	Fastigial nuclei	Motor control and execution, axial and proximal muscles
	Medial aspect of cerebellar hemispheres	Interposed (globose plus emboliform) nuclei	Motor control and execution, distal muscles
Cerebrocerebellum	Lateral cerebellar hemispheres	Dentate nuclei	Planning, timing coordinated movements

the body is controlled by the left cerebrum with the right cerebellum. Motor control of the left side of the body is controlled by the right cerebrum with the left cerebellum. Connections from the cerebrum to the cerebellum, via pons, therefore cross on entry and exit, whereas ascending connections from the spinal cord largely do not. Figure 2.2 shows a schema of the key pathways through the peduncles, and additional detail is provided in Table 2.4.

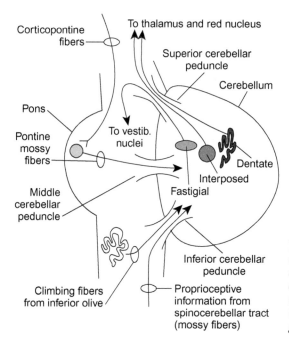

FIGURE 2.2 Schematic of the three primary afferent (inferior peduncles and middle peduncles) and efferent (superior peduncles) pathways of the cerebellum. See Table 2.4. *From lectures by Dr. T. Thach (deceased); used with permission from the Washington University School of Medicine Neuroscience Tutorial. Basal ganglia and cerebellum. Copyright 1997.*[15]

TABLE 2.4   Cerebellar Peduncles, Fiber Bundles, and Deep Cerebellar Nuclei Targets

Peduncles	Afferent and efferent fibers
Inferior	*Afferent fibers* (to cerebellum) from multiple sources: the vestibular nerve, the inferior olivary nuclei, the spinal cord (dorsal and rostral spinocerebellar, cuneocerebellar, and reticulocerebellar tracts)
	Efferent fibers (from cerebellum): fastigiobulbar tract projecting to vestibular nuclei, completing a vestibular circuit
Middle	*Afferent fibers:* from pons (crossed fibers from cerebral cortex to pontine gray matter nuclei to middle peduncle)
Superior	*Afferent fibers:* few fibers from ventral spinocerebellar, rostral spinocerebellar, and trigeminocerebellar projections
	Efferent fibers: Rubral, thalamic, reticular projections from deep cerebellar nuclei—dentate, interposed nuclei

Types of Afferent Fibers

There are two distinct types of afferent fibers that carry excitatory signals, predominantly via the inferior and middle peduncles, into the cerebellum. These are the mossy and climbing fibers, as shown in Table 2.5. Single mossy fibers project to multiple branches in multiple folia where they synapse at tens of granule cells. Climbing fibers ascend from the inferior olive to provide excitatory input at Purkinje cells. In immature cerebellum, multiple climbing fibers innervate individual Purkinje cells. These connections are pruned during development so that ultimately one climbing fiber innervates a single Purkinje cell.[16] Both of these fiber types send a few collateral axons to the deep cerebellar nuclei.

The Three Layers of Cerebellar Cortex

Three layers make up the cerebellar cortex.[17] A schema of the predominant cells and their interactions is shown in Figure 2.3, and additional detail about these layers and their predominant cell types and functional connections are shown in Table 2.6.

TABLE 2.5   Functional Anatomy of Mossy and Climbing Fibers

Mossy fibers—the primary afferents	Excitatory, originating from multiple brainstem nuclei and spinocerebellar tracts, synapse at the granule cells, carry tactile and proprioceptive information
Climbing fibers—afferent	Excitatory, originating from the inferior olivary nucleus in the cerebellum, climb up to the outer, molecular layer and synapse on the soma and dendrites of the Purkinje cells. These carry information critical for error correction

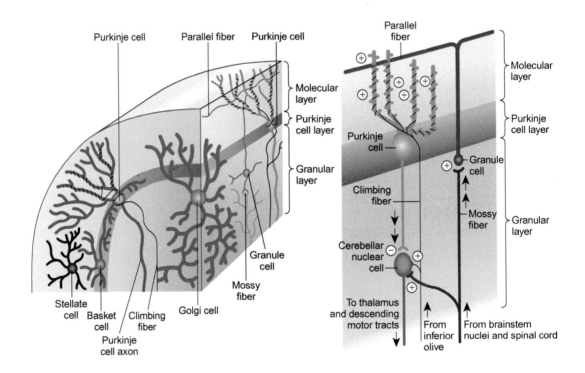

FIGURE 2.3   Schematic of the three primary cell layers (granular, molecular, and Purkinje) of the cerebellum. From Ref. [18].

TABLE 2.6 Cerebellar Layers, Cell Types, and Function

Layer	Cells	Input/output and function
Innermost—granular cell layer	Granule cells	Densely packed granule cells receive excitatory input from ascending mossy fibers. Granule cells are the only excitatory cells within the cerebellum. Axons ascend toward outer, molecular layer where they synapse and form parallel fibers.
	Golgi cells	Receive excitatory, glutamatergic[19] input from granule cells and provide negative GABAergic feedback to granule cells. Receive glycinergic and GABAergic input from the Lugaro cells.[20]
	Lugaro cells	Low prevalence interneurons, receive serotonergic input.[21] Inhibit Golgi cells.
Outermost—molecular layer	Parallel fibers	These are the bifurcated axons from granule cell layers. They have excitatory synapses directly on Purkinje cell dendrites and on stellate and basket interneurons.
	Stellate and basket cells	Excited by glutamatergic input from parallel fibers from granule cells. Output inhibitory on Purkinje cells.
Middle—Purkinje cell layer	Purkinje cells	These cells have extensive dendrites in the molecular layer. Cell bodies are in a single layer. Output is inhibitory to deep cerebellar nuclei.

NEUROTRANSMITTERS IN THE CEREBELLUM

Understanding the neurotransmitter systems provides a basis for identifying potentially beneficial pharmacological symptomatic interventions for diseases affecting the cerebellum.

Glutamate

Glutamate, the main excitatory neurotransmitter in the brain, acts at both ionotropic and metabotropic receptors. The ionotropic glutamate receptors are a diverse group classified into three types—AMPA (alpha-amino-3-hydroxy-5-methyl-4-isoxazolepropionic acid), NMDA (*N*-methyl-D-aspartic acid), and kainate. These are ligand-gated ion channels, meaning that when glutamate binds, charged ions pass through a channel in the receptor center. Both basket and stellate cells in the molecular layer express presynaptic AMPA receptors, to which overflowing glutamate from the climbing fibers can bind.[22]

The metabotropic glutamate receptors, which are G-protein–coupled receptors acting via second messengers, are expressed in a developmentally dependent fashion in the cerebellum,[23] with mGluR1 receptors playing a significant role in postsynaptic, dendritic calcium flux and Purkinje cell signaling.[5] Metabotropic glutamate receptors also mediate plasticity at the mossy fiber/granule cell/Golgi cell glomerulus (junction).[2] Developmentally, these processes are vital for short- and long-term plasticity underlying learning motor control. Pathophysiologically, this is relevant in paraneoplastic and autoimmune cerebellar diseases.[24] For example, mGluR1 antibodies, which can occur in Hodgkin's disease, cause a combination of acute, chronic/plastic, and degenerative effects in Purkinje cells.[25] In NMDA receptor encephalitis, *in vitro* methods showed that antibodies in patients' cerebrospinal fluid (CSF) bind to NMDA receptors in cerebellar granule cells and suppress calcium influx.[26]

Glutamate Transporters

Glutamate transporters are important for glutamatergic neurotransmission, as well as excitatory neuropathology. Excitatory amino acid transporters (EAAT) 1, 2, and 3 are expressed in the motor cortex, but EAAT1 predominates in the cerebellum,[27] where it is expressed in Bergmann glial cell processes and is also known as the glutamate aspartate transporter. This plays an important role in glutamate reuptake shortly after synaptic release. EAAT4 is found on extrasynaptic regions of Purkinje cell dendrites and reduces spillover of glutamate to adjacent synapses.[28] Co-localization of these transporters with perisynaptic mGluR1 receptors results in competition for glutamate, and this interaction modulates neuroplasticity in the cerebellum.[29,30]

Gamma-Aminobutyric Acid

Gamma-aminobutyric acid (GABA) is the major inhibitory neurotransmitter in the cerebellum, as well as the cerebrum. Its synthesis from glutamate is catalyzed by the enzyme glutamic acid decarboxylase (GAD). Anti-GAD antibodies have been reported in adults with ataxia.[31] GABA acts via chloride channels to hyperpolarize neurons. GABA receptors include GABA-A and GABA-C receptors, which are ionotropic, and GABA-B receptors, which are metabotropic, G-protein–coupled receptors. GABA-A receptors also have allosteric binding sites for other compounds including barbiturates, ethanol, neurosteroids, and picrotoxin. Baclofen is a GABA-B agonist.

GABA-A receptors are found in the granule cell layer,[32] where they receive GABA input from the Golgi cells, as well as molecular layer interneurons, the basket and stellate cells.[33] GABA-B receptors are predominantly in the molecular layer.[34] Ethanol affects cerebellar function via GABA-A receptor binding, but may also suppress responses in Purkinje cells to mGluR1 excitation from climbing fibers.[35]

Acetylcholine, Dopamine, Norepinephrine, and Serotonin

Acetylcholine, dopamine, norepinephrine, and serotonin[21] and their receptors occur in the cerebellum. However, the clinical effects of these neurotransmitter systems in the cerebellum are poorly understood and at this time seem not to be very helpful for ataxia. In general, the medications involving these neurotransmitter systems, when prescribed to improve mood, motor function, or cognition, do not improve or worsen ataxia. Recognition, in mixed movement disorders, of the cerebellar ataxia component can help with realistic assessment of the probable benefits of pharmacologic interventions. For example, in mixed dystonia and ataxia, the dystonia may respond to anticholinergics but cerebellar symptoms will not.

Endocannabinoids

The potential role of the endocannabinoid (endogenous cannabinoid) system and exogenous administration of various cannabinoids has been of interest for 25 years.[36–38] This system is involved in the so-called retrograde signaling in the hippocampus, basal ganglia, and cerebellum. In cerebellum, strong depolarization of Purkinje cells triggering Ca^{2+} influx or activation of metabotropic glutamate receptors (mGluR1) evokes dendritic release of endocannabinoids. These endocannabinoids bind to cannabinoid receptor 1 (CB1R) on the presynaptic terminal, resulting in a transient suppression of presynaptic neurotransmitter excitatory and inhibitory synaptic activity, a form of short-term neuroplasticity.[2,5] GABAergic basket and stellate cells, in the molecular layer, regulate presynaptic neurotransmission from excitatory parallel fibers from the granule cells. The significance of pathology within this system in children is currently unknown, although both active marijuana use and the exposure to cannabis prenatally may have adverse cognitive effects involving the cerebellum.[39-41]

NEUROPLASTICITY IN THE CEREBELLUM

Multiple forms of cerebellar plasticity have been identified and characterized in increasing physiological and molecular detail.[2] A fundamental form of plasticity in cerebellum is long-term depression (LTD) in Purkinje cells. The genesis of this involves repeated paired associated stimulation into Purkinje cells from one afferent climbing fiber plus multiple parallel fibers from granule cells. Through repeated motor performance (practice), differential induction of LTD downgrades synaptic connections associated with errors.[42]

More recently, multiple, coordinated forms of plasticity in cerebellar cortex and deep cerebellar nuclei have been identified and circuit-tested through combining physiological recording, targeted mutations, and vestibular system and other behavioral testing.[2] In addition to synaptic plasticity, there is intrinsic plasticity, involving neuronal spike- or synaptic activity-induced changes in ion channel expression in the neuron membrane.[43] Presynaptic, short-term plasticity at the parallel fiber to Purkinje cell synapse may fine-tune memory formation.[44,45] Bidirectional plasticity, i.e., both LTD and LTP, occurs in Purkinje cells guided by input from climbing fibers[46] and at the mossy fiber/granule cell synapse.[47]

The various forms of presynaptic and postsynaptic LTP and LTD may operate synergistically to create diverse and redundant systems for learning and storing for decades a vast array of procedural memories in cerebellar cortex.

CEREBELLAR STIMULATION

TMS and tDCS are forms of noninvasive stimulation that can be used to probe cerebellar projections to cerebrum. Most research to date has used this method to externally excite or inhibit cerebellar cortex and evaluate "readouts" in motor cortex or motor behaviors. The basic idea is one of quantifying cerebellar to cerebral inhibition. Cerebellar cortical output via Purkinje cells inhibits dentate/deep cerebellar nuclei which in turn send excitatory projections to thalamus and again to cortex. The extent to which these phenomena occur depends on the integrity of the pathways. So, e.g., a disease causing degeneration of Purkinje cells would reduce cerebellar to cerebral inhibition.

Noninvasive brain stimulation with TMS can be used in simple experimental paradigms to evaluate these pathways. The most basic protocol involves single pulse stimulation of motor cortex and paired pulse stimulation of cerebellum and motor cortex. The single pulses over motor cortex quantify baseline excitability by generating a motor-evoked potential, measured using surface electromyography (EMG) in an intrinsic muscle in contralateral hand. The paired pulses involve a conditioning, initial pulse over cerebellum followed by the pulse over motor cortex. If the cerebellar conditioning stimulation pulse precedes the test motor cortex stimulation by 5–7 ms, the motor cortex is less excited (due to Purkinje, dentate, thalamus, cortex output). Then the pulse over the motor cortex generates a smaller evoked potential, reflecting the evoked cerebellar inhibitory capacity.[48]

These same input/output relationships can be evaluated using neuromodulatory noninvasive brain stimulation. Repetitive TMS (rTMS) or tDCS protocols which activate cells on the surface of the cerebellum should therefore have inhibitory downstream effects in cerebrum. rTMS or tDCS protocols which inhibit cells on the surface of the cerebellum should disinhibit this pathway to cerebrum, thereby increasing cortical excitation. Various rTMS and prolonged sessions of tDCS over cerebellum have stimulatory or inhibitory effects that outlast the stimulation period.[11] These effects have been demonstrated with single and paired pulse motor cortex stimulation and are under investigation as biomarkers of cerebellar plasticity. Of additional interest is their potential as therapies, as preliminary investigations suggest specific stimulation protocols may modify locomotor adaptation,[49] improve verbal working memory,[50] improve tremor,[51] and alter behavioral function in other ways.[11]

CONCLUSION

This overview of cerebellar function provides a framework for understanding cerebellar disorders and diseases and current and future treatments.

References

1. Strick PL, Dum RP, Fiez JA. Cerebellum and nonmotor function. *Annu Rev Neurosci*. 2009;32:413–434.
2. Gao Z, van Beugen BJ, De Zeeuw CI. Distributed synergistic plasticity and cerebellar learning. *Nat Rev Neurosci*. 2012;13(9):619–635.
3. Lamont MG, Weber JT. The role of calcium in synaptic plasticity and motor learning in the cerebellar cortex. *Neurosci Biobehav Rev*. 2012;36(4):1153–1162.
4. Bostan AC, Dum RP, Strick PL. Cerebellar networks with the cerebral cortex and basal ganglia. *Trends Cogn Sci*. 2013;17(5):241–254.
5. Kitamura K, Kano M. Dendritic calcium signaling in cerebellar Purkinje cell. *Neural Netw*. 2013;47:11–17.
6. Manto M, Bower JM, Conforto AB, et al. Consensus paper: roles of the cerebellum in motor control—the diversity of ideas on cerebellar involvement in movement. *Cerebellum*. 2012;11(2):457–487.
7. Manto M, Oulad Ben Taib N. The contributions of the cerebellum in sensorimotor control: what are the prevailing opinions which will guide forthcoming studies? *Cerebellum*. 2013;12(3):313–315.
8. Holmes G. Clinical symptoms of cerebellar disease and their interpretation. The Croonian lecture III. *Lancet*. 1922;2:59–65.
9. Holmes G. The cerebellum of man. *Brain*. 1939;62:1–30.
10. Stoodley CJ, Schmahmann JD. Functional topography in the human cerebellum: a meta-analysis of neuroimaging studies. *NeuroImage*. 2009;44(2):489–501.
11. Grimaldi G, Argyropoulos GP, Boehringer A, et al. Non-invasive cerebellar stimulation—a consensus paper. *Cerebellum*. 2014;13(1):121–138.

12. Ghez C. The cerebellum. In: Kandel ER, Schwartz JH, Jessell TM, eds. *Principles of Neural Science*. 3rd ed. New York, NY: Elsevier; 1991:626–646.

13. Cerminara NL, Lang EJ, Sillitoe RV, Apps R. Redefining the cerebellar cortex as an assembly of non-uniform: Purkinje cell microcircuits. *Nat Rev Neurosci*. 2015;16(2):79–93.

14. Kandel ER. *Principles of Neuroscience*. 4th ed. McGraw Hill Medical; 2000, 630.

15. <http://web.archive.org/web/19990430001107/http://thalamus.wustl.edu/course/cerebell.html>.

16. Hashimoto K, Kano M. Functional differentiation of multiple climbing fiber inputs during synapse elimination in the developing cerebellum. *Neuron*. 2003;38(5):785–796.

17. Ito M. Cerebellar circuitry as a neuronal machine. *Prog Neurobiol*. 2006;78(3–5):272–303.

18. Apps R, Garwicz M. Anatomical and physiological foundations of cerebellar information processing. *Nature Rev Neurosci*. 2005;6:297–311.

19. Petralia RS, Wang YX, Niedzielski AS, Wenthold RJ. The metabotropic glutamate receptors, mGluR2 and mGluR3, show unique postsynaptic, presynaptic and glial localizations. *Neuroscience*. 1996;71(4):949–976.

20. Dumoulin A, Triller A, Dieudonne S. IPSC kinetics at identified GABAergic and mixed GABAergic and glycinergic synapses onto cerebellar Golgi cells. *J Neurosci*. 2001;21(16):6045–6057.

21. Dieudonne S, Dumoulin A. Serotonin-driven long-range inhibitory connections in the cerebellar cortex. *J Neurosci*. 2000;20(5):1837–1848.

22. Liu SJ. Biphasic modulation of GABA release from stellate cells by glutamatergic receptor subtypes. *J Neurophysiol*. 2007;98(1):550–556.

23. Douyard J, Shen L, Huganir RL, Rubio ME. Differential neuronal and glial expression of GluR1 AMPA receptor subunit and the scaffolding proteins SAP97 and 4.1N during rat cerebellar development. *J Comp Neurol*. 2007;502(1):141–156.

24. Hadjivassiliou M, Boscolo S, Tongiorgi E, et al. Cerebellar ataxia as a possible organ-specific autoimmune disease. *Mov Disord*. 2008;23(10):1370–1377.

25. Coesmans M, Smitt PA, Linden DJ, et al. Mechanisms underlying cerebellar motor deficits due to mGluR1-autoantibodies. *Ann Neurol*. 2003;53(3):325–336.

26. Rubio-Agusti I, Dalmau J, Sevilla T, Burgal M, Beltran E, Bataller L. Isolated hemidystonia associated with NMDA receptor antibodies. *Mov Disord*. 2011;26(2):351–352.

27. Arriza JL, Fairman WA, Wadiche JI, Murdoch GH, Kavanaugh MP, Amara SG. Functional comparisons of three glutamate transporter subtypes cloned from human motor cortex. *J Neurosci*. 1994;14(9):5559–5569.

28. Takayasu Y, Iino M, Kakegawa W, et al. Differential roles of glial and neuronal glutamate transporters in Purkinje cell synapses. *J Neurosci*. 2005;25(38):8788–8793.

29. Otis TS, Brasnjo G, Dzubay JA, Pratap M. Interactions between glutamate transporters and metabotropic glutamate receptors at excitatory synapses in the cerebellar cortex. *Neurochem Int*. 2004;45(4):537–544.

30. Wadiche JI, Jahr CE. Patterned expression of Purkinje cell glutamate transporters controls synaptic plasticity. *Nat Neurosci*. 2005;8(10):1329–1334.

31. Manto MU, Laute MA, Aguera M, Rogemond V, Pandolfo M, Honnorat J. Effects of anti-glutamic acid decarboxylase antibodies associated with neurological diseases. *Ann Neurol*. 2007;61(6):544–551.

32. Palacios JM, Young III WS, Kuhar MJ. Autoradiographic localization of gamma-aminobutyric acid (GABA) receptors in the rat cerebellum. *Proc Natl Acad Sci USA*. 1980;77(1):670–674.

33. Trigo FF, Chat M, Marty A. Enhancement of GABA release through endogenous activation of axonal GABA(A) receptors in juvenile cerebellum. *J Neurosci*. 2007;27(46):12452–12463.

34. Wilkin GP, Hudson AL, Hill DR, Bowery NG. Autoradiographic localization of GABAB receptors in rat cerebellum. *Nature*. 1981;294(5841):584–587.

35. Carta M, Mameli M, Valenzuela CF. Alcohol potently modulates climbing fiber—> Purkinje neuron synapses: role of metabotropic glutamate receptors. *J Neurosci*. 2006;26(7):1906–1912.

36. Herkenham M, Groen BG, Lynn AB, De Costa BR, Richfield EK. Neuronal localization of cannabinoid receptors and second messengers in mutant mouse cerebellum. *Brain Res*. 1991;552(2):301–310.

37. Moldrich G, Wenger T. Localization of the CB1 cannabinoid receptor in the rat brain. An immunohistochemical study. *Peptides*. 2000;21(11):1735–1742.

38. Hillard CJ, Weinlander KM, Stuhr KL. Contributions of endocannabinoid signaling to psychiatric disorders in humans: genetic and biochemical evidence. *Neuroscience*. 2012;204:207–229.

39. Chang L, Yakupov R, Cloak C, Ernst T. Marijuana use is associated with a reorganized visual-attention network and cerebellar hypoactivation. *Brain*. 2006;129(Pt 5):1096–1112.

40. Smith AM, Fried PA, Hogan MJ, Cameron I. Effects of prenatal marijuana on response inhibition: an fMRI study of young adults. *Neurotoxicol Teratol*. 2004;26(4):533–542.
41. Rodriguez-Cueto C, Benito C, Fernandez-Ruiz J, Romero J, Hernandez-Galvez M, Gomez-Ruiz M. Changes in CB(1) and CB(2) receptors in the post-mortem cerebellum of humans affected by spinocerebellar ataxias. *Br J Pharmacol*. 2014;171(6):1472–1489.
42. Ito M. Cerebellar long-term depression: characterization, signal transduction, and functional roles. *Physiol Rev*. 2001;81(3):1143–1195.
43. Pugh JR, Raman IM. Nothing can be coincidence: synaptic inhibition and plasticity in the cerebellar nuclei. *Trends Neurosci*. 2009;32(3):170–177.
44. Le Guen MC, De Zeeuw CI. Presynaptic plasticity at cerebellar parallel fiber terminals. *Funct Neurol*. 2010;25(3):141–151.
45. Salin PA, Malenka RC, Nicoll RA. Cyclic AMP mediates a presynaptic form of LTP at cerebellar parallel fiber synapses. *Neuron*. 1996;16(4):797–803.
46. Coesmans M, Weber JT, De Zeeuw CI, Hansel C. Bidirectional parallel fiber plasticity in the cerebellum under climbing fiber control. *Neuron*. 2004;44(4):691–700.
47. D'Errico A, Prestori F, D'Angelo E. Differential induction of bidirectional long-term changes in neurotransmitter release by frequency-coded patterns at the cerebellar input. *J Physiol*. 2009;587(Pt 24):5843–5857.
48. Ugawa Y, Uesaka Y, Terao Y, Hanajima R, Kanazawa I. Magnetic stimulation over the cerebellum in humans. *Ann Neurol*. 1995;37(6):703–713.
49. Jayaram G, Galea JM, Bastian AJ, Celnik P. Human locomotor adaptive learning is proportional to depression of cerebellar excitability. *Cerebral Cortex*. 2011;21(8):1901–1909.
50. Pope PA, Miall RC. Task-specific facilitation of cognition by cathodal transcranial direct current stimulation of the cerebellum. *Brain Stimul*. 2012;5(2):84–94.
51. Grimaldi G, Oulad Ben Taib N, Manto M, Bodranghien F. Marked reduction of cerebellar deficits in upper limbs following transcranial cerebello-cerebral DC stimulation: tremor reduction and re-programming of the timing of antagonist commands. *Front Syst Neurosci*. 2014;8:9.

Classification of Movement Disorders

Harvey S. Singer[1], Jonathan W. Mink[2], Donald L. Gilbert[3] and Joseph Jankovic[4]

[1]Department of Neurology, Johns Hopkins Hospital, Baltimore, MD, USA; [2]Division of Child Neurology, University of Rochester Medical Center, Rochester, NY, USA; [3]Division of Neurology, Cincinnati Children's Hospital Medical Center, Cincinnati, OH, USA; [4]Department of Neurology, Baylor College of Medicine, Houston, TX, USA

INTRODUCTION

Movement disorders are neurological syndromes that involve impaired performance of voluntary movements, dysfunction of posture, the presence of abnormal involuntary movements, or the performance of normal-appearing movements at inappropriate or unintended times. The abnormalities of movement are not due to weakness or

Movement Disorders in Childhood, Second Edition.
DOI: http://dx.doi.org/10.1016/B978-0-12-411573-6.00003-6

27

abnormal muscle tone, but may be accompanied by weakness or abnormal tone. By convention, movement disorders are divided into two major categories. The first is hyperkinetic movement disorders, sometimes referred to as dyskinesias. This term refers to abnormal, repetitive involuntary movements and includes most of the childhood movement disorders including tics, stereotypies, chorea, dystonia, myoclonus, and tremor. The second is hypokinetic movement disorders, sometimes referred to as akinetic/rigid disorders. The primary movement disorder in this category is Parkinsonism, which manifests primarily in adulthood as Parkinson disease or one of many forms of secondary parkinsonism. Hypokinetic disorders are relatively uncommon in children. Although weakness and spasticity are characterized by motor dysfunction, by common convention these entities are not included among "movement disorders."

When faced with a movement disorder, the first step is to characterize the movement phenomena. Is the pattern of movements normal or abnormal? Are there excessive movements or is there a paucity of movement? Is there decomposition or disorder of voluntary movement trajectories? Is the movement paroxysmal (sudden onset and offset), continual (repeated again and again), or continuous (without stop)? Has the movement disorder changed over time? Do environmental stimuli or emotional states modulate the movement disorder? Can the movements be suppressed voluntarily? Is the abnormal movement heralded by a premonitory sensation or urge? Are there findings on the examination suggestive of focal neurologic deficit or systemic disease? Is there a family history of a similar or related condition? Does the movement disorder abate with sleep?

In clinical practice, the diagnosis of a movement disorder requires a qualitative appreciation of the movement type and context. Abnormal movements can be difficult to define. To best classify the disorder phenomenologically, one should describe the characteristics of the movements. Even under the best circumstances, movement disorders may be difficult to characterize. However, careful observation of the spatial and temporal properties of the movement, often with the aid of video, can usually lead to appropriate identification of the phenomenology.

Movements in some contexts may be normal and in others may indicate underlying pathology. Movements that are worrisome for a degenerative disorder in adolescents (myoclonus) may be completely normal in an infant (benign neonatal myoclonus). It can be quite difficult to specifically diagnose a movement disorder without seeing the abnormal movements. Thus, obtaining video examples of the child's movement may be essential to making a correct diagnosis. The video atlas accompanying this book provides examples of the different types of movement disorders.

Many classification schemes have been used to provide a taxonomy for the wide variety of movement disorders. Disorders can be classified by phenomenology, based on the observed temporal and spatial features of the movements themselves, along with characteristic clinical features (Tables 3.1 and 3.2). They can also be classified based on presumed etiology, anatomic localization or neuropathological features, by disease course, by genetic or molecular criteria, or by other biological factors.[1-5] This chapter focuses on classification based on phenomenology. Subsequent chapters discuss the etiologies, localization, and differential diagnosis of these disorders.

TABLE 3.1   Key Features of Hyperkinetic Disorders

	Rhythmic	Repeated posture	Repeated stereotyped movement	Suppressible
Dystonia	Rarely	Yes	Sometimes	Partial or only briefly
Chorea	No	No	Rarely	No
Athetosis	No	No	No	No
Myoclonus	Sometimes	Sometimes	Usually	No
Tremor	Yes	No	Yes	Sometimes briefly
Tics	No	Yes	Yes	Usually
Stereotypies	Yes	Sometimes	Yes	Yes

From Ref. [4].

ATAXIA (CHAPTER 14)

Ataxia literally means "without order." It is defined as an inability to generate a normal or expected voluntary movement trajectory that cannot be attributed to weakness or involuntary muscle activity about the affected joints.[3] Ataxia can result from impairment of spatial pattern of muscle activity, of the timing of that activity, or both. Specific associated deficits include dysmetria (inaccurate movement to a target (undershoot or overshoot)), dyssynergia (decomposition of multijoint movements), and dysdiadochokinesis (impaired rhythmicity of rapid alternating movements). Ataxia does not occur at rest, but it may be associated with hypotonia of affected body parts at rest. Although ataxia is classically associated with dysfunction of the cerebellum, it can result from lesions in the cerebellar afferent or efferent pathways (see Chapter 2).

ATHETOSIS (CHAPTER 10)

Athetosis literally means "without position or place."[6] It is defined as slow, writhing, continuous, involuntary movements. In athetosis the same regions of the body are repeatedly involved, unlike chorea where moves appear to move from one body part to another.[4] Athetosis may worsen with attempts at movement or posture, but it can also occur at rest. Athetosis typically involves the distal extremities (hands or feet) more than the proximal extremities and it can also involve the face, neck, and trunk.

Athetosis is distinguished from dystonia by the lack of sustained postures. Athetosis differs from chorea by the lack of identifiable movement fragments. Athetosis is not rhythmic or stereotyped. There is some debate as to whether athetosis should be considered as a discrete entity, or whether it is part of the spectrum of dystonia or chorea.[6] Because athetosis is typically non-patterned and it resembles slow chorea, it may be considered to be more linked to chorea than dystonia. Although cerebral palsy is one of the most common causes of childhood athetosis,[7] athetosis may be associated with multiple etiologies.[4]

TABLE 3.2 Clinical Features of Hyperkinetic Disorders

	Dystonia	Chorea	Athetosis	Myoclonus	Tremor	Tics	Stereotypies
Distractibility	No	No	No	No	No	Yes	Yes
Suppressibility	Partial	No	No	No	Briefly	Usually	Yes
Duration	Variable	Ongoing	Ongoing	Shock like	Ongoing	Variable	Variable
Speed	Variable	Medium–fast	Slow–medium	Very fast (<1 second)	2–14 Hz	Variable	Variable
Jerkiness	Sometimes	Sometimes	No	Very	Sometimes	Sometimes	Rare
Stereotyped	Often	No	No	Usually	Yes	Yes	Yes
Rhythmic	Sometimes	No	No	Sometimes	Yes	Usually not	Yes
Intermittent	Sometimes	Sometimes	No	Sometimes	Sometimes	Yes	Yes
Ongoing	Sometimes	Yes	Yes	Sometimes	Yes	No	Yes
Flowing	No	Yes	Yes	No	No	Sometimes	Sometimes
Sub-movements	No	Yes	Maybe	No	No	Sometimes	Sometimes
Context	Movement > rest	Movement > rest	Rest > movement	All	Variable	Rest	Rest
Predictable	Sometimes	No	No	No	No	Yes	Often not aware
Normal pattern	Sometimes	Yes	Yes	No	Yes	Yes	Yes

From Ref. [4].

BALLISMUS (CHAPTER 10)

Ballismus or *ballism* refers to involuntary, high amplitude, flinging movements typically occurring proximally. These movements may be brief or continual and may occur in conjunction with chorea. Often, one side of the body is affected, i.e. *hemiballism*. In many cases, hemiballism gets milder with time and evolves into chorea. It has been suggested that because the same lesions can produce both ballismus and chorea, ballismus is likely to be part of the spectrum of chorea and not a separate entity.[8]

CHOREA (CHAPTER 10)

Chorea literally means "dance-like" and refers to an ongoing random-appearing sequence of one or more discrete involuntary movements or movement fragments.[4] Movements appear random due to variability in timing, duration, rate, direction, or anatomic location. Each movement has a distinct start and stop, but these may be difficult to identify when one movement immediately follows or overlaps with another. Chorea may be accompanied by motor impersistence (such as the inability to maintain a voluntary posture) and hypotonia. All body parts may be involved, though certain distributions may be characteristic of distinct diseases or disorders.

Chorea is distinguished from dystonia based on the apparently random, unpredictable, and continuously ongoing nature of the movements, compared with the more predictable and stereotyped movements or postures of dystonia. The movements of chorea are often more rapid than those associated with dystonia.[9] Chorea may occur at rest, but is typically worsened by voluntary movement. Chorea may be accompanied by "parakinesia," in which children incorporate the involuntary movement into a more purposeful movement in an attempt to hide the disorder.

Chorea is distinguished from athetosis by the ability to identify discrete movements or movement fragments within the ongoing sequence of chorea. The individual movement fragments in chorea are brief and often appear jerky. In contrast, the ongoing movement in athetosis is not composed of discrete movements, and athetosis thus appears to be a sinuous, continuously flowing, ongoing, random movement as opposed to the sequence of randomly selected brief movements that characterizes chorea.[4]

Chorea is distinguished from tremor by its lack of rhythmicity and predictability. Chorea is distinguished from myoclonus by the fact that in myoclonus all the movements are quick, whereas in chorea only some are. Movements due to myoclonus may appear more stereotyped, as a consistent pattern of muscles is often involved. Chorea is distinguished from tics by the fact that chorea is not voluntarily suppressible, is not preceded by an urge, and does not consist of repeated stereotyped movement.[4]

Chorea is distinguished from ataxia by the fact that ataxia accompanies voluntary movement and is not present at rest. Abnormal movements in ataxia increase near a target (intention tremor and dysmetria) and improve with stabilization of proximal joints or other interventions that lower the degrees of freedom for movement.

DYSTONIA (CHAPTER 11)

Dystonia is a movement disorder characterized by sustained or intermittent muscle contractions causing abnormal, often repetitive, movements, postures, or both. Dystonic movements are typically patterned, twisting, and may be tremulous. Dystonia is often initiated or worsened by voluntary action and associated with overflow muscle activation.[10] In most cases, dystonia combines abnormal movements and postures, but some forms of dystonia are not associated with postures. This is particularly true of dystonia involving the eyelids and larynx. Dystonic postures are repeated, and particular patterns or postures may be characteristic of each child at a given point in time. Postures can be sustained or may occur during very brief intervals.

Two clinical features commonly associated with dystonia may help distinguish it from other movement disorders. The first is "task specificity" in which dystonia may accompany specific tasks, but not others that involve the same muscles. For example, dystonia may be present during forward gait, but not during backward gait, running, or hopping. The second is the phenomenon of *geste antagoniste* (sensory trick) in which lightly touching near an affected body part may help relieve the dystonia contraction.

A hallmark of dystonia is the inability to prevent unwanted contraction of muscles antagonist or adjacent to muscles involved in voluntary movement.[11,12] Often this is referred to clinically as "overflow."

Despite the name, dystonia is not a primary disorder of muscle tone (resistance to passive stretch at attempted rest). Hypotonia may accompany many forms of dystonia, but, when severe, dystonia itself may cause hypertonia.[5]

Dystonia is distinguished from chorea based on the more sustained muscle contractions and patterned appearance. Tremor may accompany dystonia, and is called "dystonic tremor," but is usually less regular than primary tremors. Dystonia is distinguished from athetosis by the sustained patterned contractions.

MYOCLONUS (CHAPTER 12)

Myoclonus refers to a sequence of repeated, often nonrhythmic, brief shock-like jerks due to sudden involuntary contraction or relaxation of one or more muscles.[4] Myoclonus may be synchronous (several muscles contracting simultaneously), spreading (several muscles contracting in a predictable sequence), or asynchronous (several muscles contracting with varying and unpredictable timing). Myoclonus is characterized by a sudden unidirectional movement due to muscle contraction (positive myoclonus) or sudden, brief muscle relaxation (negative myoclonus).[13] *Asterixis* is a form of negative myoclonus. Myoclonus can be caused or worsened by movement. Unlike most other movement disorders, myoclonus can sometimes occur during sleep.

When myoclonus is repeated rhythmically, it is called "rhythmic myoclonus" or "myoclonic tremor." Rhythmic myoclonus is characterized by alternating fast phase and slow phase movements so that the rapid phase of the jerking occurs in a single direction with subsequent slower recovery following every jerk. The fast phase may be due to either contraction or relaxation of the involved muscle. Rhythmic myoclonus may be considered a particular form of tremor or a particular manifestation of myoclonus, and thus, it may be referred to as both *myoclonus* and *tremor*.

Myoclonus is distinguished from dystonia by the lack of identifiable postures and by the short duration of the movements. Myoclonus is distinguished from athetosis by the sudden jerks and lack of smooth flowing movements. Myoclonus is distinguished from tics by the rapidity of movements, the lack of suppressibility and the lack of a premonitory urge.

Myoclonus is distinguished from tremor by the asymmetric velocity of the jerk/relax cycle (or, for negative myoclonus, the relax/restore cycle). Thus, it may have a "sawtooth" appearance in contrast to tremor which has a "sinusoidal" appearance.

Synchronous myoclonus and myoclonic tremor can be distinguished from chorea by the predictable timing of movements. Distinction from chorea is more difficult for asynchronous multifocal myoclonus, but this distinction is usually possible due to the simpler, shock-like, unidirectional movements of myoclonus compared to the more complex and often slower movement fragments commonly seen in chorea.[4,9]

PARKINSONISM (CHAPTER 15)

Parkinsonism is a neurological syndrome characterized by the presence of two or more of the cardinal features of Parkinson Disease including tremor at rest, bradykinesia, rigidity, and postural instability. Parkinsonism is the classic "hypokinetic" movement disorder and is the only one listed in this chapter. The specific characteristics of Parkinsonism are defined in Chapter 15.

STEREOTYPIES (CHAPTER 8)

Stereotypies are broadly defined as involuntary, patterned, coordinated, rhythmic, repetitive, non-reflexive movements that occur in the same fashion with each repetition.[4,14] Stereotypies are typically rhythmic simple movements such as waving or flapping the hands or arms, but they may consist of more complex sequences or movement fragments. Stereotypies may involve fingers, wrists, or more proximal portions of the upper extremity. The lower extremity is often not involved. Stereotypies can be unilateral or bilateral but are more commonly bilateral. There is no premonitory urge, and the movements tend to occur when the child is stressed, excited, distracted or engrossed. Stereotypies can be stopped by distraction or initiation of another activity. They do not usually interfere with the ability to perform tasks. Stereotypy involves a single movement performed repeatedly, rather than a set of different recognizable movements. Each movement has a clear beginning and ending, but the duration of the stereotypy is variable and can continue for many minutes to hours at a time.

Stereotypies are distinguished from tremor and rhythmic myoclonus by the more complex nature and the ability of the child to suppress the movement voluntarily by interruption with distraction or redirection. Movements in stereotypy often involve more than one joint and can have a twisting or circular quality that is not usually present in tremor (which often affects only a single joint or muscle group).

Stereotypies are distinguished from tics by the lack of a clear premonitory urge and by the largely invariant nature of the movements over time. While stereotypies may sometimes contain sustained postures, they can be distinguished from dystonia by the absence of predictable worsening with attempted movement and by the long periods of normal movement between episodes.

Stereotypies are distinguished from chorea and athetosis by the predictability of the phenomenology and triggers of the movement.

TICS (CHAPTER 7)

Tics are involuntary, sudden, rapid, abrupt, repetitive, nonrhythmic, simple or complex motor movements or vocalizations (phonic productions).[4,15] Tics are classified into two categories (motor and phonic) with each being subdivided into a simple and complex grouping. Tics are usually preceded by an uncomfortable feeling or urge (premonitory sensation) that is relieved by carrying out the movement. Characteristic features include predictability of both the nature of the movement and its onset, worsening by stress or excitement, and brief voluntary suppressibility. The specific movements can be predicted by the patient or an observer in the sense that there is often a small and identifiable number of different tics at any time point. The duration of each tic movement is characteristic of that tic, and the duration does not vary between different repetitions. It is rare for children to fall, drop objects, or inadvertently injure themselves due to tics; however, self-injurious tics may occur.

Tics wax and wane over weeks to months to years, with different tics appearing at different times and with different severities, and others disappearing completely. The frequency of tics may change during a single day, and often tics are more frequent during stress, fatigue, anxiety, or excitement. Tics can include brief sudden jerky or shock-like movements in which case they could be termed "clonic tics." Tics can include briefly sustained postures, in which case they are classified as "dystonic tics" or "tonic tics." One distinction between dystonic tics and dystonia is that dystonia is usually triggered by and interferes with voluntary movement, whereas tics are usually suppressed by and do not interfere with voluntary movement.

Tics can be distinguished from athetosis, chorea, and myoclonus by the lack of continuity of the movement, the intervening periods of normal movement, and the lack of interference with ongoing tasks. Tics are also distinguished from chorea and myoclonus by the predictability and repeatability of the movements. Tics can be distinguished from tremor and stereotypies by the clear initiation and termination of each individual tic movement, and by the lack of rhythmicity in the timing of initiation of movement.

TREMOR (CHAPTER 13)

Tremor refers to oscillating, rhythmic back-and-forth movements about a fixed point, axis, or plane.[4] Tremor is often, but not always, due to rhythmic alternating contraction of agonist and antagonist muscles. Tremor is classified as "rest tremor," "postural tremor," or "action tremor" according to the condition associated with greatest severity. Some authors use the term "kinetic tremor" to refer to tremor that is present equally with sustained posture and movement. "Intention tremor" is a specific form of tremor associated with cerebellar dysfunction that is characterized by worsening tremor on approach to a target.

Tremor is distinguished from myoclonus by the symmetric velocity in both directions, the lack of an obvious jerk-and-release cycle, and the existence of a midpoint of the movement. We recommend use of the term "rhythmic myoclonus" rather than "myoclonic tremor" as the former is more specific to the likely etiology. Tremor can be associated with dystonia, but when prominent features of dystonia are present, it is then classified as "dystonic tremor" which is best thought of as a manifestation of dystonia. Dystonic tremor is often less rhythmic or more irregular than other forms of tremor and may involve multiple joints or different joints depending on the posture of the limb. In some cases of dystonic tremor, there may be a "null point"; a particular posture in which the tremor is minimized. One form of rhythmical movement that may resemble tremor is myorhythmia, defined as repetitive, rhythmic, slow (1–4 Hz) movement affecting chiefly cranial and limb muscles.[16]

References

1. Klein C. Movement disorders: classifications. *J Inherit Metab Dis*. 2005;28:425–439.
2. Barbeau A, Duvoisin RC, Gerstenbrand F, Lakke JP, Marsden CD, Stern G. Classification of extrapyramidal disorders. Proposal for an international classification and glossary of terms. *J Neurol Sci*. 1981;51(2):311–327.
3. Sanger TD, Chen D, Delgado MR, Gaebler-Spira D, Hallett M, Mink JW. Definition and classification of negative motor signs in childhood. *Pediatrics*. 2006;118(5):2159–2167.
4. Sanger TD, Chen D, Fehlings DL, et al. Definition and classification of hyperkinetic movements in childhood. *Mov Disord*. 2010;25(11):1538–1549.
5. Sanger TD, Delgado MR, Gaebler-Spira D, Hallett M, Mink JW. Classification and definition of disorders causing hypertonia in childhood. *Pediatrics*. 2003;111(1):e89–e97.
6. Morris JG, Jankelowitz SK, Fung VS, Clouston PD, Hayes MW, Grattan-Smith P. Athetosis I: historical considerations. *Mov Disord*. 2002;17(6):1278–1280.
7. Colver A, Fairhurst C, Pharoah PO. Cerebral palsy. *Lancet*. 2014;283(9924):1240–1249.
8. Mink JW. The basal ganglia: focused selection and inhibition of competing motor programs. *Prog Neurobiol*. 1996;50:381–425.
9. Marsden CD, Obeso JA, Rothwell JC. Clinical neurophysiology of muscle jerks: myoclonus, chorea, and tics. *Adv Neurol*. 1983;39:865–881.
10. Albanese A, Bhatia K, Bressman SB, et al. Phenomenology and classification of dystonia: a consensus update. *Mov Disord*. 2013;28:863–873.
11. Hallett M. Dystonia: abnormal movements result from loss of inhibition. *Adv Neurol*. 2004;94:1–9.
12. Mink J. The basal ganglia and involuntary movements: impaired inhibition of competing motor patterns. *Arch Neurol*. 2003;60:1365–1368.
13. Shibasaki H. Pathophysiology of negative myoclonus and asterixis. *Adv Neurol*. 1995;67:199–209.
14. Mahone EM, Bridges D, Prahme C, Singer HS. Repetitive arm and hand movements (complex motor stereotypies) in children. *J Pediatr*. 2004;145:391–395.
15. McNaught KS, Mink JW. Advances in understanding and treatment of Tourette syndrome. *Nat Rev Neurol*. 2011;7(12):667–676.
16. Baizabal-Carvallo JF, Cordoso F, Jankovic J. Myorhythmia: phenomenology, etiology, and treatment. *Mov Disord*. 2015;30:171–179.

Diagnostic Evaluation of Children with Movement Disorders

Harvey S. Singer[1], Jonathan W. Mink[2], Donald L. Gilbert[3] and Joseph Jankovic[4]

[1]Department of Neurology, Johns Hopkins Hospital, Baltimore, MD, USA;
[2]Division of Child Neurology, University of Rochester Medical Center,
Rochester, NY, USA; [3]Division of Neurology, Cincinnati Children's Hospital
Medical Center, Cincinnati, OH, USA; [4]Department of Neurology, Baylor
College of Medicine, Houston, TX, USA

OUTLINE

Movement Disorders in Childhood, Second Edition.
DOI: http://dx.doi.org/10.1016/B978-0-12-411573-6.00004-8

INTRODUCTION

Diagnosis of movement disorders involves recognition and classification of phenomenology (Chapter 3), as well as knowledge of neuroanatomy, particularly basal ganglia (Chapter 1) and cerebellum (Chapter 2). By definition, movement disorders do not result from an interruption in the terminal pathway from the primary motor cortex to muscle. For example, motor cortex strokes, spinal cord diseases, anterior horn cell diseases, neuropathies, diseases at the neuromuscular junction, and myopathies interfere with movement but are not designated as movement disorders. Rather, movement disorders result from an interruption in typical, adaptive function of subcortical and cerebellar structures and circuits, the activity of which precedes signaling via the final common pathway from motor cortex to muscle. These circuits subserve learning, planning, selection, timing, and inhibition of movement.

It is also helpful throughout the diagnostic process to recognize the importance to a patient of a normally functioning motor system and an intact sense of agency. The awareness of one's own actions and sense of full control over one's motor system for achievement of goals is taken for granted throughout mature life. Development of movement control and a sense of agency for one's actions is a basic experience of childhood. Loss of a sense of this control due to reduced efficiency of action performance, the occurrence of movements without a sense of agency, or compulsions to move repetitively without purpose have psychological consequences. Training in execution of particular, skilled actions may occupy hundreds or thousands of hours in the lives of professional musicians, artists, or athletes. Any disease or disorder that interferes with the execution of movements can cause substantial impairment, psychological distress, and reduced quality of life, in children or adults.

The most common movement disorders in childhood will be seen by any general child neurologist. These diagnoses are made reliably based on pattern recognition and generally require little time, effort, or health care resources. The diagnostic challenge for these conditions may be recognition of commonly co-occurring emotional or cognitive problems.[1] In contrast, the rarest diseases causing movement disorders will never be diagnosed by most child neurologists. However, considered collectively, the presentation of a child with some rare movement disorder is not a rare event in child neurology. These diagnoses can be time-consuming for physicians, emotionally difficult for families, and costly for the health care system. Parents want their physicians to make a specific diagnosis and to understand a specific cause for their child's problem, even if no medical treatment is available.

A systematic approach to diagnosis of both rare and common movement disorders is a pragmatic goal of this chapter and of Appendix B. The approach is based on knowledge of relevant neuroanatomy, skill in phenomenology classification, and knowing how to get the most information possible from the clinical encounter. This chapter is not an encyclopedia or a reference list of diagnoses, of variably present clinical features, and of genes. That information is left for more detailed presentation in the phenomenology-based chapters. Rather, this chapter addresses general approaches to obtaining the most comprehensive and accurate information in the clinic and applying this information to make both straightforward and difficult diagnoses. With this foundation and the approach in this chapter, a provisional diagnosis, or at least a narrowed differential diagnosis, should be achieved for most children referred for movement disorders.

The skillful recognition of movement disorder phenomenology involves training in visual pattern recognition, understanding of the neuroanatomy of motor control, and understanding of movement disorder classification systems. A unique challenge in children is that the nervous system is developing. Diseases manifest in different forms at different stages of motor system maturation. Also, of course, children may not communicate symptoms and will not always cooperate with the examination. Diagnosis through pattern recognition is greatly enhanced by clinical experience but also by the independent and group study of case videos.

This chapter is organized in the framework of a new clinic visit for a chief complaint of a movement disorder, where the initial goal is *diagnosis.* The elements of a typical outpatient visit form the chapter sections. The use of computer databases for diagnosis is discussed in the final section.

PRECLINIC

The Scheduling Process

Some institutions support clinics devoted specifically to pediatric movement disorders. This requires an appropriate triaging process where schedulers have a list of chief complaints. Essentially, the list of chapter titles in this text can provide a useful, comprehensive listing of disease categories. For children, this works well for common problems such as tremor or tics that are readily recognized by referring physicians (or self-referring parents). Other problems, such as ataxia, dystonia, or chorea, create greater difficulties because referring physicians and office staff may not know how to describe the problem or whether it is a movement disorder. However, once a clinic program becomes established and with good physician communication, the percentage of appropriate referrals improves.

Urgent Referrals

Most movement disorders are chronic and not life-threatening. Therefore, emergency room visits and medically urgent scheduling encompass a small fraction of neurological consultations for movement disorders. However, some movement disorders, including those listed in Table 4.1, may emerge and become disabling fairly rapidly. Costly emergency department visits sometimes can be avoided with flexible scheduling and supportive doctor–doctor communication about urgent visits. Recognizing both real disability in children and overwhelming distress in some parents, it is important to have mechanisms in place to facilitate rapid evaluation of patients. The successful movement disorder neurologist should be available for some form of direct communication from primary physicians who may need to advocate for children with particularly impairing movement disorders. Parents often advocate directly for their children through phone calls or electronic communication. An advantage of email and other electronic communications is that parents can provide chief complaint, videos, and history of present illness data in advance, which can help with triaging.

TABLE 4.1   Acute, Subacute Pediatric Movement Disorders Which May Present Urgently

Movement disorder phenomenology	Most common etiology or precipitant	Comment
Acute ataxia	Postinfectious/postvaccine	Usually causes significant functional interference
Akathisia, ataxia, chorea, dyskinesias, dystonia, myoclonus, rigidity with hyperthermia, tics, tremor while starting, adjusting, stopping psychiatric medications	Drug-induced, particularly related to dopamine receptor blockers	Acute akathisia or dystonic reactions, withdrawal emergent dyskinesias on rapid neuroleptic withdrawal
Chorea	Poststreptococcal (Sydenham), other immune mediated	Usually causes significant functional interference
Chorea/Ballism	Fever/illness in children with dyskinetic cerebral palsy	Can lead to rhabdomyolysis
Dystonia/status dystonicus	Variable - e.g. neurodegenerative diseases, baclofen pump failure	Can lead to rhabdomyolysis, respiratory compromise
Encephalopathy with any facial dyskinesia or mixed movement disorder	Encephalitis	Anti-NMDA receptor, other auto-immune
Functional Movement disorders: psychogenic tremor/shaking, tics, gait disturbance, dystonia	Acute stressors often not identified in children	Early diagnosis is probably critical for improving prognosis
Opsoclonus myoclonus	Unknown	Usually causes significant functional interference
Tics/Status Ticcus	Sometimes acute stressor	Tourette syndrome or Provisional Tic Disorder may present or exacerbate dramatically in the absence of an identifiable precipitant

Gathering Data before the Visit

Standardized intake questionnaires can yield essential information for the diagnostic evaluation. Much of this information can be effectively provided by parents before the visit. Emailing intake questionnaires before the visit can be cost-effective. Advance review by the nursing staff can also help identify patients who should be seen more promptly or arrange for testing to be done efficiently in concert with the visit. Video files or links may also be sent prior to the visit.

IN CLINIC

The goal of the first clinic encounter is to arrive at a specific diagnosis or to allow a plan to be put in place to find the etiology of the movement disorder. It is helpful to bear in mind that the most common movement disorder complaints in children are emotionally distressing to parents, but are not life-threatening or indicative of a progressive neurologic disease. Through history, examination, and direct observation, the clinician should obtain an accurate impression of the movement phenomenology. Another important goal is to establish a trusting relationship with the child and family to facilitate appropriate, beneficial long-term management.

In the Waiting Room/Check-in by Ancillary Personnel or Nursing

Some information about phenomenology can be gathered before entry into the clinic room. One obvious example is loud vocal tics. However, more severe problems affecting gait or involuntary movements can be observed in the waiting room or when the staff is weighing the child and checking vitals. Staff can also gauge parental anxiety and may record the primary movement disorder of concern to the family. Some parents may wish to discuss the chief complaint with the physician separately, without the child present. This is generally counterproductive, as it may reinforce or create unnecessary anxiety in the child about the problem.

The First Physician Encounter in the Clinic Room

The first minutes of the clinic room encounter with the physician are very important for both the diagnosis and the therapeutic alliance. After a brief introduction to parents, the clinician should focus on the child. This provides an important opportunity for observation, during which the chief complaint may be directly observed. For an infant this can involve complimenting the child's appearance and asking to hold him or her. For toddlers or older children who may be playing in the room, watching or participating in their play with toys can be useful. When children are engaged with cell phones or other electronic devices, quick observation of their interactions with the device, followed by handing the device to the parent is advisable.

Interviewing the Child

The diagnostic assessment is best served by opening the conversation with topics such as fun after-school activities, hobbies, sports, music participation, pets, siblings, or best friends. An age-appropriate conversation about these topics helps make the child feel comfortable, so that the history and examination are more likely to be informative. This also provides essential information for assessing symptom-related impairment and making treatment decisions later. Finally, parents and children usually appreciate kind and direct interaction by the physician with the child.

During this conversation, continuous abnormal movements will be observed if present. Also, many intermittent or paroxysmal movements may be observed. Many children are anxious in clinic and may be embarrassed about their movement disorder. Sensing this, a clinician may set the child more at ease by indicating that he or she has observed the movements during the conversation and that they resemble movements in some other boys and girls he or she knows. The reassured, less anxious child may then be able to provide additional important information and cooperation during the examination.

Data about the movement disorder to be obtained from the child include the following:

- Awareness that the movement is occurring
- Preceding/premonitory sensations, urges, or intrusive thoughts
- Volition and suppressibility
- Exacerbating or ameliorating factors
- Effect of purposeful actions using the same body area as that involved in the movement disorder
- Associated pain
- Functional interference with previously discussed fun activities
- Awareness, comments on the movement by previously discussed friends or teachers
- Associated social embarrassment/effect on peer relationships
- Historical and subjective information for movement disorder rating scales.

Interviewing the Parents/Guardians

During the remainder of the history, the parents/guardians can provide complementary and usually more detailed and accurate information. This may be efficiently provided as well on a standardized intake questionnaire. In particular, parents/guardians can provide the following information:

- Verification of the details above, provided by the child; presence of movement disorder during sleep
- Past treatments
- Past diagnostic testing
- Current and past medications
- Past medical history: Detailed prenatal and perinatal history including maternal health, diseases, medication or substance use, delivery, postnatal hospitalization, jaundice
- Other medical diagnoses
- Neurologic development: Skill acquisition—gross motor, fine motor, speech, and language

- Academic performance: e.g., whether the child reads at grade level or requires extra academic assistance for math or reading
- Emotional/behavioral and cognitive problems
- Past school testing details
- Review of systems
- Family history—movement disorders, neurologic, psychiatric, or learning disorders and diseases; at least three generations (siblings; parents, aunts, uncles; grandparents)
- Parent education and occupation
- Social history/recent stressors/substance abuse history
- Information for rating scale scores.

The family history may be critical to identifying the etiology. Neurologists must understand patterns of inheritance: autosomal dominant and recessive, X-linked, and maternal/mitochondrial. Other important concepts are penetrance, genetic anticipation, premutation status, copy number variation, toxic gain of function, and haplotype insufficiency (see Table 4.2). The examiner should be sensitive to the possibility that parents may feel guilty or sad about the role of genetics in their child's symptoms. Inquiring about consanguinity can be important and may require extra tact. Ethnic backgrounds may also narrow the differential diagnosis.

The previously described history-taking process is usually sufficient to diagnose tic disorders and stereotypies in otherwise healthy children. For these common, patterned, hyperkinetic movement disorders, the general and neurologic examinations add little or no specific diagnostic information.[2] They may provide useful, nonspecific complementary information, e.g., about fine motor coordination. However, the examination remains important for those less common instances of secondary tics and stereotypies. Another important purpose of the examination is to reassure anxious parents. It is easier (and more appropriate) to convey reassurance about the child's neurologic health and development if there has been a moderately thorough neurologic examination, even in cases where the examination adds no new information. In academic clinic settings where a trainee has been the initial examiner, it is important for the attending physician to "lay on the hands" as well. When staffing the encounter with the trainee, the attending physician should establish a friendly rapport with the parents and child and repeat key portions of the motor examination, even if she or he trusts this has been competently performed by the trainee.

The Physical and Neurologic Examination

The examination begins with observation and ideally may include observation in the waiting room, during walking into the clinic room, and in all cases during the previously described interview.

The General Physical Examination

The goal of the general examination is to identify additional features of the phenotype that provide diagnostic clues and aid in medical decision making. Characteristic findings in other organs narrow the differential diagnosis. The eye examination may require ophthalmology consultation. The presence of skin pigmentary abnormalities or dysmorphic face,

TABLE 4.2   Definitions of Genetic Terms Related to Variability in Disease Expression

Term	Definition	Example
Penetrance	The frequency of expression of an allele when it is present in the genotype; the frequency with which a heritable trait occurs in individuals carrying the principal gene(s) for that trait	The penetrance of DYT1 mutations is 30%; 30% of persons carrying the GAG deletion in the DYT1 gene develop dystonia
Genetic anticipation	When genetically transmitted diseases manifest earlier or more severely in successive generations	The biological basis for genetic anticipation in Huntington disease is expansion of trinucleotide CAG repeats in the huntingtin (HTT) gene, leading to increasingly dysfunctional protein/earlier onset
Premutation status	A genetic variation that increases the risk of disease in subsequent generations	Based on the number of CGG repeats in the FMR-1 (Fragile X) gene, the status of individuals may be classified as healthy, premutation, or full mutation
		Normal: Fewer than 54 CGG repeats
		Premutation: Male or female carrier with 54–200 CGG repeats; premutation females are unaffected or mildly affected cognitively but are at risk for affected sons with full mutation. Premutation males over age 50 are at risk for Fragile X Tremor Ataxia Syndrome
		Full mutation: Trinucleotide CGG expansion over 200 causing Fragile X Syndrome with autism, intellectual disability
Haplo-insufficiency/ haplotype insufficiency	When a mutation occurs in one gene, and the amount of protein produced by the other gene is insufficient for healthy function. This concept that disease symptoms may depend on gene dosage/ protein dosage may partially explain differences in penetrance and disease severity in autosomal dominant, single gene diseases	Haplo-insufficiency has been suggested to play a role in forms of disease expression related to potassium channel subunits and to mitochondria-regulating polymerase gamma1 (POLG1)
Copy Number Variation (CNV)	In comparative genome studies, segments of DNA have been identified where duplications, deletions, inversions, or translocations have resulted in changes in copy number. These CNVs are heritable and may affect gene expression	CNV has been suggested to play a role in susceptibility to autism, schizophrenia, Tourette syndrome, and Parkinson disease

trunk, limb structures, thyroid enlargement, cardiac murmurs, and organomegaly, e.g., can also guide diagnosis.

The Neurologic Examination

The neurologic examination should be thorough, with the goal of the best possible neuroanatomic localization, as well as fully characterizing the phenotype. A challenge is to interpret possibly abnormal findings in the context of the range of coordination and skills in typically developing young children.

Because of the dynamic, state-dependent nature of movement disorders, a critical element is to directly observe the motor system in states of rest, maintenance of postures, and actions. Specific useful maneuvers are described in the symptom-based chapters. Occasionally, if an uncooperative child does not perform these helpful tasks in clinic, parents can be instructed in how to obtain this information at home and send a digital video file.

MENTAL STATUS

The mental status should essentially be screened throughout the history-taking process. Additional information is gained through observation during the examination. As movement disorders often occur with developmental and psychiatric disorders, including autism spectrum disorder (ASD),[3] the clinician should be vigilant for this possibility. The physician concerned about the possibility of ASD should note presence of communication difficulties, atypical or immature social skills, poor eye contact, repetitive behaviors and need for sameness, inability to understand jokes, and excessively concrete interpretations. Sometimes, additional assessments may be employed. For example, the Modified Checklist of Autism in Toddlers, available at www.firstsigns.org/, is validated for screening. For adolescents exhibiting concerning signs of cognitive impairment or memory loss, the Montreal Cognitive Assessment (www.mocatest.org/) may be used. This is available free of charge for clinical purposes, is translated into many languages, and may be used to assess cognition in older children. Simple writing, reading, drawing Gesell figures, drawing freehand spirals, and math computations are also useful.

EXPRESSIVE AND RECEPTIVE LANGUAGE

This is gauged informally through conversation in most cases. Expressive language is more likely to be impaired than receptive. When language problems are present, it is important to obtain formal hearing evaluation. Sensorineural hearing loss may be a clue to the diagnosis of genetic and mitochondrial diseases.[4] Children with speech disorders commonly have subnormal motor development.[5]

Some of the more commonly described speech difficulties and their relationship to movement and developmental disorders include the following:

- *Developmental dysarthria,* with predominant problems with articulation, is common and nonspecific. Mistakes are usually consistent (e.g., difficulty with certain consonants). The expected trajectory of language acquisition is delayed.
- *Developmental apraxia/dyspraxia of speech,* manifested as difficulty generating speech sounds and putting them together consistently in the correct order to form words, is less common. There is some controversy about formal criteria. It is usually diagnosed by

speech pathologists but should be suspected by neurologists in the appropriate setting. In adults, this occurs in corticobasal degeneration[6] or strokes involving areas supporting speech. In children, this is usually nonlesional and nonspecific. It is often accompanied by fine motor skills problems.[5] It is seen in galactosemia with diffuse dysmyelination.[7]

- *Dysprosody/lack of prosody*, alterations in speech intensity and pitch, speech rate, and pauses, is a component of speech abnormalities in Parkinson's disease.[8] In children, dysprosody may be seen in autism. Infants rely on prosody for word recognition,[9] and failure to appreciate prosody or appropriately generate prosody commonly occurs in children with ASD.
- *Abnormal speech cadence*, dysrhythmic or abnormally timed speech, is classically affected in cerebellar syndromes.
- *Selective mutism*, elective speech in some environments but not others, is usually related to anxiety.[10]
- *Cerebellar mutism*, part of a syndrome of ataxia, reduced speech output, emotional lability, and hypotonia, is well described after midline cerebellar tumor resections in children.[11]
- *Foreign accent syndrome* is a condition involving development or acquisition of speech patterns and pronunciation that fellow native language speakers judge to be nonnative. Although this is only sparsely documented in the pediatric literature,[12] this phenomenon is readily observed in clinics where children with ASD are evaluated.

Cranial Nerves

Key points of this section of the examination include the following: (1) brainstem signs of conditions affecting the posterior fossa that may affect both cerebellar and brainstem function; (2) eye movements; and (3) weakness, as a portion of the general motor examination (brain, brainstem, root, nerve, junction, muscle), as well as abnormal movements. Dystonia, chorea, myoclonus, and tics may all be manifest in the face. Nystagmus, other abnormal eye movements, slow saccades, saccadic pursuits, and oculomotor apraxia are also important to characterize.

Motor Examination

Assessments of bulk, tone, strength, and reflexes are standard. In children with movement disorders, these assessments also afford an opportunity to identify adventitious movements. Finger tapping and sequential finger movements should also be assessed. Many movement disorders are mixed, and may also be accompanied by weakness due to dysfunction or lesions within the corticospinal tract or nerves. Many children spontaneously exhibit tics or stereotypies. Direct observation of stereotypies in young children may also be induced by "maneuvers" such as bringing out an exciting toy. Not all involuntary movements observed in a child are abnormal. For example, many children have low-amplitude choreic movements in their fingers and hands when their arms are outstretched and held in a horizontal position in front of their bodies. This phenomenon is present in typically developing children, and is more common in children with developmental neuropsychiatric conditions such as Attention-Deficit Hyperactivity Disorder. Characterizing hypertonia in mixed spasticity and dystonia can be challenging (see Chapters 16 and 20). Children with severe, secondary generalized dystonia may become extremely dystonic due to the stimulation of the clinic room setting. This level of extreme dystonia then masks underlying tone and reflexes. The parental report of tone during sleep is helpful, as dystonic hypertonia disappears in sleep. Any procedures in which sedation is used offer a useful opportunity to examine such children in a state where dystonia is not present. In toddlers, the assessment of strength is mainly functional. For example, patterns of proximal and distal weakness in legs can be assessed through observation of rising from the floor, walking, running, and jumping or hopping. Other important maneuvers include tongue protrusion for darting tongue, sustaining grip for "milkmaid's sign," and arms and hands up over head, for involuntary pronation (see Chapter 10).

Sensory Examination

A detailed, multimodal sensory examination has low yield in children as it may provide ambiguous or uninterpretable information. Comparisons of intensity of sensation side to side, e.g., may not be accurate. Young children may simply be unable to accurately interpret and describe sensations comparing distal versus proximal or left versus right. Generally, young children can report presence of light touch and vibration, and, with practice, may be able to report proprioception. Older children with Tourette syndrome, obsessive-compulsive disorder, anxiety, ASD, or functional disorders may ruminate over examination details and provide conflicting, nonanatomic reports. A detailed sensory examination is generally most useful when a specific localization hypothesis is being tested.

Cerebellar Examination

This is discussed extensively in Chapter 2. The clinician should have the full range of cerebellar bedside tests at his or her disposal to be used in cases where careful characterization of coordination and cerebellar function is needed.

Tremor Examination

The child should be observed at rest, in several postures with arms and hands outstretched and with elbows flexed and fingers facing each other, and on finger-to-nose testing. Additional discussion is found in Chapter 13.

Video-Enhanced Examination

If the examination does not reveal the movement disorder described by the parents, either because the child is not exhibiting the abnormal movements at the time of the visit, is trying to suppress or camouflage it, or is simply not cooperating with the examination, the parents should be instructed to take home videos of their children. This is especially important in patients with paroxysmal movements such as tics, stereotypies, paroxysmal dyskinesias or ataxias, and repetitive leg and pelvic movements in girls with self-stimulatory (masturbatory) behavior. This can also be helpful when seizures are in the differential diagnosis.

The following instructions should be provided to the parents on how to take the best videos: Instructions to patients and their family members and/or caregivers how to use mobile device for home videos:

1. Turn on the video mode of your mobile device (smartphone, etc.) and position the device into a horizontal (not vertical) position.
2. To capture the affected area as clearly as possible, initially establish a distant view before bringing the device up close to the affected body area.
3. Ensure lighting is adequate.
4. Ensure sound volume is adequate and if possible eliminate any ambient noise.
5. Hold the device steady or use a tripod or flat, stabilizing surface.

THE DIAGNOSIS

This section reviews three general strategies for diagnosis, given the information obtained in the previous sections.

Strategy 1: Recognize Patterns Based on Phenomenology and Time Course

Experienced clinicians can correctly identify common and some rare diagnoses in clinic, using information described previously, without further medical diagnostic testing. Some diagnoses may literally be made in the doorway to the clinic room. The most common diagnoses in each chapter of this book are usually not difficult for child neurologists to make. Particularly straightforward diagnoses made accurately in most cases by pattern recognition include tic disorders, chorea, stereotypies, developmental tremor, and mild motor symptoms caused by static encephalopathies.

These common diagnoses may be very stressful for a family. When appropriate, it is important to make the clinical diagnosis confidently and steer families away from obtaining unnecessary diagnostic tests.[13–16] For example, in most movement disorder cases, electroencephalograms will not provide useful information.[17]

Strategy 2: Focus on Proximate Causes as Possible Etiologies for Acute- and Subacute-Onset, Acquired Movement Disorders

For acute and subacute manifestations, it is helpful to think in terms of categories:

- Infectious
- Inflammatory: postinfection, postvaccine, para-neoplastic, other autoimmune
- Iatrogenic: drug-induced
- Ingestion/intoxication
- Electrolyte, Endocrine, other organ system (renal, liver)
- Migrainous
- Epileptic
- Traumatic
- Vascular
- Metabolic/mitochondrial
- Paroxysmal or episodic genetic

The phenomenology, the age of the child, and the history of present illness usually narrow this list substantially, and this guides diagnostic decision making. In many cases, the diagnostic process will involve neuroimaging or laboratory testing. Specific acute and subacute diseases and diagnostic strategies are discussed in the phenomenology-based chapters in this book.

Strategy 3: Have a Stepwise, Organized Approach to More Difficult Chronic Diagnoses

For more difficult diagnoses, many pieces of data can be important, and sometimes arriving at the precise diagnosis requires days, months, or even years.[18,19] Patients with no molecular diagnosis for years may still acquire one as clinical and basic science advance.

The following is a useful, stepwise approach for more difficult diagnoses:

1. Classify the phenomenology.
2. Identify the most likely anatomic substrate, bearing in mind that many disorders in children are mixed movement disorders, and that classic phenomenology/brain substrate relationships do not always apply.
3. Review the time course: acute, subacute, paroxysmal, chronic static, chronic progressive, continuous but waxing and waning, relapsing and remitting.
4. Use the three-generation family history to consider heritability and to narrow the differential diagnosis.
5. Use other key features of the history or physical examination including findings outside of the nervous system.
6. Use helpful online resources. For any suspected disease that is not clearly secondary or environmentally induced, there are an enormous number of genetic possibilities. Use of online resources, as described later in this chapter and in Appendix B, is recommended. Note that the boundaries of the phenotypes of rare genetic diseases are probably known only imprecisely. For example, the range of age of onset in rare diseases reflects ascertainment bias in the few reported cases. Intra-familial heterogeneity is common, so inter-familial heterogeneity should be expected as well.

These six steps are considered in detail next.

Step 1: Classify the Phenomenology

Phenomenology classification is the critical first step. This is discussed in greater detail in Chapter 3. Classification aids in limiting the list of possible diagnoses, based on probable anatomic substrate for symptoms. This may allow targeted laboratory testing rather than more expensive testing with a genetic panel or exome sequencing. For example, dystonia or chorea often points toward basal ganglia and ataxia toward cerebellum and its inflow and outflow pathways. Most often, determination of phenomenology is based on skilled visual pattern recognition of movements observed spontaneously or elicited during the examination.

In cases where several phenomenological terms may seem appropriate, the determination may require supplementation of visual impressions by details from the history or careful repeat examination over time. After the initial examination, review of videotape of the child's movements and collaborative discussion in movement disorder video rounds may clarify or correct impressions from the real-time observation. A partial list of overlapping phenomena that can be difficult to distinguish visually appears in Table 4.3.

TABLE 4.3   Selected Challenging Classifications

Movement disorders with overlapping phenomenologies	Keys to differentiation based on history, examination
Brief tics; myoclonus	*Tics:* The child interview is critical. The child should be aware of some tics and of urges to perform tics, particularly when stressed or in other predictable situations. Tics are usually at least partly suppressible. Both tics and subcortical myoclonus may diminish during purposeful activity, but this is more universally characteristic of tics.
	Myoclonus: The child may be unaware of movement. If aware, the child experiences myoclonus as involuntary. Action may enhance myoclonus.
Complex tics; compulsions; stereotypies	*Tics:* The child should sometimes be aware of an urge to perform the tic. Tics usually begin with simple movements, after age 3 years, with waxing and waning and increasing complexity over time. Young children with complex tics often ultimately manifest obsessive-compulsive disorder.
	Compulsions: The urge to perform these commonly corresponds to an obsession (e.g., obsession with germs/compulsions with washing, obsessions with safety/compulsions with checking). This is not always true in children who may have compulsions and rituals but not articulate a fear or obsession. Query for set number of repetitions, "evening up", or making "just right."
	Stereotypies: Complex, patterned, with earlier onset than tics, usually before age 3. Characteristic of autism and a relatively small number of serious neurologic diagnoses, but occurs often in typical children.
Multifocal and truncal myoclonus; truncal ataxia and titubation; jerky chorea	*Myoclonus* of muscles of limbs and trunk, when frequent, may fairly continuously move the trunk, creating an appearance of titubation. This is particularly true in toddlers. Myoclonus may occur at multiple levels of the neuraxis, so detailed neurologic examination may provide additional clues. Opsoclonus is an ominous finding.
	Titubation and *ataxia* are characteristic of cerebellar disease, for which other cerebellar findings and nystagmus may be clues.
	Jerky chorea, as in benign hereditary chorea, may be difficult to distinguish from ataxia or myoclonus. Expert consensus cannot always be achieved in individual cases.
Akathisia; chorea	*Akathisia* is characterized by restless movements and subjective sensory hypersensitivity and discomfort. It most often occurs as a side effect of psychiatric medication.
	Chorea is involuntary restlessness, with jerky or flowing, random-appearing movement fragments occurring fairly continuously. It causes aggravation but not sensory discomfort. Both movement disorders may be drug-induced but subacute chorea is more likely autoimmune.

(Continued)

TABLE 4.3   (Continued)

Movement disorders with overlapping phenomenologies	Keys to differentiation based on history, examination
Ataxic gait; choreic gait; progressive spastic gait	*Ataxic gait:* Fairly consistently broad-based. Other signs including positive Romberg, dysmetria on heel to shin and finger to nose often present.
	Choreic gait: Less consistently broad-based. Choreic intrusions may lead to lurching intermittently rather than a stably broad-based gait. Upper limb chorea should be readily distinguishable from ataxia.
	Spastic gait: Can be difficult to characterize in gradually progressive parapareses and leukodystrophies. When scissoring/hip adduction is not prominent, consistent or intermittent hypertonic extensions during walking may produce broad-based gait and poor balance mimicking ataxia. Careful motor examination often clarifies the picture.
Seizure; not-seizure: Clonic movements and automatisms in simple and complex partial seizures versus paroxysmal movement disorders	*Simple partial seizures:* Brief-patterned clonic movements may occur, with preserved consciousness. These cannot be suppressed by the patient or observer.
	Epileptic automatisms: Blinking, patterned movements may resemble tics. Awareness is limited or absent. In contrast to tics, there is no urge to perform these and no ability to suppress. These cannot be interrupted by the observer, in contrast to stereotypies, which can be interrupted.
	Paroxysmal movement disorders: Dyskinesias, tics, stereotypies—no loss of consciousness, no "postictal" confusion or fatigue; phenomenology, subjective experience, interruptibility all help distinguish from epilepsies.

Step 2: Localize the Anatomic Substrate

The neurological examination and classification of phenomenology in many cases allow for localization. Neuroimaging is sometimes needed. Additional details about neuroanatomy of basal ganglia and cerebellum and associated normal and abnormal function are presented in the first two chapters. Mixed movement disorders pose a special challenge, as do movement disorders in infancy, because the examination is relatively insensitive at that stage of neurodevelopment. Once the clinician has localized the disease, it is important not to be too dogmatic in narrowing the differential diagnosis. The examination in children can be difficult to interpret, and diseases manifest in uncommon or unexpected ways. For example, Huntington disease in young children manifests with dystonia and Parkinsonism, not chorea. Spinocerebellar ataxias and ataxia telangiectasia may manifest with chorea or dystonia, not ataxia.

Step 3: Incorporate the Time Course into the Diagnostic Process

Time course includes age of onset and acute, subacute, paroxysmal, waxing and waning, chronic-static, or chronic-progressive history. These assist with identifying probable etiologic categories for primary and secondary movement disorders.

Step 4: Use the Family History of Neurologic and Psychiatric Conditions

When heritability is suspected, a three-generation family pedigree, including cousins and siblings of parents and grandparents, can clarify an inheritance pattern. Examples of common inheritance patterns are shown in Figure 4.1.

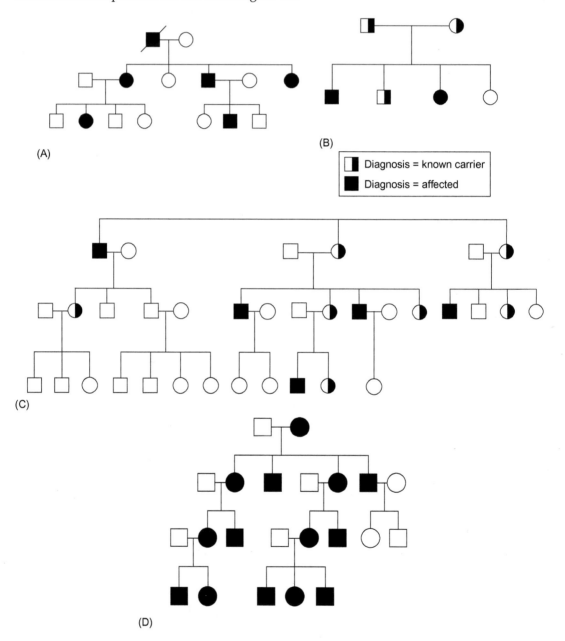

FIGURE 4.1   Patterns of inheritance. Individuals affected by the disease are indicated by darker colors; squares = males; circles = females. (A) Autosomal dominant (AD): Autosomal—the disease-causing gene is located on an

In selected situations, presence of nonneurologic diseases is also worth noting on the pedigree. For example, family history of autoimmune, thrombotic, endocrine, or psychiatric diseases can be informative. The family history helps narrow the search. However, the absence of a family history does not mean the disease is not heritable.

Challenges to obtaining and interpreting the family history include genetic, neurologic, and social factors:

- Spontaneous, new mutations
- Incomplete penetrance
- Genetic anticipation—the child may become symptomatic at a much younger age than the parent did
- Age-related disease expression—the child's phenotype may differ because of younger age of onset
- X-linked diseases or those with greater penetrance in males, such that carrier mother may be asymptomatic
- Single-gene diseases with substantial intra-familial variability in phenotype
- Unknown but important modifier genes
- Environmental or epigenetic factors
- Mitochondrial diseases with heteroplasmy
- Nonpaternity
- Absence of information on one or both biologic parents
- Guilt/denial leading to inaccurate reporting
- Prior misdiagnoses or lack of precise knowledge of problems in family members

---

"autosome" (chromosomes 1 through 22) and not a sex chromosome (X, Y). Males and females are equally likely to inherit and pass on these genes. Dominant—one copy of the disease-causing gene suffices to produce disease. Probability that an affected parent will pass the disease-causing gene to each child is 50%. Note that in pedigrees for diseases with incomplete penetrance such as DYT1 (i.e., some individuals have the disease-causing gene but remain unaffected), there will be more disease-gene carriers than affected individuals. AD heritability may be suspected when males or females in multiple generations are affected, including pedigrees with male-to-male or male-to-female transmission. (B) Autosomal recessive (AR): Recessive—one copy of the disease-carrying gene does not suffice to produce disease. Individuals with one copy are not affected and usually are unaware of the presence of the gene. They are designated as "carriers." Two copies of the disease-carrying gene yield the disease, in either males or females. The probability that a child of two carrier-parents will be homozygous for the disease-carrying gene and have the disease is 25%. AR heritability may be suspected when siblings in one generation only are affected. (C) X-linked recessive (XR): the disease-causing gene is on the X chromosome. No male-to-male transmission is possible. Only males may be affected, or carrier females may have mild phenotype. Probability that a male child of a carrier-mother will inherit the disease-carrying gene is 50%. XR heritability may be suspected when only males, related through common females, are affected. (D) Mitochondrial DNA (mtDNA): The disease-causing gene is located in mitochondrial DNA. Mitochondria are passed to children through the egg, not the sperm, so affected males cannot pass on mtDNA diseases. Affected females can pass diseases on to some or all male or female offspring. Note that mitochondria contain multiple copies of DNA, and cells contain multiple mitochondria, so there is a mixture of more than one type of mtDNA within cells, a phenomenon referred to as heteroplasmy. Sorting of disease-causing mtDNA occurs during cell division, meaning there is vast potential for variability in organ involvement as well as age of onset of mitochondrial diseases. MtDNA inheritance may be suspected when both males and females in multiple generations are affected, with no male-to-offspring transmission.

As our understanding of disease inheritance and genotype/phenotype interactions has evolved, a simple understanding of Mendelian genetics has become insufficient for neurologists. An abbreviated list of important and relatively recent genetic concepts is found in Table 4.3.

Step 5: Identify and Consider Nonneurologic, Key Features of History or Physical Examination

Involvement of other organ systems in the disease may assist in identifying the diagnosis. For example, short stature, migraine, and hearing loss may narrow the search to mitochondrial disease. Hepatomegaly or splenomegaly may increase the likelihood of lysosomal or other storage diseases. Unique or unusual facial features may also provide useful clues. Combining these with the movement disorder phenomenology may vastly narrow the differential diagnosis.

Step 6: Use Online Resources

Multiple websites can provide assistance in the complex process of diagnosis. Several particularly useful ones are:

1. Online Mendelian Inheritance in Man (OMIM) (http://www.omim.org)
2. Simulconsult (http://www.simulconsult.com/)
3. Genetic Testing Registry (https://www.ncbi.nlm.nih.gov/gtr/)
4. Genetests (http:// www.genetests.org).

Further discussion of diagnostic search strategies is found in Appendix B.

Education about the diagnosis, referrals to psychology for coping skills, and referrals to high-quality websites for education and advocacy are often very helpful. For genetic diseases, the Genetics Home Resource (http://ghr.nlm.nih.gov/) is a great starting point.

SUMMARY

Diagnosis begins with a careful history and a thorough physical examination, with the goal of classifying the phenomenology first. If the movement disorder is not present at the time of the examination, parents should be instructed to take home or school videos (see above) and these should often be reviewed prior to decisions about medical diagnostic testing. Even experts may fail to reach consensus in some clinical situations.[20] Advances in molecular understanding can ultimately provide clarification,[21,22] although there are still cases where a molecular diagnosis remains elusive.[23]

More difficult cases may require a review of relevant neuroanatomy, as presented in the first two chapters of this book, or as reviewed on useful websites or other textbooks. There are myriad opportunities for second opinions from colleagues through in-person clinic visits, teleconferences, meeting presentations, or emailing videos.

Repeated searching of databases such as OMIM, as described in Appendix B, is also helpful, because these are regularly updated based on new discoveries. Once a diagnosis is made, treatment remains, in most cases, at best symptomatic. However, education about the diagnosis, advocacy, and obtaining appropriate services for a child can have profound benefits for the child and family. Increasing knowledge of the molecular basis of diseases will eventually yield more rational and effective therapies.

References

1. Bitsko RH, Danielson M, King M, Visser SN, Scahill L, Perou R. Health care needs of children with Tourette syndrome. *J Child Neurol*. 2013;28(12):1626–1636.
2. Dooley JM, Gordon KE, Wood EP, Camfield CS, Camfield PR. The utility of the physical examination and investigations in the pediatric neurology consultation. *Pediatr Neurol*. 2003;28(2):96–99.
3. Canitano R, Vivanti G. Tics and Tourette syndrome in autism spectrum disorders. *Autism*. 2007;11(1):19–28.
4. Leveque M, Marlin S, Jonard L, et al. Whole mitochondrial genome screening in maternally inherited non-syndromic hearing impairment using a microarray resequencing mitochondrial DNA chip. *Eur J Hum Genet*. 2007;15(11):1145–1155.
5. Visscher C, Houwen S, Scherder EJ, Moolenaar B, Hartman E. Motor profile of children with developmental speech and language disorders. *Pediatrics*. 2007;120(1):e158–163.
6. Zadikoff C, Lang AE. Apraxia in movement disorders. *Brain*. 2005;128(Pt 7):1480–1497.
7. Ridel KR, Leslie ND, Gilbert DL. An updated review of the long-term neurological effects of galactosemia. *Pediatr Neurol*. 2005;33(3):153–161.
8. Skodda S, Rinsche H, Schlegel U. Progression of dysprosody in Parkinson's disease over time—A longitudinal study. *Mov Disord*. 2009;24(5):716–722.
9. Johnson EK, Seidl AH. At 11 months, prosody still outranks statistics. *Dev Sci*. 2009;12(1):131–141.
10. Sharp WG, Sherman C, Gross AM. Selective mutism and anxiety: a review of the current conceptualization of the disorder. *J Anxiety Disord*. 2007;21(4):568–579.
11. Robertson PL, Muraszko KM, Holmes EJ, et al. Incidence and severity of postoperative cerebellar mutism syndrome in children with medulloblastoma: a prospective study by the Children's Oncology Group. *J Neurosurg*. 2006;105(6):444–451.
12. Marien P, Verhoeven J, Wackenier P, Engelborghs S, De Deyn PP. Foreign accent syndrome as a developmental motor speech disorder. *Cortex*. 2009;45(7):870–878.
13. Espay AJ, Goldenhar LM, Voon V, Schrag A, Burton N, Lang AE. Opinions and clinical practices related to diagnosing and managing patients with psychogenic movement disorders: an international survey of movement disorder society members. *Mov Disord*. 2009;24(9):1366–1374.
14. Gilbert DL. Treatment of children and adolescents with tics and Tourette syndrome. *J Child Neurol*. 2006;21:690–700.
15. Zinner SH, Mink JW. Movement disorders I: tics and stereotypies. *Pediatr Rev*. 2010;31(6):223–233.
16. Mink JW, Zinner SH. Movement disorders II: chorea, dystonia, myoclonus, and tremor. *Pediatr Rev*. 2010;31(7):287–294. quiz 295.
17. Gilbert DL, Gartside PS. Factors affecting the yield of pediatric EEGs in clinical practice. *Clin Pediatr*. 2002;41(1):25–32.
18. Gospe Jr. SM, Caruso RD, Clegg MS, et al. Paraparesis, hypermanganesaemia, and polycythaemia: a novel presentation of cirrhosis. *Arch Dis Child*. 2000;83(5):439–442.
19. Tuschl K, Clayton PT, Gospe Jr. SM, et al. Syndrome of hepatic cirrhosis, dystonia, polycythemia, and hypermanganesemia caused by mutations in SLC30A10, a manganese transporter in man. *Am J Hum Genet*. 2012;90(3):457–466.
20. Schrag A, Quinn NP, Bhatia KP, Marsden CD. Benign hereditary chorea—entity or syndrome? *Mov Disord*. 2000;15(2):280–288.
21. Breedveld GJ, Percy AK, MacDonald ME, et al. Clinical and genetic heterogeneity in benign hereditary chorea. *Neurology*. 2002;59(4):579–584.
22. Breedveld GJ, van Dongen JW, Danesino C, et al. Mutations in TITF-1 are associated with benign hereditary chorea. *Hum Mol Genet*. 2002;11(8):971–979.
23. Neveling K, Feenstra I, Gilissen C, et al. A post-hoc comparison of the utility of sanger sequencing and exome sequencing for the diagnosis of heterogeneous diseases. *Hum Mutat*. 2013;34(12):1721–1726.

Motor Assessments

Harvey S. Singer[1], Jonathan W. Mink[2],
Donald L. Gilbert[3] and Joseph Jankovic[4]

[1]Department of Neurology, Johns Hopkins Hospital, Baltimore, MD, USA;
[2]Division of Child Neurology, University of Rochester Medical Center,
Rochester, NY, USA; [3]Division of Neurology, Cincinnati Children's Hospital
Medical Center, Cincinnati, OH, USA; [4]Department of Neurology, Baylor
College of Medicine, Houston, TX, USA

INTRODUCTION

Clinical assessment of movement disorders requires visual observation. The definitions presented in Chapter 3 and detailed characteristics of individual movement disorders provided in Chapters 7–8 and 10–17 rely on descriptions of characteristic spatial and temporal properties of both voluntary and involuntary movements in the specific disorders. Pattern recognition can be helpful, but in many cases a systematic approach to evaluating specific features is necessary to assure that a correct diagnosis is made. Many movement disorders can be evaluated during a face-to-face clinic visit, but in other cases the movements may not be observed. In those cases, video capture of the movements can be essential for correct diagnosis. The widespread availability of smart phones or tablets with high-quality video capability has greatly enhanced the ability of physicians to witness movements in order to make more accurate diagnoses. Indeed, some movement disorders neurologists are now using telemedicine to evaluate and treat patients with movement disorders.[1,2]

Although visual assessment of movement patterns by an experienced clinician is sufficient to classify movement disorders, there are limitations. Some patients have more than one movement disorder. Other patients have one or more movement disorders in association with other neurological signs. In these situations it is usually possible to diagnose the movement disorders clinically, but it is often difficult to separate out the relative contribution of each to the patient's disability. And sometimes it is difficult to be certain of the correct classification of the movements when they are at the extremes of the characteristic range. For example, very brief choreic movements may resemble myoclonus. The use of technology to measure movements (kinematics), muscle contractions (electromyography), or central nervous system signals associated with individual movements (evoked potentials) may assist in making an accurate diagnosis. Technology has also been used to investigate the pathophysiology of movement disorders in children; those applications will be discussed in chapters on the specific movement disorders.

Beyond diagnosis, there is often a need to assess the severity of the movement disorder in order to gauge disease progression or response to treatment. Although certain technologies can also be used for this, clinical rating scales have greater utility in a routine clinical setting. Several valid and reliable clinical rating scales are available for use in children with movement disorders.

QUANTITATIVE MEASUREMENT IN MOVEMENT DISORDERS

Kinematics

Kinematic analysis of movement involves the measurement of position, velocity, and acceleration of one or more body parts. Linear measurements of specific parts, angular measurements at joints, or a combination can be performed in order to quantify the special and temporal properties of movements of multiple body parts simultaneously. It is generally best for kinematic measurements to be made in three dimensions, but two-dimensional measures can also be useful. Kinematic methods have been employed in a large number of adult studies, but some methods are less practical for young children. However, kinematic methods have been used in children to quantify the pattern, severity, or impact of several disorders including ataxia,[3,4] dystonia,[5–7] parkinsonism,[8] stereotypies,[9] tics,[9] and tremor.[8] Moreover, these methods have been applied to discriminate among multiple movement disorders occurring within or across individual patients.[5,8,9]

Electromyography

Surface electromyography (EMG) has been used in adults to define the temporal features of myoclonus, chorea, dystonia, and tics.[10] Similar studies have not been performed in children. However, EMG has been used to assess hypothesized features of childhood dystonia.[11] EMG can be helpful in distinguishing organic movement disorders from psychogenic (also referred to functional or conversion) disorders in some cases.[12–15]

Cortical Potentials

Measurement of cortical electrical potentials with surface EEG electrodes may help assess the pathophysiology of certain movement disorders. Simultaneous measurement of the cortical electrical potentials and EMG may be helpful in determining whether myoclonus is originating in cerebral cortex or in subcortical regions.[10] The "readiness potential" (Bereitschaftspotential), which precedes voluntary movement, may be useful in some cases to distinguish organic from functional movement disorders.[16]

Transcranial Magnetic Stimulation

Transcranial magnetic stimulation (TMS) can be used to study excitability of motor cortex, cortical inhibitory mechanisms, and interactions between brain regions in different disorders.[17,18] It is safe to use as an investigative tool in children, and has been used in several studies of Tourette syndrome[19–23] and cerebral palsy.[24,25] TMS has revealed differences in children with Tourette syndrome with or without accompanying ADHD.[19,21] It is not known whether TMS has the potential to inform diagnosis of children with movement disorders.

RATING SCALES FOR PEDIATRIC MOVEMENT DISORDERS

Rating scales are clinical instruments that are designed to measure the presence and severity of clinical features. Rating scales can be disease specific, encompassing many features of the disease. The Unified Parkinson Disease Rating Scale (UPDRS)[26] and the Unified Huntington Disease Rating Scale (UHDRS)[27] are multidimensional scales that were designed to rate the key features of the relevant disease. One axis for each scale is a "motor" subscale that specifically rates the key features of the movement disorders. These scales have been used widely in clinical studies of Parkinson's disease and Huntington's disease in adults. Although these scales were designed to be disease specific, neither scale is a diagnostic instrument. In other words, a nonzero score on the motor subscale of the UPDRS does not mean that the patient being evaluated has Parkinson's disease. Other scales are restricted to a specific sign or symptoms. For example, the Ashworth scale rates spasticity only.[28]

Most published movement disorders rating scales were designed for the evaluation of movement disorders in adults. Some of these scales have been applied in studies of children, but their use may be confounded by the impact of development on understanding of instructions and on motor control.[29,30] Other scales have been developed and tested for use in children.

An ideal clinical rating meets certain criteria including validity, reliability, internal consistency, utility, and responsiveness to treatment. *Validity* is the ability of a scale to actually measure what it was designed to measure. There are several types of validity. The most common type of validity demonstrated by clinical rating scales is *construct (face) validity*: Does the measure seem reasonable based on what is known of the disorder and is it likely to yield the type of information it was designed to obtain? *Convergent validity* is the property of performing comparably to a previously validated scale. *Discriminative validity* is the property of not correlating with a measure of an unrelated variable. *Predictive validity* is the ability of a scale to predict response to future disease course or response to treatment. *Reliability* is the degree to which repeated application of the scale within a narrow time window yields the same results. It is a measure of reproducibility. Clinical scales are often evaluated for interrater reliability, agreement between examiners evaluating the same subject, and intrarater reliability, the ability of a single examiner to arrive at the same answer with repeated administration. *Internal consistency* is the ability of items that should measure the same general construct to produce similar scores. *Utility* is the ability of a scale to be administered without undue burden to examiner or to subject: Can it be used in a routine clinical setting? *Responsiveness to treatment* is the ability of scale to measure a response to treatment when one exists. Few movement disorders rating scales have met all of these criteria in adults;[31,32] even fewer have been shown to have good clinic-metric properties in children.

A comprehensive and critical review of movement disorders rating scales for children is beyond the intended scope of this chapter. Many scales designed to assess function, quality of life, care-giver burden, pain, and other aspects of disability or health, have used in studies of movement disorders, but they are not specific to any one particular disorder. In the remainder of this chapter, available scales that are specific to individual movement disorders and that have been used in children with movement disorders will be described under specific movement disorders below. Two unique instruments that were not developed for a specific movement disorder are discussed at the end of this chapter.

Ataxia

Three main ataxia scales have been used in children: the Scale for the Assessment and Rating of Ataxia (SARA), the International Cooperative Ataxia Rating Scale (ICARS), and the Friedreich Ataxia Rating Scale (FARS). All three are inter-correlated, but there are some differences that may favor one over the others in specific situations.[33,34] All three have been tested in children and all three have been shown to have limitations in children below 12 years of age due to developmental factors.[33]

SARA

The SARA was developed for use in patients with autosomal dominant inherited ataxias (ADA).[35] It is the simplest of the ataxia rating scales, consisting of eight items and has been shown to be valid and reliable.[35] It correlates well with scores on the ICARS and FARS in patients with Friedreich ataxia (FRDA), but can be administered more quickly.[34]

ICARS

The ICARS is a 100-point scale that assesses postural and stance disturbances, limb movement disturbances, speech, and oculomotor dysfunction. It was designed for use in studies of pharmacologic treatment of ataxias and has been shown to be valid and reliable in studies of ADA and FRDA.[36,37] It correlates with scores on the ICARS and FARS in patients with FRDA.[34] The ICARS is sensitive to change with disease progression, but demonstrates ceiling effects that reduce its sensitivity in advanced disease.[38]

FARS

The FARS is a disease-specific rating scale that includes multiple parts to characterize FRDA.[39] It is valid and reliable. The clinical examination component (part III) is a 122-point scale that assesses bulbar, upper limb, lower limb, peripheral nerve, and upright stability/gait functions. Separate scoring of function stage and activities of daily living are included in other parts. The FARS correlates well with the SARA and the ICARS in patients with FRDA.[34] The FARS is sensitive to disease progression at 1- and 2-year follow-up evaluations, but there is a ceiling effect that may limit its validity in patients with advanced disease.[40] The ataxia in FRDA is due, at least in large part, to afferent dysfunction and some evidence suggests that the FARS may be more appropriate for use in patients with "sensory" ataxia.[41]

Chorea

No single rating scale has been developed specifically for the evaluation of chorea. However, two disease-specific rating scales include rating of chorea as a component of a more comprehensive evaluation. The UHDRS has been shown to be valid and reliable in Huntington's disease and to be sensitive to change with disease progression.[27] However, its use in children for the assessment of chorea severity is limited due to the fact that children with Huntington's disease rarely manifest chorea.

The Universidade Federal de Minas Gerais Sydenham Chorea Rating Scale (USCRS) rates the several signs and symptoms of patients with Sydenham's chorea (SC).[42] It is a 108-point scale that provides assessment of motor function, activities of daily living, and behavioral abnormalities, and motor function of subjects with SC. It has good face validity and has been shown to have interrater reliability and internal consistency.

Dystonia

There are many clinical rating scales for dystonia,[31] but few have been studied in children. The Burke–Fahn–Marsden Dystonia Rating Scale (BFMDRS), the Unified Dystonia Rating Scale (UDRS), and the Global Dystonia Rating Scale (GDRS) have been validated for the assessment of dystonia in adults.[43,44] These have been shown to have reasonable agreement when compared in the same subjects.[43] Of these, only the BFMDRS has been evaluated in children. Another scale, the Barry–Albright Dystonia (BAD) Scale was developed for use in children with acquired dystonia (secondary dystonia) or dystonia accompanied by spasticity.[45] A feature common to all of these scales is the assignment of a numerical score to individual body regions, with higher numbers indicating more severe dystonia in the corresponding region.

BFMDRS

The BFMDRS is composed of two clinician-rated subscales: a movement subscale, based on patient examination, and a disability subscale, based on the patient's report of disability in activities of daily living.[46] The 120-point movement subscale rates dystonia severity and provoking factors in nine body areas, including eyes, mouth, speech and swallowing, neck, trunk, and both arms and legs.

The 30-point disability subscale is composed of seven items for activities of daily living, such as speech, writing, feeding, eating, hygiene, dressing, and walking.[46] The BFMDRS is the most frequently used in children with genetic dystonias,[47–50] but its clinicometric properties have not been established in children. Further, the dependence on provoking factors limits its validity in young children.

BAD

The BAD was developed for use in children with reduced capacity for voluntary control of movement, specifically those with cerebral palsy.[45] It emphasizes the impact of abnormal posturing on positioning and activities of daily living, rather than on provoking factors. It has been shown to have good validity, reliability, and is responsive to treatment. The BAD has not been validated in children dystonia due to genetic causes.

Myoclonus

A myoclonus rating scale has been developed, but has not been evaluated specifically in children.[51]

Parkinsonism

The UPDRS is the most studied and utilized movement disorders rating scale. It rates aspects of Parkinson's disease on four subscales: (1) evaluation of mentation, behavior, and mood; (2) evaluation of activities of daily living; (3) motor examination; and (4) complications of therapy. Although the UPDRS has been applied to assess the severity of parkinsonism in juvenile neuronal ceroid lipofuscinosis (Batten disease),[52] its clinicometric properties have not been evaluated in children.

Stereotypies

The *Stereotypy Severity Scale* (SSS) is a 5-item caregiver questionnaire consisting of two components (motor and impairment) for the ranking of motor stereotypies (Miller et al. 2006). The *motor* severity component (maximum = 18 points), rates the movement along four discriminate dimensions including number (0–3 points), frequency (0–5 points), intensity (0–5 points), and interference (0–5 points). An independent rating of *impairment*, caused by the movement (up to 50 points) is added to obtain the *total* score (maximum 68 points). The validity of the SSS has been confirmed in the study by Freeman (2010).[53,54]

Tics

Several rating scales have been developed for tics. These include the Yale Global Tic Severity Scale (YGTSS), the Motor tics, Obsessions and compulsions, Vocal tics Evaluation Survey (MOVES), and the Modified Rush Video-based Tic Rating Scale (RVTRS). All were developed for use in patients with Tourette syndrome, but their validity is not limited to that disorder. The YGTSS is based on clinician rating from interview and observation, the MOVES is a patient self-report scale, and the RVTRS is a clinician scored video-based observation scale.

YGTSS

The YGTSS is the most widely used tic rating scale and has the most extensive data supporting validity, reliability, utility, and sensitivity to change.[55–58] The YGTSS is score by a clinician based on interview about tics over the previous week. It consists of two parts: a Total Tic Score and an Impairment Score. The Total Tic Score includes for both motor and vocal tics scores of tic number, tic frequency, tic intensity, tic complexity, and tic interference for a maximum possible 50 points. The Impairment Score is a 0–50 rating of the impairment due to tics. The Total Tic Score has stronger clinicometric properties than does the Impairment Score.

MOVES

The MOVES is a self-report scale for symptoms of Tourette syndrome that can be completed by children, adolescents, or adults.[59] It is a 20-item scale that includes four items each for motor tics, phonic tics, obsessions, compulsions, and "associated symptoms." The MOVES correlates well with the YGTSS and appears to be sensitive to change.

RVTRS

The RVTRS involves video recording of tics during a clinic visit.[60,61] The video protocol involves a 10-minute recording the patient in a quiet room. Two body views are recorded: full frontal body and zoomed in to include the head and shoulders only. Video segments of 2.5-minute duration are recorded with each view with the examiner in the room and with the patient alone. The recordings with the patient alone are scored for number of body areas, frequency of motor tics, frequency of phonic tics, severity of motor tics, and severity of phonic tics. The RVTRS is valid and reliable. It correlates well with the YGTSS Total Tic Score.[60] A modification of the RVTRS has been proposed to allow its use with home video.[62]

Tremor

The Fahn–Tolosa–Marin Tremor Rating Scales (TRS) was developed for the evaluation of essential tremor, but has been used in other forms of tremor in adults.[63] It consists of two parts: Part A scores the magnitude of tremor in different body parts and Part B scores tremor in writing and drawings. It has good face validity and reliability in adults. It has not been evaluated in children, but has good face validity for use in children who are old enough to write. Another tremor rating scale, The Essential Tremor Rating Scale (TETRAS), developed by the Tremor Research Group, has been validated against the TRS.[68]

Scales for Combined Movement Disorders

The Hypertonia Assessment Tool (HAT) is a discriminative tool to ascertain the presence of spasticity, dystonia, parkinsonian rigidity, or a combination in children with mixed movement disorders.[64,65] The revised version of the HAT has six items that are scored as present or absent, with each being a characteristic property of spasticity, dystonia, or rigidity.[64] The HAT has good clinicometric properties in children.

The Movement Disorder Childhood Rating Scale evaluated the severity of movement disorders in children regardless of the specific movement disorder present.[66] It describes the clinical features of different types of movement disorders, evaluates the intensity of movement disorders in different body regions at rest and during specific tasks, and assesses the influence of movement disorders on motor function and daily living activities. Scoring is based on a 20-minute standardized video protocol. It has been shown to have good reliability and internal consistency. Its major shortcoming is the lack of ability to discriminate among movement disorders and their individual contribution to severity. A separate version for use in children less than 3 years of age has also been developed.[67]

References

1. Biglan KM, Voss TS, Deuel LM, et al. Telemedicine for the care of nursing home residents with Parkinson's disease. *Mov Disord*. 2009;24(7):1073–1076.
2. Dorsey ER, Venkataraman V, Grana MJ, et al. Randomized controlled clinical trial of "virtual house calls" for Parkinson disease. *JAMA Neurol*. 2013;70(5):565–570.
3. Bastian A, Mink J, Kaufman B, Thach W. Posterior vermal split syndrome. *Ann Neurol*. 1998;44:601–610.
4. Ramos E, Latash MP, Hurvitz EA, Brown SH. Quantification of upper extremity function using kinematic analysis. *Arch Phys Med Rehabil*. 1997;78(5):491–496.
5. Gordon LM, Keller JL, Stashinko EE, Hoon AH, Bastian AJ. Can spasticity and dystonia be independently measured in cerebral palsy? *Pediatr Neurol*. 2006;35(6):375–381.
6. de Campos AC, Kukke SN, Hallett M, Alter KE, Damiano DL. Characteristics of bilateral hand function in individuals with unilateral dystonia due to perinatal stroke: sensory and motor aspects. *J Child Neurol*. 2014;29(5):623–632.
7. Kawamura A, Klejman S, Fehlings D. Reliability and validity of the kinematic dystonia measure for children with upper extremity dystonia. *J Child Neurol*. 2012;27(7):907–913.
8. Hsu AW, Piboolnurak PA, Floyd AG, et al. Spiral analysis in Niemann-Pick disease type C. *Mov Disord*. 2009;24(13):1984–1990.
9. Crosland KA, Zarcone JR, Schroeder S, Zarcone T, Fowler S. Use if an antecedent analysis and a force sensitive platform to compare stereotyped movements and motor tics. *Am J Mental Retard*. 2005;110(3):181–192.
10. Marsden CD, Obeso JA, Rothwell JC. Clinical neurophysiology of muscle jerks: myoclonus, chorea, and tics. *Adv Neurol*. 1983;39:865–881.
11. Malfait N, Sanger TD. Does dystonia always include co-contraction? A study of unconstrained reaching in children with primary and secondary dystonia. *Exp Brain Res*. 2007;176(2):206–216.
12. Monday K, Jankovic J. Psychogenic myoclonus. *Neurology*. 1993;43:349–352.
13. Erro R, Edwards MJ, Bhatia KP, Esposito M, Farmer SF, Cordivari C. Psychogenic axial myoclonus: clinical features and long-term outcome. *Parkinsonism Relat Disord*. 2014;20(6):596–599.
14. Brown P, Thompson P. Electrophysiological aids to the diagnosis of psychogenic jerks, spasms, and tremor. *Mov Disord*. 2001;16:595–599.
15. Kenney C, Diamond A, Mejia N, Davidson A, Hunter C, Jankovic J. Distinguishing psychogenic and essential tremor. *J Neurol Sci*. 2007;263:94–99.
16. van der Salm SM, Erro R, Cordivari C, et al. Propriospinal myoclonus: clinical reappraisal and review of literature. *Neurology*. 2014;83(20):1862–1870.
17. Ferreri F, Rossini PM. TMS and TMS-EEG techniques in the study of the excitability, connectivity, and plasticity of the human motor cortex. *Rev Neurosci*. 2013;24(4):431–442.

18. Rossini PM, Burke D, Chen R, et al. Non-invasive electrical and magnetic stimulation of the brain, spinal cord, roots and peripheral nerves: basic principles and procedures for routine clinical and research application. An updated report from an I.F.C.N. Committee. *Clin Neurophysiol.* 2015;126(6):1071–1107.

19. Gilbert DL, Sallee FR, Zhang J, Lipps TD, Wassermann EM. Transcranial magnetic stimulation-evoked cortical inhibition: a consistent marker of attention-deficit/hyperactivity disorder scores in tourette syndrome. *Biol Psychiatry.* 2005;57(12):1597–1600.

20. Jackson SR, Parkinson A, Manfredi V, Millon G, Hollis C, Jackson GM. Motor excitability is reduced prior to voluntary movements in children and adolescents with Tourette syndrome. *J Neuropsychol.* 2013;7(1):29–44.

21. Orth M, Rothwell JC. Motor cortex excitability and comorbidity in Gilles de la Tourette syndrome. *J Neurol Neurosurg Psychiatry.* 2009;80(1):29–34.

22. Wu SW, Gilbert DL. Altered neurophysiologic response to intermittent theta burst stimulation in Tourette syndrome. *Brain Stimul.* 2012;5(3):315–319.

23. Wu SW, Maloney T, Gilbert DL, et al. Functional MRI-navigated repetitive transcranial magnetic stimulation over supplementary motor area in chronic tic disorders. *Brain Stimul.* 2014;7(2):212–218.

24. Juenger H, Kuhnke N, Braun C, et al. Two types of exercise-induced neuroplasticity in congenital hemiparesis: a transcranial magnetic stimulation, functional MRI, and magnetoencephalography study. *Dev Med Child Neurol.* 2013;55(10):941–951.

25. Kuhnke N, Juenger H, Walther M, Berweck S, Mall V, Staudt M. Do patients with congenital hemiparesis and ipsilateral corticospinal projections respond differently to constraint-induced movement therapy? *Dev Med Child Neurol.* 2008;50(12):898–903.

26. Fahn S, Elton RL. Members of the UPDRS Development Committee. Unified Parkinson's Disease Rating Scale. In: Fahn S, Marsden CD, Calne DB, Goldstein M, eds. *Recent Developments in Parkinson's Disease*, vol. 2. Floram Park: MacMillan Health Care Information; 1987:153–164.

27. Huntington Study Group Unified Huntington's Disease Rating Scale: reliability and consistency. *Mov Disord.* 1996;11(2):136–142.

28. Ashworth B. Preliminary trial of carisopordal in multiple sclerosis. *Practitioner.* 1964;192:540–542.

29. Mink JW. Special concerns in defining, studying, and treating dystonia in children. *Mov Disord.* 2013;28(7):921–925.

30. Mink JW. The impact of development on the interpretation of movement disorders rating scales. *Dev Med Child Neurol.* 2014;56(6):511–512.

31. Albanese A, Sorbo FD, Comella C, et al. Dystonia rating scales: critique and recommendations. *Mov Disord.* 2013;28(7):874–883.

32. Goetz CG, Tilley BC, Shaftman SR, et al. Movement Disorder Society-sponsored revision of the Unified Parkinson's Disease Rating Scale (MDS-UPDRS): scale presentation and clinimetric testing results. *Mov Disord.* 2008;23(15):2129–2170.

33. Brandsma R, Spits AH, Kuiper MJ, et al. Ataxia rating scales are age-dependent in healthy children. *Dev Med Child Neurol.* 2014;56(6):556–563.

34. Burk K, Malzig U, Wolf S, et al. Comparison of three clinical rating scales in Friedreich ataxia (FRDA). *Mov Disord.* 2009;24(12):1779–1784.

35. Schmitz-Hubsch T, du Montcel ST, Baliko L, et al. Scale for the assessment and rating of ataxia: development of a new clinical scale. *Neurology.* 2006;66(11):1717–1720.

36. Cano SJ, Hobart JC, Hart PE, Korlipara LV, Schapira AH, Cooper JM. International Cooperative Ataxia Rating Scale (ICARS): appropriate for studies of Friedreich's ataxia? *Mov Disord.* 2005;20(12):1585–1591.

37. Schmitz-Hubsch T, Tezenas du Montcel S, Baliko L, et al. Reliability and validity of the International Cooperative Ataxia Rating Scale: a study in 156 spinocerebellar ataxia patients. *Mov Disord.* 2006;21(5):699–704.

38. Metz G, Coppard N, Cooper JM, et al. Rating disease progression of Friedreich's ataxia by the International Cooperative Ataxia Rating Scale: analysis of a 603-patient database. *Brain.* 2013;136(Pt 1):259–268.

39. Lynch DR, Farmer JM, Tsou AY, et al. Measuring Friedreich ataxia: complementary features of examination and performance measures. *Neurology.* 2006;66(11):1711–1716.

40. Regner SR, Wilcox NS, Friedman LS, et al. Friedreich ataxia clinical outcome measures: natural history evaluation in 410 participants. *J Child Neurol.* 2012;27(9):1152–1158.

41. Schwabova J, Maly T, Laczo J, et al. Application of a Scale for the Assessment and Rating of Ataxia (SARA) in Friedreich's ataxia patients according to posturography is limited. *J Neurol Sci.* 2014;341(1–2):64–67.

42. Teixeira Jr. AL, Maia DP, Cardoso F. UFMG Sydenham's chorea rating scale (USCRS): reliability and consistency. *Mov Disord.* 2005;20(5):585–591.

43. Comella CL, Leurgans S, Wuu J, Stebbins GT, Chmura T. Rating scales for dystonia: a multicenter assessment. *Mov Disord*. 2003;18(3):303–312.
44. Krystkowiak P, du Montcel ST, Vercueil L, et al. Reliability of the Burke-Fahn-Marsden scale in a multicenter trial for dystonia. *Mov Disord*. 2007;22(5):685–689.
45. Barry MJ, VanSwearingen JM, Albright AL. Reliability and responsiveness of the Barry-Albright Dystonia Scale. *Dev Med Child Neurol*. 1999;41(6):404–411.
46. Burke RE, Fahn S, Marsden CD, Bressman SB, Moskowitz C, Friedman J. Validity and reliability of a rating scale for the primary torsion dystonias. *Neurology*. 1985;35(1):73–77.
47. Isaias IU, Alterman RL, Tagliati M. Outcome predictors of pallidal stimulation in patients with primary dystonia: the role of disease duration. *Brain*. 2008;131(Pt 7):1895–1902.
48. Borggraefe I, Mehrkens JH, Telegravciska M, Berweck S, Botzel K, Heinen F. Bilateral pallidal stimulation in children and adolescents with primary generalized dystonia--report of six patients and literature-based analysis of predictive outcomes variables. *Brain Dev*. 2010;32(3):223–228.
49. Cif L, Vasques X, Gonzalez V, et al. Long-term follow-up of DYT1 dystonia patients treated by deep brain stimulation: an open-label study. *Mov Disord*. 2010;25(3):289–299.
50. Markun LC, Starr PA, Air EL, Marks Jr. WJ, Volz MM, Ostrem JL. Shorter disease duration correlates with improved long-term deep brain stimulation outcomes in young-onset DYT1 dystonia. *Neurosurgery*. 2012;71(2):325–330.
51. Frucht SJ, Leurgans SE, Hallett M, Fahn S. The unified myoclonus rating scale. *Adv Neurol*. 2002;89:361–376.
52. Aberg LE, Rinne JO, Rajantie I, Santavuori P. A favorable response to antiparkinsonian treatment in juvenile neuronal ceroid lipofuscinosis. *Neurology*. 2001;56(9):1236–1239.
53. Miller JM, Singer HS, Bridges DD, Waranch HR. Behavioral therapy for treatment of stereotypic movements in nonautistic children. *J Child Neurol*. 2006;21:119–125.
54. Freeman RD, Soltanifar A, Baer S. Stereotypic movement disorderL easily missed. *Develop Med Child Neurol*. 2010;52:733–738.
55. Kircanski K, Woods DW, Chang SW, Ricketts EJ, Piacentini JC. Cluster analysis of the Yale Global Tic Severity Scale (YGTSS): symptom dimensions and clinical correlates in an outpatient youth sample. *J Abnorm Child Psychol*. 2010;38(6):777–788.
56. Leckman JF, Riddle MA, Hardin MT, et al. The Yale Global Tic Severity Scale: initial testing of a clinician-rated scale of tic severity. *J Am Acad Child Adolesc Psychiatry*. 1989;28(4):566–573.
57. Storch EA, De Nadai AS, Lewin AB, et al. Defining treatment response in pediatric tic disorders: a signal detection analysis of the Yale Global Tic Severity Scale. *J Child Adolesc Psychopharmacol*. 2011;21(6):621–627.
58. Storch EA, Murphy TK, Geffken GR, et al. Reliability and validity of the Yale Global Tic Severity Scale. *Psychol Assess*. 2005;17(4):486–491.
59. Gaffney GR, Sieg K, Hellings J. The MOVES: A Self-Rating Scale for Tourette's Syndrome. *J Child Adolesc Psychopharmacol*. 1994;4(4):269–280.
60. Goetz CG, Pappert EJ, Louis ED, Raman R, Leurgans S. Advantages of a modified scoring method for the Rush Video-Based Tic Rating Scale. *Mov Disord*. 1999;14(3):502–506.
61. Goetz CG, Tanner CM, Wilson RS, Shannon KM. A rating scale for Gilles de la Tourette's syndrome: description, reliability, and validity data. *Neurology*. 1987;37(9):1542–1544.
62. Goetz CG, Leurgans S, Chmura TA. Home alone: methods to maximize tic expression for objective videotape assessments in Gilles de la Tourette syndrome. *Mov Disord*. 2001;16(4):693–697.
63. Stacy MA, Elble RJ, Ondo WG, Wu SC, Hulihan J. Assessment of interrater and intrarater reliability of the Fahn-Tolosa-Marin Tremor Rating Scale in essential tremor. *Mov Disord*. 2007;22(6):833–838.
64. Knights S, Datoo N, Kawamura A, Switzer L, Fehlings D. Further evaluation of the scoring, reliability, and validity of the Hypertonia Assessment Tool (HAT). *J Child Neurol*. 2014;29(4):500–504.
65. Jethwa A, Mink J, Macarthur C, Knights S, Fehlings T, Fehlings D. Development of the Hypertonia Assessment Tool (HAT): a discriminative tool for hypertonia in children. *Dev Med Child Neurol*. 2010;52(5):e83–e87.
66. Battini R, Sgandurra G, Petacchi E, et al. Movement disorder-childhood rating scale: reliability and validity. *Pediatr Neurol*. 2008;39(4):259–265.
67. Battini R, Guzzetta A, Sgandurra G, et al. Scale for evaluation of movement disorders in the first three years of life. *Pediatr Neurol*. 2009;40(4):258–264.
68. Elble R, Bain P, João Forjaz M, et al. Task force report: Scales for screening and evaluating tremor: Critique and recommendations. Mov Disord. 2013;28:1793–1800.

DEVELOPMENTAL MOVEMENT DISORDERS

Transient and Developmental Movement Disorders in Children

Harvey S. Singer[1], Jonathan W. Mink[2], Donald L. Gilbert[3] and Joseph Jankovic[4]

[1]Department of Neurology, Johns Hopkins Hospital, Baltimore, MD, USA;
[2]Division of Child Neurology, University of Rochester Medical Center,
Rochester, NY, USA; [3]Division of Neurology, Cincinnati Children's Hospital
Medical Center, Cincinnati, OH, USA; [4]Department of Neurology, Baylor
College of Medicine, Houston, TX, USA

The presence of a movement disorder in a child usually raises concerns about an underlying serious, progressive, degenerative, or metabolic disease. However, many movement disorders are benign and related to normal stages of development. In fact, it may be difficult to

TABLE 6.1   Transient Developmental Movement Disorders of Infancy and Childhood

Disorder	Age at onset	Age at resolution	Treatment
Benign neonatal sleep myoclonus	Less than 1 month	6 months	Reassurance
Benign myoclonus of early infancy	3–9 months	Typically by 15 months	Reassurance
Jitteriness	First week of life	Typically before 6 months	Reassurance
Shuddering	Infancy, early childhood	Unknown	Reassurance
Paroxysmal tonic upgaze (downgaze) of infancy	Usually first year of life	Usually age 1–4 years	Levodopa may be effective
Spasmus nutans	3–12 months	Within a few months, but subtle nystagmus may persist for years	Reassurance
Head nodding	Before age 3 years	May persist for years	Reassurance
Benign paroxysmal torticollis	First year of life	By 5 years	Reassurance
Benign idiopathic dystonia of infancy	Before 5 months	By 1 year	Reassurance
Infantile masturbation	Before 3 years	Becomes more covert	Reassurance

justify the term "disorder" in describing many of these movements. The developing nervous system may produce a variety of motor patterns that would be pathological in older children and adults, but are simply a manifestation of CNS immaturity. Like many of the neonatal reflexes (e.g., grasping, rooting, placing, tonic neck reflexes), these motor patterns disappear as neuron connectivity and myelination matures. Examples include the minimal chorea of infants and young children ("chorea minima"), the mild action dystonia commonly seen in toddlers, and the overflow movements that are commonly seen in young children. Other transient or developmental movement disorders may be manifestations of abnormal neural function, but do not correlate with serious underlying pathology. These are typically associated with complete resolution of the abnormal movements and ultimately normal development and neurological function. Most of these conditions occur during infancy or early childhood (Table 6.1). It is important to recognize these transient developmental movement disorders, distinguish them from more serious disorders, and be able to provide reassurance when appropriate.

BENIGN NEONATAL SLEEP MYOCLONUS

Benign neonatal sleep myoclonus is characterized by repetitive myoclonic jerks occurring during sleep.[1–3] The myoclonic jerks typically occur in the distal more than proximal limbs and are more prominent in the upper than the lower extremities. In some cases, jerks of axial or facial muscles can be seen. The myoclonus can be focal, multifocal, unilateral, or bilateral. The movements can be rhythmic or nonrhythmic. Typically, the movements occur in clusters of jerks at 1–5 Hz over a period of several seconds. Benign neonatal sleep myoclonus begins during the first month of life, diminishes in the second month, and is usually gone before 6 months of age, but has been reported to persist as long as 3 years in one patient.[4,5] Ictal and interictal electroencephalograms (EEGs) are typically normal.[6] The movements are most likely to occur during quiet (non-REM) sleep.[7] They can also be triggered by noise.[3] Waking the baby causes the movements to cease. Episodes of myoclonus can be exacerbated by treatment with benzodiazepines.[8] Familial cases have been reported.[5,9] Treatment is not required and neurological outcome is typically normal.[5]

BENIGN MYOCLONUS OF EARLY INFANCY (BENIGN INFANTILE SPASMS)

Benign myoclonus of early infancy (BMEI) was initially characterized as episodes of myoclonic spasms involving flexion of the trunk, neck, and extremities in a manner resembling the infantile spasms of West syndrome.[10,11] The myoclonic spasms typically occur in clusters. There is no change in consciousness during the spells. Unlike benign neonatal sleep myoclonus, the movements in BMEI only occur in the waking state. Because of their resemblance to infantile spasms, a video EEG including awake and sleeping states is warranted to rule out infantile spasms.

In BMEI, the onset of these spells is usually between ages 3 and 9 months, but they may begin in the first month of life. The spells usually cease within 2 weeks to 8 months of onset,[12] but may persist for 1–2 years.[10] Both ictal and interictal EEGs are normal, distinguishing this entity from infantile spasms. Treatment is not required. Development and neurological outcome are normal.

Although the original descriptions of BMEI emphasized the similarity to infantile spasms, a more recent review has advocated for inclusion of a variety of somewhat similar spells under the category of BMEI. These include (1) myoclonus, (2) spasms and brief tonic contractions, (3) shuddering, (4) atonia or negative myoclonus, or (5) more than one type of motor phenomenon.[13] While it is true that normal infants may manifest a variety of benign nonepileptic paroxysmal movements, as described in this chapter, it remains useful to approach these entities systematically based initially on the phenomenology of the spells.

JITTERINESS

Jitteriness is a movement disorder that is commonly observed in the neonatal period. Jitteriness manifests as generalized, symmetric, rhythmic oscillatory movements that resemble tremor or clonus. Up to 50% of term infants exhibit jitteriness during the first few days of life, especially when stimulated or crying. Jitteriness usually disappears shortly after birth, but can persist for months or recur after being gone for several weeks.[14,15] Persistent jitteriness has been associated with hypoxic-ischemic injury, hypocalcemia, hypoglycemia, and drug withdrawal. Jitteriness is highly stimulus sensitive. It can be precipitated by startle and suppressed by gentle passive flexion of the limb. Unlike seizures, there are no associated abnormal eye movements or autonomic changes.[16] Idiopathic jitteriness is usually associated with normal development and neurologic outcome. The outcome of infants with symptomatic jitteriness depends on the underlying cause.

SHUDDERING

Shuddering episodes are characterized by periods of rapid tremor of the head, shoulders, and arms that resemble shivering.[17,18] Shuddering is often accompanied by facial grimacing. Onset is in infancy or early childhood, but can occur as late as 10 years of age. The episodes last several seconds and can occur up to 100 times/day. During a spell, there is no change in consciousness. Ictal and interictal EEGs are normal. However, seizures with a shuddering semiology have been described[19] and an EEG may be warranted. The preservation of consciousness and normal EEG distinguish this entity from seizures. Shuddering attacks may be differentiated from neonatal jitteriness in that shuddering attacks last only a few seconds and jitteriness is often more prolonged in duration. Jitteriness typically involves the limbs more than the trunk and neck, can be suppressed with passive limb flexion, and is more likely to occur in neonates.[20] Similarity to BMEI has been suggested.[13,17,21] Shuddering attacks are similar to BMEI in their frequency, duration, and clinical course; however, they differ in the semiology of the events. Shuddering attacks typically consist of fine tremor. In contrast, BMEI typically involves paroxysms of myoclonic limb contractions often associated with an atonic head drop that mimics the infantile spasms of West syndrome.

There may be similarity or overlap between shuddering episodes and stereotypies (see Chapter 8). Typical stereotypies are rhythmic, patterned, and repetitive involuntary movements such as body rocking, hand flapping or clapping, or head nodding. Parallels to shuddering attacks include their age of onset in infancy and early childhood, their rhythmic component, and the presence of facial grimacing. However, the movement frequency is usually lower in stereotypies, the duration of stereotypies tends to be longer (up to minutes), and stereotypies tend to persist into late childhood, or longer.

Shuddering episodes typically abate as the child grows older. The prognosis for development and neurological function is uniformly good. Treatment is usually not warranted, but one case of benefit from propranolol has been reported.[22] Some authors have suggested that "shuddering attacks" of infancy might be the initial manifestation of essential tremor[17,73], but others have failed to find an association.[23]

PAROXYSMAL TONIC UPGAZE OF INFANCY

Paroxysmal tonic upgaze (PTU) of infancy is a disorder characterized by repeated episodes of upward gaze deviation,[24,25] though downward gaze has also been reported.[26,27] Onset is usually in the first year of life but may present as late as 7 years of age.[28]

PTU is characterized by episodes of variably sustained conjugate upward deviation of the eyes that is often accompanied by neck flexion. The gaze deviation can be sustained or intermittent during an episode. The typical episode may be brief (seconds to minutes) or prolonged (hours to days).[25,28] Episodes may occur several times per day. Attempts to look downward are accompanied by down-beating nystagmus. Horizontal eye movements are normal during an episode. Spells may resolve with sleep and be aggravated by fatigue or infection. Some infants may have ataxia during some episodes.

PTU is usually idiopathic, but has been reported to have autosomal dominant inheritance. Paroxysmal upgaze has been reported in association with mutation in *CACNA1A* in one large family that also had members affected by episodic ataxia, benign paroxysmal torticollis,[29] and in three other individuals who also had developmental delay and ataxia.[30] It is uncommonly associated with structural lesions, but reported conditions have included hypomyelination,[31] periventricular leukomalacia, Vein of Galen malformation, or pinealoma.[25] In the absence of other neurological signs or symptoms, imaging is unlikely to be revealing. There is no specific treatment, but there have been a few reports of improvement with levodopa treatment.[24,32] There is a report of PTU developing in relation to valproate treatment of absence seizures.[33] The condition typically remits spontaneously and completely within a 1–4 years.[28,34] Outcome is good in most cases, but persistent ataxia, cognitive impairment, and residual minor oculomotor disorders have been reported.[25]

SPASMUS NUTANS

Spasmus nutans is a condition beginning in late infancy (3–8 months) that is characterized by a slow head tremor (approximately 2 Hz) that can be horizontal ("no–no") or vertical ("yes–yes"). The head movements are accompanied by a small-amplitude nystagmus that can be dysconjugate, conjugate, or uniocular.[35] The nystagmus is typically pendular with high frequencies (up to 15 Hz) and low amplitudes (0.5–3°) and is most commonly dysconjugate.[36] When the child is looking at an object, the nodding may increase. If the head is held, the nystagmus typically increases. These observations have led to the suggestion that the head nodding is compensatory for the nystagmus.[37] Spasmus nutans generally resolves within several months, but the majority of patients continue to have a fine, subclinical, nystagmus until at least 5–12 years of age.[38] Long-term outcome for visual acuity is good.

Spasmus nutans must be distinguished from congenital nystagmus.[39] Indeed, head nodding has been reported in association with congenital nystagmus.[40] In those cases, it appears that the head nodding serves no function. Congenital nystagmus usually begins in the newborn period before 6 months of age. Congenital nystagmus is usually bilaterally symmetric where spasmus nutans is often asymmetric. Congenital nystagmus persists beyond a few months. Visual acuity is abnormal in about 90% of children with congenital nystagmus. While these features are useful in distinguishing congenital nystagmus from spasmus nutans, children who clinically appear to have spasmus nutans at the time of presentation have been found to have retinal[41,42] or chiasmatic abnormalities.[43] Thus, ophthalmologic evaluation, including electroretinogram, is recommended for children with spasmus nutans. Neuroimaging abnormalities, including tumor Chiari type I malformation, and aplasia of the cerebellar vermis, have been described in patients with spasmus nutans, but this is an uncommon association.[42,44,45] Routine neuroimaging in the absence of other evidence for intracranial pathology has limited yield.[46]

HEAD NODDING

Head nodding without accompanying nystagmus can occur as paroxysmal events in older infants and toddlers.[47] These head movements can be lateral ("no–no"), vertical ("yes–yes"), or oblique. The episodes may occur several times a day. The frequency (1–2 Hz) is slower than that of shuddering. The movements do not occur when the child is lying, but can occur in the sitting or standing position. The movements typically resolve within months, but can persist longer. Some children with head nodding have a prior history of shuddering spells; others may have a family history of essential tremor.[20] However, it is unclear whether there is any etiological relationship with these other conditions. An unusual head nodding epileptic syndrome has been described in sub-Saharan Africa. This head nodding epilepsy syndrome appears to be associated with hippocampal sclerosis and may be related to infection with *Onchocerca volvulus*.[48] Head nodding may also occur as a benign stereotypy that can persist through adolescence (see Chapter 8). Developmental and neurological outcome are benign in idiopathic head nodding.

Head nodding may also occur with visual impairment, oculomotor dysfunction, or brain malformations. It also must be differentiated from the more serious bobble-head doll syndrome (see Chapter 8). Thus, a thorough history and examination are required to rule out other associated abnormalities in infants with head nodding.

BENIGN PAROXYSMAL TORTICOLLIS

Benign paroxysmal torticollis is an episodic disorder starting in the first year of life. It typically manifests as a head tilt to one side for a few hours or days. Spells can last as little as 10 min or as long as 2 months, but this is uncommon.[49] The torticollis may occur without any associated symptoms, or may be accompanied by pallor, vomiting, irritability, or ataxia. The direction of the torticollis may differ across episodes. Episodes typically recur with some regularity, up to twice a month initially and becoming less frequent as the child grows older. The spells abate spontaneously, usually by 2–3 years of age but always by age 5. The child is normal between spells. Interictal and ictal EEGs are normal.

It has been suggested that benign paroxysmal torticollis is a migraine variant.[50] There is often a family history of migraine.[51] Some older children complain of headache during a spell, and many children go on to develop typical migraine after they have "outgrown" the paroxysmal torticollis.[52,53]

Benign paroxysmal torticollis is idiopathic in most cases, but has been reported in association with mutations in *CACNA1A*[29,49,54] or *PRRT2*.[55,56]

The differential diagnosis is broad and diagnosis of benign paroxysmal torticollis is one of exclusion. Torticollis can be seen as an acute dystonic reaction to medication, as a symptom of a posterior fossa or cervical cord lesion, or cervical vertebral abnormalities. In the case of structural lesions, the torticollis tends to be persistent and not paroxysmal. Torticollis can also be a sign of IV nerve palsy. Congenital muscular torticollis is present from birth, is nonparoxysmal, and is associated with palpable tightness or fibrosis of the sternocleidomastoid muscle unilaterally (see Video 6.1).[74]

Outcome of benign paroxysmal torticollis is likely related to the underlying cause, especially in the case of specific genetic mutations. Idiopathic cases may be associated with mild developmental delays that are likely to improve over time.[51]

BENIGN IDIOPATHIC DYSTONIA OF INFANCY

Benign idiopathic dystonia of infancy is a rare disorder characterized by a segmental dystonia, usually of one upper extremity, that can be intermittent or persistent.[57,58] The syndrome usually appears before 5 months of age and disappears by 1 year of age. The characteristic posture is of shoulder abduction, pronation of the forearm, and flexion of the wrist. The posture occurs when the infant is at rest and goes away completely with volitional movement. Occasionally, both arms, an arm and leg on one side of the body, or the trunk can be involved. In some infants, the posture is only apparent with relaxation or in certain positions. In others it may be present during all waking hours. The rest of the neurological examination is normal and the developmental and neurologic outcome is normal. Exclusion of progressive dystonia, brachial plexus injury, infantile hemiplegia, and orthopedic abnormalities is important, but can be based on history and examination.

SANDIFER SYNDROME

Sandifer syndrome involves flexion of the neck, arching of the back, or opisthotonic posturing, associated with either gastroesophageal reflux or the presence of hiatal hernia. Sandifer syndrome was first described by Kinsbourne[59] as "hiatus hernia with contortions of the neck." In the initial report, five patients ranging in age from 4 to 14 years presented with abnormal head and neck postures with neck extension, rotation and side flexion worsened by eating. All patients had subjective swallowing difficulties and weight loss, but were otherwise neurologically normal. These patients were found to have hiatus hernia and the movements were thought to be associated in some way to the hernia.[59] It was later found that the syndrome occurred with gastroesophageal reflux and esophagitis, even in the absence of hiatus hernia.[60,61]

The exact incidence is not known, but in children with gastroesophageal reflux, Sandifer's syndrome occurred in 7.9% of cases.[62] In a study of paroxysmal nonepileptic events in children, Sandifer's syndrome was diagnosed in 15% of children under 5 years of age.[63] Diagnosis is often delayed and children often undergo extensive investigations before the diagnosis is reached.

In the original five cases, surgical repair of the hiatus hernia led to complete resolution of the involuntary neck movements.[59] In subsequent patients, medical treatment of the gastroesophageal reflux and esophagitis relieved symptoms.[60,61] Treatment of gastroesophageal reflux disease by medical or surgical means results in resolution of the symptoms in 94% of patients.[64]

POSTURING DURING MASTURBATION

Masturbation (gratification behavior) is a normal behavior that occurs in the majority of both boys and girls. While masturbation occurs at all ages and has even been observed *in utero*, it is most common at about 4 years of age and during adolescence.[65] Masturbation in young children may involve unusual postures or movements,[66] which may be mistaken for abdominal pain or seizures.[67,68] Masturbatory movements in boys are usually obvious to the observer due to direct genital manipulation. In girls, they are more subtle and often involves adduction of the thighs, or sitting on a hand or foot and rocking. When the movements are accompanied by posturing of the limbs they are often mistaken for paroxysmal dystonia. Several characteristic features of masturbating girls who present for diagnosis have been identified[67–70]: (1) onset after 2 months of age and before 3 years of age; (2) stereotyped posturing with pressure applied to the pubic area; (3) quiet grunting, diaphoresis, or facial flushing; (4) episode duration of less than a minute to several hours; (5) no alteration of consciousness; (6) normal findings on examination; and (7) cessation with distraction or engagement of the child in another activity. Several of these also occur in boys during masturbation. Unnecessary diagnostic tests are commonly performed before the true nature of the behavior is recognized. No imaging or laboratory evaluation is required if the movements abate when the child is distracted; the movements involve irregular rocking, the child remains interactive, there is some degree of volitional control, direct genital stimulation is involved, and the neurologic and physical examinations are normal (see Video 6.2). There appears to be no association with sexual thoughts in the child. Instead, it is probably better to view these movements on the spectrum of other self-comforting behaviors such as thumb sucking or rocking, which have no concerning connotations for the parents.[69,71] Masturbation is a normal human behavior, so there is no expectation that this behavior will cease as the child grows older. However, the frequency of the behavior usually decreases as the child gets older and the behavior is less likely to occur under the observation of the parents. Neurological and developmental outcome is normal in most cases.[72] No treatment is required, but it is important to educate the parents about the behavior. Reassurance for the family is the key to management, with recommendation for behavioral redirection should the behavior prove to be embarrassing for the family.[65,67,69] The parents should be educated that this is a normal behavior resulting from random exploration of the body by the infant.

References

1. Coulter D, Allen R. Benign neonatal myoclonus. *Arch Neurol.* 1982;39:191–192.
2. Paro-Panjan D, Neubauer D. Benign neonatal sleep myoclonus: experience from the study of 38 infants. *Eur J Paediatr Neurol.* 2008;12:14–18.
3. Maurer VO, Rizzi M, Bianchetti MG, Ramelli GP. Benign neonatal sleep myoclonus: a review of the literature. *Pediatrics.* 2010;125(4):e919–e924.
4. Egger J, Grossmann G, Auchterlonie IA. Lesson of the week: benign sleep myoclonus in infancy mistaken for epilepsy. *BMJ.* 2003;326:975–976.
5. Suzuki Y, Toshikawa H, Kimizu T, et al. Benign neonatal sleep myoclonus: our experience of 15 Japanese cases. *Brain Dev.* 2015;37(1):71–75.
6. DiCapua M, Fusco L, Ricci S, Vigevano F. Benign neonatal sleep myoclonus: clinical features and videopolygraphic recordings. *Mov Disord.* 1993;8:191–194.
7. Resnick TJ, Moshe SL, Perotta L, Chambers HJ. Benign neonatal sleep myoclonus. Relationship to sleep states. *Arch Neurol.* 1986;43:266–268.
8. Reggin J, Johnson M. Exacerbation of benign sleep myoclonus by benzodiazepine treatment. *Ann Neurol.* 1989;26:455.
9. Afawi Z, Bassan H, Heron S, et al. Benign neonatal sleep myoclonus: an autosomal dominant form not allelic to KCNQ2 or KCNQ3. *J Child Neurol.* 2012;27(10):1260–1263.
10. Lombroso C. Early myoclonic encephalopathy, early infantile epileptic encephalopathy, and benign and severe infantile myoclonic epilepsies: a critical review and personal contributions. *J Clin Neurophysiol.* 1990;7:380–408.
11. Lombroso C, Fejerman N. Benign myoclonus of early infancy. *Ann Neurol.* 1977;1:138–148.

12. Maydell BV, Berenson F, Rothner AD, Wyllie E, Kotagal P. Benign myoclonus of early infancy: an imitator of West's syndrome. *J Child Neurol.* 2001;16:109–112.
13. Caraballo RH, Capovilla G, Vigevano F, Beccaria F, Specchio N, Fejerman N. The spectrum of benign myoclonus of early infancy: clinical and neurophysiologic features in 102 patients. *Epilepsia.* 2009;50(5):1176–1183.
14. Kramer U, Nevo Y, Harel S. Jittery babies: a short term follow-up. *Brain Devel.* 1994;16:112–114.
15. Shuper A, Zalzberg J, Weitz R, Mimouni M. Jitteriness beyond the neonatal period: a benign pattern of movement in infancy. *J Child Neurol.* 1991;6:243–245.
16. Volpe J. *Neurology of the Newborn.* 3rd ed. Philadelphia, PA: WB Saunders; 1995.
17. Kanazawa O. Shuddering attacks-report of four children. *Pediatr Neurol.* 2000;23:421–424.
18. Holmes G, Russman B. Shuddering attacks. Evaluation using electroencephalographic frequency modulation radiotelemetry and videotape monitoring. *Am J Dis Child.* 1986;140:72–73.
19. Jahodova A, Krsek P, Komarek V, et al. Frontal lobe epilepsy with atypical seizure semiology resembling shuddering attacks or wet dog shake seizures. *Epileptic Disord.* 2012;14(1):69–75.
20. DiMario FJ. Childhood head tremor. *J Child Neurol.* 2000;15:22–25.
21. Pachatz C, Fusco L, Vigevano F. Benign myoclonus of early infancy. *Epileptic Disord.* 1999;1:57–62.
22. Barron TF, Younkin DP. Propranolol therapy for shuddering attacks. *Neurology.* 1992;42(1):258–259.
23. Jan MM. Shuddering attacks are not related to essential tremor. *J Child Neurol.* 2010;25(7):881–883.
24. Ouvrier R, Billson F. Benign paroxysmal upgaze of childhood. *J Child Neurol.* 1988;3:177–180.
25. Ouvrier R, Billson F. Paroxysmal tonic upgaze of childhood—a review. *Brain Dev.* 2005;27(3):185–188.
26. Wolsey DH, Warner JE. Paroxysmal tonic downgaze in two healthy infants. *J Neuroophthalmol.* 2006;26(3):187–189.
27. Tzoufi M, Sixlimiri P, Makis A, Siamopoulou-Mavridou A. Another case of paroxysmal tonic downgaze in infancy. *J Neuroophthalmol.* 2009;29(1):74–75.
28. Salmina C, Taddeo I, Falesi M, Weber P, Bianchetti MG, Ramelli GP. Paroxysmal tonic upgaze in normal children: a case series and a review of the literature. *Eur J Paediatr Neurol.* 2012;16(6):683–687.
29. Roubertie A, Echenne B, Leydet J, et al. Benign paroxysmal tonic upgaze, benign paroxysmal torticollis, episodic ataxia and CACNA1A mutation in a family. *J Neurol.* 2008;255(10):1600–1602.
30. Blumkin L, Leshinsky-Silver E, Michelson M, et al. Paroxysmal tonic upward gaze as a presentation of de-novo mutations in CACNA1A. *Eur J Paediatr Neurol.* 2015;19(3):292–297.
31. Blumkin L, Lev D, Watemberg N, Lerman-Sagie T. Hypomyelinating leukoencephalopathy with paroxysmal tonic upgaze and absence of psychomotor development. *Mov Disord.* 2007;22(2):226–230.
32. Campistol J, Prats J, Garaizar C. Benign paroxysmal tonic upgaze of childhood with ataxia. A neuroophthalmological syndrome of familial origin? *Devel Med Child Neurol.* 1993;35:436–439.
33. Luat AF, Asano E, Chugani HT. Paroxysmal tonic upgaze of childhood with co-existent absence epilepsy. *Epileptic Disord.* 2007;9(3):332–336.
34. Verrotti A, Trotta D, Blasetti A, Lobefalo L, Gallenga P, Chiarell F. Paroxysmal tonic upgaze of childhood: effect of age-of-onset on prognosis. *Acta Paediatr.* 2001;90:1343–1345.
35. Anthony J, Ouvrier R, Wise G. Spasmus nutans, a mistaken entity. *Arch Neurol.* 1980;37:373–375.
36. Weissman BM, Dell'Osso LF, Abel LA, Leigh RJ. Spasmus nutans. A quantitative prospective study. *Arch Ophthalmol.* 1987;105:525–528.
37. Gottlob I, Zubcov A, Wizov S, Reinecke R. Head nodding is compensatory in spasmus nutans. *Ophthalmology.* 1992;99(7):1024–1031.
38. Gottlob I, Wizov S, Reinecke R. Spasmus nutans. A long-term follow-up. *Invest Ophthalmol Vis Sci.* 1995;36:2768–2771.
39. Gottlob I, Zubcov A, Catalano R, et al. Signs distinguishing spasmus nutans (with and without central nervous system lesions) from infantile nystagmus. *Ophthalmology.* 1990;97:1166–1175.
40. Carl JR, Optican LM, Chu FC, Zee DS. Head shaking and vestibulo-ocular reflex in congenital nystagmus. *Invest Ophthalmol Vis Sci.* 1985;26:1043–1050.
41. Smith D, Fitzgerald K, Stass-Isern M, Cibis G. Electroretinography is necessary for spasmus nutans diagnosis. *Pediatr Neurol.* 2000;23:33–36.
42. Kiblinger GD, Wallace BS, Hines M, Siatkowski RM. Spasmus nutans-like nystagmus is often associated with underlying ocular, intracranial, or systemic abnormalities. *J Neuroophthalmol.* 2007;27(2):118–122.
43. Brodsky MC, Keating GF. Chiasmal glioma in spasmus nutans: a cautionary note. *J Neuroophthalmol.* 2014;34(3):274–275.

44. Unsold R, Ostertag C. Nystagmus in suprasellar tumors: recent advances in diagnosis and therapy. *Strabismus*. 2002;10:173–177.
45. Kim JS, Park SH, Lee KW. Spasmus nutans and congenital ocular motor apraxia with cerebellar vermian hypoplasia. *Arch Neurol*. 2003;60:1621–1624.
46. Arnoldi K, Tychsen L. Prevalence of intracranial lesions in children initially diagnosed with disconjugate nystagmus (spasmus nutans). *J Pediatr Ophthalmol Strabismus*. 1995;32:296–301.
47. Nellhaus G. Abnormal head movements of young children. *Devel Med Child Neurol*. 1983;25:384–389.
48. Winkler AS, Friedrich K, Konig R, et al. The head nodding syndrome—clinical classification and possible causes. *Epilepsia*. 2008;49(12):2008–2015.
49. Giffin NJ, Benton S, Goadsby PJ. Benign paroxysmal torticollis of infancy: four new cases and linkage to CACNA1A mutation. *Dev Med Child Neurol*. 2002;44:490–493.
50. Al-Twaijri W, Shevell M. Pediatric migraine equivalents: occurrence and clinical features in practice. *Pediatr Neurol*. 2002;26:365–368.
51. Rosman NP, Douglass LM, Sharif UM, Paolini J. The neurology of benign paroxysmal torticollis of infancy: report of 10 new cases and review of the literature. *J Child Neurol*. 2009;24(2):155–160.
52. Deonna T, Martin D. Benign paroxysmal torticollis in infancy. *Arch Dis Child*. 1981;56:956–959.
53. Roulet E, Deonna T. Benign paroxysmal torticollis in infancy. *Devel Med Child Neurol*. 1988;30:409–410.
54. Vila-Pueyo M, Gene GG, Flotats-Bastardes M, et al. A loss-of-function CACNA1A mutation causing benign paroxysmal torticollis of infancy. *Eur J Paediatr Neurol*. 2014;18(3):430–433.
55. Dale RC, Gardiner A, Antony J, Houlden H. Familial PRRT2 mutation with heterogeneous paroxysmal disorders including paroxysmal torticollis and hemiplegic migraine. *Dev Med Child Neurol*. 2012;54(10):958–960.
56. Meneret A, Gaudebout C, Riant F, Vidailhet M, Depienne C, Roze E. PRRT2 mutations and paroxysmal disorders. *Eur J Neurol*. 2013;20(6):872–878.
57. Deonna T, Ziegler A, Nielsen J. Transient idiopathic dystonia in infancy. *Neuropediatrics*. 1991;22:220–224.
58. Willemse J. Benign idiopathic dystonia in the first year of life. *Devel Med Child Neurol*. 1986;28:355–363.
59. Kinsbourne M. Hiatus hernia with contortions of the neck. *Lancet*. 1964;13:1058–1061.
60. Murphy WJ, Gellis SS. Torticollis with hiatus hernia in infancy. Sandifer syndrome. *Am J Dis Child*. 1977;131(5):564–565.
61. Bray PF, Herbst JJ, Johnson DG, Book LS, Ziter FA, Condon VR. Childhood gastroesophageal reflux. Neurologic and psychiatric syndromes mimicked. *JAMA*. 1977;237(13):1342–1345.
62. Shepherd RW, Wren J, Evans S, Lander M, Ong TH. Gastroesophageal reflux in children. Clinical profile, course and outcome with active therapy in 126 cases. *Clin Pediatr (Phila)*. 1987;26(2):55–60.
63. Kotagal P, Costa M, Wyllie E, Wolgamuth B. Paroxysmal nonepileptic events in children and adolescents. *Pediatrics*. 2002;110(4):e46.
64. Leape LL, Ramenofsky ML. Surgical treatment of gastroesophageal reflux in children. Results of Nissen's fundoplication in 100 children. *Am J Dis Child*. 1980;134(10):935–938.
65. Leung AKC, Robson WLM. Childhood masturbation. *Clin Pediatr*. 1993;32:238–241.
66. Bower B. Fits and other frightening or funny turns in young people. *Practitioner*. 1981;225:297–304.
67. Fleisher DR, Morrison A. Masturbation mimicking abdominal pain or seizures in young girls. *J Pediatr*. 1990;116:810–814.
68. Nechay A, Ross LM, Stephenson JB, O'Regan M. Gratification disorder ("infantile masturbation"): a review. *Arch Dis Child*. 2004;89(3):225–226.
69. Yang ML, Fullwood E, Goldstein J, Mink JW. Masturbation in infancy and early childhood presenting as a movement disorder: 12 cases and a review of the literature. *Pediatrics*. 2005;116(6):1427–1432.
70. Hansen JK, Balslev T. Hand activities in infantile masturbation: a video analysis of 13 cases. *Eur J Paediatr Neurol*. 2009;13(6):508–510.
71. Mink J, Neil J. Masturbation mimicking paroxysmal dystonia or dyskinesia in a young girl. *Mov Disord*. 1995;10:518–520.
72. Jan MM, Al Banji MH, Fallatah BA. Long-term outcome of infantile gratification phenomena. *Can J Neurol Sci*. 2013;40(3):416–419.
73. Vanasse M, Bedard P, Andermann F. Shuddering attacks in children: an early clinical manifestation of essential tremor. Neurology. 1976;11:1027–1030.
74. Collins A, Jankovic J. Botulinum toxin injection for congenital muscular torticollis presenting in children and adults. *Neurology*. 2006;67(6):1083–1085.

PAROXYSMAL MOVEMENT DISORDERS

Tics and Tourette Syndrome

Harvey S. Singer[1], Jonathan W. Mink[2],
Donald L. Gilbert[3] and Joseph Jankovic[4]

[1]Department of Neurology, Johns Hopkins Hospital, Baltimore, MD, USA;
[2]Division of Child Neurology, University of Rochester Medical Center,
Rochester, NY, USA; [3]Division of Neurology, Cincinnati Children's Hospital
Medical Center, Cincinnati, OH, USA; [4]Department of Neurology, Baylor
College of Medicine, Houston, TX, USA

OUTLINE

Movement Disorders in Childhood, Second Edition.
DOI: http://dx.doi.org/10.1016/B978-0-12-411573-6.00007-3

INTRODUCTION

Tourette syndrome (TS) is named after the French physician Georges Gilles de la Tourette, who in 1885 reported nine patients with a condition he referred to as "maladie of tics."[1] Although credited with making the diagnosis, this disorder was previously described in the medical literature by Jean Itard in 1825.[2] This syndrome, characterized by the presence of involuntary motor and phonic tics, represents only one entity in a spectrum of disorders that have tics as their cardinal feature, ranging from a provisional form to those associated with general medical conditions. In addition to tics, children with tic disorders often suffer from a variety of concomitant psychopathologies, including attention-deficit hyperactivity disorder (ADHD), obsessive-compulsive disorder (OCD), anxiety, mood disorder, anger outbursts, learning difficulties, and sleep abnormalities. Although some tics may be mild, others can be more severe and result in psychosocial, physical, and functional difficulties that can, in turn, affect one's social and academic functions and achievements.

TIC PHENOMENOLOGY

Formal definitions of tics include sudden, rapid, recurrent, nonrhythmic motor movements or vocalizations (phonic productions). The term stereotyped has been eliminated to avoid confusion and the misdiagnosis of motor stereotypies (see Chapter 8). Nevertheless, observation either directly in the office or via homemade video is essential for the correct diagnosis. Tics are classified into two categories (motor and phonic) with each being subdivided into a simple and complex grouping. Brief rapid movements that involve only a single muscle or localized group are considered "simple" (eye blink, head jerk, shoulder shrug), whereas complex tics involve either a cluster of simple actions or a more coordinated sequence of movements (Videos 7.1–7.8). Complex motor tics can be nonpurposeful (facial or body contortions), appear purposeful but actually serve no purpose (touching, hitting, smelling, jumping, imitating gestures (echopraxia), touching one's genitalia (copropraxia)), have a tonic character (prolonged tensing of abdominal movements), or a dystonic quality (oculogyric movements, sustained mouth opening, torticollis) (Video 7.9). Simple phonations include various sounds and noises (grunts, barks, sniffs, and throat clearing) (Videos 7.10, 7.11 and 7.12), whereas complex vocalizations involve the repetition of words, i.e., syllables, phrases, echolalia (repeating other people's words), palilalia (repeating one's own words), or coprolalia (obscene words or profanity) (Video 7.13). It should be noted that many believe the division between motor and vocal tics is arbitrary, since vocalizations represent motor tics that involve nasal, laryngeal, pharyngeal, or respiratory abnormalities.

It has been stated that almost any movement or sound could become a tic. Unique tics have included vomiting and retching,[3] anterior–posterior displacement of the external ear,[4] sign language tics,[5] air swallowing,[6] palatal movements,[7] and in individuals who stutter, an array of nonspeech motor behaviors (eye blinking or deviation, head jerks, limb and trunk movements).[8] Some complex motor tics may be repetitive and appear stereotypic. Features of catatonia, including classic negative symptoms such as immobility, staring, and posturing, are referred to as "blocking" tics.[9] Nontic movements, that need to be distinguished, include those that are drug-induced (akathisia, dystonia, stereotypy, Parkinsonism), associated with common comorbidities such as OCD, ADHD, impulsive and antisocial behaviors, or are motor stereotypies.[10,11]

Tics have several characteristics that are useful in identifying their presence including a waxing and waning pattern, the intermixture of new and old tics, a fluctuating frequency, and variable intensity. Brief exacerbations are often provoked by stress, anxiety, excitement, anger, fatigue, or infections,[12,13] however the mechanism for prolonged tic exacerbations, whether environmental or biological, remains to be determined. Although stress influences tics, in general, life events do not account for changes in tic severity.[14] Tic reduction often occurs when the affected individual is concentrating, focusing, emotionally pleased, or sleeping. The absence of tics during sleep is commonly reported by observers/parents. Polysomnograms of TS subjects, however, demonstrate tics in all phases of sleep.[15] About 90% of adults[16] and 37% of children[17] report a premonitory urge/sensation just before a motor or phonic tic. Whether the failure to identify a preceding urge in children less than age 10 years is due to its absence, difficulty to describe, or presence of OC urges in adults is unknown. Vaguely defined as an urge, tension, pressure, itch, or feeling, it is generally localized to the region of the tic.[18] If the sensation recurs in a specific body part, it is sometimes referred to as a sensory tic.[16] At times, an attempt to voluntarily suppress a tic often triggers an exacerbation of premonitory sensations or a sense of increased internal tension. Both of these conditions resolve when the tic is permitted to occur. The intensity of premonitory urges correlates with interoceptive awareness and the presence of more severe tics. The pathophysiology of this sensory alteration is not well understood,[19] although some have suggested an alteration of sensorimotor gating.[20]

Misdiagnoses are common; e.g., eye blinking tics may be thought to stem from ophthalmologic problems, ocular tics are confused with opsoclonus, throat-clearing tics are thought to be due to sinusitis or allergic conditions, involuntary sniffing frequently results in referral to an allergist, and a chronic persistent cough-like bark is incorrectly labeled as asthma. Tic-like psychogenic movement disorders have prominent distractibility, the presence of other functional movements, and tend to lack a premonitory sense, suppressibility, and family history.[21] Speech pauses, hesitations, word interjections, changes in tone, and prolongations of words are common in TS and can usually be differentiated from developmental stuttering.[22]

TIC DISORDERS

The diagnosis of a tic disorder is based on historical features and a clinical examination that confirms their presence and eliminates other conditions. There is currently no definitive

TABLE 7.1   Tic Classifications

DSM-5 classification
Provisional tic disorder
Chronic motor or vocal tic disorder
Tourette's disorder (Tourette syndrome)
Tic disorder, not otherwise specified
Substance-induced tic disorder
Tic disorder due to a general medical condition

diagnostic blood test, brain imaging alteration, or genetic screen. TS represents only one entity in a spectrum of disorders that have tics as their cardinal feature. The *Diagnostic and Statistical Manual of Mental Disorders, Fifth Edition* (DSM-5),[26] now classifies tics into six categories including Provisional, Chronic motor or vocal tic disorder, Tourette's disorder (TD), Tic disorder, not otherwise specified, Substance-induced tic disorder, and Tic disorder due to a general medical condition (Table 7.1). A previous entity labeled transient tic disorder has been eliminated. In each category, a tic is a sudden, rapid, recurrent, nonrhythmic, motor movement or vocalization. Tics may wax and wane in frequency, but there are requirements for tic duration from the first tic onset, the physiological consequence of a general medical condition, and substance use.

Provisional Tic Disorder

This category is used to designate an individual with ongoing single or multiple motor and/or vocal tics that have been present for less than 1 year since first tic onset. A provisional diagnosis is required because it is impossible to predict whether an individual's tics will persist for the requisite 1-year time interval required for a "chronic" designation or resolve.

Chronic Motor or Vocal Tic Disorder (CMVTD)

CMVTD requires that a single or multiple motor or vocal tic, but not both, be present for greater than 1 year after first onset, without regard for tic frequency. Several studies have documented that chronic motor tic disorder represents a mild form of TS and both are transmitted as inherited traits in the same family.[23,24]

Tourette Syndrome and Tourette's Disorder

Formal criteria for TS, based on the definition provided by the Tourette Syndrome Classification Study Group,[25] are very similar to TD, as outlined by the DSM-5.[26] One difference remaining is the actual required age of onset; TD requires an age of onset of less than 18 years whereas for TS onset is prior to age 21 years. Since 93% of patients are symptomatic by age 10 years,[27] this is not considered a significant difference. Two previously required criteria have been eliminated, including statements that no tic-free interval lasts longer than

3 months' duration and the necessity that tics be causing an impairment. Coprolalia, one of the most socially distressing symptoms, is not a diagnostic criterion, and studies have suggested its presence in 19.3% of males and 14.6% of females.[28] The mean age of onset for coprolalia is 11.0 years.

Tic Disorder; Not Otherwise Specified

This category is for disorders characterized by tics that do not meet criteria for a specific tic disorder because the movements or vocalizations are atypical in terms of age of onset or clinical presentation.

Substance-Induced Tic Disorder

This category requires evidence from the history, physical examination, or laboratory that motor and/or vocal tics developed (a) during or within 1 month of substance intoxication or withdrawal or (b) substance use is etiologically related to the disturbance. Examples in this group include cocaine-induced tics and individuals who developed tics following the use of neuroleptics.[29–31] Stimulant medications are not considered a precipitating agent for tics.

Tic Disorder Due to a General Medical Condition

Within this group are a variety of entities that have tics resulting from the direct consequence of a medical condition.[32] For example, tics are reported in association with a variety of sporadic, genetic, and neurodegenerative disorders, such as neuroacanthocytosis, Huntington's disease, Neurodegeneration with Brain Iron Accumulation, neurocutaneous syndromes, and Creutzfeldt–Jakob disease.[33–35] Tics have also been reported in medical conditions such as infection (encephalitis, Sydenham's chorea),[36–39] drugs,[40–42] toxins (carbon monoxide),[43] stroke,[44,45] head trauma,[46–49] peripheral trauma,[48,49] and surgery.[50,51]

EPIDEMIOLOGY

TS occurs worldwide with increasing evidence for common features in all cultures and races. The current prevalence figure (number of cases in population at a given time) for tics in childhood is about 6–12% (range 4–24%).[52–54] The precise prevalence of chronic motor and vocal tics (TS) is unknown, with estimates for moderately severe cases being about 1–10 per 1000 children and adolescents. One meta-analysis of 13 studies identified a TS prevalence 0.77% in children and adolescents[55] a second including 21 populations based studies showed a prevalence estimate of 0.52%.[297] Another estimate is that an additional 10–30 per 1000 children and adolescents have a mild unidentified form.[52,55–57] TS is more common in males than in females (more than 3:1), the mean age of onset is typically between 4 and 8 years, and most patients develop tics before their teenage years.[54,58,59] Tic phenomenology and severity appear to be similar between children and adults.[60] Adult-onset tic disorders have been reported and are often associated with potential environmental triggers, severe symptoms, greater social morbidity, and a poorer response to medications.[61] Other studies in adults have suggested a reemergence or exacerbation of a childhood disorder with prominent facial, neck, and trunk tics.[62] TS is common in children with autism, Asperger syndrome, fragile X syndrome,[63] and other autistic spectrum disorders,[64] but its presence appears to be unrelated to the severity of autistic symptoms.[65] Tics and related behaviors have not been found to be overrepresented among adult inpatients with psychiatric illnesses.[66] Neurological examination and neuroradiographical studies are typically normal. "Soft" signs, including abnormalities of coordination and fine motor performance, synkinesis, and motor restlessness, are often observed in affected children especially those with ADHD.

SCALES

The Yale Global Tic Severity Scale (YGTSS), a semistructured clinical interview, is the most widely used tic-severity ranking instrument.[67] This scale consists of two components: (1) The Total Tic Score (TTS) consisting of five separate ratings (number, frequency, intensity, complexity, and interference) for both motor and vocal tics made along five dimensions on a scale of 0 to 5 and (2) The Tic Impairment Score (TIS) representing a ranking of impairment, with a maximum of 50 points. The latter subjective component is scored based on the impact of the tic disorder on self-esteem, family life, and social acceptance. A Gilles de la Tourette Syndrome-Quality of Life (GTS-QOL) scale has been developed and validated.[68] This is a 27-item patient-reported TS-specific scale with four subscales (psychological, physical, obsessional, and cognitive).

OUTCOME

Although TS was originally proposed to be a lifelong disorder, its course can be highly variable, with most patients having a spontaneous remission or marked improvement over time. The maximum severity of tics tends to be between ages 8 and 12.5 years.[69,70] Most long-term studies support a decline in symptoms during the teenage–early adulthood years.[69,71,72] The "rule of thirds," i.e., one third disappear, one third are better, and one third continue, is a reasonable estimate of outcome.[73] Although tic resolution is reported by many adults, whether they fully resolve has been questioned.[74] Proposed predictors of severity and longevity remain controversial.[75] Included in this list are factors such as tic severity, fine motor control, and the volumetric size of brain regions such as caudate and subgenual areas.[76,77] The presence of coexisting neuropsychiatric issues has a significant effect on impairment in children; individuals solely with chronic tics are less impaired than those with OCD, ADHD, mood disorders, and other associated behaviors.[78–80]

ASSOCIATED BEHAVIORS AND PSYCHOPATHOLOGIES IN TIC DISORDERS

Georges Gilles de la Tourette, in his early descriptions, noted the presence of a variety of comorbid neurobehavioral problems, including obsessive compulsive symptoms, anxieties, and phobias.[1] As the list of associated problems has expanded, it has become clear that psychopathology occurs in 86–90% of children with TS[81,82] and its clinical impact may be more significant than the tics.[80,83,84] For example, health-related quality of life (HR-QOL), as measured by HR-QOL scales, confirms that outcome is predicted by comorbidities such as ADHD and OCD rather than tic severity.[68,80,85,86] On QOL measures, high ADHD symptom scores relate to poorer outcomes within the Self and Relationship domains, whereas high OCD symptom scores produce difficulties in the Self, Relationship, Environment, and General domains.[87] Hence, it is essential that the physician caring for an individual with a tic disorder be aware of potential psychopathologies, be able to differentiate comorbidities from tics, continually assess patients to determine their presence, and be part of a comprehensive treatment program. TS rarely leads to criminal behavior, but individuals with TS and comorbidities are at risk for involvement with the legal system.[88]

Attention-Deficit Hyperactivity Disorder

ADHD is characterized by impulsivity, hyperactivity, and a decreased ability to maintain attention. Symptoms usually precede the onset of tics by 2–3 years. ADHD is reported to affect about 50% (range 21–90%) of referred cases with TS.[89] Attentional impairments in TS + ADHD subjects differ from those with ADHD only, the latter having greater impairment on tests that measure visual search and mental flexibility, slower reaction times, and fewer corrective responses on simple and choice reaction time tasks.[90] In patients with tics, the addition of ADHD symptoms correlates with increased psychosocial difficulties, disruptive behavior, emotional problems, functional impairment, learning disabilities, and school problems.[91–94] TS and ADHD are not alternate phenotypes of a single underlying genetic cause but there is likely a shared genetic susceptibility and overlap in their underlying neurobiology.[82,95]

Obsessive-Compulsive Disorder

Obsessions are recurrent ideas, thoughts, images, or impulses that intrude on conscious thought, are persistent, and are unwelcome (ego dystonic). Compulsions are repetitive, seemingly purposeful behaviors usually performed in response to an obsession, or in accord with certain rules, or in a stereotyped fashion. Obsessive-compulsive behaviors (OCBs) become OCD when activities are sufficiently severe to cause marked distress, take up more than 1 h of the day, or have a significant impact on normal routine, function, social activities, or relationships. A genetic association has been identified between OCD and TS.[96–98]

OCBs generally emerge several years after the onset of tics, usually during early adolescence, although one study has suggested an earlier age of onset.[82] Behaviors occur in 20–89% of patients with TS and typically become more severe at a later age.[99–101] Two subtypes of OCD, based on differences in prevalence in age groups and implied etiologic relationships, have been proposed: a juvenile subtype and one related to tics.[102,103] In patients with TS, OCBs usually include a need for order or routine and a requirement for things to be symmetric or "just right," e.g., arranging, ordering, hoarding, touching, tapping, rubbing, counting, checking for errors, and performing activities until things are symmetric or feel/look just right ("evening-up" rituals). In contrast, OCD subjects without tics typically have fear of contamination and cleaning compulsions. Differentiating OCBs from tics may be difficult, with clues favoring OCB including the following: a cognitive-based drive and need to perform the action in a particular fashion, i.e., a certain number of times, until it feels "just right," or equally on both sides of the body. Children with tic-related OCD do not differ from those with nontic-related OCD in terms of age, OCD severity, related impairment, or comorbidity.[104]

Anxiety and Depression

The incidence of generalized anxiety disorder in TS subjects ranges from 19% to 80%.[105,106] In a large cohort, the high risk period for anxiety disorder began at age 4 and for a mood disorder at age 7 years.[82] TS patients are likely to be more depressed than controls, and depression has correlated positively with earlier onset and longer duration of tics.[105,106] It has been suggested that anxiety and disruptive behavioral disorder are mediated by ADHD whereas mood disorder is influenced by comorbid OCD.[82] Genetic studies show that major depressive disorder (MDD) is genetic but that TS and MDD are unrelated.[107]

Episodic Outbursts (Rage), Disruptive Behavior, and Self-Injurious Behavior

Rage attacks, disruptive behaviors, difficulty with aggression, and self-injurious behaviors are common in patients with TS.[82,108,109] In clinical TS populations, 25–70% experience episodic behavioral outbursts and anger control problems.[83] Whether these behaviors are due to the presence of other disruptive psychopathology, such as obsessions, compulsions, ADHD-related impulsivity, risk-taking behaviors, or affective disorders, is unclear.

Other Psychopathologies

Antisocial behaviors, oppositional behaviors, and personality disorders are more frequent in TS, but the cause of this increase may be attributed to childhood ADHD, OCD, family, or economic issues.[110] Schizotypal traits are relatively common in TS.[111] A variety of other behavioral/emotional problems have been identified in patients with TS. For example, in studies based on the Child Behavior Checklist (CBCL), up to two thirds of TS subjects had abnormal scores, with clinical problems including OCBs, aggressiveness, hyperactivity, immaturity, withdrawal, and somatic complaints.[112–114] Antisocial personality, coupled with impulsivity, occasionally leads to actions that involve the legal system, although there is no evidence that TS patients are more likely to engage in criminal behavior than those without TS.[88]

Academic Difficulties

Poor school performance in children with tics can be secondary to several factors, including severe tics, psychosocial problems, ADHD, OCD, learning disabilities, or medications.[115] For example, poor arithmetic performance was found only in children with TS who had attentional deficits.[93] Individuals with TS typically have normal intellectual functioning, although there may be concurrent executive dysfunction, discrepancies between performance and verbal IQ testing, impairment of visual-perceptual achievement, and decrease in visual-motor skills.[78,116–119]

Sleep Disorders

Problems associated with sleep have been reported in about 20–50% of children and young adults with TS. Common symptoms include difficulties falling asleep, difficulties staying asleep, restless sleep, increased movement-related arousals, and parasomnias.[15,120] Sleep deficits may be associated with the presence of other comorbidities such as ADHD, anxiety, mood disorders, or OCD.[121,122]

ETIOLOGY

Genetic Basis

Despite Georges Gilles de la Tourette's suggestion of an inherited nature for TS, the precise pattern of transmission and the identification of the gene remains elusive. A positive family history for tics is present in about one-half of patients and studies of monozygotic twins show an 86% concordance rate with chronic tic disorder compared to 20% in dizygotic twins.[123–125] A complex genetic etiology is further supported by a study of unbiased estimates of familial risk and heritability of tic disorders at the population level.[126] A genetic predisposition is also felt to increase tic severity, rate of comorbidities, and psychosocial and educational difficulties.[127] Nevertheless, despite the efforts of international collaborative groups and genome-wide association studies, a specific causative gene mutation or risk allele has not been identified.[128] One possible explanation is the phenotypic and genotypic heterogeneity in this disorder.[129] Others have suggested a complex multifactorial and polygenetic background that is complicated by the effects of genomic imprinting (sex of the transmitting parent affects the clinical phenotype), bilineal transmission (genetic contribution from both sides of the family),[130–132] genetic heterogeneity, epigenetic factors, and gene–environment interactions.[133,134]

Several approaches have been used to identify the genetic site, including linkage analysis, cytogenetics, candidate gene studies, and molecular genetic studies.[135,136] Recognizing the importance of neurotransmitter abnormalities in TS, several candidate genes involving the dopaminergic and serotonergic pathways have been supported by independent studies including involvement of the dopamine 2 receptor, the dopamine transporter, and monoamine oxidase A (MAO-A).[136] Chromosomal studies have suggested abnormalities at various loci, many with unidentified genes.[135,136] An abnormality of the *SLITRK1* gene, located at 13q31.1, received much attention, but suggestions of an association with TS[137] have not been confirmed in additional populations.[138,139] A genome-wide scan of a two-generation pedigree with TS identified a premature termination codon in the gene that encodes histidine decarboxylase, the rate limiting enzyme in histamine biosynthesis.[140] Once again, however, subsequent investigations failed to identify this mutation in larger population studies. In the first genome-wide association study for TS, although no single marker attained significance (5×10^{-8}), the single-nucleotide polymorphism (SNP) with the strongest signal, rs7868992 located on chromosome 9q32, is close to a collagen gene.[139] In another study, the top TS-associated SNP (rs2060546) was an intergenic region on chromosome 12q22, 32kb distal to Netrin 4 (NTN4).[141] NTN4 belongs to a family of extracellular proteins that interact with other axon guidance proteins (e.g., SLIT and WNT), direct axon outgrowth and guidance, and are expressed in developing striatum.[142] A combined primary SNP and meta-analysis study with 4200 TS cases and 9000 controls has identified one genome-wide significant result ($p = 3.8 \times 10^{-9}$) on chromosome 2 that is not within a known gene (Scharf et al., personal communication). Since OCD and TS are clinically closely associated and both highly heritable, they have long been suspected to share genetic liability.[143] Although specific gene variants have been difficult to identify, one study suggested distinct components to the genetic architectures of these disorders[144] whereas another implicated 16p13.11 deletions in OCD, with weaker evidence for a role in TS.[145]

Potential epigenetic risk factors that have been suggested include timing of perinatal care, severity of mother's nausea and vomiting during the pregnancy, low proband birth weight, the Apgar score at 5 min, thimerosal,[146] nonspecific maternal emotional stress,[147] and prenatal maternal smoking.[148] Further replication of these latter studies is necessary recognizing that existing studies have limitations including the use of clinic rather than epidemiologically derived samples, retrospective data collection, and multiple hypothesis testing.[149] In summary, TS is thought to arise from a complex genetic background interacting with additional environmental factors, which will ultimately require the need for large-scale genetic studies and the replication of results in independent cohorts.

Autoimmune Disorder

Several investigators have proposed that, in a subset of children, tic symptoms are caused by a preceding group A β-hemolytic streptococcal infection, labeled as pediatric autoimmune neuropsychiatric disorder associated with streptococcal infection (PANDAS).[140,141] This controversial disorder is discussed further in chapter 18.

PATHOPHYSIOLOGY OF TIC DISORDERS

Physiological Studies

Bereitschafts potentials (BPs) are recordable slow-rising electrical negativity potentials that occur prior to a voluntary movement; an early component arising from both medial and lateral area 6, the supplementary motor area (SMA), and premotor cortex and a late component over the motor cortex contralateral to the moving limb.[155] Hence, if tics are voluntary, one would expect the presence of a BP prior to a tic. Unfortunately, results in TS are variable, with reports of no BP,[156] just a late component,[157] or a combination of no BP and others with early/late findings.[158] In TS patients, despite reports of increased sensory stimulation to a variety of factors, formal sensory threshold measurements are normal.[159]

Neuroanatomic Localization

A series of parallel cortico-striatal-thalamocortical (CSTC) circuits provide a unifying framework for understanding the interconnected neurobiological relationships that exist between movement disorders and associated behaviors.[150–152] The motor circuit, proposed to be abnormal in the production of tic symptoms, originates primarily from the SMA and projects to the putamen in a somatotopic distribution. The oculomotor circuit, possibly influencing ocular tics, begins principally in the frontal eye fields and connects to the central region of the caudate. The dorsolateral prefrontal circuit links Brodmann's areas 9 and 10 with the dorsolateral head of the caudate and appears to be involved with "executive functions" (flexibility, organization, constructional strategy, verbal and design fluency) and "motor planning" (sequential and alternating reciprocal motor tasks). The lateral orbitofrontal circuit originates in the inferior lateral prefrontal cortex (areas 11 and 12) and projects to the ventral medial caudate. This circuit is associated with OCBs, personality changes, mania, disinhibition, and irritability. The anterior cingulate circuit arises in the cingulate gyrus and projects to the ventral striatum, which also receives input from the amygdala, hippocampus, medial orbitofrontal cortex, entorhinal, and perirhinal cortex. Hence, as described, the basal ganglia is involved in cognitive and motivational functions as well as motor control.[298] Although direct and indirect evidence suggests that components of CSTC circuits are involved in the expression of tic disorders, identification of the primary abnormality remains an area of active research.[153,154,299]

Striatum

Associations between basal ganglia dysfunction and movements in other disorders, as well as numerous neuroimaging studies,[76,160–167] have led some investigators to emphasize the striatal component in TS. For example, one magnetic resonance imaging (MRI) volumetric investigation suggested that caudate volume correlated inversely with the severity of tics in early adulthood.[74] Diffusion-tensor MRI (DT-MRI), sensitive to the diffusion of water, has suggested reduced white matter integrity bilaterally in the putamen and decreased uneven diffusion (anisotropy) in the right thalamus.[168] Others suggest a striatal compartment abnormality at the level of striosome-matrix organization based on anatomic, physiologic, and lesion studies,[169,170] the clinical response to dopamine-receptor agonists,[171] and the association of stereotypies with variations in the inducibility of immediate-early genes for the Fos/Fra family of transcription factors within the striosomes and matrix.[172] Postmortem investigations of TS brains have identified a reduced number and density of parvalbumin-positive neurons in the caudate and globus pallidus externa (GPe), and an increased number in globus pallidus interna (GPi).[173] Other investigators have focused on the ventral striatum, based on its role in sequential learning and habit formation[174] and imaging studies indicating monoaminergic hyperinnervation. For example, positron emission tomography (PET) imaging studies have shown a ventral-to-dorsal gradient of increased striatal dopaminergic innervation using a ligand for type-2 vesicular monoamine transporters.[175] PET studies with ^{11}C-raclopride and amphetamine have also shown robust increases in dopamine release in the ventral striatum of TS subjects as compared with controls.[176] Evidence supporting basal ganglia involvement in tic formation also comes from animal models. For example, disinhibition of the sensorimotor portion of the striatum, by use of local $GABA_A$ antagonist injections in both rodent and non-human primates produced contralateral motor tic behaviors.[299] In addition, using a primate model, projection neurons in the striatum were shown to have earlier bursting activity than in the motor cortex.[300,301]

Cortical

Clinically, children with TS have cortically related executive dysfunction[117,118] and cognitive inhibitory deficits.[177] Numerous neuroimaging studies have been published with results showing larger dorsolateral prefrontal regions on volumetric MRI,[178] larger hippocampal regions,[179] controversial alterations of amygdala volume and morphology,[179,180] increased cortical white matter in the right frontal lobe[181] or decreases in the deep left frontal region,[182] and alterations in size of the corpus callosum.[183,184] DT-MRI studies of the corpus callosum in TS have shown lower fractional anisotropy, suggesting reduced white matter connectivity in this interhemispheric pathway.[185] Imaging has identified frontal and parietal cortical thinning, most prominent in ventral portions of the sensory and motor homunculi.[186] Using DTI to compute probalistic tracts between regions, enhanced connectivity has been identified between cortical regions (primary motor and sensory cortex and SMA) and the striatum.[187] Several studies have reported differences in fractional anisotropy in white matter; increased in white matter adjacent to somatosensory cortex[188] and decreased in medial and inferior frontal gyri, cingulate and premotor cortex.[189] In a large neuroimaging study, the TS group had lower white matter volume bilaterally in the orbital prefrontal cortex and anterior cingulate (Williams et al., personal communication). Direct evidence also comes from semiquantitative immunoblotting investigations on postmortem tissue that shows a greater number of changes in prefrontal centers (BA9) than in caudate, putamen, or ventral striatum.[190,191]

Evidence that the generation of tics arises in cortical structures is strongly supported by the results of several event-related functional MRI studies. In one study, containing 10 adults (6 women, 4 men), 2 seconds (s) prior to a tic, activation was prominent in the mesial and lateral premotor areas, the anterior cingulate cortex, and insula bilaterally; and at tic onset, a neural network formed by sensorimotor areas, the superior parietal lobule bilaterally and cerebellum was activated.[192] In a second study with 10 adults (8 men, 2 women) with moderate-to-severe TS, 2s before a tic, the SMA, ventral primary motor cortex, primary sensorimotor cortex and parietal operculum were activated; 1s before a tic, the anterior cingulate, putamen, insula, amygdala, cerebellum, and the extrastriatal visual cortex exhibited activation; and with tic onset, the thalamus, central operculum, primary motor and somatosensory cortices exhibited activation.[153] The early activation in the insula, (especially the right dorsal anterior insula) during the urge,[302] plus the presence of increased resting state connectivity between the insula and sensorimotor cortex,[193] has led to the suggestion that the insula directly influences the motor cortex (bypassing premotor areas) to produce tics.[155] Tic production is also likely enhanced by the presence of reduced brain inhibition. This hypothesis is supported by transcranial magnetic stimulation (TMS) studies demonstrating several forms of reduced inhibition in motor cortex[194,195] and by the presence of immature patterns of connectivity in adolescent TS patients, particularly in the frontoparietal network.[196] Lastly, some have suggested that the primary dysfunction lies not in these circuits but rather in the midbrain. For example, building on early work by Devinsky,[38] a single MRI study has shown increased left midbrain gray matter volume in TS patients as compared with controls.[197]

Neurotransmitter Abnormalities

Neurochemical hypotheses tend to be based on clinical responses to specific classes of medications; from cerebrospinal fluid (CSF), blood, and urine studies in relatively small numbers of patients; from neurochemical assays on a few postmortem brain tissues; and from PET or single-photon emission computed tomography (SPECT) studies.[198] Although the dopaminergic system may play a dominant role, the serotoninergic, glutamatergic, GABAergic, cholinergic, noradrenergic, and opioid neurotransmitter systems may have additional important effects.

Dopamine

With some variations, studies of the striatum have shown a slight increase in the number of striatal[199] or cortical[190,191] dopamine receptors, greater binding to dopamine transporters (DAT),[200–202] altered DAT-binding ratio after methylphenidate,[203] an increased release of dopamine following amphetamine stimulation,[176,204] and altered D2 receptor availability in meso-limbo-cortical areas.[205] These findings have led to a potentially unifying hypothesis involving the tonic-phasic release of dopamine,[176,204] first proposed by Grace for schizophrenia.[206,207] The phasic dopamine hypothesis is further supported by clinical findings, including (1) the possible exacerbation of tics by stimulant medications, likely secondary to enhanced dopamine release from the axon terminal; (2) tic exacerbation by environmental stimuli, such as stress, anxiety, and medications, events shown to increase phasic bursts of dopamine; and (3) tic suppression with very low doses of dopamine agonists, likely due to presynaptic reduction of phasic dopamine release. Although the dopaminergic tonic-phasic model hypothesis could exist in either the cortex or striatum, a frontal dopaminergic abnormality is favored based on the presence of dopaminergic abnormalities in this area.[190,191] Other hypotheses have suggested a developmental hypofunction of dopamine neurons resulting in dopamine-receptor hypersensitivity[208] or altered interactions between dopamine and either glutamate[209] or gamma-aminobutyric acid (GABA).[210,211] An association has been identified between a polymorphism of the dopamine transporter gene, DAT DdeI, and TS.[212]

GABA

GABA is the primary neurotransmitter of striatal medium-sized spiny neurons and interneurons located within both the striatum and cortex. In animal models, disruption of striatal GABAergic connectivity by local injections of the $GABA_A$ antagonist bicuculline produced tic-like behaviors.[213–215] In individuals with TS, a deficiency of cortical inhibitory interneurons is suggested by a reduction of short-interval intracortical inhibition measured by TMS[195] and a reduction of GABA measured by magnetic resonance spectroscopy in the primary sensorimotor cortex that inversely correlated with motor tic severity.[216] In contrast, 7T-MRS paradoxically showed elevated concentrations of GABA within the supplementary motor area,[217] a region associated with tics. It is suggested that tic suppression may result from a localized tonic inhibition mediated by extracellular GABA within this area. An alteration of striatal GABA is supported by both postmortem and PET studies. Anatomically, two postmortem studies have identified a reduction of GABAergic parvalbumin-containing interneurons in TS caudate and putamen.[218,219] PET imaging of $GABA_A$ receptors using [^{11}C]flumazenil showed decreased binding bilaterally in the ventral striatum, globus pallidus, thalamus, amygdala, and right insula.[220] Other supporting evidence for GABA involvement includes the beneficial effect of benzodiazepines, which enhance the inhibitory effect of GABA, on tic suppression[221] and an association between GABA-related genes and tic severity.[222]

Glutamate

Glutamate is the primary excitatory neurotransmitter in the mammalian brain, with approximately 60% of brain neurons using glutamate as their primary neurotransmitter.[223] Several lines of evidence suggest that a dysfunction of the glutamatergic system may have a role in TS: reduced levels of this amino acid have been identified in the GPi, GPe, and substantia nigra pars reticulata (SNpr) regions of four TS brains[224]; glutamate has an essential role in pathways involved with CSTC circuits[225]; there is an extensive interaction between the glutamate and dopamine neurotransmitter systems,[173,209,227] and glutamate-altering medications have a beneficial therapeutic effect on obsessive-compulsive symptoms.[209,226] In a small study, tic suppression following treatment with a glutamate agonist (D-serine) or a glutamate antagonist (riluzole) did not differ from the placebo-control group.[228]

Serotonin

Direct evidence for a serotoninergic role in TS comes from serum studies in TS patients that show decreased levels of serum serotonin and tryptophan.[229] Although 5-HIAA (a serotonin metabolite) levels in TS subjects were normal in the cortex,[230] levels in basal ganglia[225] and CSF[231] were reduced. Investigators have reported a negative correlation between vocal tics and [^{123}I]βCIT binding to the serotonin transporter (SERT) in the midbrain thalamus,[232] suggesting that serotoninergic neurotransmission in the midbrain and serotoninergic or noradrenergic neurotransmission in the thalamus may be important factors in the expression of TS. [^{123}I]βCIT and SPECT studies investigating SERT-binding capacity in TS patients have also shown reduced binding in TS, but findings appear to be associated with the presence of OCD.[232] The combined finding of diminished SERT and elevated serotonin 2A receptor binding in some patients has suggested a possible serotonergic modulatory effect.[176] PET of tryptophan metabolism has demonstrated abnormalities in cortical and subcortical regions.[233] The finding of increased dopamine release, decreased SERT-binding potential, and possible elevation of 5-HT2A-receptor binding in individuals with TS + OCD has suggested a condition of increased phasic dopamine release modulated by low 5-HT in TS + OCD.[176] Polymorphic variants of tryptophan hydroxylase 2 and the serotonin receptor HTR2C have been associated with TS.[234,235]

TREATMENT

General Principles

The initial step in establishing a therapeutic plan for individuals with tic disorders is the careful evaluation of all potential issues and the determination of their resulting impairment. In conjunction with the patient, family, and school personnel, it is essential to identify whether tics or associated problems, e.g., ADHD, OCD, school problems, or behavioral disorders, represent the greatest handicap. The discussion of tics and comorbid symptoms as separate entities frequently enables families and health-care specialists to focus on the patient's immediate needs more effectively. Therapy should be targeted and reserved for those problems that are functionally disabling and not remediable by nondrug interventions. Providing clear and accurate information and allowing adequate time for questions and answers enhances the ability of patients and family members to cope with issues surrounding this disorder. For many, education about the diagnosis, outcome, genetic predisposition, underlying pathophysiologic mechanisms, and availability of tic-suppressing pharmacotherapy often obviates or delays the need for medication. The treatment of a child with

TS requires a chronic commitment and often a comprehensive multidisciplinary approach, especially in those individuals with academic or psychiatric difficulties.

Tic Suppression

There is no cure for tics, and all pharmacotherapy is symptomatic. Physicians considering pharmacologic treatment should be aware of the natural waxing and waning course of tics and the influence of psychopathologies on outcome. Specific criteria for initiating tic-suppressing medication include the presence of psychosocial (i.e., loss of self-esteem; peer problems; difficulty participating in academic, work, family, social, and after-school activities; and disruption of classroom settings) and/or musculoskeletal/physical difficulties. The goal of treatment is not complete suppression of tics, but rather their reduction to a level where they no longer cause significant psychosocial or physical disturbances.

Nonpharmacological Treatments

Over the years, behavioral therapeutic approaches have been evaluated in TS including assertiveness training,[236] biofeedback,[237] massed negative practice,[238] exposure and response prevention,[239] and habit reversal training (HRT).[240] Randomized, blinded, controlled trials have definitively established the safety and efficacy of HRT for tics.[242,243] American, European and Canadian practice guidelines suggest that HRT should be the front-line intervention for tics.[239,240] HRT was subsequently expanded into the treatment program now known as Comprehensive Behavioral Intervention for Tics (CBIT)[242]: the latter containing core components including psychoeducation, inconvenience review, awareness training, self-monitoring, competing response training, relaxation training, and contingency management. CBIT has been shown to be beneficial in several large studies with an overall effectiveness equal to that of several tic-suppressing pharmacotherapeutic agents.[242,244-246] Unfortunately, there remain an insufficient number of trained behaviorists to provide either HRT or CBIT to Tourette patients. For example, a survey of urban-based mental/behavioral health-care providers found that less than 10% reported knowing how to implement HRT.[247] The use of telemedicine (telehealth), with techniques such as videoconferencing to deliver therapeutic or consultation services, has also been considered a possible means to circumvent the deficiency of behavioral practitioners,[247,248] as has parent-directed home-based therapy (Singer, personal communication). Other concerns about behavioral approaches include the time and effort required on the part of both parent and child, its effectiveness in controlling more severe tics, and its long-term effectiveness.

Preliminary studies using repetitive TMS (rTMS) have been beneficial when the supplemental motor area is targeted,[249] but of little success stimulating motor or premotor regions.[250,251] In two patients, transcranial direct current stimulation was beneficial.[252] Reports have suggested a worsening of symptoms associated with caffeinated beverages[253] and a beneficial tic response to the use of alternative dietary therapies (i.e., vitamin B_6, magnesium)[254] and self-hypnosis.[255] To date, however, there is no scientific evidence to support the use of diets, food restrictions, or general use of minerals or vitamin preparations. Acupuncture was beneficial in a single study,[256] but has not received much attention in the scientific literature. A randomized controlled trial with biofeedback did not produce a clinical effect greater than placebo.[257]

TABLE 7.2   Approach to the Treatment of Tics

1. Education

2. Behavioral therapy:

   HRT, CBIT

3. Pharmacotherapy

1st Tier	2nd Tier	Other
Guanfacine	Pimozide	Dopamine agonists
Clonidine	Fluphenazine	Tetrabenazine
Topiramate	Risperidone	Ecopipam
	Aripiprazole	Delta-9-tetrahydrocannabinol
	Olanzapine	Botulinum toxin
	Haloperidol	
	Ziprasidone	
	Quetiapine	
	Sulpiride	
	Tiapride	

4. Deep brain stimulation

Pharmacotherapy

A two-tiered approach is recommended: for milder tics, nonneuroleptic medications (tier 1), and for more severe tics, typical and atypical neuroleptics (tier 2) (Table 7.2). Therapeutic agents should be prescribed at the lowest effective dosage, the regimen be given an adequate trial, and the patient carefully followed with periodic determinations made about the need for continued therapy. Generally, after several months of successful treatment, consider a gradual taper of the medication during a nonstressful time, typically during vacation time. If significant symptoms reemerge, treatment is reinstituted. Only three medications, pimozide, haloperidol, and aripiprazole are approved by the Food and Drug Administration (FDA) for tic suppression. The extent of supporting evidence for many of the medications has been documented.[258,259]

TIER ONE MEDICATIONS

In general, there is fair evidence for the use of alpha-adrenergics for tic suppression as initial medications for tic suppression. Medications in this category include clonidine[260] and guanfacine.[261] The anticonvulsant topiramate has been shown to be beneficial,[262,263] whereas data for valproic acid[264] is very limited, and for levetiracetam[265] is controversial.[258,266,267] There is minimal evidence for use of baclofen[268] or long-term clonazepam[221] for tic suppression.

TIER TWO MEDICATIONS

Medications in this category include those that act as dopamine-receptor antagonists (antipsychotics). Although tic-suppressing agents are often effective, side effects from the use of typical and atypical neuroleptics frequently limit their usefulness. The development of tardive dyskinesia is not limited to typical neuroleptics[30] and there is a low remission rate of tardive syndromes even after the offending agent has been removed.[269] The sequence of drug usage varies among physicians, and the order listed in Table 7.2 represents that of the authors. Pimozide and fluphenazine[270] are preferred to haloperidol because of reduced side effects. A new D1-receptor antagonist, ecopipam, has been shown to be beneficial for the treatment of tics in adults.[271] Atypical neuroleptics (aripiprazole, risperidone, olanzapine, ziprasidone, quetiapine) are characterized by a relatively greater affinity for 5HT2 receptors than for D2 receptors and a reduced potential for extrapyramidal side effects. In this group, risperidone has been studied most extensively.[272,273] Several small studies have confirmed the clinical effectiveness of olanzapine,[274–276] ziprasidone,[277,278] quetiapine,[279,280] and aripiprazole.[281–283] Tetrabenazine, a benzoquinolizine derivative that depletes the presynaptic stores of monoamines and blocks postsynaptic dopamine receptors, may also be effective.[284,285] Sulpiride and tiapride, substituted benzamides, have been beneficial in European trials, but neither is available in the United States.

OTHER MEDICATIONS AND BOTULINUM TOXIN

The dopamine agonists, pergolide and ropinirole, prescribed at lower doses than used in treating Parkinson's disease, have been beneficial, but ergot-containing medications should be avoided because of side effects.[171,286] Delta-9-tetrahydrocannabinol, the major psychoactive ingredient of marijuana, has been effective,[287,288] but lacks rigorously conducted studies. Botulinum toxin (Botox), a focal chemodenervator has a beneficial effect on both dystonic motor and vocal tics as well as reducing the premonitory sensory component.[289–294]

Surgical Approaches

Deep brain stimulation (DBS), a stereotactic treatment, has had preliminary success in treating tics. As of 2014,[295] several DBS studies have been published including approximately 120 patients from 23 countries. The most appropriate brain region for individual symptoms remains unknown. At least seven different brain target sites have been used, the most common being the centromedian-parafascicular complex of the thalamus followed by various pallidal regions. Although most reports describe a beneficial effect, interpretation is confounded by variations in methodologies, differences in complications, variable use of standard outcome measures, and the lack of a control population. All prospective patients should be evaluated by a multidisciplinary team and suggested criteria have been published.[295] At a minimum, the individual should have failed therapeutic trials with tic-suppressing medications from three pharmacological classes: an alpha–adrenergic agonist, two dopamine antagonists (including one typical and atypical), and a drug from another class (preferably tetrabenazine). CBIT should also have been tried, if available. DBS for individuals less than age 18 years should have additional institutional approval. Other neurosurgical approaches, with target sites including the frontal lobe (bimedial frontal leucotomy and prefrontal lobotomy), limbic system (anterior cingulotomy and limbic leucotomy), cerebellum, and thalamus, have been tried in attempts to reduce severe tics.[303]

References

1. Tourette GDL. Étude sur une affection nerveuse caractérisée par l'incoordination motrice accompagnée d'écholalie et de copralalie. *Arch Neurol.* 1885;9:19–42, 158–200.
2. Kushner HI. Medical fictions: the case of the cursing marquise and the (re) construction of Gilles de la Tourette's syndrome. *Bulletin of the History of Medicine.* 1995;69(2):224–254.
3. Rickards H, Robertson MM. Vomiting and retching in Gilles de la Tourette syndrome: a report of ten cases and a review of the literature. *Mov Disord.* 1997;12(4):531–535.
4. Cardoso F, Faleiro R. Tourette syndrome: another cause of movement disorder of the ear. *Mov Disord.* 1999;14(5):888–889.
5. Morris HR, Thacker AJ, Newman PK, Lees AJ. Sign language tics in a prelingually deaf man. *Mov Disord.* 2000;15(2):318–320.
6. Weil RS, Cavanna AE, Willoughby JM, Robertson MM. Air swallowing as a tic. *J Psychosom Res.* 2008;65(5):497–500.
7. Rizzo R, Cath D, Pavone P, Tijssen M, Robertson MM. Three Cases of Palatal Tics and Gilles De La Tourette Syndrome. *Journal of child neurology.* 2014. http://dx.doi.org/0883073814546687.
8. Abwender DA, Trinidad KS, Jones KR, Como PG, Hymes E, Kurlan R. Features resembling Tourette's syndrome in developmental stutterers. *Brain Lang.* 1998;62(3):455–464.
9. Cavanna AE, Robertson MM, Critchley HD. Catatonic signs in Gilles de la Tourette syndrome. *Cogn Behav Neurol.* 2008;21(1):34–37.
10. Kompoliti K, Goetz CG. Hyperkinetic movement disorders misdiagnosed as tics in Gilles de la Tourette syndrome. *Movement Disorders.* 1998;13(3):477–480.
11. Mahone EM, Bridges D, Prahme C, Singer HS. Repetitive arm and hand movements (complex motor stereotypies) in children. *J Pediatr.* 2004;145(3):391–395.
12. Lin H, Katsovich L, Ghebremichael M, et al. Psychosocial stress predicts future symptom severities in children and adolescents with Tourette syndrome and/or obsessive-compulsive disorder. *J Child Psychol Psychiatry.* 2007;48(2):157–166.
13. Hoekstra P, Steenhuis M, Kallenberg C, Minderaa R. Association of small life events with self reports of tic severity in pediatric and adult tic disorder patients: a prospective longitudinal study. *J Clin Psychiatry.* 2004;65(3):426–431.
14. Horesh N, Zimmerman S, Steinberg T, Yagan H, Apter A. Is onset of Tourette syndrome influenced by life events? *J Neural Transm.* 2008;115(5):787–793.
15. Cohrs S, Rasch T, Altmeyer S, et al. Decreased sleep quality and increased sleep related movements in patients with Tourette's syndrome. *J Neurol Neurosurg Psychiatry.* 2001;70(2):192–197.
16. Kwak C, Dat Vuong K, Jankovic J. Premonitory sensory phenomenon in Tourette's syndrome. *Mov Disord.* 2003;18(12):1530–1533.
17. Banaschewski T, Woerner W, Rothenberger A. Premonitory sensory phenomena and suppressibility of tics in Tourette syndrome: developmental aspects in children and adolescents. *Dev Med Child Neurol.* 2003;45(10):700–703.
18. Prado HS, Rosario MC, Lee J, Hounie AG, Shavitt RG, Miguel EC. Sensory phenomena in obsessive-compulsive disorder and tic disorders: a review of the literature. *CNS Spectr.* 2008;13(5):425–432.
19. Patel N, Jankovic J, Hallett M. Sensory aspects of movement disorders. *Lancet Neurol.* 2014;13(1):100–112.
20. Rajagopal S, Seri S, Cavanna AE. Premonitory urges and sensorimotor processing in Tourette syndrome. *Behavioural neurology.* 2013;27(1):65–73.
21. Baizabal-Carvallo JF, Jankovic J. The clinical features of psychogenic movement disorders resembling tics. *J Neurol Neurosurg Psychiatry.* 2013;85(5):573–575.
22. Van Borsel J, Tetnowski JA. Fluency disorders in genetic syndromes. *Journal of fluency disorders.* 2007;32(4):279–296.
23. Diniz JB, Rosario-Campos MC, Hounie AG, et al. Chronic tics and Tourette syndrome in patients with obsessive-compulsive disorder. *J Psychiatr Res.* 2006;40(6):487–493.
24. Saccomani L, Fabiana V, Manuela B, Giambattista R. Tourette syndrome and chronic tics in a sample of children and adolescents. *Brain Dev.* 2005;27(5):349–352.
25. The Tourette Syndrome Classification Study Group. Definitions and classification of tic disorders. *Arch Neurol.* 1993;50(10):1013–1016.

26. Association AP [text revision] *Diagnostic and statistical manual of mental disorders: DSM-V, 5th ed.* Washington, D.C.: American Psychiatric Association; 2013.

27. Freeman RD, Fast DK, Burd L, Kerbeshian J, Robertson MM, Sandor P. An international perspective on Tourette syndrome: selected findings from 3,500 individuals in 22 countries. *Dev Med Child Neurol.* 2000;42(7):436–447.

28. Freeman RD, Zinner SH, Muller-Vahl KR, et al. Coprophenomena in Tourette syndrome. *Dev Med Child Neurol.* 2009;51(3):218–227.

29. Singer WD. Transient Gilles de la Tourette syndrome after chronic neuroleptic withdrawal. *Dev Med Child Neurol.* 1981;23(4):518–521.

30. Fountoulakis KN, Panagiotidis P. Tardive Tourette-like syndrome in a patient treated with paliperidone. *J Neuropsychiatry Clin Neurosci.* 2011;23(4):E35–36.

31. Attig E, Amyot R, Botez T. Cocaine induced chronic tics. *J Neurol Neurosurg Psychiatry.* 1994;57(9):1143–1144.

32. Mejia NI, Jankovic J. Secondary tics and tourettism. *Rev Bras Psiquiatr.* 2005;27(1):11–17.

33. Jankovic J, Ashizawa T. Tourettism associated with Huntington's disease. *Mov Disord.* 1995;10(1):103–105.

34. Scarano V, Pellecchia M, Filla A, Barone P. Hallervorden-Spatz syndrome resembling a typical Tourette syndrome. *Movement Disorders.* 2002;17(3):618–620.

35. Sacks OW. Acquired Tourettism in adult life. *Adv Neurol.* 1982;35:89–92.

36. Northam RS, Singer HS. Postencephalitic acquired Tourette-like syndrome in a child. *Neurology.* 1991;41(4):592–593.

37. Riedel M, Straube A, Schwarz MJ, Wilske B, Muller N. Lyme disease presenting as Tourette's syndrome. *Lancet.* 1998;351(9100):418–419.

38. Devinsky O. Neuroanatomy of Gilles de la Tourette's syndrome. Possible midbrain involvement. *Arch Neurol.* 1983;40(8):508–514.

39. Luo F, Leckman JF, Katsovich L, et al. Prospective longitudinal study of children with tic disorders and/or obsessive-compulsive disorder: relationship of symptom exacerbations to newly acquired streptococcal infections. *Pediatrics.* 2004;113(6):e578–585.

40. Klawans HL, Falk DK, Nausieda PA, Weiner WJ. Gilles de la Tourette syndrome after long-term chlorpromazine therapy. *Neurology.* 1978;28(10):1064–1066.

41. Lombroso C. Lamotrigine-induced tourettism. *Neurology.* 1999;52(6):1191–1194.

42. Moshe K, Iulian I, Seth K, Eli L, Joseph Z. Clomipramine-induced tourettism in obsessive-compulsive disorder: clinical and theoretical implications. *Clin Neuropharmacol.* 1994;17(4):338–343.

43. Ko S, Ahn T, Kim J, Kim Y, Jeon B. A case of adult onset tic disorder following carbon monoxide intoxication. *Can J Neurol Sci.* 2004;31(2):268–270.

44. Kwak CH, Jankovic J. Tourettism and dystonia after subcortical stroke. *Mov Disord.* 2002;17(4):821–825.

45. Gomis M, Puente V, Pont-Sunyer C, Oliveras C, Roquer J. Adult onset simple phonic tic after caudate stroke. *Mov Disord.* 2008;23(5):765–766.

46. Majumdar A, Appleton RE. Delayed and severe but transient Tourette syndrome after head injury. *Pediatr Neurol.* 2002;27(4):314–317.

47. Krauss J, Jankovic J. Tics secondary to craniocerebral trauma. *Movement Disorders.* 1997;12(5):776–782.

48. O'Suilleabhain P, Dewey Jr. RB. Movement disorders after head injury: diagnosis and management. *J Head Trauma Rehabil.* 2004;19(4):305–313.

49. Erer S, Jankovic J. Adult onset tics after peripheral injury. *Parkinsonism Relat Disord.* 2008;14(1):75–76.

50. Singer HS, Dela Cruz PS, Abrams MT, Bean SC, Reiss AL. A Tourette-like syndrome following cardiopulmonary bypass and hypothermia: MRI volumetric measurements. *Mov Disord.* 1997;12(4):588–592.

51. Chemali Z, Bromfield E. Tourette's syndrome following temporal lobectomy for seizure control. *Epilepsy Behav.* 2003;4(5):564–566.

52. Kurlan R, McDermott MP, Deeley C, et al. Prevalence of tics in schoolchildren and association with placement in special education. *Neurology.* 2001;57(8):1383–1388.

53. Robertson MM. The prevalence and epidemiology of Gilles de la Tourette syndrome. Part 2: tentative explanations for differing prevalence figures in GTS, including the possible effects of psychopathology, aetiology, cultural differences, and differing phenotypes. *J Psychosom Res.* 2008;65(5):473–486.

54. Scahill L, Bitsko R, Visser S, Blumberg S. Prevalence of diagnosed tourette syndrome in persons aged 6-17 years-United States, 2007. *Morbidity and Mortality Weekly Report.* 2009;58(21):581–585.

55. Knight T, Steeves T, Day L, Lowerison M, Jette N, Pringsheim T. Prevalence of tic disorders: a systematic review and meta-analysis. *Pediatric neurology.* 2012;47(2):77–90.

III. PAROXYSMAL MOVEMENT DISORDERS

56. Robertson MM. Diagnosing Tourette syndrome: is it a common disorder? *J Psychosom Res*. 2003;55(1):3–6.

57. Khalifa N, von Knorring AL. Prevalence of tic disorders and Tourette syndrome in a Swedish school population. *Dev Med Child Neurol*. 2003;45(5):315–319.

58. Robertson MM. The prevalence and epidemiology of Gilles de la Tourette syndrome. Part 1: the epidemiological and prevalence studies. *J Psychosom Res*. 2008;65(5):461–472.

59. Robertson MM, Stern JS. Gilles de la Tourette syndrome: symptomatic treatment based on evidence. *Eur Child Adolesc Psychiatry*. 2000;9(suppl 1):I60–75.

60. Cubo E, Chmura T, Goetz CG. Comparison of tic characteristics between children and adults. *Mov Disord*. 2008;23(16):2407–2411.

61. Eapen V, Lees A, Lakke J, Trimble M, Robertson M. Adult-onset tic disorders. *Movement Disorders*. 2002;17(4):735–740.

62. Jankovic J, Gelineau-Kattner R, Davidson A. Tourette's syndrome in adults. *Movement Disorders*. 2010;25(13):2171–2175.

63. Schneider SA, Robertson MM, Rizzo R, Turk J, Bhatia KP, Orth M. Fragile X syndrome associated with tic disorders. *Mov Disord*. 2008;23(8):1108–1112.

64. Canitano R, Vivanti G. Tics and Tourette syndrome in autism spectrum disorders. *Autism*. 2007;11(1):19–28.

65. Baron-Cohen S, Mortimore C, Moriarty J, Izaguirre J, Robertson M. The prevalence of Gilles de la Tourette's syndrome in children and adolescents with autism. *J Child Psychol Psychiatry*. 1999;40(2):213–218.

66. Eapen V, Laker M, Anfield A, Dobbs J, Robertson MM. Prevalence of tics and Tourette syndrome in an inpatient adult psychiatry setting. *J Psychiatry Neurosci*. 2001;26(5):417–420.

67. Leckman JF, Riddle MA, Hardin MT, et al. The Yale Global Tic Severity Scale: initial testing of a clinician- rated scale of tic severity. *J Am Acad Child Adolesc Psychiatry*. 1989;28(4):566–573.

68. Cavanna AE, Schrag A, Morley D, et al. The Gilles de la Tourette syndrome-quality of life scale (GTS-QOL): development and validation. *Neurology*. 2008;71(18):1410–1416.

69. Bloch MH, Peterson BS, Scahill L, et al. Adulthood outcome of tic and obsessive-compulsive symptom severity in children with Tourette syndrome. *Arch Pediatr Adolesc Med*. 2006;160(1):65–69.

70. Shprecher DR, Gannon K, Agarwal N, Shi X, Anderson JS. Elucidating the nature and mechanism of tic improvement in Tourette syndrome: a pilot study. *Tremor and Other Hyperkinetic Movements*. 2014;4:217.

71. Hassan N, Cavanna AE. The prognosis of Tourette syndrome: implications for clinical practice. *Functional neurology*. 2012;27(1):23.

72. Leckman JF, Zhang H, Vitale A, et al. Course of tic severity in Tourette syndrome: the first two decades. *Pediatrics*. 1998;102(1 Pt 1):14–19.

73. Erenberg G, Cruse RP, Rothner AD. The natural history of Tourette syndrome: a follow-up study. *Ann Neurol*. 1987;22(3):383–385.

74. Pappert EJ, Goetz CG, Louis ED, Blasucci L, Leurgans S. Objective assessments of longitudinal outcome in Gilles de la Tourette's syndrome. *Neurology*. 2003;61(7):936–940.

75. Singer HS. Discussing outcome in tourette syndrome. *Arch Pediatr Adolesc Med*. 2006;160(1):103–105.

76. Bloch MH, Leckman JF, Zhu H, Peterson BS. Caudate volumes in childhood predict symptom severity in adults with Tourette syndrome. *Neurology*. 2005;65(8):1253–1258.

77. Bloch MH, Sukhodolsky DG, Leckman JF, Schultz RT. Fine-motor skill deficits in childhood predict adulthood tic severity and global psychosocial functioning in Tourette's syndrome. *J Child Psychol Psychiatry*. 2006;47(6):551–559.

78. Channon S, Pratt P, Robertson MM. Executive function, memory, and learning in Tourette's syndrome. *Neuropsychology*. 2003;17(2):247–254.

79. Sukhodolsky DG, Scahill L, Zhang H, et al. Disruptive behavior in children with Tourette's syndrome: association with ADHD comorbidity, tic severity, and functional impairment. *J Am Acad Child Adolesc Psychiatry*. 2003;42(1):98–105.

80. Cavanna AE, Rickards H. The psychopathological spectrum of Gilles de la Tourette syndrome. *Neuroscience & Biobehavioral Reviews*. 2013;37(6):1008–1015.

81. Cohen SC, Leckman JF, Bloch MH. Clinical assessment of Tourette syndrome and tic disorders. *Neuroscience & Biobehavioral Reviews*. 2013;37(6):997–1007.

82. Hirschtritt ME, Lee PC, Pauls DL, et al. Lifetime prevalence, age of risk, and genetic relationships of comorbid psychiatric disorders in tourette syndrome. *JAMA psychiatry*. 2015;72(4):325–333.

83. Mol Debes NM. Co-morbid disorders in Tourette syndrome. *Behavioural neurology*. 2013;27(1):7–14.

84. Pringsheim T, Lang A, Kurlan R, Pearce M, Sandor P. Understanding disability in Tourette syndrome. *Dev Med Child Neurol*. 2008;51(6):468–472.

85. Storch EA, Merlo LJ, Lack C, et al. Quality of life in youth with Tourette's syndrome and chronic tic disorder. *J Clin Child Adolesc Psychol*. 2007;36(2):217–227.

86. Gutierrez-Colina AM, Eaton CK, Lee JL, LaMotte J, Blount RL. Health-related quality of life and psychosocial functioning in children with Tourette syndrome: parent-child agreement and comparison to healthy norms. *J Child Neurol*. 2015;30(3):326–332.

87. Eddy CM, Cavanna AE, Gulisano M, Calì P, Robertson MM, Rizzo R. The effects of comorbid obsessive-compulsive disorder and attention-deficit hyperactivity disorder on quality of life in Tourette syndrome. *The Journal of neuropsychiatry and clinical neurosciences*. 2012;24(4):458–462.

88. Jankovic J, Kwak C, Frankoff R. Tourette's syndrome and the law. *J Neuropsychiatry Clin Neurosci*. 2006;18(1):86–95.

89. Comings DE, Comings BG. A controlled study of Tourette syndrome. I. Attention-deficit disorder, learning disorders, and school problems. *Am J Hum Genet*. 1987;41(5):701–741.

90. Silverstein SM, Como PG, Palumbo DR. Multiple sources of attentional dysfunction in adults with Tourette syndrome: comparison with attention-decifit hyperactivity disorder. *Neuropsychol*. 1995;9:157.

91. Hoekstra PJ, Steenhuis MP, Troost PW, Korf J, Kallenberg CG, Minderaa RB. Relative contribution of attention-deficit hyperactivity disorder, obsessive-compulsive disorder, and tic severity to social and behavioral problems in tic disorders. *J Dev Behav Pediatr*. 2004;25(4):272–279.

92. Freeman RD. Tic disorders and ADHD: answers from a world-wide clinical dataset on Tourette syndrome. *Eur Child Adolesc Psychiatry*. 2007;16(suppl 1):15–23.

93. Huckeba W, Chapieski L, Hiscock M, Glaze D. Arithmetic performance in children with Tourette syndrome: relative contribution of cognitive and attentional factors. *J Clin Exp Neuropsychol*. 2008;30(4):410–420.

94. Mol Debes NM, Hjalgrim H, Skov L. Validation of the presence of comorbidities in a Danish clinical cohort of children with Tourette syndrome. *J Child Neurol*. 2008;23(9):1017–1027.

95. Stewart SE, Illmann C, Geller DA, Leckman JF, King R, Pauls DL. A controlled family study of attention-deficit/hyperactivity disorder and Tourette's disorder. *J Am Acad Child Adolesc Psychiatry*. 2006;45(11):1354–1362.

96. Pauls DL, Alsobrook II JP, Goodman W, Rasmussen S, Leckman JF. A family study of obsessive-compulsive disorder. *Am J Psychiatry*. 1995;152(1):76–84.

97. Nestadt G, Samuels J, Riddle M, et al. A family study of obsessive-compulsive disorder. *Arch Gen Psychiatry*. 2000;57(4):358–363.

98. Grados MA, Riddle MA, Samuels JF, et al. The familial phenotype of obsessive-compulsive disorder in relation to tic disorders: the Hopkins OCD family study. *Biol Psychiatry*. 2001;50(8):559–565.

99. Gaze C, Kepley HO, Walkup JT. Co-occurring psychiatric disorders in children and adolescents with Tourette syndrome. *J Child Neurol*. 2006;21(8):657–664.

100. Lombroso PJ, Scahill L. Tourette syndrome and obsessive-compulsive disorder. *Brain Dev*. 2008;30(4):231–237.

101. Mula M, Cavanna AE, Critchley H, Robertson MM, Monaco F. Phenomenology of obsessive compulsive disorder in patients with temporal lobe epilepsy or tourette syndrome. *J Neuropsychiatry Clin Neurosci*. 2008;20(2):223–226.

102. Scahill L, Kano Y, King RA, et al. Influence of age and tic disorders on obsessive-compulsive disorder in a pediatric sample. *J Child Adolesc Psychopharmacol*. 2003;13(Suppl 1):S7–17.

103. Jaisoorya TS, Reddy YC, Srinath S, Thennarasu K. Obsessive-compulsive disorder with and without tic disorder: a comparative study from India. *CNS Spectr*. 2008;13(8):705–711.

104. Conelea CA, Walther MR, Freeman JB, et al. Tic-related obsessive-compulsive disorder (OCD): phenomenology and treatment outcome in the Pediatric OCD Treatment Study II. *J Am Acad Child Adolesc Psychiatry*. 2014;53(12):1308–1316.

105. Rickards H, Robertson M. A controlled study of psychopathology and associated symptoms in Tourette syndrome. *World J Biol Psychiatry*. 2003;4(2):64–68.

106. Coffey BJ, Park KS. Behavioral and emotional aspects of Tourette syndrome. *Neurol Clin*. 1997;15(2):277–289.

107. Pauls DL, Leckman JF, Cohen DJ. Evidence against a genetic relationship between Tourette's syndrome and anxiety, depression, panic and phobic disorders. *Br J Psychiatry*. 1994;164(2):215–221.

108. Budman CL, Rockmore L, Stokes J, Sossin M. Clinical phenomenology of episodic rage in children with Tourette syndrome. *J Psychosom Res*. 2003;55(1):59–65.

109. Mathews CA, Waller J, Glidden D, et al. Self injurious behaviour in Tourette syndrome: correlates with impulsivity and impulse control. *J Neurol Neurosurg Psychiatry*. 2004;75(8):1149–1155.
110. Robertson MM, Banerjee S, Hiley PJ, Tannock C. Personality disorder and psychopathology in Tourette's syndrome: a controlled study. *Br J Psychiatry*. 1997;171:283–286.
111. Cavanna AE, Robertson MM, Critchley HD. Schizotypal personality traits in Gilles de la Tourette syndrome. *Acta Neurol Scand*. 2007;116(6):385–391.
112. Singer HS, Rosenberg LA. Development of behavioral and emotional problems in Tourette syndrome. *Pediatr Neurol*. 1989;5(1):41–44.
113. Rosenberg LA, Brown J, Singer HS. Self-reporting of behavior problems in patients with tic disorders. *Psychol Rep*. 1994;74(2):653–654.
114. Ghanizadeh A, Mosallaei S. Psychiatric disorders and behavioral problems in children and adolescents with Tourette syndrome. *Brain Dev*. 2009;31(1):15–19.
115. Singer HS, Schuerholz LJ, Denckla MB. Learning difficulties in children with Tourette syndrome. *J Child Neurol*. 1995;10(Suppl 1):S58–61.
116. Brand N, Geenen R, Oudenhoven M, et al. Brief report: cognitive functioning in children with Tourette's syndrome with and without comorbid ADHD. *J Pediatr Psychol*. 2002;27(2):203–208.
117. Schuerholz LJ, Singer HS, Denckla MB. Gender study of neuropsychological and neuromotor function in children with Tourette syndrome with and without attention-deficit hyperactivity disorder. *J Child Neurol*. 1998;13(6):277–282.
118. Harris EL, Schuerholz LJ, Singer HS, et al. Executive function in children with Tourette syndrome and/or attention deficit hyperactivity disorder. *J Int Neuropsychol Soc*. 1995;1(6):511–516.
119. Schuerholz LJ, Baumgardner TL, Singer HS, Reiss AL, Denckla MB. Neuropsychological status of children with Tourette's syndrome with and without attention deficit hyperactivity disorder. *Neurology*. 1996;46(4):958–965.
120. Kostanecka-Endress T, Banaschewski T, Kinkelbur J, et al. Disturbed sleep in children with Tourette syndrome: a polysomnographic study. *J Psychosom Res*. 2003;55(1):23–29.
121. Allen RP, Singer HS, Brown JE, Salam MM. Sleep disorders in Tourette syndrome: a primary or unrelated problem? *Pediatr Neurol*. 1992;8(4):275–280.
122. Kirov R, Kinkelbur J, Banaschewski T, Rothenberger A. Sleep patterns in children with attention-deficit/hyperactivity disorder, tic disorder, and comorbidity. *J Child Psychol Psychiatry*. 2007;48(6):561–570.
123. Price RA, Kidd KK, Cohen DJ, Pauls DL, Leckman JF. A twin study of Tourette syndrome. *Arch Gen Psychiatry*. 1985;42(8):815–820.
124. Hyde TM, Aaronson BA, Randolph C, Rickler KC, Weinberger DR. Relationship of birth weight to the phenotypic expression of Gilles de la Tourette's syndrome in monozygotic twins. *Neurology*. 1992;42(3 Pt 1):652–658.
125. Robertson MM. The Gilles de la Tourette syndrome: the current status. Archives of disease in childhood. *Education and practice edition*. 2012;97(5):166–175.
126. Mataix-Cols D, Isomura K, Pérez-Vigil A, et al. Familial risks of tourette syndrome and chronic tic disorders: a population-based cohort study. *JAMA Psychiatry*. 2015;72(8):787–793.
127. Eysturoy AN, Skov L, Debes NM. Genetic predisposition increases the tic severity, rate of comorbidities, and psychosocial and educational difficulties in children with Tourette syndrome. *J Child Neurol*. 2015;30(3):320–325.
128. Dietrich A, Fernandez TV, King RA, et al. The Tourette International Collaborative Genetics (TIC Genetics) study, finding the genes causing Tourette syndrome: objectives and methods. *Eur Child Adolesc Psychiatry*. 2015;24(2):141–151.
129. Grados MA, Mathews CA. Latent class analysis of gilles de la tourette syndrome using comorbidities: clinical and genetic implications. *Biol Psychiatry*. 2008;64(3):219–225.
130. Eapen V, O'Neill J, Gurling HM, Robertson MM. Sex of parent transmission effect in Tourette's syndrome: evidence for earlier age at onset in maternally transmitted cases suggests a genomic imprinting effect. *Neurology*. 1997;48(4):934–937.
131. Lichter DG, Dmochowski J, Jackson LA, Trinidad KS. Influence of family history on clinical expression of Tourette's syndrome. *Neurology*. 1999;52(2):308–316.
132. Hanna PA, Janjua FN, Contant CF, Jankovic J. Bilineal transmission in Tourette syndrome. *Neurology*. 1999;53(4):813–818.

133. Walkup JT, LaBuda MC, Singer HS, Brown J, Riddle MA, Hurko O. Family study and segregation analysis of Tourette syndrome: evidence for a mixed model of inheritance. *Am J Hum Genet.* 1996;59(3):684–693.

134. Seuchter SA, Hebebrand J, Klug B, et al. Complex segregation analysis of families ascertained through Gilles de la Tourette syndrome. *Genet Epidemiol.* 2000;18(1):33–47.

135. Deng H, Gao K, Jankovic J. The genetics of Tourette syndrome. *Nature Reviews Neurology.* 2012;8(4):203–213.

136. Paschou P. The genetic basis of Gilles de la Tourette Syndrome. *Neuroscience & Biobehavioral Reviews.* 2013;37(6):1026–1039.

137. Abelson JF, Kwan KY, O'Roak BJ, et al. Sequence variants in SLITRK1 are associated with Tourette's syndrome. *Science.* 2005;310(5746):317–320.

138. Scharf JM, Moorjani P, Fagerness J, et al. Lack of association between SLITRK1var321 and Tourette syndrome in a large family-based sample. *Neurology.* 2008;70(16 Pt 2):1495–1496.

139. Scharf JM, Yu D, Mathews CA, et al. Genome-wide association study of Tourette's syndrome. *Molecular psychiatry.* 2013;18(6):721–728.

140. Ercan-Sencicek AG, Stillman AA, Ghosh AK, et al. L-histidine decarboxylase and Tourette's syndrome. *New England Journal of Medicine.* 2010;362(20):1901–1908.

141. Paschou P, Yu D, Gerber G, et al. Genetic association signal near NTN4 in Tourette syndrome. *Annals of neurology.* 2014;76(2):310–315.

142. Sun KLW, Correia JP, Kennedy TE. Netrins: versatile extracellular cues with diverse functions. *Development.* 2011;138(11):2153–2169.

143. Browne HA, Hansen SN, Buxbaum JD, et al. Familial clustering of tic disorders and obsessive-compulsive disorder. *JAMA psychiatry.* 2015;72(4):359–366.

144. Yu D, Mathews CA, Scharf JM, et al. Cross-Disorder Genome-Wide Analyses Suggest a Complex Genetic Relationship Between Tourette's Syndrome and OCD. *American Journal of Psychiatry.* 2015;172:82–93.

145. McGrath LM, Yu D, Marshall C, et al. Copy number variation in obsessive-compulsive disorder and tourette syndrome: a cross-disorder study. *Journal of the American Academy of Child & Adolescent Psychiatry.* 2014;53(8):910–919.

146. Thompson WW, Price C, Goodson B, et al. Early thimerosal exposure and neuropsychological outcomes at 7 to 10 years. *N Engl J Med.* 2007;357(13):1281–1292.

147. Burd L, Severud R, Klug MG, Kerbeshian J. Prenatal and perinatal risk factors for Tourette disorder. *J Perinat Med.* 1999;27(4):295–302.

148. Mathews CA, Bimson B, Lowe TL, et al. Association between maternal smoking and increased symptom severity in Tourette's syndrome. *Am J Psychiatry.* 2006;163(6):1066–1073.

149. Chao T-K, Hu J, Pringsheim T. Prenatal risk factors for Tourette Syndrome: a systematic review. *BMC pregnancy and childbirth.* 2014;14(1):53.

150. Alexander GE, DeLong MR, Strick PL. Parallel organization of functionally segregated circuits linking basal ganglia and cortex. *Annu Rev Neurosci.* 1986;9:357–381.

151. Alexander GE, Crutcher MD. Functional architecture of basal ganglia circuits: neural substrates of parallel processing. *Trends Neurosci.* 1990;13(7):266–271.

152. Cummings JL. Frontal-subcortical circuits and human behavior. *Arch Neurol.* 1993;50(8):873–880.

153. Neuner I, Werner CJ, Arrubla J, et al. Imaging the where and when of tic generation and resting state networks in adult Tourette patients. *Front Hum Neurosci.* 2014;8:362.

154. Ganos C, Roessner V, Munchau A. The functional anatomy of Gilles de la Tourette syndrome. *Neurosci Biobehav Rev.* 2013;37(6):1050–1062.

155. Hallett M. Tourette Syndrome: Update. *Brain Dev.* 2015.

156. Obeso JA, Rothwell JC, Marsden CD. Simple tics in Gilles de la Tourette's syndrome are not prefaced by a normal premovement EEG potential. *J Neurol Neurosurg Psychiatry.* 1981;44(8):735–738.

157. Karp BI, Porter S, Toro C, Hallett M. Simple motor tics may be preceded by a premotor potential. *J Neurol Neurosurg Psychiatry.* 1996;61(1):103–106.

158. van der Salm SM, Tijssen MA, Koelman JH, van Rootselaar AF. The bereitschaftspotential in jerky movement disorders. *J Neurol Neurosurg Psychiatry.* 2012;83(12):1162–1167.

159. Belluscio BA, Jin L, Watters V, Lee TH, Hallett M. Sensory sensitivity to external stimuli in Tourette syndrome patients. *Mov Disord.* 2011;26(14):2538–2543.

160. Hall M, Costa DC, Shields J. Brain perfusion patterns with 99Tcm -HMPAO/SPECT in patients with Gilles de la Tourette syndrome-short report *Nucleur Medicine: The State of the Art of Nuclear Medicine in Europe*. Stuttgart: Schattauer; 1991: 243–245.

161. Riddle MA, Rasmusson AM, Woods SW, Hoffer PB. SPECT imaging of cerebral blood flow in Tourette syndrome. *Adv Neurol*. 1992;58:207–211.

162. Baxter Jr. LR, Schwartz JM, Guze BH, Bergman K, Szuba MP. PET imaging in obsessive compulsive disorder with and without depression. *J Clin Psychiatry*. 1990;51(suppl 1):61–69. [discussion 70].

163. Jeffries KJ, Schooler C, Schoenbach C, Herscovitch P, Chase TN, Braun AR. The functional neuroanatomy of Tourette's syndrome: an FDG PET study III: functional coupling of regional cerebral metabolic rates. *Neuropsychopharmacology*. 2002;27(1):92–104.

164. Singer HS, Reiss AL, Brown JE, et al. Volumetric MRI changes in basal ganglia of children with Tourette's syndrome. *Neurology*. 1993;43(5):950–956.

165. Moriarty J, Varma AR, Stevens J, Fish M, Trimble MR, Robertson MM. A volumetric MRI study of Gilles de la Tourette's syndrome. *Neurology*. 1997;49(2):410–415.

166. Stern E, Silbersweig DA, Chee KY, et al. A functional neuroanatomy of tics in Tourette syndrome. *Arch Gen Psychiatry*. 2000;57(8):741–748.

167. Peterson BS, Thomas P, Kane MJ, et al. Basal Ganglia volumes in patients with Gilles de la Tourette syndrome. *Arch Gen Psychiatry*. 2003;60(4):415–424.

168. Makki MI, Behen M, Bhatt A, Wilson B, Chugani HT. Microstructural abnormalities of striatum and thalamus in children with Tourette syndrome. *Mov Disord*. 2008;23(16):2349–2356.

169. Mink JW. The basal ganglia: focused selection and inhibition of competing motor programs. *Prog Neurobiol*. 1996;50(4):381–425.

170. Mink JW, Thach WT. Basal ganglia intrinsic circuits and their role in behavior. *Curr Opin Neurobiol*. 1993;3(6):950–957.

171. Gilbert DL, Dure L, Sethuraman G, Raab D, Lane J, Sallee FR. Tic reduction with pergolide in a randomized controlled trial in children. *Neurology*. 2003;60(4):606–611.

172. Canales JJ, Graybiel AM. Patterns of gene expression and behavior induced by chronic dopamine treatments. *Ann Neurol*. 2000;47(Suppl 1):S53–59.

173. Canales J, Capper-Loup C, Hu D, Choe E, Upadhyay U, Graybiel A. Shifts in striatal responsivity evoked by chronic stimulation of dopamine and glutamate systems. *Brain*. 2002;125(10):2353–2363.

174. Seymour B, O'Doherty JP, Dayan P, et al. Temporal difference models describe higher-order learning in humans. *Nature*. 2004;429(6992):664–667.

175. Albin RL, Mink JW. Recent advances in Tourette syndrome research. *Trends Neurosci*. 2006;29(3):175–182.

176. Wong DF, Brasic JR, Singer HS, et al. Mechanisms of dopaminergic and serotonergic neurotransmission in Tourette syndrome: clues from an in vivo neurochemistry study with PET. *Neuropsychopharmacology*. 2008;33(6):1239–1251.

177. Stern ER, Blair C, Peterson BS. Inhibitory deficits in Tourette's syndrome. *Dev Psychobiol*. 2008;50(1):9–18.

178. Peterson BS, Staib L, Scahill L, et al. Regional brain and ventricular volumes in Tourette syndrome. *Arch Gen Psychiatry*. 2001;58(5):427–440.

179. Peterson BS, Choi HA, Hao X, et al. Morphologic features of the amygdala and hippocampus in children and adults with Tourette syndrome. *Arch Gen Psychiatry*. 2007;64(11):1281–1291.

180. Ludolph AG, Pinkhardt EH, Tebartz van Elst L, et al. Are amygdalar volume alterations in children with Tourette syndrome due to ADHD comorbidity? *Dev Med Child Neurol*. 2008;50(7):524–529.

181. Fredericksen KA, Cutting LE, Kates WR, et al. Disproportionate increases of white matter in right frontal lobe in Tourette syndrome. *Neurology*. 2002;58(1):85–89.

182. Kates WR, Frederikse M, Mostofsky SH, et al. MRI parcellation of the frontal lobe in boys with attention deficit hyperactivity disorder or Tourette syndrome. *Psychiatry Res*. 2002;116(1-2):63–81.

183. Baumgardner TL, Singer HS, Denckla MB, et al. Corpus callosum morphology in children with Tourette syndrome and attention deficit hyperactivity disorder. *Neurology*. 1996;47(2):477–482.

184. Plessen KJ, Wentzel-Larsen T, Hugdahl K, et al. Altered Interhemispheric Connectivity in Individuals With Tourette's Disorder. *Am J Psychiatry*. 2004;161(11):2028–2037.

185. Plessen KJ, Gruner R, Lundervold A, et al. Reduced white matter connectivity in the corpus callosum of children with Tourette syndrome. *J Child Psychol Psychiatry*. 2006;47(10):1013–1022.

186. Sowell ER, Kan E, Yoshii J, et al. Thinning of sensorimotor cortices in children with Tourette syndrome. *Nat Neurosci.* 2008;11(6):637–639.

187. Worbe Y, Marrakchi-Kacem L, Lecomte S, et al. Altered structural connectivity of cortico-striato-pallido-thalamic networks in Gilles de la Tourette syndrome. *Brain.* 2015;138(Pt 2):472–482.

188. Thomalla G, Siebner HR, Jonas M, et al. Structural changes in the somatosensory system correlate with tic severity in Gilles de la Tourette syndrome. *Brain.* 2009;132(Pt 3):765–777.

189. Muller-Vahl KR, Grosskreutz J, Prell T, Kaufmann J, Bodammer N, Peschel T. Tics are caused by alterations in prefrontal areas, thalamus and putamen, while changes in the cingulate gyrus reflect secondary compensatory mechanisms. *BMC Neurosci.* 2014;15:6.

190. Minzer K, Lee O, Hong JJ, Singer HS. Increased prefrontal D2 protein in Tourette syndrome: a postmortem analysis of frontal cortex and striatum. *J Neurol Sci.* 2004;219(1-2):55–61.

191. Yoon DY, Gause CD, Leckman JF, Singer HS. Frontal dopaminergic abnormality in Tourette syndrome: a post-mortem analysis. *J Neurol Sci.* 2007;255(1-2):50–56.

192. Peterson BS, Skudlarski P, Anderson AW, et al. A functional magnetic resonance imaging study of tic suppression in Tourette syndrome. *Arch Gen Psychiatry.* 1998;55(4):326–333.

193. Tinaz S, Belluscio BA, Malone P, van der Veen JW, Hallett M, Horovitz SG. Role of the sensorimotor cortex in Tourette syndrome using multimodal imaging. *Hum Brain Mapp.* 2014;35(12):5834–5846.

194. Moll GH, Wischer S, Heinrich H, Tergau F, Paulus W, Rothenberger A. Deficient motor control in children with tic disorder: evidence from transcranial magnetic stimulation. *Neurosci Lett.* 1999;272(1):37–40.

195. Gilbert DL, Bansal AS, Sethuraman G, et al. Association of cortical disinhibition with tic, ADHD, and OCD severity in Tourette syndrome. *Mov Disord.* 2004;19(4):416–425.

196. Church JA, Fair DA, Dosenbach NU, et al. Control networks in paediatric Tourette syndrome show immature and anomalous patterns of functional connectivity. *Brain.* 2009;132(Pt 1):225–238.

197. Garraux G, Goldfine A, Bohlhalter S, Lerner A, Hanakawa T, Hallett M. Increased midbrain gray matter in Tourette's syndrome. *Ann Neurol.* 2006;59(2):381–385.

198. Singer HS, Minzer K. Neurobiology of Tourette syndrome: concepts of neuroanatomical localization and neurochemical abnormalities. *Brain and Development.* 2003;25(suppl 1):S70–S84.

199. Wong DF, Singer HS, Brandt J, et al. D2-like dopamine receptor density in Tourette syndrome measured by PET. *J Nucl Med.* 1997;38(8):1243–1247.

200. Singer HS, Hahn IH, Moran TH. Abnormal dopamine uptake sites in postmortem striatum from patients with Tourette's syndrome. *Ann Neurol.* 1991;30(4):558–562.

201. Serra-Mestres J, Ring HA, Costa DC, et al. Dopamine transporter binding in Gilles de la Tourette syndrome: a [123I]FP-CIT/SPECT study. *Acta Psychiatr Scand.* 2004;109(2):140–146.

202. Choen KA, Ryu YH, Namkoong K, Kim CH, Kim JJ, Lee JD. Dopamine transporter density of the basal ganglia assessed with [123I]IPT SPECT in drug-naive children with Tourette's disorder. *Psychiatry Res.* 2004;130(1):85–95.

203. Yeh CB, Lee CS, Ma KH, Lee MS, Chang CJ, Huang WS. Phasic dysfunction of dopamine transmission in Tourette's syndrome evaluated with 99mTc TRODAT-1 imaging. *Psychiatry Res.* 2007;156(1):75–82.

204. Singer HS, Szymanski S, Giuliano J, et al. Elevated intrasynaptic dopamine release in Tourette's syndrome measured by PET. *Am J Psychiatry.* 2002;159(8):1329–1336.

205. Gilbert DL, Christian BT, Gelfand MJ, Shi B, Mantil J, Sallee FR. Altered mesolimbocortical and thalamic dopamine in Tourette syndrome. *Neurology.* 2006;67(9):1695–1697.

206. Grace AA. The tonic/phasic model of dopamine system regulation: its relevance for understanding how stimulant abuse can alter basal ganglia function. *Drug Alcohol Depend.* 1995;37(2):111–129.

207. Grace AA. Phasic versus tonic dopamine release and the modulation of dopamine system responsivity: a hypothesis for the etiology of schizophrenia. *Neuroscience.* 1991;41(1):1–24.

208. Nomura Y, Segawa M. Neurology of Tourette's syndrome (TS) TS as a developmental dopamine disorder: a hypothesis. *Brain Dev.* 2003;25(suppl 1):S37–42.

209. Singer HS, Morris C, Grados M. Glutamatergic modulatory therapy for Tourette syndrome. *Medical hypotheses.* 2010;74(5):862–867.

210. Marenco S, Savostyanova AA, van der Veen JW, et al. Genetic modulation of GABA levels in the anterior cingulate cortex by GAD1 and COMT. *Neuropsychopharmacology.* 2010;35(8):1708–1717.

211. Seamans JK, Gorelova N, Durstewitz D, Yang CR. Bidirectional dopamine modulation of GABAergic inhibition in prefrontal cortical pyramidal neurons. *J Neurosci.* 2001;21(10):3628–3638.

212. Yoon DY, Rippel CA, Kobets AJ, et al. Dopaminergic polymorphisms in Tourette syndrome: association with the DAT gene (SLC6A3). *Am J Med Genet B Neuropsychiatr Genet.* 2007;144(5):605–610.

213. Bronfeld M, Yael D, Belelovsky K, Bar-Gad I. Motor tics evoked by striatal disinhibition in the rat. *Frontiers in systems neuroscience.* 2013;7:50.

214. Worbe Y, Malherbe C, Hartmann A, et al. Functional immaturity of cortico-basal ganglia networks in Gilles de la Tourette syndrome. *Brain.* 2012;135(Pt 6):1937–1946.

215. Worbe Y, Baup N, Grabli D, et al. Behavioral and movement disorders induced by local inhibitory dysfunction in primate striatum. *Cereb Cortex.* 2009;19(8):1844–1856.

216. Puts NA, Harris AD, Crocetti D, et al. Reduced GABAergic inhibition and abnormal sensory symptoms in children with Tourette Syndrome. *J Neurophysiol.* 2015. http://dx.doi.org/10.1152/jn.00060.2015.

217. Draper A, Stephenson MC, Jackson GM, et al. Increased GABA contributes to enhanced control over motor excitability in Tourette syndrome. *Curr Biol.* 2014;24(19):2343–2347.

218. Kalanithi PS, Zheng W, Kataoka Y, et al. Altered parvalbumin-positive neuron distribution in basal ganglia of individuals with Tourette syndrome. *Proc Natl Acad Sci USA.* 2005;102(37):13307–13312.

219. Kataoka Y, Kalanithi PS, Grantz H, et al. Decreased number of parvalbumin and cholinergic interneurons in the striatum of individuals with Tourette syndrome. *J Comp Neurol.* 2010;518(3):277–291.

220. Lerner A, Bagic A, Simmons JM, et al. Widespread abnormality of the gamma-aminobutyric acid-ergic system in Tourette syndrome. *Brain.* 2012;135(Pt 6):1926–1936.

221. Gonce M, Barbeau A. Seven cases of Gilles de la tourette's syndrome: partial relief with clonazepam: a pilot study. *Can J Neurol Sci.* 1977;4(4):279–283.

222. Tian Y, Gunther JR, Liao IH, et al. GABA- and acetylcholine-related gene expression in blood correlate with tic severity and microarray evidence for alternative splicing in Tourette syndrome: a pilot study. *Brain Res.* 2011;1381:228–236.

223. Nieuwenhuys R. The neocortex. An overview of its evolutionary development, structural organization and synaptology. *Anat Embryol (Berl).* 1994;190(4):307–337.

224. Harris K, Singer HS. Tic disorders: neural circuits, neurochemistry, and neuroimmunology. *J Child Neurol.* 2006;21(8):678–689.

225. Anderson GM, Pollak ES, Chatterjee D, Leckman JF, Riddle MA, Cohen DJ. Postmortem analysis of subcortical monoamines and amino acids in Tourette syndrome. *Adv Neurol.* 1992;58:123–133.

226. Kushner MG, Kim SW, Donahue C, et al. D-cycloserine augmented exposure therapy for obsessive-compulsive disorder. *Biol Psychiatry.* 2007;62(8):835–838.

227. Wu Y, Pearl S, Zigmond M, Michael A. Inhibitory glutamatergic regulation of evoked dopamine release in striatum. *Neuroscience.* 2000;96(1):65–72.

228. Lemmon ME, Grados M, Kline T, Thompson CB, Ali SF, Singer HS. Efficacy of glutamate modulators in tic suppression: a double-blind, randomized control trial of d-serine and riluzole in tourette syndrome. *Pediatr Neurol.* 2015;52(6):629–634.

229. Comings DE. Blood serotonin and tryptophan in Tourette syndrome. *Am J Med Genet.* 1990;36(4):418–430.

230. Singer HS, Hahn IH, Krowiak E, Nelson E, Moran T. Tourette's syndrome: a neurochemical analysis of postmortem cortical brain tissue. *Ann Neurol.* 1990;27(4):443–446.

231. Butler IJ, Koslow SH, Seifert Jr. WE, Caprioli RM, Singer HS. Biogenic amine metabolism in Tourette syndrome. *Ann Neurol.* 1979;6(1):37–39.

232. Muller-Vahl KR, Meyer GJ, Knapp WH, et al. Serotonin transporter binding in Tourette Syndrome. *Neurosci Lett.* 2005;385(2):120–125.

233. Behen M, Chugani HT, Juhasz C, et al. Abnormal brain tryptophan metabolism and clinical correlates in Tourette syndrome. *Mov Disord.* 2007;22(15):2256–2262.

234. Mossner R, Muller-Vahl KR, Doring N, Stuhrmann M. Role of the novel tryptophan hydroxylase-2 gene in Tourette syndrome. *Mol Psychiatry.* 2007;12(7):617–619.

235. Dehning S, Muller N, Matz J, et al. A genetic variant of HTR2C may play a role in the manifestation of Tourette syndrome. *Psychiatr Genet.* 2010;20(1):35–38.

236. Mansdorf IJ. Assertiveness training in the treatment of a child's tics. *Journal of behavior therapy and experimental psychiatry.* 1986;17(1):29–32.

237. Tansey MA. A simple and a complex tic (Gilles de la Tourette's syndrome): Their response to EEG sensorimotor rhythm biofeedback training. *International Journal of Psychophysiology.* 1986;4(2):91–97.

238. Storms L. Massed negative practice as a behavioral treatment for Gilles de la Tourette's syndrome. *American journal of psychotherapy*. 1985;39(2):277–281.

239. Verdellen C, van de Griendt J, Hartmann A, Murphy T. European clinical guidelines for Tourette syndrome and other tic disorders. Part III: behavioural and psychosocial interventions. *European child & adolescent psychiatry*. 2011;20(4):197–207.

240. Azrin NH, Peterson AL. Treatment of Tourette syndrome by habit reversal: A waiting-list control group comparison. *Behav Ther*. 1990;21:305–318.

241. Murphy TK, Lewin AB, Storch EA, Stock S. Practice parameter for the assessment and treatment of children and adolescents with tic disorders. *J Am Acad Child Adolesc Psychiatry*. 2013;52(12):1341–1359.

242. Piacentini J, Woods DW, Scahill L, et al. Behavior therapy for children with Tourette disorder: a randomized controlled trial. *JAMA*. 2010;303(19):1929–1937.

243. Cook CR, Blacher J. Evidence-based psychosocial treatments for tic disorders. *Clinical Psychology: Science and Practice*. 2007;14(3):252–267.

244. Scahill L, Woods DW, Himle MB, et al. Current controversies on the role of behavior therapy in Tourette syndrome. *Movement Disorders*. 2013;28(9):1179–1183.

245. Wile DJ, Pringsheim TM. Behavior therapy for Tourette syndrome: a systematic review and meta-analysis. *Current Treatment Options in Neurology*. 2013;15(4):385–395.

246. Wilhelm S, Peterson AL, Piacentini J, et al. Randomized trial of behavior therapy for adults with Tourette syndrome. *Archives of general psychiatry*. 2012;69(8):795–803.

247. Himle MB, Olufs E, Himle J, Tucker BT, Woods DW. Behavior therapy for tics via videoconference delivery: an initial pilot test in children. *Cognitive and Behavioral Practice*. 2010;17(3):329–337.

248. Himle MB, Freitag M, Walther M, Franklin SA, Ely L, Woods DW. A randomized pilot trial comparing videoconference versus face-to-face delivery of behavior therapy for childhood tic disorders. *Behaviour research and therapy*. 2012;50(9):565–570.

249. Mantovani A, Leckman JF, Grantz H, King RA, Sporn AL, Lisanby SH. Repetitive Transcranial Magnetic Stimulation of the Supplementary Motor Area in the treatment of Tourette Syndrome: report of two cases. *Clin Neurophysiol*. 2007;118(10):2314–2315.

250. Munchau A, Bloem BR, Thilo KV, Trimble MR, Rothwell JC, Robertson MM. Repetitive transcranial magnetic stimulation for Tourette syndrome. *Neurology*. 2002;59(11):1789–1791.

251. Orth M, Kirby R, Richardson MP, et al. Subthreshold rTMS over pre-motor cortex has no effect on tics in patients with Gilles de la Tourette syndrome. *Clin Neurophysiol*. 2005;116(4):764–768.

252. Mrakic-Sposta S, Marceglia S, Mameli F, Dilena R, Tadini L, Priori A. Transcranial direct current stimulation in two patients with Tourette syndrome. *Mov Disord*. 2008;23(15):2259–2261.

253. Muller-Vahl KR, Buddensiek N, Geomelas M, Emrich HM. The influence of different food and drink on tics in Tourette syndrome. *Acta Paediatr*. 2008;97(4):442–446.

254. Garcia-Lopez R, Romero-Gonzalez J, Perea-Milla E, Ruiz-Garcia C, Rivas-Ruiz F, de Las Mulas Bejar M. [An open study evaluating the efficacy and security of magnesium and vitamin B(6) as a treatment of Tourette syndrome in children.]. *Med Clin (Barc)*. 2008;131(18):689–692.

255. Lazarus JE, Klein SK. Nonpharmacological treatment of tics in Tourette syndrome adding videotape training to self-hypnosis. *J Dev Behav Pediatr*. 2010;31(6):498–504.

256. Wu L, Li H, Kang L. 156 cases of Gilles de la Tourette's syndrome treated by acupuncture. *J Tradit Chin Med*. 1996;16(3):211–213.

257. Nagai Y, Cavanna AE, Critchley HD, Stern JJ, Robertson MM, Joyce EM. Biofeedback treatment for Tourette syndrome: a preliminary randomized controlled trial. *Cognitive and Behavioral Neurology*. 2014;27(1):17–24.

258. Scahill L, Erenberg G, Berlin Jr. CM, et al. Contemporary assessment and pharmacotherapy of Tourette syndrome. *NeuroRx*. 2006;3(2):192–206.

259. Shprecher D, Kurlan R. The management of tics. *Mov Disord*. 2009;24(1):15–24.

260. Gaffney GR, Perry PJ, Lund BC, Bever-Stille KA, Arndt S, Kuperman S. Risperidone versus clonidine in the treatment of children and adolescents with Tourette's syndrome. *J Am Acad Child Adolesc Psychiatry*. 2002;41(3):330–336.

261. Scahill L, Chappell PB, Kim YS, et al. A placebo-controlled study of guanfacine in the treatment of children with tic disorders and attention deficit hyperactivity disorder. *Am J Psychiatry*. 2001;158(7):1067–1074.

262. Yang C-S, Zhang L-L, Zeng L-N, Huang L, Liu Y-T. Topiramate for Tourette's Syndrome in Children: A Meta-Analysis. *Pediatric neurology*. 2013;49(5):344–350.
263. Jankovic J, Jimenez-Shahed J, Brown LW. A randomised, double-blind, placebo-controlled study of topiramate in the treatment of Tourette syndrome. *J Neurol Neurosurg Psychiatry*. 2010;81(1):70–73.
264. Ye L, Lippmann S. Tourette Disorder Treated With Valproic Acid. *Clinical neuropharmacology*. 2014;37(1):36–37.
265. Awaad Y, Michon AM, Minarik S. Use of levetiracetam to treat tics in children and adolescents with Tourette syndrome. *Mov Disord*. 2005;20(6):714–718.
266. Smith-Hicks CL, Bridges DD, Paynter NP, Singer HS. A double blind randomized placebo control trial of levetiracetam in Tourette syndrome. *Mov Disord*. 2007;22(12):1764–1770.
267. Hedderick EF, Morris CM, Singer HS. Double-blind, crossover study of clonidine and levetiracetam in Tourette syndrome. *Pediatr Neurol*. 2009;40(6):420–425.
268. Singer HS, Wendlandt J, Krieger M, Giuliano J. Baclofen treatment in Tourette syndrome: a double-blind, placebo- controlled, crossover trial. *Neurology*. 2001;56(5):599–604.
269. Zutshi D, Cloud LJ, Factor SA. Tardive Syndromes are Rarely Reversible after Discontinuing Dopamine Receptor Blocking Agents: Experience from a University-based Movement Disorder Clinic. *Tremor and other hyperkinetic movements (New York, NY)*. 2014;4:266.
270. Wijemanne S, Wu LJ, Jankovic J. Long-term efficacy and safety of fluphenazine in patients with Tourette syndrome. *Movement Disorders*. 2014;29(1):126–130.
271. Gilbert DL, Budman CL, Singer HS, Kurlan R, Chipkin RE. A D1 Receptor Antagonist, Ecopipam, for Treatment of Tics in Tourette Syndrome. *Clinical neuropharmacology*. 2014;37(1):26–30.
272. Scahill L, Leckman JF, Schultz RT, Katsovich L, Peterson BS. A placebo-controlled trial of risperidone in Tourette syndrome. *Neurology*. 2003;60(7):1130–1135.
273. Dion Y, Annable L, Sandor P, Chouinard G. Risperidone in the treatment of tourette syndrome: a double-blind, placebo-controlled trial. *J Clin Psychopharmacol*. 2002;22(1):31–39.
274. Stephens RJ, Bassel C, Sandor P. Olanzapine in the treatment of aggression and tics in children with Tourette's syndrome--a pilot study. *J Child Adolesc Psychopharmacol*. 2004;14(2):255–266.
275. Mogwitz S, Buse J, Ehrlich S, Roessner V. Clinical pharmacology of dopamine-modulating agents in Tourette's syndrome. *Int Rev Neurobiol*. 2013;112:281–349.
276. McCracken JT, Suddath R, Chang S, Thakur S, Piacentini J. Effectiveness and tolerability of open label olanzapine in children and adolescents with Tourette syndrome. *J Child Adolesc Psychopharmacol*. 2008;18(5):501–508.
277. Sallee FR, Kurlan R, Goetz CG, et al. Ziprasidone treatment of children and adolescents with Tourette's syndrome: a pilot study. *J Am Acad Child Adolesc Psychiatry*. 2000;39(3):292–299.
278. Sallee FR, Gilbert DL, Vinks AA, Miceli JJ, Robarge L, Wilner K. Pharmacodynamics of ziprasidone in children and adolescents: impact on dopamine transmission. *J Am Acad Child Adolesc Psychiatry*. 2003;42(8):902–907.
279. Mukaddes NM, Abali O. Quetiapine treatment of children and adolescents with Tourette's disorder. *J Child Adolesc Psychopharmacol*. 2003;13(3):295–299.
280. Copur M, Arpaci B, Demir T, Narin H. Clinical effectiveness of quetiapine in children and adolescents with Tourette's syndrome : a retrospective case-note survey. *Clin Drug Investig*. 2007;27(2):123–130.
281. Yoo HK, Kim JY, Kim CY. A pilot study of aripiprazole in children and adolescents with Tourette's disorder. *J Child Adolesc Psychopharmacol*. 2006;16(4):505–506.
282. Seo WS, Sung HM, Sea HS, Bai DS. Aripiprazole treatment of children and adolescents with Tourette disorder or chronic tic disorder. *J Child Adolesc Psychopharmacol*. 2008;18(2):197–205.
283. Yee HA, Loh HS, Ng CG. The prevalence and correlates of alcohol use disorder amongst bipolar patients in a hospital setting, Malaysia. *International journal of psychiatry in clinical practice*. 2013;17(4):292–297.
284. Kenney CJ, Hunter CB, Mejia NI, Jankovic J. Tetrabenazine in the treatment of Tourette syndrome. *Journal of Pediatric Neurology*. 2007;5(1):9–13.
285. Porta M, Sassi M, Cavallazzi M, Fornari M, Brambilla A, Servello D. Tourette's syndrome and role of tetrabenazine: review and personal experience. *Clin Drug Investig*. 2008;28(7):443–459.
286. Anca MH, Giladi N, Korczyn AD. Ropinirole in Gilles de la Tourette syndrome. *Neurology*. 2004;62(9):1626–1627.
287. Muller-Vahl KR. Treatment of Tourette syndrome with cannabinoids. *Behav Neurol*. 2013;27(1):119–124.

288. Muller-Vahl KR, Schneider U, Koblenz A, et al. Treatment of Tourette's syndrome with Delta 9-tetrahydrocan-nabinol (THC): a randomized crossover trial. *Pharmacopsychiatry*. 2002;35(2):57–61.

289. Awaad Y. Tics in Tourette syndrome: new treatment options. *J Child Neurol*. 1999;14(5):316–319.

290. Kwak C, Jankovic J. Tics in Tourette syndrome and botulinum toxin. *J Child Neurol*. 2000;15(9):631–634.

291. Kwak CH, Hanna PA, Jankovic J. Botulinum toxin in the treatment of tics. *Arch Neurol*. 2000;57(8):1190–1193.

292. Marras C, Andrews D, Sime E, Lang AE. Botulinum toxin for simple motor tics: a randomized, double-blind, controlled clinical trial. *Neurology*. 2001;56(5):605–610.

293. Trimble MR, Whurr R, Brookes G, Robertson MM. Vocal tics in Gilles de la Tourette syndrome treated with botulinum toxin injections. *Mov Disord*. 1998;13(3):617–619.

294. Vincent Jr. DA. Botulinum toxin in the management of laryngeal tics. *J Voice*. 2008;22(2):251–256.

295. Schrock LE, Mink JW, Woods DW, et al. Tourette syndrome deep brain stimulation: A review and updated rec-ommendations. *Mov Disord*. 2015;30(4):448–471.

296. Ganos C, Garrido A, Navalpotro-Gomez I, et al. Premonitory urge to tic in tourette's is associated with intero-ceptive awareness. *Mov Disord*. 2015.

297. Scharf JM, Miller LL, Gauvin CA, Alabiso J, Mathews CA, Ben-Shlomo Y. Population prevalence of Tourette syndrome: a systematic review and meta-analysis. *Mov Disord*. 2015;30(2):221–228.

298. Tremblay L, Worbe Y, Thobois S, Sgambato-Faure V, Feger J. Selective dysfunction of basal ganglia subterrito-ries: From movement to behavioral disorders. *Mov Disord*. 2015.

299. Yael D, Vinner E, Bar-Gad I. Pathophysiology of tic disorders. *Mov Disord*. 2015.

300. McCairn KW, Bronfeld M, Belelovsky K, Bar-Gad I. The neurophysiological correlates of motor tics following focal striatal disinhibition. *Brain*. 2009;132(Pt 8):2125–2138.

301. Bronfeld M, Belelovsky K, Bar-Gad I. Spatial and temporal properties of tic-related neuronal activity in the cortico-basal ganglia loop. *J Neurosci*. 2011;31(24):8713–8721.

302. Tinaz S, Malone P, Hallett M, Horovitz SG. Role of the right dorsal anterior insula in the urge to tic in tourette syndrome. *Mov Disord*. 2015.

303. Temel Y, Visser-Vandewalle V. Surgery in Tourette syndrome. *Mov Disord*. 2004;19(1):3–14.

Motor Stereotypies

Harvey S. Singer[1], Jonathan W. Mink[2],
Donald L. Gilbert[3] and Joseph Jankovic[4]

[1]Department of Neurology, Johns Hopkins Hospital, Baltimore, MD, USA;
[2]Division of Child Neurology, University of Rochester Medical Center,
Rochester, NY, USA; [3]Division of Neurology, Cincinnati Children's Hospital
Medical Center, Cincinnati, OH, USA; [4]Department of Neurology, Baylor
College of Medicine, Houston, TX, USA

OUTLINE

Movement Disorders in Childhood, Second Edition.
DOI: http://dx.doi.org/10.1016/B978-0-12-411573-6.00008-5

INTRODUCTION

Despite not being a new disorder, the definition, classification, treatment, and underlying pathophysiology of motor stereotypies continue to evolve. Historically, stereotypic movement disorders have been linked to autism and impaired cognitive deficiency, although they commonly occur in typically developing children. Motor stereotypies can be readily classified into two groups: "primary," indicating a physiologic basis, and "secondary," for those associated with other neurodevelopmental problems. Both types of stereotypies usually begin in early childhood, frequently persist into adulthood, and are often a source of concern for parents. Although viewed by some as behaviors produced to alter a state of arousal, there is increasing evidence to support a neurobiological mechanism. Accumulating evidence includes the use of behavioral therapy whereas there is only limited support for the use of pharmacologic treatment.

DEFINITION

Stereotypies have been variably defined. Two often cited definitions include "involuntary, rhythmic, repetitive, fixed (fashion, form, amplitude, and location) movements that appear purposeful, but are purposeless (serve no obvious adaptive function or purpose), and stop with distraction"[1] and "a non-goal-directed movement pattern that is repeated continuously for a period of time in the same form and on multiple occasions, and which is typically distractible."[2] Both of the aforementioned emphasize hand/arm flapping/waving/wiggling activities and exclude brief intermittent movements (tics). Also rejected are movements that arise from the physiologic effect of a substance, delusional beliefs or obsessive thoughts, mannerisms, dyskinesia, and actions typically performed in situations of boredom (drumming fingers and tapping feet). The aforementioned differ from the *Diagnostic and Statistical Manual of Mental Disorders, Fifth Edition* (DSM-V), criteria which requires that the repetitive motor behavior interferes with social, academic, or other activities or possibly causes self-injury. Stereotypic movements come in a variety of forms (e.g., arm flapping, finger wiggling, body rocking, and head nodding) and may be initially misdiagnosed as normal mannerisms, habits, tics, or mere nervousness. Suggested definitions are broadly descriptive and visualization of the movements is essential for proper diagnosis. Motor stereotypies should also be considered distinct from the multiple domains of repetitive behaviors often mentioned with autism, e.g., restricted interests and routines, cognitive rigidity symptoms, unusual sensory responses, social communication difficulties, preoccupations, circumscribed interest patterns, abnormal object attachments, cognitive rigidity, unusual sensory responses, and social communication difficulties.[3–5]

Motor stereotypies typically begin before age 3 years. Movements occur in bursts, last from seconds to minutes, appear many times per day, have a fixed pattern, and are associated with periods of engrossment, excitement, stress, fatigue, or boredom. Each child typically has his or her own repertoire that may evolve over time. Several primary movements, such as bilateral flapping or rotating the hands, fluttering fingers in front of the face, flapping/waving arm movements, and head nodding, tend to predominate. It is not unusual to add other activities onto the primary movement. For example, flapping and waving arm/hand movements may be accompanied by mouth opening, tilting one's head back, jumping or pacing around the room. Vocalizations may accompany the patterned movements and are not considered to be vocal tics unless the latter occur independently of the stereotyped behavior. Stereotypies can be readily suppressed by a sensory stimulus or distraction, especially in children with normal cognition. There are no associated premonitory urges, contrary to what is frequently seen in tic disorders. Occasionally, patients report that they enjoy their movements or it makes them feel good. Some children have also reported engaging in visual imagery while performing the movements, e.g., envision participating in computer games or reenacting scenes from a favorite TV program.[6] Stereotypies are frequently upsetting to parents due to concerns about disruptions and social stigmatization. They are, however, usually of little concern for the child whose daily routine may not be impacted. The incidence of attention-deficit hyperactivity disorder (ADHD), learning disabilities, tics, and obsessive-compulsive behaviors is increased in typically developing children with complex arm and hand movements.[7] Suggestions that behaviors resolve in early childhood are often incorrect.[7–9] Several scales have been used for the assessment stereotypy severity include the Stereotypy Severity Scale,[10] the Repetitive Behavior Scale—Revised,[11] and the Behavior Problems Inventory.[12]

DIFFERENTIATING STEREOTYPIES FROM OTHER DISORDERS

The diagnosis of stereotypies requires the exclusion of other disorders such as habits, mannerisms, complex motor tics, obsessive-compulsive behaviors, paroxysmal dyskinesias, and seizures. Most frequently, stereotypies are misdiagnosed as complex motor tics.

1. *Mannerisms* are gestures or individual flourishes/embellishments that are attached to a normal activity (e.g., a baseball player's routine while awaiting a pitch). These movements that tend to be unique to the individual can be repetitive, do not appear in clusters, are of brief duration, and are less complex than stereotypies.
2. *Complex motor tics* are quick, rapid movements that involve either a cluster of simple motor tics or a more coordinated sequence of movements. Complex tics have several features in common with stereotypies; e.g., they are often repetitive, patterned, and intermittent and may be precipitated by excitement. In contrast, other characteristics are helpful in differentiating stereotypies from complex motor tics. Stereotypies have an earlier age of onset (<3 years) than do tics (mean onset 4–8 years). They are consistent and fixed in their pattern as compared to the frequent addition and subtraction of tics. In terms of body location, stereotypies frequently involve arms, hands, or the entire body rather than the more common tic locations of eyes, face, head, and shoulders. Stereotypies are more fixed, rhythmic, and prolonged in duration than are tics which, except for the occasional dystonic tic, are brief, rapid, random, and fluctuating. Stereotypies, in contrast to tics, are not associated with premonitory urges, preceding sensations, or an internal desire to perform. Both occur during periods of anxiety, excitement, or fatigue, but stereotypic movements are also common when the child is engrossed in an activity. Both tics and stereotypic movements are reduced by distraction, but the effect on stereotypic movements is more instantaneous and dramatic. Lastly, using a force sensitive platform, temporal measures and spectral analysis, stereotyped

TABLE 8.1   Factors Distinguishing Stereotypies from Tics

	Tics	**Stereotypies**
Age at onset	4–8 years	<3 years
Pattern	Variable, wax, and wane	Fixed, identical, patterned, predictable
Movements	Blink, grimace, twist, shrug	Arms/hands (flap, wave), body rock/head nod
Vocalizations	Sniffing, throat clearing	Moan, humming with movement
Rhythm	Rapid, sudden, random	Rhythmic
Duration	Intermittent, brief, abrupt	Intermittent, continuous, prolonged
Premonitory urge	Yes	No
Precipitant	Excitement, stress	Excitement, stress, also when engrossed
Suppression	Brief, voluntary (but have increased "inner tension")	With distraction, rare conscious effort
Distraction	Reduction of tics	Stops
Family history	Frequently positive	Positive, 25%
Force sensitive platform analysis[13]	Brief, less rhythmic	Longer duration: more rhythmic qualities
Treatment	Clonidine, guanfacine, D2 receptor antagonists	Behavioral therapy

Adapted from Ref. [14].

movements differ from tics both quantitatively and qualitatively.[13] Again, it is important to note that both stereotypies and tics may occur in the same individual (Table 8.1).

3. *Compulsions* are repetitive behaviors or mental acts that are performed to prevent or reduce distress or some dreaded event or situation, and are driven by an obsessive thought or by intrinsic rules that must be applied rigidly. The compulsion is either (a) unrealistically connected to distress reduction or contingency prevention or (b) clearly excessive.[15] Compulsions are often associated with obsessive thoughts that intrude into consciousness and are typically experienced as senseless or alien.

4. *Paroxysmal dyskinesias* are generally shorter in duration and usually occur as dystonic or choreoathetoid movements that are precipitated by voluntary movement (paroxysmal kinesigenic dyskinesias), exertion of exercise (paroxysmal exertional dyskinesia), or are less predictable, arising from normal background activity (paroxysmal nonkinesigenic dyskinesias) (see Chapter 9).

5. *Masturbation*, or self-stimulation of the genitalia, is a normal part of human sexual behavior that occurs in both males and females. In some infants and young children such self-gratifying behavior can manifest as patterned, coordinated, repetitive movements, usually consisting of crossing and extending of legs or repetitive pelvic movements that may be classified as a stereotypy.[16,17] Observation of movements on a video can often clarify the diagnosis and eliminate the need for unnecessary diagnostic tests.[18] The most

challenging aspect of this form of stereotypy is to help the parents understand the benign and self-remitting nature of this behavior.

6. Seizures, or more specifically automatisms in the context of epileptic seizures, are also within the differential diagnosis of stereotypies.[2] In 17 patients, motor stereotypies were associated with prefrontal cortex seizure activity.[19] Although not mentioned, it is assumed that the seizure was not aborted by a sensory stimulation.

PATHOPHYSIOLOGY

The underlying pathophysiological mechanism for stereotypies in both primary and secondary categories is unknown, with hypotheses ranging from psychological concerns to neurobiological abnormalities. In the former, the observation of a higher frequency of stereotyped behaviors in situations characterized by tedium or an altered state of arousal has led some investigators to suggest that these movements act to maintain an optimal state of arousal.[20] Proponents of a psychogenic mechanism tend to suggest several possibilities: (1) a form of self-stimulation or automatic reinforcement designed to compensate for a deficit of external arousal (e.g., congenital blindness, caging, autism, or mental retardation); (2) an attempt to deplete aversive stimuli, use up excess attention capacity or to reduce external distractions by channeling thoughts and actions into movements[21]; (3) the substitution of behaviors to take the place of imagined activities[6,22]; and (4) a relationship to obsessive-compulsive disorder (OCD)[23]; a general anxiety disorder[24]; and perfectionism or impulse dyscontrol.[3,25]

Accumulating lines of evidence, however, support a neurobiological basis for stereotypies, including its correlation with the severity of autism and cognitive impairment,[26] association with disorders such as Rett syndrome (RS),[27,28] pharmacological induction in animal models and in humans, and abnormal findings on neuroimaging. Primary CMS likely involve cortico-striatal thalamocortical (CSTC) circuits and their interconnecting brain regions (see Chapter 1). An electrophysiological study of children with primary CMS found that unlike voluntary movements, complex stereotypies were not preceded by premotor movement-related cortical potentials.[29] These findings suggest that stereotypies utilize different pathways from those involved in voluntary movements. Recent animal and human studies have identified distinct separate cortical-striatal pathways in goal-directed and habitual behavioral activities.[32–35] More specifically, habitual behaviors, like motor stereotypies, are supported by a (pre)motor to putamen connection. In contrast, flexible goal-directed behavior, mediated by goal anticipation and evaluation, involves ventromedial prefrontal to caudate pathways. Animal studies of drug-induced stereotypies have suggested involvement of the ventral striatum and a differential activation of the striatal striosomal compartment.[29–31] Two small magnetic resonance volumetric neuroimaging studies have been performed in children with primary CMS. In the first, involving six participants, reductions were identified in the caudate and frontal white matter.[36] In a second study, 20 children with primary CMS, compared to an equal number of typically developing controls, showed significant volumetric reductions in putamen (total), and posterior cerebellar vermis white matter (lobules VI-VII and VIII-X), and with increased gray matter in anterior vermis (lobules I-V). There were no significant group differences in total cerebral volume or in gray or white matter volumes in any lobar cortical regions (Mahone, Singer, Kline personal communication). The detection of motor and executive dysfunction in children with primary CMS also raises the possibility of involvement of brain regions such as the cerebellum, which has direct connections to CSTC pathways.[38] In other studies, stereotypic movements have spontaneously appeared in a patient after meningoencephalitis with bilateral frontoparietal cortical lesions[39] and in association with strokes involving the right putamen,[40] right lenticular nucleus,[41] and bilateral paramedian thalamic and midbrain regions.[42] In patients with Down syndrome, cerebellar white matter volumes positively correlated with the severity of stereotypic behaviors.[43] Volumetric studies in autistic children, with stereotyped behaviors have been variable. In some, movements negatively correlated with the size of the cerebellar vermal lobules VI and VII, and positively correlated with frontal lobe volumes[44] whereas in others there was no specific structural alteration.[45]

Although numerous neurotransmitter systems coexist within cortical-striatal pathways, some evidence suggests involvement of the dopaminergic system. In rodent models, repetitive sequences of behaviors, such as sniffing, chewing, rearing, or grooming, can be induced by low doses of stimulants (release dopamine) and cocaine (block dopamine reuptake).[46–48] Stereotyped behaviors characterized by a fascination with repetitive, meaningless movements (punding), have been linked to stimulation of dopamine receptors with levodopa, dopamine agonists, and rarely dopamine receptor blockers.[49,50] Further, plasma concentrations of homovanillic acid, a dopamine metabolite, are reduced in adults with high rates of body rocking.[51] Other hypotheses have suggested cortical or striatal hyperexcitability as represented by elevated glutamatergic or reduced GABAergic neurotransmission. Using single-voxel 7T MR spectroscopy, in 19 children with primary CMS, GABA was reduced in the anterior cingulate and striatum, but not prefrontal cortex.[52] In contrast, no group differences were observed for glutamate.

A pattern of Mendelian inheritance has been suggested for primary stereotypies based on a report of one hundred typically developing children with CMS.[7] Seventeen had a first-degree relative (parent or siblings) with similar movements and 25 had at least one relative with motor stereotypies. A second study with 49 subjects showed that approximately 40% of participants reported a family history of stereotypies and 29% had an affected first-degree relative.[9] Whole exome sequencing on 121 trios (individuals with CMS and their unaffected parents) has identified two independent *de novo* nonsense variants in *KDM5B* carried by two unrelated CMS probands. A finding that is highly unlikely to be seen by chance (Thomas Fernandez, personal communication). *KDM5B* is a member of the histone lysine demethylase (KDM) family, and alterations within related genes have been observed in children with neurodevelopmental disorders including autistic spectrum disorder (ASD) and RS.[53–55]

CLASSIFICATION OF MOTOR STEREOTYPIES

Repetitive motor stereotypic behaviors are common in children with autism, mental retardation, or sensory deprivation, as well as typically developing children. A favored classification subdivides by etiology into primary and secondary categories, dependent on the existence of other behavioral or neurologic findings (Table 8.2). Whereas some investigators have suggested that a particular movement, complexity, duration, frequency, or accompanying vocalization may be more indicative of a secondary type,[56] others have emphasized that there is considerable overlap between the two subdivisions.

TABLE 8.2   Classification of Stereotypies Based on Etiology

I. *Primary* (otherwise developmentally normal)

Common type

Head nodding

Complex motor

II. *Secondary* (in the presence of other pathologies)

Autism: infantile autism, Asperger's syndrome, pervasive developmental disability, Rett syndrome

Mental retardation

Sensory deprivation: congenital blindness/deafness, caging, constraints

Inborn errors of metabolism: Lesch–Nyhan syndrome

Genetic: Angelman, Cornelia de Lange, Cri-du-Chat, Fragile X, Prader–Willi, Lowe, Smith–Magenis, neuroacanthocytosis

Drug-induced: psychostimulants, tardive dyskinesia

Infection: encephalitis

Tumor/cyst: bobble-headed doll syndrome

Trauma

Psychiatric: OCD, schizophrenia, catatonia, functional

Primary

This category implies that there is no specific cause for the stereotypy as it occurs in an otherwise normal individual; mild delays in either language or motor development may be present.[7,14,57] Primary stereotypies can be readily classified into three groups: *common behaviors* (e.g., rocking, head banging, finger drumming, pencil tapping, hair twisting) and two forms that contain atypical or complex behaviors, i.e., *head nodding*, or those with *complex motor movements* (e.g., hand and arm flapping/waving) (Videos 8.1, 8.5–8.9). Precise estimates of the prevalence of stereotypic movements in the typically developing child are unknown; approximations ranging from 2% to 10%. In part, difficulties quantifying primary stereotypies are related to the definition of which movements should be included within the tally, e.g., thumb and hand sucking, nail biting, and foot tapping.[58,59] Few studies have attempted to clarify whether outcome, comorbidities, or other features differ among the three subgroups.

Common Stereotypies

Behaviors such as thumb sucking, nail/lip biting, hair twirling, body rocking, self-biting, and head banging, sometimes called habits, are relatively common in childhood and generally most regress.[59–63] In some children, stereotypic behaviors evolve with thumb and hand sucking in the younger child replaced by body rocking and head banging, and later by nail biting, finger tapping, and foot tapping.[58] It has been estimated that about 20% of healthy children exhibit these stereotypies.[59] Investigation of stereotypies in college students has identified a variety of common movements (touch face; play with hair, pens, or jewelry; shake leg, tap fingers, scratch head, etc.), but most were not time-consuming or disruptive.[25] The prevalence of body rocking has varied between 3% and 25% depending on the identifying methodology.[64] In the college population, since stereotypies were often accompanied by general distress, anxiety, obsessive-compulsive symptoms, and impulsive aggressive traits, some investigators have suggested that common stereotypies may lie on a spectrum with other neuropsychiatric disorders, especially obsessive-compulsive phenomena.[23,24] Whether body rocking should be considered as a separate entity, based on a high frequency in first-degree relatives with similar movements and without evidence of mental retardation or autism,[23,24] is controversial. A leg stereotypies disorder has been reported occurring in seated individuals consisting of repetitive, stereotypical, 1-4 Hz flexion-extension, abduction-adduction, movement of the proximal legs (hips) when feet rest on the floor.[65]

Head-Nodding Stereotypies

Rhythmic regular head movements (either a side-to-side, "no" movement; an up-and-down, "yes" movement; or a shoulder-to-shoulder movement) with a frequency of 1–2 per second, that can be stopped voluntarily, have been reported in normal children as a form of stereotypy.[7,66] Up-gaze eye deviations or movements of the hands or feet occasionally accompany the head shaking. In a study following eight children with typical development and head nodding, three stopped entirely, suggesting that outcome may differ in this category as compared to children with CMS.[7] Repetitive head nodding can also occur in children with problems ranging from visual or oculomotor dysfunction to developmental brain malformations. Persistent stereotyped figure-8 and side-to-side head shaking has been reported to be a common feature in children with rhombencephalosynapsis, a brain malformation characterized by partial or complete absence of the cerebellar vermis with continuity of the cerebellar hemispheres across the midline.[67] Other entities to be considered in the differential diagnosis include Sandifer's syndrome, spasmus nutans, bobble-head doll syndrome, congenital nystagmus, oculomotor apraxia, and jactatio capitis nocturna (rhythmic movement disorder/nocturnal head banging).

The bobble-head doll syndrome is characterized by stereotypic antero-posterior (yes–yes) and rarely side–side (no–no) head movements at a frequency of 2–3 Hz.[68–70] The movements tend to increase with activity and excitement and decrease with concentration. This phenomenon is usually associated with lesions of the third ventricle but has been reported in association with aqueductal stenosis, Dandy–Walker Syndrome,[71] and large suprasellar arachnoid cysts.[72] The precise pathophysiological mechanism is unknown. Surgical treatment of the underlying lesion typically results in complete resolution of the abnormal head movement.

Complex Hand and Arm Movement Stereotypies

Movements in this group include hand shaking, posturing, flapping or waving, opening and closing of the hands, finger wiggling, arm flapping, and flexion and extension of the wrists. Additional movement patterns may occur in conjunction (e.g., body rocking, leg shaking or kicking, facial grimacing, mouth opening, neck extension, and involuntary noises), but the hand/arm movements are dominant.[7,14] Although several small studies have attempted to compare and contrast stereotypic movements of children in the general population to those in autistic children,[63,73] most investigators suggest that the complex stereotypies seen in typical children can be prolonged, include complex motor patterns, and resemble those in the autistic population.

Primary CMS typically appear before the age of 3 years and have a persistent course. Episodes last for periods of seconds to minutes, occur in clusters, and may appear many times per day. They are associated with periods of excitement, engrossment, stress, fatigue, and boredom, and are readily suppressed by sensory stimuli or distraction.[7,14]

Similar to other childhood movement disorders, such as Tourette syndrome, motor stereotypies are associated with a variety of comorbidities that often have a greater functional impact than the stereotypic behavior. Common comorbid issues, based on parent report, include ADHD, tics, OCD, and anxiety. The frequency for some of these difficulties appears to increase as the child gets older. For example, in subjects between 7 and 12 years of age, i.e., beyond the expected age for symptom appearance, 30% had ADHD, 18% had tics, and 9% OCD.[7] In contrast, in individuals between 9 and 19 years, clinical levels of comorbidity were ADHD (63%), tics/TS (22%), OCD (35%), and anxiety (73%).[9] It is of note that in another study fewer children were diagnosed with ADHD and OCD,[37] discrepancies possibly being related to differences in methodology to obtain data.

A case-control study has been performed examining neuropsychological function in children with primary CMS, including IQ, reading, attention, language, and motor and executive functions. Findings suggest that this group has largely intact neuropsychological profiles, with the exception of difficulties with motor coordination and speed, an increased rate of motor subtle signs, and one third of the group having signs of developmental motor coordination difficulties. Parent report of stereotypy severity was significantly associated with their assessment of inattention and executive dysfunction.[37] Behavioral and social difficulties are present in children with primary CMS. In a study examining the relationships between stereotypy severity and functional impairment,[74] girls with CMS were rated as having significantly greater social impairments than boys, even after controlling for ADHD symptoms. In this cross-sectional study, stereotypy severity increased significantly with age and was associated with social cognition deficits as well as inattentive and hyperactive ADHD symptoms.

The outcome of stereotypies in primary CMS was previously controversial, with some investigators suggesting that they increase by 3 years of age and decline after age 4.[59] In contrast, there is now increasing evidence that the majority of complex motor behaviors persist.[7–9,14] Consistent with prior reports suggesting only a limited resolution of stereotypic movements, e.g., 3–20% of affected individuals,[7,14,57,75] an extended longitudinal follow-up in 9- to 20-year-olds confirmed that most motor stereotypies were persistent, i.e., only 2% stopped.[9] Most individuals reported a reduction in frequency and duration and all denied any current functional impairment related specifically to their movements.

Secondary

Associated with Autism and Intellectual Disabilities

Repetitive behaviors are a major diagnostic feature of autistic disorder, i.e., "restricted repetitive and stereotyped patterns of behavior, interests, and activities."[15] Some authors have attempted to divide repetitive and stereotyped behaviors of autism into narrow subgroups (e.g., repetitive movements, motor sequencing, sensory behaviors, inflexibility, and complex repetitive behaviors),[65,76] whereas others have devised less complex systems. Stereotypic motor behaviors are common in the vast majority of autistic children and in many are complex and variable in nature.[77,78] Attempts, however, to identify specific behavioral markers that can assist in the identification of a neurodevelopmental origin have been unsuccessful. Children with autism have more stereotypies than do equally intellectually impaired children without autism,[79] and their severity and frequency positively relate to severity of illness,[11,80] cognitive deficiency,[76,81] impairment of adaptive functioning,[82,83] and symbolic play.[22] In neurodevelopmentally delayed populations, the differentiation of stereotypies, tics, repetitive behaviors, and compulsions has been variable and often depended on the bias of the evaluator.[84,85] Repetitive behaviors are variable across genetic syndromes such as Angelman, Cornelia de Lange, Cri-du-Chat, Prader–Willi, Fragile X, Smith–Magenis, and Norrie's syndrome.[86] Based on scoring of motor stereotypies observed on videos of standardized play sessions, children with autism or those with a low nonverbal IQ had a greater number and variety of movements than controls (Videos 8.4 and 8.10).[85] These authors further suggested that the stereotypy of gazing atypically at fingers or objects was almost entirely found in cognitively impaired autistic children. Other investigators have suggested that "hands to ears" (abducting and externally rotating the arms with the hands close to the ears) was more common in children with autistic spectrum disorder than controls,[26] whereas visual fixation/staring at objects was more common in children with developmental delay than autism.[87] Nevertheless, despite these individual suggestions of a possible behavioral marker, most researchers emphasize the considerable overlap in repertoire of stereotypic movements among autistic, intellectually disabled, and typically developing children.

Rett Syndrome

Classic RS occurs in girls who have had a normal prenatal and perinatal history, normal head circumference, and normal psychomotor development through the first 6–12 months of life.[88] The course is then one of developmental arrest or regression, with deterioration of communicative skills, social withdrawal, and loss of fine finger function. The RS child continues to deteriorate over the next few years, resulting in a loss of language, poor motor function (truncal and gait apraxia/ataxia), and a deceleration of head growth. RS is caused in most girls by a mutation in the *MECP2* gene. Bilateral hand washing movements are a hallmark of this syndrome, but have been identified in a group of children without the *MECP2* mutation.[89] In addition to the hand movements, individuals with RS also have a variety of other rhythmic movements (Videos 8.2 and 8.3).[27,28,90–94] Hair pulling, bruxism, and cervical retropulsion have been found to occur more frequently in mutation-positive individuals.[89] Stereotypic movements may begin before or after the loss of purposeful hand movements or the onset of developmental regression.[27,28,91,92,95] Video-polygraphic recordings have been beneficial in differentiating movement disorders in RS from seizures.[96]

Associated with Sensory Deprivation

Stereotypic motor behaviors occur frequently in vision-impaired children, e.g., eye rubbing, pressing, or poking ("oculodigital phenomena").[95,97,98] In this group, it has been suggested that voluntary stimulation of the optic nerve evokes sensations of light at the cortical level, termed *phosphenes*.[99] Other interpretations for these behaviors include a desire to produce certain insensitivity to pain. Blind children also have a variety of additional stereotypies including, in descending order of frequency, body rocking, repetitive handling of objects, hand and finger movements, lying face down, and jumping.[100] These activities have been variably attributed to a lack of stimulation or as a means of reducing tension. Deaf children frequently have rocking behaviors, but fewer self-injurious behaviors.[101] Stereotypies also occur in association with imprisonment in close quarters.[102]

Associated with Inborn Errors of Metabolism/Genetic

Lesch–Nyhan disease is characterized by hyperuricemia, self-injurious behaviors, and neurologic problems. In these patients, common stereotypic movements include self-biting, head banging, eye poking, and arm flinging. Neuroacanthocytosis is characterized by the presence of acanthocytes, orofacial dyskinesias, extrapyramidal movements, and tics. Affected individuals often have stereotypic movements and self-injurious behaviors.

Drug-Induced

The classic features of tardive dyskinesia (repetitive orolingual and facial movements) have been considered by some to be classic examples of stereotypies.[103] For example, experienced raters comparing videotapes of children with autistic-related stereotypies to neuroleptic-related dyskinesias were unable to reliably differentiate between the two disorders.[101] Besides the typical oro-facial-lingual chewing movements, other stereotypies present in tardive dyskinesia include leg crossings/swinging, pacing, hair and face rubbing, finger tapping, arm grasping, picking, thumb twiddling, and a variety of sensory symptoms such as burning pain in the mouth and vaginal area.[104] Intense fascination with repetitive handling of objects or compulsive picking occurs as part of a syndrome (punding) following the use of cocaine, amphetamines, or L-dopa.[105,106]

Associated with Psychiatric Disorders

Anxiety disorders, OCD, and borderline personality disorders have all been reported to have associated stereotypies.[107] Psychiatric symptoms may be the initial presentation of anti-NMDAR encephalitis, which is often associated with a variety of stereotypies.[107A]

THERAPY

Treatment for children with motor stereotypies is often not necessary. In fact, evidence-based therapy for the suppression of motor stereotypies is generally limited.

Behavioral treatment: Various behavioral interventions have been used to treat repetitive behaviors in autistic children.[108,109] In a small number of primary CMS children, the combination of two behavior-modifying techniques, habit reversal and differential reinforcement of other behaviors, was beneficial in reducing motor stereotypies.[110] In a study of 54 children, using a home-based, parent-directed instructional video mirroring the aforementioned published treatment, improvement was noted in the Stereotypy Severity Scale (SSS) Motor, SSS Impairment, and Linear Analog Scale scores (15%, 24%, and 20% respectively). Improvement obtained at one month was maintained in those individuals for at least an additional two months. (Specht, et al, submitted). In both of the aforementioned primary CMS studies, the intervention was generally well tolerated and adherence to study procedures appeared to predict treatment response.

Pharmacotherapy: In the autistic or retarded population, many with associated self-injurious behaviors, risperidone and aripiprazole have been shown to be effective for treating repetitive behaviors.[111] The suggested beneficial effect of serotonin receptor inhibitors has been questioned,[112] and citalopram, guanfacine, levetiracetam, and atomoxetine have not been beneficial.[111] No formal studies have been performed in children with primary CMS. However, based on patient report, a variety of pharmacotherapeutic agents including methylphenidate, atomoxetine, amphetamine mixed salts, lisdexamfetamine, dexmethylphenidate, guanfacine, fluoxetine, lamotrigine, topiramate, and escitalopram were not effective.[9]

PATIENT AND FAMILY RESOURCES

An educational video for children with primary complex motor stereotypies (CMS) and their families is available at www.motorstreotypiesandyou.org.

References

1. Singer H. Stereotypic movement disorders. *Handb Clin Neurol*. 2011;100:631–639.
2. Edwards MJ, Lang AE, Bhatia KP. Stereotypies: a critical appraisal and suggestion of a clinically useful definition. *Mov Disord*. 2012;27(2):179–185.
3. Carcani-Rathwell I, Rabe-Hasketh S, Santosh PJ. Repetitive and stereotyped behaviours in pervasive developmental disorders. *J Child Psychol Psychiatry*. 2006;47(6):573–581.
4. Leekam S, Tandos J, McConachie H, et al. Repetitive behaviours in typically developing 2-year-olds. *J Child Psychol Psychiatry*. 2007;48(11):1131–1138.
5. Symons FJ, Sperry LA, Dropik PL, Bodfish JW. The early development of stereotypy and self-injury: a review of research methods. *J Intellect Disabil Res*. 2005;49(Pt 2):144–158.
6. Robinson S, Woods M, Cardona F, Baglioni V, Hedderly T. Intense imagery movements: a common and distinct paediatric subgroup of motor stereotypies. *Dev Med Child Neurol*. 2014;56(12):1212–1218.
7. Harris KM, Mahone EM, Singer HS. Nonautistic motor stereotypies: clinical features and longitudinal follow-up. *Pediatr Neurol*. 2008;38(4):267–272.
8. Oakley C, MorrisBerry C, French B, Singer H. Nonautistic complex motor stereotypies in 40 older children and adolescents: clinical features and longitudinal follow-up. *Abstract Child Neurol Soc Ann Neurol*. 2012;72:S188–S189.
9. Oakley C, Mahone EM, Morris-Berry C, Kline T, Singer HS. Primary complex motor stereotypies in older children and adolescents: clinical features and longitudinal follow-up. *Pediatr Neurol*. 2015;52(4):398–403.
10. Miller JM, Singer HS, Bridges DD, Waranch HR. Behavioral therapy for treatment of stereotypic movements in nonautistic children. *J Child Neurol*. 2006;21(2):119–125.
11. Bodfish JW, Symons FJ, Parker DE, Lewis MH. Varieties of repetitive behavior in autism: comparisons to mental retardation. *J Autism Dev Disord*. 2000;30(3):237–243.
12. Rojahn J. Self-injurious and stereotypic behavior of noninstitutionalized mentally retarded people: prevalence and classification. *Am J Ment Defic*. 1986;91(3):268–276.
13. Crosland KA, Zarcone JR, Schroeder S, Zarcone T, Fowler S. Use of an antecedent analysis and a force sensitive platform to compare stereotyped movements and motor tics. *Am J Ment Retard*. 2005;110(3):181–192.
14. Mahone EM, Bridges D, Prahme C, Singer HS. Repetitive arm and hand movements (complex motor stereotypies) in children. *J Pediatr*. 2004;145(3):391–395.
15. American Psychiatric Association. (text revision). *Diagnostic and Statistical Manual of Mental Disorders: DSM-IV-TR*. 4th ed. Washington, DC: American Psychiatric Association; 2000.
16. Yang ML, Fullwood E, Goldstein J, Mink JW. Masturbation in infancy and early childhood presenting as a movement disorder: 12 cases and a review of the literature. *Pediatrics*. 2005;116(6):1427–1432.
17. Mink JW, Neil JJ. Masturbation mimicking paroxysmal dystonia or dyskinesia in a young girl. *Mov Disord*. 1995;10(4):518–520.

18. Casteels K, Wouters C, Van Geet C, Devlieger H. Video reveals self-stimulation in infancy. *Acta Paediatr.* 2004;93(6):844–846.

19. McGonigal A, Chauvel P. Prefrontal seizures manifesting as motor stereotypies. *Mov Disord.* 2013;29(9):1181–1185.

20. Zentall SS, Zentall TR. Optimal stimulation: a model of disordered activity and performance in normal and deviant children. *Psychol Bull.* 1983;94(3):446–471.

21. Hutt C. Specific and diversive exploration. *Adv Child Dev Behav.* 1970;5:119–180.

22. Honey E, Leekam S, Turner M, McConachie H. Repetitive behaviour and play in typically developing children and children with autism spectrum disorders. *J Autism Dev Disord.* 2007;37(6):1107–1115.

23. Castellanos FX, Ritchie GF, Marsh WL, Rapoport JL. DSM-IV stereotypic movement disorder: persistence of stereotypies of infancy in intellectually normal adolescents and adults. *J Clin Psychiatry.* 1996;57(3):116–122.

24. Rafaeli-Mor N, Foster L, Berkson G. Self-reported body-rocking and other habits in college students. *Am J Ment Retard.* 1999;104(1):1–10.

25. Niehaus DJ, Emsley RA, Brink P, Stein DJ. Stereotypies: prevalence and association with compulsive and impulsive symptoms in college students. *Psychopathology.* 2000;33(1):31–35.

26. Goldman S, Wang C, Salgado MW, Greene PE, Kim M, Rapin I. Motor stereotypies in children with autism and other developmental disorders. *Dev Med Child Neurol.* 2009;51(1):30–38.

27. Temudo T, Maciel P, Sequeiros J. Abnormal movements in Rett syndrome are present before the regression period: a case study. *Mov Disord.* 2007;22(15):2284–2287.

28. Temudo T, Oliveira P, Santos M, et al. Stereotypies in Rett syndrome—analysis of 83 patients with and without detected MECP2 mutations. *Neurology.* 2007;68(15):1183–1187.

29. Houdayer E, Walthall J, Belluscio BA, Vorbach S, Singer HS, et al. Absent movement-related cortical potentials in children with primary motor stereotypies. *Mov Disord.* 2014;29(9):1134–1140.

30. Canales JJ. Stimulant-induced adaptations in neostriatal matrix and striosome systems: transiting from instrumental responding to habitual behavior in drug addiction. *Neurobiol Learn Mem.* 2005;83(2):93–103.

31. Saka E, Goodrich C, Harlan P, Madras BK, Graybiel AM. Repetitive behaviors in monkeys are linked to specific striatal activation patterns. *J Neurosci.* 2004;24(34):7557–7565.

32. Tanaka SC, Balleine BW, O'Doherty JP. Calculating consequences: brain systems that encode the causal effects of actions. *J Neurosci.* 2008;28(26):6750–6755.

33. Tricomi E, Balleine BW, O'Doherty JP. A specific role for posterior dorsolateral striatum in human habit learning. *Eur J Neurosci.* 2009;29(11):2225–2232.

34. de Wit S, Watson P, Harsay HA, Cohen MX, van de Vijver I, Ridderinkhof KR. Corticostriatal connectivity underlies individual differences in the balance between habitual and goal-directed action control. *J Neurosci.* 2012;32(35):12066–12075.

35. Balleine BW, O'Doherty JP. Human and rodent homologies in action control: corticostriatal determinants of goal-directed and habitual action. *Neuropsychopharmacology.* 2010;35(1):48–69.

36. Kates WR, Lanham DC, Singer HS. Frontal white matter reductions in healthy males with complex stereotypies. *Pediatr Neurol.* 2005;32(2):109–112.

37. Mahone EM, Ryan M, Ferenc L, Morris-Berry C, Singer HS. Neuropsychological function in children with primary complex motor stereotypies. *Dev Med Child Neurol.* 2014;56(10):1001–1008.

38. DeLong M, Wichmann T. Update on models of basal ganglia function and dysfunction. *Parkinsonism Relat Disord.* 2009;15(suppl 3):S237–S240.

39. Sato S, Hashimoto T, Nakamura A, Ikeda S. Stereotyped stepping associated with lesions in the bilateral medial frontoparietal cortices. *Neurology.* 2001;57(4):711–713.

40. Maraganore DM, Lees AJ, Marsden CD. Complex stereotypies after right putaminal infarction: a case report. *Mov Disord.* 1991;6(4):358–361.

41. Kulisevsky J, Berthier ML, Avila A, Roig C. Unilateral parkinsonism and stereotyped movements following a right lenticular infarction. *Mov Disord.* 1996;11(6):752–754.

42. Yasuda Y, Akiguchi I, Ino M, Nabatabe H, Kameyama M. Paramedian thalamic and midbrain infarcts associated with palilalia. *J Neurol Neurosurg Psychiatry.* 1990;53(9):797–799.

43. Carter JC, Capone GT, Kaufmann WE. Neuroanatomic correlates of autism and stereotypy in children with Down syndrome. *Neuroreport.* 2008;19(6):653–656.

44. Pierce K, Courchesne E. Evidence for a cerebellar role in reduced exploration and stereotyped behavior in autism. *Biol Psychiatry.* 2001;49(8):655–664.

45. Goldman S, O'Brien LM, Filipek PA, Rapin I, Herbert MR. Motor stereotypies and volumetric brain alterations in children with autistic disorder. *Res Autism Spectr Discord.* 2013;7(1):82–92.

46. Druhan JP, Deschamps SE, Stewart J. D-amphetamine-like stimulus properties are produced by morphine injections into the ventral tegmental area but not into the nucleus accumbens. *Behav Brain Res.* 1993;59(1–2):41–51.

47. Graybiel AM, Canales JJ. The neurobiology of repetitive behaviors: clues to the neurobiology of Tourette syndrome. *Adv Neurol.* 2001;85:123–131.

48. Kelley AE, Lang CG, Gauthier AM. Induction of oral stereotypy following amphetamine microinjection into a discrete subregion of the striatum. *Psychopharmacology.* 1988;95(4):556–559.

49. Evans AH, Costa DC, Gacinovic S, et al. L-Dopa-responsive Parkinson's syndrome in association with phenylketonuria: in vivo dopamine transporter and D2 receptor findings. *Mov Disord.* 2004;19(10):1232–1236.

50. Miwa H, Morita S, Nakanishi I, Kondo T. Stereotyped behaviors or punding after quetiapine administration in Parkinson's disease. *Parkinsonism Relat Disord.* 2004;10(3):177–180.

51. Lewis MH, Bodfish JW, Powell SB, Wiest K, Darling M, Golden RN. Plasma HVA in adults with mental retardation and stereotyped behavior: biochemical evidence for a dopamine deficiency model. *Am J Ment Retard.* 1996;100(4):413–418.

52. Harris AD, Singer HS, Horska A, Kline T, et al. GABA and glutamate in children with primary complex motor stereotypies: a 1H MRS study at 7T. *J Neuroradiology.* In press.

53. Wynder C, Stalker L, Doughty ML. Role of H3K4 demethylases in complex neurodevelopmental diseases. *Epigenomics.* 2010;2(3):407–418.

54. Mencarelli M, Spanhol-Rosseto A, Artuso R, et al. Novel FOXG1 mutations associated with the congenital variant of Rett syndrome. *J Med Genet.* 2010;47(1):49–53.

55. Papa FT, Mencarelli MA, Caselli R, et al. A 3 Mb deletion in 14q12 causes severe mental retardation, mild facial dysmorphisms and Rett-like features. *Am J Med Genet A.* 2008;146(15):1994–1998.

56. Ghosh PS, Friedman NR, Ghosh D. Pitt-Hopkins syndrome in a boy with Charcot Marie Tooth disease type 1A: a rare co-occurrence of 2 genetic disorders. *J Child Neurol.* 2012;27(12):1602–1606.

57. Tan A, Salgado M, Fahn S. The characterization and outcome of stereotypical movements in nonautistic children. *Mov Disord.* 1997;12(1):47–52.

58. Kravitz H, Boehm JJ. Rhythmic habit patterns in infancy: their sequence, age of onset, and frequency. *Child Dev.* 1971;42(2):399–413.

59. Sallustro F, Atwell CW. Body rocking, head banging, and head rolling in normal children. *J Pediatr.* 1978;93(4):704–708.

60. Abe K, Oda N, Amatomi M. Natural history and predictive significance of head-banging, head-rolling and breath-holding spells. *Dev Med Child Neurol.* 1984;26(5):644–648.

61. Werry JS, Carlielle J, Fitzpatrick J. Rhythmic motor activities (stereotypies) in children under five: etiology and prevalence. *J Am Acad Child Psychiatry.* 1983;22(4):329–336.

62. Foster LG. Nervous habits and stereotyped behaviors in preschool children. *J Am Acad Child Adolesc Psychiatry.* 1998;37(7):711–717.

63. MacDonald R, Green G, Mansfield R, et al. Stereotypy in young children with autism and typically developing children. *Res Dev Disabil.* 2007;28(3):266–277.

64. Berkson G, Rafaeli-Mor N, Tarnovsky S. Body-rocking and other habits of college students and persons with mental retardation. *Am J Ment Retard.* 1999;104(2):107–116.

65. Jankovic J. Leg stereotypy disorder. J Neurol Neurosurg Psychiatry. Published online July 2015.

66. Hottinger-Blanc PM, Ziegler AL, Deonna T. A special type of head stereotypies in children with developmental (?cerebellar) disorder: description of 8 cases and literature review. *Eur J Paediatr Neurol.* 2002;6(3):143–152.

67. Tully HM, Dempsey JC, Ishak GE, et al. Persistent figure-eight and side-to-side head shaking is a marker for rhombencephalosynapsis. *Movement Disord.* 2013;28(14):2019–2023.

68. Hagebeuk EE, Kloet A, Grotenhuis JA, Peeters EA. Bobble-head doll syndrome successfully treated with an endoscopic ventriculocystocisternostomy: case report and review of the literature. *J Neurosurg.* 2005;103(3):253–259.

69. Benton JW, Nellhaus G, Huttenlocher PR, Ojemann RG, Dodge PR. The bobble-head doll syndrome report of a unique truncal tremor associated with third ventricular cyst and hydrocephalus in children. *Neurology.* 1966;16(8):725.

70. Ishihara M, Nonaka M, Oshida N, Hamada Y, Nakajima S, Yamasaki M. "No–No" type bobble-head doll syndrome in an infant with an arachnoid cyst of the posterior fossa: a case report. *Pediatr Neurol.* 2013;49(6):474–476.

71. de Brito HJ, Henriques K, Fonseca L, Cardoso F, Da Silva M. Bobble-head doll syndrome associated with Dandy–Walker syndrome. Case report. *J Neurosurg*. 2007;107(suppl 3):248–250.
72. Reddy OJ, Gafoor JA, Suresh B, Prasad PO. Bobble head doll syndrome: a rare case report. *J Pediatr Neurosci*. 2014;9(2):175.
73. Smith EA, Van Houten R. A comparison of the characteristics of self-stimulatory behaviors in "normal" children and children with developmental delays. *Res Dev Disabil*. 1996;17(4):253–268.
74. McCurdy MA, Bellows A, Ferrand J, et al. Social cognition, repetitive behavior, and ADHD symptoms among children with primary complex motor stereotypies [abstract]. *J Int Neuropsychol Soc*. 2014;20(S1):12–13.
75. Freeman RD, Soltanifar A, Baer S. Stereotypic movement disorder: easily missed. *Dev Med Child Neurol*. 2010;52(8):733–738.
76. Militerni R, Bravaccio C, Falco C, Fico C, Palermo MT. Repetitive behaviors in autistic disorder. *Eur Child Adolesc Psychiatry*. 2002;11(5):210–218.
77. Goldman S, Greene PE. Stereotypies in autism: a video demonstration of their clinical variability. *Front Integr Neurosci*. 2013;6:121.
78. Harris JC. *Developmental Neuropsychiatry*. New York, NY: Oxford University Press; 1995.
79. Frith CD, Done DJ. Stereotypy in psychiatry. In: Cooper SJ, Dourish CT, eds. *Neurobiology of Stereotyped Behavior*. Oxford: Oxford Science Publications; 1990:232–259.
80. Campbell M, Locascio JJ, Choroco MC, et al. Stereotypies and tardive dyskinesia: abnormal movements in autistic children. *Psychopharmacol Bull*. 1990;26(2):260–266.
81. Bishop SL, Richler J, Lord C. Association between restricted and repetitive behaviors and nonverbal IQ in children with autism spectrum disorders. *Child Neuropsychol*. 2006;12(4–5):247–267.
82. Gabriels RL, Cuccaro ML, Hill DE, Ivers BJ, Goldson E. Repetitive behaviors in autism: relationships with associated clinical features. *Res Dev Disabil*. 2005;26(2):169–181.
83. Matson JL, Kiely SL, Bamburg JW. The effect of stereotypies on adaptive skills as assessed with the DASH-II and Vineland Adaptive Behavior Scales. *Res Dev Disabil*. 1997;18(6):471–476.
84. Vitiello B, Spreat S, Behar D. Obsessive-compulsive disorder in mentally retarded patients. *J Nerv Ment Dis*. 1989;177(4):232–236.
85. Bodfish JW, Newell KM, Sprague RL, Harper VN, Lewis MH. Akathisia in adults with mental retardation: development of the Akathisia Ratings of Movement Scale (ARMS). *Am J Ment Retard*. 1997;101(4):413–423.
86. Moss J, Oliver C, Arron K, Burbidge C, Berg K. The prevalence and phenomenology of repetitive behavior in genetic syndromes. *J Autism Dev Disord*. 2009;39(4):572–588.
87. Loh A, Soman T, Brian J, et al. Stereotyped motor behaviors associated with autism in high-risk infants: a pilot videotape analysis of a sibling sample. *J Autism Dev Disord*. 2007;37(1):25–36.
88. Smeets E, Pelc K, Dan B. Rett syndrome. *Mol Syndromol*. 2012;2(3–5):113–127.
89. Singer HS, Naidu S. Rett syndrome: "we'll keep the genes on for you". *Neurology*. 2001;56(5):582–584.
90. Wales L, Charman T, Mount RH. An analogue assessment of repetitive hand behaviours in girls and young women with Rett syndrome. *J Intellect Disabil Res*. 2004;48(Pt 7):672–678.
91. FitzGerald P, Jankovic J, Glaze D, Schultz R, Percy A. Extrapyramidal involvement in Rett's syndrome. *Neurology*. 1990;40(2):293.
92. FitzGerald PM, Jankovic J, Percy AK. Rett syndrome and associated movement disorders. *Mov Disord*. 1990;5(3):195–202.
93. Nomura Y, Segawa M. Characteristics of motor disturbances of the Rett syndrome. *Brain Dev*. 1990;12(1):27–30.
94. Nomura Y, Segawa M. Clinical features of the early stage of the Rett syndrome. *Brain Dev*. 1990;12(1):16–19.
95. Einspieler C, Kerr AM, Prechtl HF. Abnormal general movements in girls with Rett disorder: the first four months of life. *Brain Dev*. 2005;27(suppl 1):S8–S13.
96. d'Orsi G, Trivisano M, Luisi C, et al. Epileptic seizures, movement disorders, and breathing disturbances in Rett syndrome: diagnostic relevance of video-polygraphy. *Epilepsy Behav*. 2012;25(3):401–407.
97. Davenport RK, Berkson G. Stereotyped movements of mental defective: III Situation effects. *Am J Ment Defic*. 1963;67:879–882.
98. Fazzi E, Lanners J, Danova S, et al. Stereotyped behaviours in blind children. *Brain Dev*. 1999;21(8):522–528.
99. Troster H, Brambring M, Beelmann A. Prevalence and situational causes of stereotyped behaviors in blind infants and preschoolers. *J Abnorm Child Psychol*. 1991;19(5):569–590.
100. Jan JE, Freeman RD, McCormick AQ, Scott EP, Robertson WD, Newman DE. Eye-pressing by visually impaired children. *Dev Med Child Neurol*. 1983;25(6):755–762.

III. PAROXYSMAL MOVEMENT DISORDERS

101. Bachara GH, Phelan WJ. Rhythmic movement in deaf children. *Percept Mot Skills*. 1980;50(3 Pt 1):933–934.
102. Ridley RM, Baker HF. Stereotypy in monkeys and humans. *Psychol Med*. 1982;12(1):61–72.
103. Stacy M, Cardoso F, Jankovic J. Tardive stereotypy and other movement disorders in tardive dyskinesias. *Neurology*. 1993;43(5):937–941.
104. Burke RE, Kang UJ, Jankovic J, Miller LG, Fahn S. Tardive akathisia: an analysis of clinical features and response to open therapeutic trials. *Mov Disord*. 1989;4(2):157–175.
105. Fernandez HH, Friedman JH. Punding on L-dopa. *Mov Disord*. 1999;14(5):836–838.
106. Oliveira M, Oliveira JR, da Cunha JEG. Punding as a transient symptom in a patient with an early-onset form of dementia. *J Neuropsychiatry Clin Neurosci*. 2013;25(3):E08–E10.
107. Hymas N, Lees A, Bolton D, Epps K, Head D. The neurology of obsessional slowness. *Brain*. 1991;114(Pt 5): 2203–2233.
107A. Baizabal-Carvallo JF, Stocco A, Muscal E, Jankovic J. The spectrum of movement disorders in children with anti-NMDA receptor encephalitis. *Mov Disord*. 2013;28(4):543–547.
108. Boyd BA, McDonough SG, Bodfish JW. Evidence-based behavioral interventions for repetitive behaviors in autism. *J Autism Dev Disord*. 2012;42(6):1236–1248.
109. Giles AF, St Peter CC, Pence ST, Gibson AB. Preference for blocking or response redirection during stereotypy treatment. *Res Dev Disabil*. 2012;33(6):1691–1700.
110. Rapp JT, Vollmer TR. Stereotypy I: a review of behavioral assessment and treatment. *Res Dev Disabil*. 2005;26(6):527–547.
111. Rajapakse T, Pringsheim T. Pharmacotherapeutics of Tourette syndrome and stereotypies in autism. *Semin Pediatr Neurol*. 2010;17(4);254–260.
112. Carrasco M, Volkmar FR, Bloch MH. Pharmacologic treatment of repetitive behaviors in autism spectrum disorders: evidence of publication bias. *Pediatrics*. 2012;129(5):e1301–e1310.

Paroxysmal Dyskinesias

Harvey S. Singer[1], Jonathan W. Mink[2],
Donald L. Gilbert[3] and Joseph Jankovic[4]

[1]Department of Neurology, Johns Hopkins Hospital, Baltimore, MD, USA;
[2]Division of Child Neurology, University of Rochester Medical Center,
Rochester, NY, USA; [3]Division of Neurology, Cincinnati Children's Hospital
Medical Center, Cincinnati, OH, USA; [4]Department of Neurology, Baylor
College of Medicine, Houston, TX, USA

INTRODUCTION

Paroxysmal dyskinesias represent a group of movement disorders that are characterized by episodes of abnormal movements arising from a baseline of normal or nearly normal movement. They are defined by their episodic nature, usually arising out of a background of normal movement and behavior. The specific type of dyskinesia can be dystonia, chorea,

Movement Disorders in Childhood, Second Edition.
DOI: http://dx.doi.org/10.1016/B978-0-12-411573-6.00009-7

or a combination. Many movement disorders in childhood are paroxysmal, but paroxysmal dyskinesias comprise a specific set of disorders. Other paroxysmal movement disorders are considered in other chapters including episodic ataxia (Chapter 14), hyperekplexia (Chapter 12), tics (Chapter 7), stereotypies (Chapter 8), and a variety of transient disorders that are related to specific periods during development (Chapter 6). Most paroxysmal dyskinesias begin during childhood and continue into adulthood.[1,2]

Paroxysmal dyskinesias may be classified as primary (usually genetic), or secondary (caused by identifiable disorders)[1]. They are further classified based on the specific clinical features of the disorders. The terminology used to describe and classify paroxysmal dyskinesia has varied over the years and has led to confusion about whether there were multiple entities, each with characteristic presentation, or few entities, each with wide phenotypic variability. Recent genetic advances, aided by a concise descriptive classification scheme, have provided important insights into the mechanisms underlying these disorders and have resulted in better diagnostic and treatment strategies.

CLINICAL CHARACTERISTICS

The term "paroxysmal choreoathetosis" first appeared in a report by Mount and Reback of a family in which the proband had infantile onset of periodic but prolonged dyskinesia that could be induced by alcohol and other agents.[3] The episodes were characterized by an aura of a tight sensation in the neck and abdomen and a sense of fatigue followed by involuntary flexion of the arms and extension of the legs (dystonia). Spells typically progressed to involuntary choreoathetosis and dysarthria with preservation of consciousness. Mount and Reback called the condition "familial paroxysmal choreoathetosis." Subsequently, Kertesz described a group of patients who had childhood onset of paroxysmal choreoathetosis that was precipitated by sudden movement.[4] Kertesz highlighted the kinesigenic component and called the condition "paroxysmal kinesigenic choreoathetosis," suggesting that it was a specific entity within the paroxysmal choreoathetosis syndrome. A striking feature of the kinesigenic form was the brief (seconds to minutes) duration of the episode, whereas the episodes described by Mount and Reback were lasting longer (minutes to hours). To better distinguish these forms, Richards and Barnett coined the term "paroxysmal dystonic choreoathetosis of Mount and Reback" to help delineate it from "paroxysmal kinesigenic choreoathetosis."[5] A third form of paroxysmal dyskinesia was reported by Lance in a family with intermediate-duration attacks that were precipitated by prolonged exercise.[6] These attacks that were provoked by exertion were differentiated from paroxysmal dystonic choreoathetosis and paroxysmal kinesigenic choreoathetosis.

The clinical manifestations of paroxysmal dyskinesias can be complex. The movements may be dystonic, choreic, athetotic, or a combination. The duration of attacks may be highly variable. Although the historic distinction between "paroxysmal kinesigenic choreoathetosis" and "paroxysmal dystonic choreoathetosis," included differences in attack duration, this was not a reliable differentiating factor. Further, "paroxysmal dystonic choreoathetosis" was not always "dystonic" and neither form always included "choreoathetosis." In 1995, Demirkiran and Jankovic proposed a descriptive classification scheme that was based primarily on the precipitating event, arguing that the precipitant was the best predictor

TABLE 9.1   Paroxysmal Dyskinesias

Paroxysmal kinesigenic dyskinesia

A. Short (less than 5 min)
  1. Idiopathic—familial/sporadic
  2. Secondary
B. Long (more than 5 min)
  1. Idiopathic—familial/sporadic
  2. Secondary

Paroxysmal nonkinesigenic dyskinesia

A. Short
  1. Idiopathic—familial/sporadic
  2. Secondary
B. Long
  1. Idiopathic—familial/sporadic
  2. Secondary

Paroxysmal exertion-induced dyskinesia

A. Short
  1. Idiopathic—familial/sporadic
  2. Secondary
B. Long
  1. Idiopathic—familial/sporadic
  2. Secondary

Modified from Demirkiran and Jankovic.[7]

of clinical course and response to specific medications (Table 9.1).[7] This empiric classification scheme helped objectify the identification of different forms of paroxysmal dyskinesia. They proposed four categories based upon precipitating factors: (1) kinesigenic, (2) nonkinesigenic, (3) exertion-induced, and (4) hypnogenic (also known as paroxysmal nocturnal dystonia of sleep). Paroxysmal nocturnal dystonia of sleep is a form of frontal lobe epilepsy, and is discussed in Chapter 19. After the precipitant is identified, secondary categorization is based on duration: less than or equal to 5 min (short) or greater than 5 min (long). Tertiary classification is based on presumed etiology: primary (familial versus sporadic) or secondary. Currently, most authors and movement disorder neurologists follow this classification scheme, which may be the most reliable predictor of the underlying genetic cause.[8] The typical features of paroxysmal dyskinesias are listed in Tables 9.1 and 9.2.

SPECIFIC DISORDERS

Paroxysmal Kinesigenic Dyskinesia

Paroxysmal kinesigenic dyskinesia (PKD) is often inherited in an autosomal dominant manner, but a quarter of the cases are sporadic. Males are affected more often than females (male:female = 4:1).[9,10] The age at onset is in the first or second decade of life in familial cases but may be variable in sporadic cases. The attacks are typically precipitated by the individual

TABLE 9.2 Distinguishing Features of Kinesigenic, Nonkinesigenic, and Exertion-Induced Paroxysmal Dyskinesias

Feature	PKD	PNKD	PED
Trigger	Movement	ETOH, caffeine	Prolonged exercise, hyperventilation
Duration	Seconds to minutes	Minutes to hours	Minutes to hours
Lateralization	Unilateral or bilateral	Unilateral or bilateral	Unilateral or bilateral
Male:Female ratio	2:1	1.5:1	1:1
Age at onset	1–40 years	1–30 years	2–30 years
Frequency	Up to hundreds per day	Up to a few per day	One per day
Aura	Sometimes	Sometimes	No
Improvement with age	Sometimes	Sometimes	Unknown
Major gene	PRRT2	PNKD	SLC2A1

being startled or making a sudden movement after a period of rest. There is often a refractory period after an attack during which sudden movement will not provoke another attack. Patients may only have an abnormal sensation in the involved limbs, or the sensation may precede motor manifestation. Most patients have dystonia, but some have a combination of chorea and dystonia (Videos 9.1–9.4). The attacks may be limited to one side of the body or even to one limb. The attacks decrease in frequency during adulthood.[4] The patients typically respond well to anticonvulsants. The attacks occur frequently—up to 100 per day. The duration is short, usually a few seconds to a few minutes. However, long-lasting attacks may occur rarely.[7]

In a study of 121 individuals with PKD 95 subjects had "classic" PKD. Sixty-four of the 95 had a family history of PKD. Nearly 100% of familial cases and 79% of the total sample had a homogeneous phenotype that included: (1) identified trigger for the attacks, (2) short duration of attacks, (3) no loss of consciousness or pain during attacks, (4) clinical response to antiepileptic drugs, and (5) age at onset between 1 and 20 years (Figure 9.1). The typical trigger was sudden movement. Most episodes lasted less than 1 min. Dystonia was the most common form of dyskinesia, occurring in 57%, with chorea occurring in 6%, and a combination of different forms of dyskinesia in 33%. Attacks were unilateral in 36%, bilateral in 35%, and variable in the remainder. In those subjects with a family history of PKD, the male:female ratio was approximately 1:1, but in sporadic cases, the male:female ratio was > 2:1. This is consistent with, but less pronounced than what has been reported previously.[9] Infantile convulsions were reported in 48% of kindreds with familial PKD, and in 10% of kindreds with sporadic PKD. The authors also described two sets of outliers: 12 subjects with onset before 1 year of age, and 14 subjects with onset after 1 year of age but with atypical features.[1] One of the 12 infants had onset at 10 months of age of hemi-dystonia induced by walking with a response to carbamazepine and a family history of PKD. The other 11 almost certainly had other paroxysmal events that were distinct from PKD. Two of the 14 outliers with onset after 1 year of age were atypical because of age at onset greater than

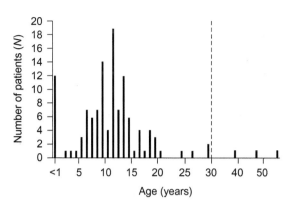

FIGURE 9.1   Age of onset of first attack in 121 individuals referred with PKD. Children with onset at less than 1 year of age are most likely to have another disorder. *From Ref. [1].*

20 years. The others were later determined to have paroxysmal nonkinesigenic dyskinesia (PNKD), paroxysmal exertion-induced dyskinesia (PED), or psychogenic disorders.

Etiology

Most cases of PKD are genetic and are related to mutations in the *PRRT2* (proline-rich trans-membrane protein 2) gene.[11,12] *PRRT2* has also been identified as the causative gene in the previously described "familial infantile convulsions and paroxysmal choreoathetosis" (ICCA) syndrome.[13] Although epilepsy and paroxysmal dyskinesia had been described as occurring within the same families and even within an individual prior to identification of the causative gene, mutations in *PRRT2* can cause a variety of paroxysmal symptoms in addition to PKD and infantile epilepsy. These include familial hemiplegic migraine,[14–16] episodic ataxia,[15] and febrile seizures.[17] In one study, penetrance was estimated to be 61% if only PKD was considered, but was almost complete when infantile convulsions were included.[76] Thus, the spectrum of paroxysmal disorders caused by *PRRT2* mutations is broader than initially thought.

Clinical characteristics of 374 individuals with paroxysmal dyskinesia associated with *PRRT2* mutations has been reported recently in a comprehensive review.[8] The mean age at onset was 9.9 years (range, 1–40 years). Only 4% of patients had onset after 18 years of age. The movement disorder during attacks was chorea in 15% of patients, dystonia in 18%, and both in 67%. The anatomic distribution of attacks was bilateral in 56%. The face was affected in 24%. In that series, 26% of patients had a personal history of infantile convulsions (ICCA). In addition to PKD, both PNKD and PED were reported in almost 2% of patients. The attack frequency ranged from 1 to 2 per year to over 100 per day; the majority (80%) had tens to hundreds of attacks per day. Attacks were very brief, lasting on average about 30s. Only 4% of patients had attacks lasting longer than 1min. About half of patients had an "aura" consisting of paresthesia or muscle tightness prior to the onset of dyskinesia. The male:female ratio was approximately 2:1, similar to that reported by Bruno et al.[1] Thirty-five percent of patients had a family history of a paroxysmal dyskinesia, 2% had a family history of epilepsy, and 37% had a family history of both paroxysmal dyskinesia and epilepsy. Thus, up to 25% of PKD cases due to *PRRT2* mutation appear to be sporadic.

PKD can also occur in association with other identifiable disorders.[18] Secondary PKD should be considered in all atypical cases, such as onset below 1 year of age, prolonged duration of attacks, and when there are associated interictal neurologic deficits. In secondary PKD, episodes are kinesigenic, but they usually differ from typical PKD in some way.

Demyelinating disease: The most common cause of secondary PKD in adults is demyelinating disease; there are no such reports in children. Paroxysmal hemidystonia may be the presenting manifestation of multiple sclerosis or may occur in established disease.[19] The attacks may be kinesigenic but are most consistently precipitated by hyperventilation and can be extremely painful. Attacks typically involve one side of the body with or without the face but may occur bilaterally. Each attack lasts from a few seconds to a few minutes, and multiple attacks may occur during the day. The attacks tend to subside spontaneously over many weeks in spite of continuing disease activity.

Cerebral palsy: PKD has been described as a delayed manifestation after perinatal hypoxic encephalopathy.[20] The age at onset was 12 years and the attacks were precipitated by being bumped from behind rather than by a sudden voluntary movement. These were short lasting (5–30 s) and occurred 5–20 times a day.

Metabolic and toxic disorders: PKD has been reported with hypoparathyroidism[21] and with pseudohypoparathyroidism.[22,23] Basal ganglia calcifications may be seen in these cases and PKD has also been reported in idiopathic basal ganglia calcification.[24] In addition, PKD has been reported in association with severe global mental retardation and thyroid hormone abnormalities as an X-linked condition due to mutations in the thyroid hormone transporter gene *MCT8*.[25] PKD has been also reported in association with methylphenidate therapy.[26] It is likely, however, that the PKD in that patient was idiopathic as it persisted even after discontinuation of methylphenidate and it responded to carbamazepine.

Differential Diagnosis and Evaluation

PKD must be distinguished from nonparoxysmal action dystonia, seizures, pseudoseizures, masturbation, and tics. Many individuals with dystonia have little or no involuntary movement when at rest and the dystonia is only present with action. Sometimes, the dystonia is associated with specific actions (see Chapter 12). However, action dystonia is present with specific movements and is not precipitated by sudden movements. In addition, action dystonia persists as long as the action is being performed, but PKD typically resolves quickly. Reflex epilepsies may resemble PKD superficially, although sudden movement is a rare precipitant of seizures. Tics are commonly preceded by an "urge," although they are rarely precipitated by sudden movement. They are also rarely seen in isolation without other tics, and rarely involve dystonia or chorea of multiple body parts (see Chapter 7).

A detailed history and videotape documentation are most important in the differential diagnosis of paroxysmal dyskinesias. A detailed family history should be obtained. In children with typical features of PKD, with a family history of PKD, and with good response to treatment, no further evaluation may be necessary. Genetic testing for *PRRT2* mutations may be confirmatory. In children with atypical features but with no other neurological signs or symptoms, an EEG, brain MRI, serum glucose, serum electrolytes, and serum calcium are recommended. In those with atypical features and an abnormal interictal exam or abnormal development, further evaluation is warranted as determined by the coexisting features.

Pathophysiology

Paroxysmal dyskinesia has some features in common with epilepsy, including presence of an aura for many patients, the paroxysmal nature of events, remarkable responsiveness to anticonvulsants, normalization of neurologic exam between events, and familial association.[27] As noted, many families contain individuals with infantile convulsions alone or who had infantile convulsions prior to development of PKD. Some patients have abnormal baseline EEGs.[9]

Most pathophysiologic studies in PKD were performed prior to identification of *PRRT2* as the most important causative gene. Most of these reports implicate basal ganglia dysfunction in PKD. In five patients with PKD, proton magnetic resonance spectroscopy revealed decreased basal ganglia levels of choline in two patients and decreased myoinositol in one patient.[28] In one case of PKD, ictal single-photon emission computed tomography (SPECT) revealed increased perfusion of the basal ganglia.[29] A study of 16 patients with idiopathic PKD and 18 controls demonstrated significant interictal hypoperfusion in the posterior regions of the caudate nuclei bilaterally.[30] But in a subsequent study of two patients with idiopathic PKD compared to six age-matched controls, the interictal and ictal perfusion changes were different in each of the patients and there were no consistent anatomic substrates observed, suggesting that there is no single brain structure involved in PKD.[31]

Although it was long believed that PKD was likely a channelopathy, it is now known that PRRT2 is a synaptic protein that interacts with SNAP 25, a synaptosomal membrane protein.[13] *PRRT2* is expressed in brain and spinal cord, with negligible expression in other tissues.[11] It is highly expressed in cerebral cortex, hippocampus, and cerebellum.

Treatment and Outcome

PKD responds best to anticonvulsants including phenytoin, carbamazepine, phenobarbital,[9,32] levetiracetam,[33] gabapentin,[34] valproic acid,[8] oxcarbazepine,[35] lamotrigine,[36] and topiramate.[37] PKD is exquisitely sensitive to phenytoin and carbamazepine at doses that are usually much less than the dosages used to treat epilepsy.[38,39] Carbamazepine and oxcarbazepine appear to be equally effective.[40] Treatment with levodopa has also been reported to be successful in rare patients.[41]

Outcome is good for patients with typical PKD. The great majority have excellent response to treatment.[8] In addition, many patients report marked spontaneous improvement (25%) or complete remission (27%) in adulthood[1,8]; most patients remit by age 20.

Paroxysmal Nonkinesigenic Dyskinesia

PNKD is also usually inherited as an autosomal dominant trait. The attacks occur more often in males (male:female = 2:1). The age at onset can be in early childhood, but attacks may not start until the early 20s. The frequency varies from 3 per day to 2 per year. The usual precipitating factors are fatigue, alcohol, caffeine, and emotional excitement. The attack may start with involuntary movements of one limb but may spread to involve all extremities and the face. The usual duration is minutes to 3–4h. During the attack the patient may be unable to communicate, but the patient remains conscious and continues to breathe normally. Some families have predominant dystonia,[42] whereas others have predominant choreoathetosis.[3] The attacks are relieved by sleep and in some cases respond to pharmacologic intervention.

Identification of an association of PNKD with mutation in the myofibrillogenesis regulator 1 (MR-1) gene, later renamed PNKD gene, on chromosome 2[43] has provided more precise specification of the phenotype associated with this mutation.[2] In a study of 49 patients with PNKD who were positive for a PNKD mutation and 22 patients with PNKD who did not have MR-1 mutation, several common features were found in the MR-1 mutation positive subjects. These findings have been largely confirmed in a recent review of the literature describing 73 patients (including the 49 described by Bruno et al.) with PNKD and PNKD mutations.[8] Patients with PNKD mutations had: (1) onset in infancy or early childhood, typically in the first decade of life with 25–33% having onset in the first year of life; (2) a mixture of chorea and dystonia in the limbs, face, and trunk; 70–88% had a mixture of chorea and dystonia, 12–27% had dystonia alone; (3) typical attack duration between 10 min and 1 h, but could be as long as 12 h. Only 5% of attacks lasted less than 1 min; (4) precipitation by caffeine, alcohol, fatigue, or emotional stress; and (5) favorable response to benzodiazepines. Families without PNKD mutations had more variable age at onset, precipitants, clinical features, and response to medications. Forty-one percent of those with MR-1 mutation had a premonitory sensation localized to a limb (80%) or a sense of anxiety (20%).[2] Alcohol and caffeine precipitated spells in 98% of subjects with an MR-1 mutation. Unlike PKD, there was no benefit from typical antiepileptic medications, but there was moderate benefit from diazepam or clonazepam.[2]

Although PNKD is typically genetic in origin, it has been also reported in a patient with familial ataxia.[44] In one family, PNKD was accompanied by myokymia.[45] Some families also have exertional cramping[8,46] or may represent PED (see Section "Paroxysmal Exertion-Induced Dyskinesia"). Unlike PRRT-2, PNKD mutations have not been associated with other paroxysmal disorders such as migraine or epilepsy.

Etiology

Prior to association of PNKD with mutations in PNKD, it was thought that PNKD was most likely due to channelopathy. The function of MR-1 is not known, but it is not an ion channel protein. It has substantial homology with hydroxyacylglutathione hydrolase (HAGH).[47] HAGH catalyzes the final step in the conversion of methylglyoxal to lactic acid and reduced glutathione. Interestingly, methylglyoxal is found in coffee and in alcoholic beverages,[48] both of which reliably precipitate attacks of PNKD.[2] However, MR1 protein does not catalyze these reactions, but may play a role in cellular redox reactions.[49]

An autosomal dominant syndrome of generalized epilepsy and PNKD has been described in a single large family in association with mutation on chromosome 10q22 in the alpha subunit of the large conductance calcium-sensitive potassium (BK) channel.[50] The family included 16 affected individuals over four generations. Of 13 individuals for which detailed clinical information was reported, 12 had PNKD either alone ($n = 7$) or in combination with seizures ($n = 5$). One affected individual had seizures alone. The characteristics of the PNKD are not fully described in this family. It is not known if the episodes were precipitated by caffeine or alcohol. At least two family members benefitted from benzodiazepines. Most seizures in this family were absence in type and when EEG abnormalities were present, there were 3–3.5 Hz generalized spike-wave discharges. This BK mutation is associated with increased neuronal excitability by causing rapid repolarization of action potentials.[50] Thus, this form of PNKD is due to a channelopathy.

As described for PKD, PNKD can also occur secondary to other disorders.[18] Similar to PKD, the most common cause of secondary PNKD is multiple sclerosis. Most disorders causing PKD have also been associated with PNKD, and in some reports it is unclear whether the patient had PKD, PNKD, or both. However, PNKD has been reported specifically in a child with maple syrup urine disease[51] and in one child with GLUT1 deficiency.[52] PNKD is more likely to be a presentation of a conversion disorder than is PKD.[2,7]

Differential Diagnosis and Evaluation

It is more difficult to separate PNKD from other episodic movement disorders than is PKD because of the lack of a temporally clear precipitant. PNKD must be differentiated from the other paroxysmal dyskinesias, dopa-responsive dystonia, seizures, pseudoseizures, and tics. Dopa-responsive dystonia usually presents in childhood and may have marked diurnal fluctuations, with the patient improving with rest and worsening with exercise.[53] However, discrete paroxysms do not occur. Other differential diagnostic considerations are discussed in the section on PKD earlier.

In children with typical features of PNKD and with a family history of PNKD, no further evaluation may be necessary. In children with atypical features but with no other neurological signs or symptoms, an EEG, brain MRI, serum glucose, serum electrolytes, and serum calcium are recommended. In those with atypical features and an abnormal interictal exam or abnormal development, further evaluation is warranted as determined by the coexisting features.

Pathophysiology

Several reports implicate the basal ganglia in PNKD. PET scanning revealed abnormalities in the basal ganglia metabolism of a patient with posttraumatic PNKD.[54] One patient with PNKD showed decreased [18]FDOPA uptake and increased ^{11}C raclopride binding in the striatum, but no metabolic abnormalities with [18]FDG PET.[55] Invasive electrophysiology showed no cortical discharges associated with the episodes of PNKD, but showed an abnormal discharge in the caudate nucleus.

Treatment and Outcome

Since alcohol, caffeine, and sleep deprivation can precipitate attacks in PNKD, avoidance of those precipitants can reduce attacks.[8] PNKD tends to respond better to benzodiazepines than to other medications.[2,8] Clonazepam and diazepam are mostly commonly used, but other benzodiazepines have been reported to be beneficial including lorazepam[56] and alternate-day oxazepam.[57] Benefit has also been reported in individual cases with haloperidol,[58] levetiracetam,[59] valproate,[58] or anticholinergics.[60] Carbamazepine is ineffective in most cases. Deep brain stimulation of thalamus[61] and globus pallidus internal segment[62] has been reported to be effective in single adult cases.

Outcome is variable, but there is a tendency toward decreased attacks with age.[2] Complete remission is uncommon.

Paroxysmal Exertion-Induced Dyskinesia

PED is characterized by attacks that are triggered by prolonged exercise,[6] in contrast to the sudden movement that triggers PKD. The frequency varies from 1 per day to 2 per month. The usual duration is 5–30 min. The clinical features may be indistinguishable from PNKD of long-lasting type, but legs are usually more affected. However, exercise limited to the upper extremity may provoke an attack in the upper extremity alone.[63] Of note, 68% of the *PNKD* negative PNKD patients described by Bruno et al.[2] had attacks of dyskinesia provoked by exercise. Thus, there may be some phenotypic overlap between different conditions manifested by exertion-induced dystonia such as "runner's dystonia".[77]

Etiology

PED is usually inherited in an autosomal dominant fashion, although sporadic cases have been described.[63,64] PED has been associated with mutations in the *SLC2A1* gene that encodes the glucose transporter 1 (GLUT1). Many of these patients also have epilepsy and mild developmental delay and it is thought to be on the milder end of the phenotypic spectrum of GLUT1 deficiency.[52,65] One family also had hemolytic anemia with echinocytosis and altered erythrocyte ion concentrations. Over 65% of patients with PED due to *SLC2A1* mutations also have epilepsy, learning difficulties, ataxia, pyramidal signs, hemolytic anemia, or a combination.[8,66]

Autosomal dominant paroxysmal choreoathetosis/spasticity, an exercise-induced dyskinesia frequently including spastic paraplegia during the episode, has been mapped to a 12 cM region on chromosome 1p in the vicinity of a potassium channel gene cluster.[67] Another family has been described with PED and migraine that was not linked to the PNKD locus on chromosome 2, the PKD locus on chromosome 16, or the familial hemiplegic migraine locus on chromosome 19.[68] Another family with autosomal dominant PED, generalized epilepsy, developmental delay, and migraines has been described in which linkage to chromosomes 2 and 16 were excluded.[69] Thus, it appears that at least three phenotypic forms of PED exist with possibly as many genetic bases. PED has been reported following trauma.[7,70]

Pathophysiology

In two patients with PED, SPECT scanning revealed decreased ictal perfusion of the frontal cortex during the motor attacks. In contrast, increased cerebellar perfusion was observed. The perfusion of the basal ganglia also decreased.[71] No cortical hyperperfusion indicative of an epileptic nature was seen. Cerebellar hyperactivity in connection with prominent frontal hypoactivity has also been described in both the idiopathic and the symptomatic forms of PED.

Treatment and Outcome

Avoidance of prolonged exercise may help diminish the frequency of attacks. Drug therapy is often ineffective but there are isolated reports of improvement with levodopa[7] and acetazolamide.[64] Like other forms of GLUT1 deficiency, PED may respond to the ketogenic diet[72–74] or the modified Atkins diet.[75]

Outcome appears to be variable, but has not been studied systematically.

References

1. Waln O, Jankovic J. Paroxysmal movement disorders. *Neurol Clin.* 2015;33(1):137–152.
2. Bruno MK, Lee HY, Auburger GWJ, et al. Genotype-phenotype correlation of paroxysmal nonkinesigenic dyskinesia. *Neurology.* 2007;68(21):1782–1789.

3. Mount LA, Reback S. Familial paroxysmal choreoathetosis. *Arch Neurol Psych*. 1940;44:841–847.
4. Kertesz A. Paroxysmal kinesigenic choreoathetosis. *Neurology*. 1967;17:680–690.
5. Richards RN, Barnett HJM. Paroxysmal dystonic choreoathetosis; a family study and review of the literature. *Neurology*. 1968;18:461–469.
6. Lance JW. Familial paroxysmal dystonic choreoathetosis and its differentiation from related syndromes. *Ann Neurol*. 1977;2:285–293.
7. Demirkiran M, Jankovic J. Paroxysmal dyskinesias: clinical features and classification. *Ann Neurol*. 1995;38:571–579.
8. Erro R, Sheerin U-M, Bhatia KP. Paroxysmal dyskinesias revisited: a review of 500 genetically proven cases and a new classification. *Mov Disord*. 2014;29:1108–1116.
9. Goodenough DJ, Fariello RG, Annis BL, Chun RW. Familial and acquired paroxysmal dyskinesias. A proposed classification with delineation of clinical features. *Arch Neurol*. 1978;35:827–831.
10. Lotze T, Jankovic J. Paroxysmal kinesigenic dyskinesias. *Semin Pediatr Neurol*. 2003;10:68–79.
11. Chen WJ, Lin Y, Xiong ZQ, et al. Exome sequencing identifies truncating mutations in PRRT2 that cause paroxysmal kinesigenic dyskinesia. *Nat Genet*. 2011;43(12):1252–1255.
12. Wang JL, Cao L, Li XH, et al. Identification of PRRT2 as the causative gene of paroxysmal kinesigenic dyskinesias. *Brain*. 2011;134(Pt 12):3493–3501.
13. Lee HY, Huang Y, Bruneau N, et al. Mutations in the gene PRRT2 cause paroxysmal kinesigenic dyskinesia with infantile convulsions. *Cell Rep*. 2012;1(1):2–12.
14. Cloarec R, Bruneau N, Rudolf G, et al. PRRT2 links infantile convulsions and paroxysmal dyskinesia with migraine. *Neurology*. 2012;79(21):2097–2103.
15. Gardiner AR, Bhatia KP, Stamelou M, et al. PRRT2 gene mutations: from paroxysmal dyskinesia to episodic ataxia and hemiplegic migraine. *Neurology*. 2012;79(21):2115–2121.
16. Silveira-Moriyama L, Gardiner AR, Meyer E, et al. Clinical features of childhood-onset paroxysmal kinesigenic dyskinesia with PRRT2 gene mutations. *Dev Med Child Neurol*. 2013;55(4):327–334.
17. Scheffer IE, Grinton BE, Heron SE, et al. PRRT2 phenotypic spectrum includes sporadic and fever-related infantile seizures. *Neurology*. 2012;79(21):2104–2108.
18. Blakeley J, Jankovic J. Secondary paroxysmal dyskinesias. *Mov Disord*. 2002;17:726–734.
19. Berger JR, Sheremata WA, Melamed E. Paroxysmal dystonia as the initial manifestation of multiple sclerosis. *Arch Neurol*. 1984;41:747–750.
20. Rosen J. Paroxysmal choreoathetosis associated with perinatal hypoxic encephalopathy. *Arch Neurol*. 1964;11:385–387.
21. Kato H, Kobayashi K, Kohari S, Okita N, Iijima K. Paroxysmal kinesigenic choreoathetosis and paroxysmal dystonic choreoathetosis in a patient with familial idiopathic hypoparathyroidism. *Tohoku J Exp Med*. 1987;151:233–239.
22. Dure LS, Mussell HG. Paroxysmal dyskinesia in a patient with pseudohypoparathyroidism. *Mov Disord*. 1998;13:746–748.
23. Mahmud FH, Linglart A, Bastepe M, Juppner H, Lteif AN. Molecular diagnosis of pseudohypoparathyroidism type Ib in a family with presumed paroxysmal dyskinesia. *Pediatrics*. 2005;115(2):e242–244.
24. Diaz GE, Wirrell EC, Matsumoto JY, Krecke KN. Bilateral striopallidodentate calcinosis with paroxysmal kinesigenic dyskinesia. *Pediatr Neurol*. 2010;43(1):46–48.
25. Brockmann K, Dumitrescu A, Best T, Hanefeld F, Refetoff S. X-linked paroxysmal dyskinesia and severe global retardation caused by defective MCT8 gene. *J Neurol*. 2005;252:663–666.
26. Gay CT, Ryan SG. Paroxysmal kinesigenic dystonia after methylphenidate administration. *J Child Neurol*. 1994;9:45–46.
27. Schlaggar BL, Mink JW. A 16-year-old with episodic hemisdystonia. *Semin Pediatr Neurol*. 1999;6(3):210–215.
28. Kim MO, Im J-H, Choi DG, Lee MC. Proton MR spectroscopic findings in paroxysmal kinesigenic dyskinesia. *Mov Disord*. 1998;13:570–575.
29. Koh C, Kong C, Ngai W, Ma K. Ictal (99m)Tc ECD SPECT in paroxysmal kinesigenic choreoathetosis. *Pediatr Neurol*. 2001;24:225–227.
30. Joo E, Hong S, Tae W, et al. Perfusion abnormality of the caudate nucleus in patients with paroxysmal kinesigenic choreoathetosis. *Eur J Nucl Med Mol Imaging*. 2005;32:1205–1209.
31. Kim YD, Kim JS, Chung YA, et al. Alteration of ictal and interictal perfusion in patients with paroxysmal kinesigenic dyskinesia. *Neuropediatrics*. 2011;42(6):245–248.

32. Li HF, Chen WJ, Ni W, et al. PRRT2 mutation correlated with phenotype of paroxysmal kinesigenic dyskinesia and drug response. *Neurology*. 2013;80(16):1534–1535.

33. Chatterjee A, Louis ED, Frucht S. Levetiracetam in the treatment of paroxysmal kinesiogenic choreoathetosis. *Mov Disord*. 2002;17:614–615.

34. Chudnow RS, Mimbela RA, Owen DB, Roach ES. Gabapentin for familial paroxysmal dystonic choreoathetosis. *Neurology*. 1997;49(5):1441–1442.

35. Tsao CY. Effective treatment with oxcarbazepine in paroxysmal kinesigenic choreoathetosis. *J Child Neurol*. 2004;19(4):300–301.

36. Uberall MA, Wenzel D. Effectiveness of lamotrigine in children with paroxysmal kinesigenic choreoathetosis. *Dev Med Child Neurol*. 2000;42(10):699–700.

37. Huang Y, Chen Y, Du F, et al. Topiramate therapy for paroxysmal kinesigenic choreoathetosis. *Mov Disord*. 2005;20:75–77.

38. Homan R, Vasko M, Blaw M. Phenytoin plasma concentrations in paroxysmal kinesigenic choreoathetosis. *Neurology*. 1980;30:673–676.

39. Wein T, Andermann F, Silver K, et al. Exquisite sensitivity of paroxysmal kinesigenic choreathetosis to carbamazepine. *Neurology*. 1996;47:1104–1106.

40. Yang Y, Su Y, Guo Y, et al. Oxcarbazepine versus carbamazepine in the treatment of paroxysmal kinesigenic dyskinesia. *Int J Neurosci*. 2012;122(12):719–722.

41. Loong SC, Ong YY. Paroxysmal kinesigenic choreoathetosis. Report of a case relieved by L-dopa. *J Neurol Neurosurg Psychiatry*. 1973;36(6):921–924.

42. Forssman H. Hereditary disorder characterized by attacks of muscular contraction, induced by alcohol amongst other factors. *Acta Med Scand*. 1961;170:517–533.

43. Rainier S, Thomas D, Tokarz D, et al. Myofibrillogenesis regulator 1 gene mutations cause paroxysmal dystonic choreoathetosis. *Arch Neurol*. 2004;61(7):1025–1029.

44. Mayeux R, Fahn S. Paroxysmal dystonic choreoathetosis in a patient with familial ataxia. *Neurology*. 1982;32:1184–1186.

45. Byrne E, White O, Cook M. Familial dystonic choreoathetosis with myokymia; a sleep responsive disorder. *J Neurol Neurosurg Psychiatry*. 1991;54:1090–1092.

46. Kurlan R, Behr J, Medved L, Shoulson I. Familial paroxysmal dystonic choreoathetosis: a family study. *Mov Disord*. 1987;2:187–192.

47. Lee HY, Xu Y, Huang Y, et al. The gene for paroxysmal non-kinesigenic dyskinesia encodes an enzyme in a stress response pathway. *Hum Mol Genet*. 2004;13(24):3161–3170.

48. Hayashi T, Shibamoto T. Analysis of methylglyoxal in foods and beverages. *J Agric Food Chem*. 1985;33:1090–1093.

49. Shen Y, Lee HY, Rawson J, et al. Mutations in PNKD causing paroxysmal dyskinesia alters protein cleavage and stability. *Hum Mol Genet*. 2011;20(12):2322–2332.

50. Du W, Bautista JF, Yang H, et al. Calcium-sensitive potassium channelopathy in human epilepsy and paroxysmal movement disorder. *Nat Genet*. 2005;37(7):733–738.

51. Temudo T, Martins E, Pocas F, Cruz R, Vilarinho L. Maple syrup disease presenting as paroxysmal dystonia. *Ann Neurol*. 2004;56:749–750.

52. Zorzi G, Castellotti B, Zibordi F, Gellera C, Nardocci N. Paroxysmal movement disorders in GLUT1 deficiency syndrome. *Neurology*. 2008;71(2):146–148.

53. Nygaard T. Dopa-responsive dystonia. *Curr Opin Neurol*. 1995;8:310–313.

54. Perlmutter JS, Raichle ME. Pure hemidystonia with basal ganglion abnormalities on positron emission tomography. *Ann Neurol*. 1984;15(3):228–233.

55. Lombroso CT, Fischman A. Paroxysmal non-kinesigenic dyskinesia: pathophysiological investigations. *Epileptic Disord*. 1999;1:187–193.

56. Dooley JM, Brna PM. Sublingual lorazepam in the treatment of familial paroxysmal nonkinesigenic dyskinesia. *Pediatr Neurol*. 2004;30(5):365–366.

57. Kurlan R, Shoulson I. Familial paroxysmal dystonic choreoathetosis and response to alternate-day oxazepam therapy. *Ann Neurol*. 1983;13(4):456–457.

58. Przuntek H, Monninger P. Therapeutic aspects of kinesiogenic paroxysmal choreoathetosis and familial paroxysmal choreoathetosis of the Mount and Reback type. *J Neurol*. 1983;230(3):163–169.

59. Alemdar M, Iseri P, Selekler M, Komsuoglu SS. Levetiracetam-responding paroxysmal nonkinesigenic dyskinesia. *Clin Neuropharmacol*. 2007;30(4):241–244.
60. Micheli F, Fernandez Pardal M, de Arbelaiz R, Lehkuniec E, Giannaula R. Paroxysmal dystonia responsive to anticholinergic drugs. *Clin Neuropharmacol*. 1987;10:365–369.
61. Loher TJ, Krauss JK, Burgunder JM, Taub E, Siegfried J. Chronic thalamic stimulation for treatment of dystonic paroxysmal nonkinesigenic dyskinesia. *Neurology*. 2001;56(2):268–270.
62. Yamada K, Goto S, Soyama N, et al. Complete suppression of paroxysmal nonkinesigenic dyskinesia by globus pallidus internus pallidal stimulation. *Mov Disord*. 2006;21(4):576–579.
63. Plant GT, Williams AC, Earl CJ, Marsden CD. Familial paroxysmal dystonia induced by exercise. *J Neurol Neurosurg Psychiatry*. 1984;47(3):275–279.
64. Bhatia KP, Soland VL, Bhatt MH, Quinn NP, Marsden CD. Paroxysmal exercise-induced dystonia: eight new sporadic cases and a review of the literature. *Mov Disord*. 1997;12:1007–1012.
65. Weber YG, Storch A, Wuttke TV, et al. GLUT1 mutations are a cause of paroxysmal exertion-induced dyskinesias and induce hemolytic anemia by a cation leak. *J Clin Invest*. 2008;118(6):2157–2168.
66. Weber YG, Kamm C, Suls A, et al. Paroxysmal choreoathetosis/spasticity (DYT9) is caused by a GLUT1 defect. *Neurology*. 2011;77(10):959–964.
67. Auburger G, Ratzlaff T, Lunkes A, et al. A gene for autosomal dominant paroxysmal choreoathetosis/spasticity (CSE) maps to the vicinity of a potassium channel gene cluster on chromosome 1p, probably within 2 cM between D1S443 and D1S197. *Genomics*. 1996;31:90–94.
68. Munchau A, Valente EM, Shahidi GA, et al. A new family with paroxysmal exercise induced dystonia and migraine: a clinical and genetic study. *J Neurol Neurosurg Psychiatr*. 2000;68:609–614.
69. Kamm C, Mayer P, Sharma M, Niemann G, Gasser T. New family with paroxysmal exercise-induced dystonia and epilepsy. *Mov Disord*. 2007;22(6):873–877.
70. Lim EC, Wong YS. Post-traumatic paroxysmal exercise-induced dystonia: case report and review of the literature. *Parkinsonism Relat Disord*. 2003;9(6):371–373.
71. Kluge A, Kettner B, Zschenderlein R, et al. Changes in perfusion pattern using ECD-SPECT indicate frontal lobe and cerebellar involvement in exercise-induced paroxysmal dystonia. *Mov Disord*. 1998;13:124–134.
72. Alter AS, Engelstad K, Hinton VJ, et al. Long-Term clinical course of Glut1 deficiency syndrome. *J Child Neurol*. 2015;30(2):160–169.
73. Urbizu A, Cuenca-Leon E, Raspall-Chaure M, et al. Paroxysmal exercise-induced dyskinesia, writer's cramp, migraine with aura and absence epilepsy in twin brothers with a novel SLC2A1 missense mutation. *J Neurol Sci*. 2010;295(1–2):110–113.
74. Ramm-Pettersen A, Nakken KO, Skogseid IM, et al. Good outcome in patients with early dietary treatment of GLUT-1 deficiency syndrome: results from a retrospective Norwegian study. *Dev Med Child Neurol*. 2013;55(5):440–447.
75. Leen WG, Mewasingh L, Verbeek MM, Kamsteeg EJ, van de Warrenburg BP, Willemsen MA. Movement disorders in GLUT1 deficiency syndrome respond to the modified Atkins diet. *Mov Disord*. 2013;28(10):1439–1442.
76. van Vliet R, Breedveld G, de Rijk-van Andel J, et al. PRRT2 phenotypes and penetrance of paroxysmal kinesigenic dyskinesia and infantile convulsions. Neurology. 2012;79(8):777–784.
77. Wu LJ, Jankovic J. Runner's dystonia. *J Neurol Sci*. 2006;251:73–76.

HYPERKINETIC AND HYPOKINETIC MOVEMENT DISORDERS

Chorea, Athetosis, and Ballism

Harvey S. Singer[1], Jonathan W. Mink[2],
Donald L. Gilbert[3] and Joseph Jankovic[4]

[1]Department of Neurology, Johns Hopkins Hospital, Baltimore, MD, USA;
[2]Division of Child Neurology, University of Rochester Medical Center,
Rochester, NY, USA; [3]Division of Neurology, Cincinnati Children's Hospital
Medical Center, Cincinnati, OH, USA; [4]Department of Neurology, Baylor
College of Medicine, Houston, TX, USA

OUTLINE

Movement Disorders in Childhood, Second Edition.
DOI: http://dx.doi.org/10.1016/B978-0-12-411573-6.00010-3

143

INTRODUCTION AND OVERVIEW

Chorea, athetosis, and ballism are nonpatterned, hyperkinetic movement disorders which overlap in many patients and cannot be differentiated as mutually exclusive phenomena. However, they are characterized by some salient features. Some authors place these hyperkinetic disorders on a continuum based on amplitude, velocity, and distribution: ballism → chorea → athetosis.

In practice, many children with hyperkinetic movement disorders have a combination of chorea, athetosis, or ballism. To complicate matters, dystonia, tics, or myoclonus may also be present. Moreover, the relative predominance of one type of phenomenology may be state dependent. For example, athetosis may evolve into ballism when children are stimulated or excited.

Anatomically, *chorea* classically results from disturbances in the striatum but can also have thalamic or cortical origin. *Ballism* often localizes to subthalamic nucleus. *Athetosis* often accompanies basal ganglia diseases that also produce chorea or dystonia. It is seen in children with globus pallidus interna (GPi) injury due to bilirubin toxicity in infancy (kernicterus). Thus, despite phenomenologic distinctions, clinicians may use the presence of any of these dyskinetic movements as key factors in directing diagnostic and therapeutic decision making toward the basal ganglia.

DEFINITIONS OF CHOREA, ATHETOSIS, AND BALLISM

Chorea refers to an involuntary, random-appearing sequence of one or more discrete involuntary movements or movement fragments which appear random due to variable timing, duration, rate, direction, or location. All body parts may be involved, with certain distributions being more characteristic of distinct diseases or disorders. Choreic movements usually worsen during attempted voluntary action. Individuals with chorea may generate so-called *parakinesias*, semi-volitional movements that attempt to mask the involuntary choreic movements or incorporate them into seemingly purposeful movements, such as touching the face.

Ballism refers to involuntary, high-amplitude, flinging movements typically generated proximally. These movements may be brief or continual and may occur in conjunction with chorea. Often, one side of the body is affected, i.e., *hemiballism*. In many cases, hemiballism becomes milder and evolves into chorea, athetosis, or dystonia.[1] Severe continuous ballism can cause rhabdomyolysis.

Athetosis is defined as slow, writhing, continuous, involuntary movements. This may be historically referred to as choreoathetosis. In contrast to dystonia, in which there is a sustained, twisting, patterned movement, athetosis is typically a continual, nonsustained form of movement. It may have a rotary component with finger flexion and extension. Athetosis sometimes occurs as part of a mixed spastic, hyperkinetic movement disorder in children with static encephalopathy (cerebral palsy). Some experts view athetosis on a spectrum with dystonia and chorea.

CLINICAL CHARACTERISTICS—PHENOMENOLOGY OF CHOREA, ATHETOSIS, AND BALLISM IN CHILDREN

Chorea

Patient History

In childhood, chorea is most often acquired acutely or subacutely, and thus parents can describe the onset and the way in which the child's speech and purposeful movements have changed. Acquired chorea usually interferes with purposeful movement, causing functional impairment. In subtle cases, particularly in young children with underdeveloped motor coordination or speech articulation, a parent's report that coordination or speech has changed must be relied on.

In contrast, when chorea occurs as a late or minor feature of chronic neurologic disease, parents may not accurately report onset. In diseases where the child has a global encephalopathy, the impact of the chorea on the child's quality of life is unclear but is probably limited. Diagnostically, the presence of chorea may have some localizing and etiologic value. Detailed past medical and family history is vital.

Examination

The child with chorea may have generalized or localized adventitious movements, but usually the face and upper limbs are involved. There is an appearance of restlessness and randomness as movements flow continually around the body. Speech may be slurred or slow because of involvement of tongue and facial muscles. Involvement of upper limbs is usually bilateral but also may be asymmetric. Choreic movements can occur in both proximal and distal muscles.

Action and certain postures usually exacerbate or enhance chorea, and therefore chorea usually interferes with coordination of purposeful movements. Careful observation in the presence of certain actions or postures may demonstrate the involvement of areas less affected at rest.

The motor function problems in chorea should be readily distinguished from ataxia. Close observation demonstrates that the choreic movements intrude on the trajectory of the purposeful movement. Thus, when chorea involves the legs, for example, the child may lurch intermittently when walking, but it is not the consistent broad-based or unsteady gait as seen in ataxia. Similarly, there may be difficulty with finger-to-nose and rapid alternating movement testing, but the problem is much more irregular than one sees with cerebellar disease.

Children with chorea, particularly Sydenham chorea (SC) (see later discussion), often have motor impersistence, described by Gowers in 1888 as "unintended relaxation."[2] Motor impersistence is the inability to maintain a posture or stable motor command.

The appearance is one of intermittent interruption of the intended, sustained signal from motor cortex to muscle. For example, two classic signs in SC are "darting tongue" caused by inability to keep the tongue protruded and "milkmaid's grip" caused by inability to maintain a steady grip force. In both cases, in response to the examiner's command, the cooperative patient reactivates the muscles repeatedly, leading to these back-and-forth activation/relaxation patterns. Choreic intrusions, unintended relaxations, or both may contribute to the phenomenon of motor impersistence. The abnormal movements tend to occur reproducibly during attempts to maintain certain postures. They cannot be entrained, which helps distinguish them from psychogenic chorea.[3]

Some degree of hypotonia is also apparent in many cases. This leads to hyperextensibility across joints. Another sign is "hung up" muscle stretch reflexes. This is best seen at the knee with the patient sitting and leg unsupported. Repeated tapping of the quadriceps tendon may elicit a brief period of sustained leg extension against gravity.

Ballism

In childhood, ballism usually does not occur in isolation. Ballismus or ballism refers to involuntary, high-amplitude, flinging movements typically occurring proximally. These movements may be brief or continual and may occur in conjunction with chorea. It can occur in children with static encephalopathies such as choreoathetoid cerebral palsy. Such children have action-induced choreoathetoid movements at baseline but may develop severe, forceful, flinging, high-amplitude movements during febrile illnesses. In severe cases, these movements can lead to rhabdomyolysis, renal failure, and death.[4–7] Hemiballism is occasionally described as the result of an acute process such as a vascular insult in or adjacent to the subthalamic nucleus, and hyperglycemia. Flinging, ballistic movements sometimes occur in SC.

Athetosis

The child with athetoid movements has problems similar to the child with chorea. If the athetosis is symptomatic of a chronic global encephalopathy, the movement alone usually causes little functional difficulty, relative to the encephalopathy. If the athetosis is acquired acutely or subacutely, the difficulties related solely to athetosis may be more prominent.

LOCALIZATION AND PATHOPHYSIOLOGY

Neuroanatomy of Chorea, Athetosis, and Ballism

Based on many examples of localized metabolic, vascular, and hereditary neurodegenerative diseases, it is reasonable to conclude that the primary substrate for choreic movements is disturbance in structure or function of striatum, particularly the putamen, the caudate, and/or pallidum, or their inflow or outflow pathways. These neuroanatomic pathways are described in more detail in Chapter 1. The most common form of acquired chorea in children worldwide is poststreptococcal SC (see also Chapter 18 on autoimmune diseases).[8,9] A case control study of persons with SC showed subtle increases in size of caudate, putamen, and globus pallidus, suggesting an inflammatory process in the basal ganglia.[10]

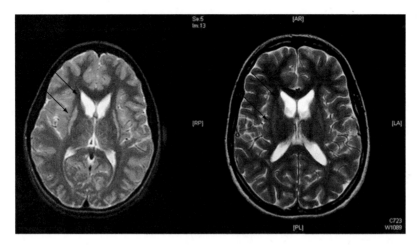

FIGURE 10.1   MRI T2 axial images of two children with HD. Both children were symptomatic at the time of genetic testing and both had affected fathers. At left, caudate volume loss and signal change in caudate and putamen in an 11-year-old boy with childhood-onset HD (Westphal variant), with dystonia and Parkinsonism, progressive for several years; CAG repeat count 84. By age 17, this boy had progressive myoclonic epilepsy, dementia, and had lost ambulation. Similar imaging findings at right in a 17-year-old girl with early-onset HD, mild depression, and mild chorea on examination manifested functionally with clumsiness, and CAG copy number 65.

Other forms of autoimmune chorea also show preferential involvement of striatum.[11] In adults, degeneration of the caudate and putamen in Huntington's disease (HD) is associated with chorea. This is also true for early-onset HD, which becomes apparent in later teenage years; however, childhood-onset HD, the Westphal variant, usually manifests with Parkinsonism, dementia, myoclonus, and seizures rather than chorea.[12–14] In children, lesions in the parietal cortex or thalamus may also be associated with chorea.

Figures 10.1–10.5 demonstrate several anatomic localizations and etiologies of chorea in children.

Neurophysiology of Chorea, Athetosis, and Ballism

Clinically, neither peripheral nor central neurophysiologic studies are helpful in diagnosis or treatment decisions for chorea, athetosis, or ballism. Electromyography of muscle shows that muscle activity differs in chorea versus normal voluntary movement. The normal initial agonist burst in a voluntary movement usually lasts less than 100 ms. However, in SC, the initial burst duration may be longer.[15] Routine EEGs show at most nonspecific abnormalities which are not helpful for diagnosis or treatment.

DISEASES AND DISORDERS

Etiologic Categories of Diseases Producing Chorea, Athetosis, and Ballism

Choreiform, athetoid, or ballistic movements can emerge as a consequence of a vast number of disease processes, including genetic and metabolic diseases, endocrine abnormalities,

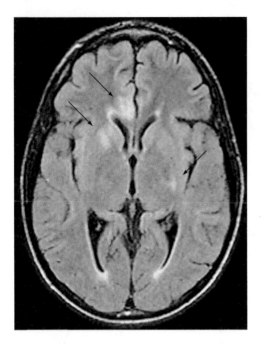

FIGURE 10.2　Subtle focal areas of signal change with no mass effect seen in MRI axial FLAIR imaging of 10-year-old boy with fever, chorea, and encephalopathy. Chorea lasted for 6 months, responded well to typical neuroleptics, and full recovery subsequently occurred. A specific etiology was not identified, but the monophasic clinical course with encephalopathy after fever and multiple focal areas of signal change in gray and white matter supported a diagnosis of form of acute disseminated encephalomyelitis (ADEM).

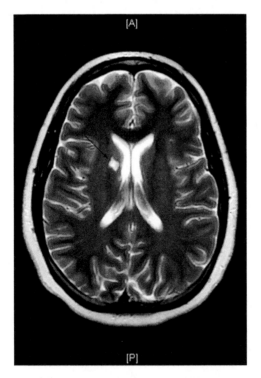

FIGURE 10.3　Axial T2 MRI shows one of several small basal ganglia lesions seen in a 20-year-old woman imaged because of headaches, 6 years after diagnosis of SC. This finding was not present or seen on MRI performed at the time of chorea presentation but likely represent encephalomalacia from small vessel ischemic changes.

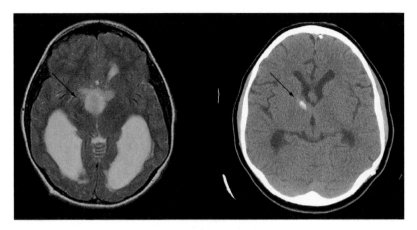

FIGURE 10.4   At left, neuroimaging of 9-year-old boy with precocious puberty, cognitive decline over several months, escalating headaches. Preoperative MRI showed a thalamic pilocytic astrocytoma (arrow). He underwent partial resection and cranial irradiation. Eight months later, the patient had acute-onset headache and left-sided hemichorea. CT scan at right showed dystrophic calcification and a small focus of radiation necrosis in right thalamus (arrow). Chorea responded to neuroleptics and resolved within several months.

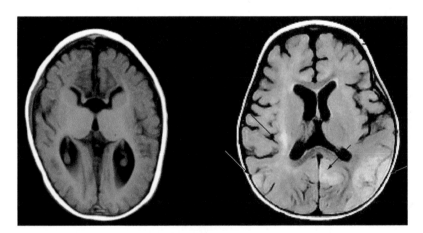

FIGURE 10.5   Axial MRI of two infants who developed continuous choreiform movements between 6 and 12 months of age. At left, 11-month-old infant with microcephaly, agenesis of corpus callosum, and elevated lactate consistent with metabolic disorder. At right, infant with acute-onset encephalopathy and severe choreiform movements. Imaging shows multifocal areas of signal change, most prominent in parietal lobe, consistent with a mitochondrial disease. Muscle biopsy testing showed a severe complex IV, electron transport chain deficiency. Treatments targeting mitochondrial dysfunction and suppression of chorea were not beneficial.

infections, autoimmune conditions, cerebrovascular disease, neoplasms, neurodegenerative diseases, toxins, and trauma. This is partly due to the vulnerability of the basal ganglia to a wide variety of pathologies. In many of these diseases, the hyperkinetic movement disorder is not the sole or predominant neurologic problem. Table 10.1 shows key etiologic categories and important diagnoses. Additional detail is provided in the remainder of this section.

TABLE 10.1   Etiological Categories of Chorea

PHYSIOLOGIC CHOREA

Infancy

Choreiform movements in neurobehavioral disorders

PRIMARY CHOREAS

Benign hereditary chorea (including syndrome of choreoathetosis, hypothyroidism, neonatal respiratory distress)

SYMPTOMATIC, SECONDARY CHOREAS

Auto immune (see chapter 18)

Poststreptococcal, Sydenham Chorea (SC)

Chorea secondary to systemic lupus erythematosus (SLE)

Chorea secondary to antiphospholipid antibody syndrome (APS)

Acute disseminated encephalomyelitis (ADEM)

Anti-N-methyl-D-aspartate (NMDA) receptor encephalitis, other paraneoplastic

Other infections and encephalitides: Lyme, human immunodeficiency virus, mycoplasma

Vascular/Hypoxic ischemic

Stroke, Moya Moya, vascular malformations/hemorrhages

Third trimester/perinatal hypoxic ischemic injuries leading to choreoathetoid cerebral palsy (see chapter 20)

Postcardiac transplant—"postpump chorea"

Toxin induced

Carbon dioxide

Methyl alcohol

Manganese

Toluene

Iatrogenic chorea/dyskinesia (see chapter 22)

Psychostimulants, dopamine agonists, levodopa

Dopamine receptor blocking agents/neuroleptics/antipsychotics

Selective serotonin reuptake inhibitors

Psychiatric polypharmacy

Anticonvulsants: carbamazepine, phenytoin, tiagabine

CHOREAS IN NEURODEGENERATIVE DISEASES AND SEVERE ENCEPHALOPATHIES (SEE CHAPTER 17)

Biopterin-dependent hyperphenylalaninemia (type VI)

Gangliosidosis

Mitochondrial encephalopathies/Leigh's disease

TABLE 10.1   Continued

Glutaric aciduria

Lesch–Nyhan disease

Phenylketonuria

Wilson's disease

Neuroacanthocytoses

Early (adolescent, not childhood-onset) Huntington Disease (HD)

DISEASES WITH CHOREA AS A MINOR OR LATE FEATURE

Alternating hemiplegia of childhood

Bilateral striatal necrosis

Ceroid lipofuscinosis

Neurodegeneration with brain iron accumulation

Rasmussen's encephalitis

Succinate semialdehyde dehydrogenase deficiency

Cerebral creatine deficiency secondary to guanidineoacetate methyltransferase deficiency

Hypoparathyroidism

CHOREA IN ATAXIAS (SEE CHAPTER 14)

Friedreich's ataxia

Ataxia telangiectasia

Ataxia with oculomotor apraxia 1 and 2

Dentatorubropallidoluysian atrophy

Spinocerebellar Ataxias (SCAs) 1, 2, 3, 6, 17 (adult onset more common)

PAROXYSMAL CHOREAS (SEE CHAPTER 9)

Paroxysmal nonkinesigenic dyskinesia 1 (PNKD)

PSYCHOGENIC CHOREA (SEE CHAPTER 23)

Physiologic Chorea

Chorea in Infancy

The decomposed or immature movements of infants may sometimes be described as choreiform. These do not generally indicate neurologic disease. In the context of a normally developing child with normal head circumference, these movements can be monitored through regular follow-up clinic visits. Brain magnetic resonance imaging (MRI) and other testing may be deferred.

Chorea Minor

Mild chorea, referred to as "chorea minima" or "chorea minor," typically manifested in hands and fingers when arms are held in an outstretched position in front of the body, may be seen in typically developing children. Children diagnosed with neurobehavioral disorders such as attention-deficit/hyperactivity disorder (ADHD) are more likely to manifest some subtle difficulties with motor control, including motor overflow and mild choreiform movements.[16]

Primary Choreas

The main primary chorea is benign hereditary chorea (BHC). The term *primary* is applied here because the disease is genetic and chorea is the predominant neurologic symptom. BHC is also sometimes referred to as brain-thyroid-lung syndrome.

Benign Hereditary Chorea

CLINICAL FEATURES

BHC, described by Haerer and colleagues in 1967, is a rare, autosomal dominant, childhood-onset, nonprogressive, hyperkinetic movement disorder characterized by onset of chorea before age 5.[17,18] While most BHC cases are caused by mutations in *NKX2-1*, another form of autosomal dominant, early childhood onset chorea, with or without facial myokymia, has recently been linked to mutations in *ADCY5*, which encodes adenylate cyclase 5.[19]

The most typical neurological course involves hypotonia in infancy followed by onset of chorea between 8 months and 5 years, with a fairly stable course in childhood. Chorea may be isolated or accompanied by myoclonus, dystonia, or tics. Chorea may improve after puberty and resolve in some adults, but other adults have developed disabling myoclonus. Cognition is believed to be broadly normal. However, in one of the largest published case series, learning disabilities occurred in 72% (20 of 28) individuals and ADHD in 25%.[20]

In approximately 80% of BHC cases, thyroid disease, lung disease, or both occur. Congenital and other forms of hypothyroidism are most common. Lung diseases include surfactant metabolism disorder which can be fatal, recurrent pulmonary infections, asthma, and lung cancer.[20] Skeletal anomalies may also occur more frequently than expected.[21]

PATHOPHYSIOLOGY

BHC usually results from deletion of or mutations in the *NKX2-1* gene, a member of the *NKX2* homeodomain transcription factor family, which encodes thyroid transcription factor 1 (called both TITF1 and TTF1).[22,23] Transmission is autosomal dominant. The severity of the chorea varies substantially within and between families.[24-26] A variety of mutations and deletions in this gene have been identified.[20,27] TITF1 protein binds to transcriptional regulatory elements of a number of genes in lung related to surfactant and in thyroid related to thyroglobulin and thyroperoxidase, however, less is known about its role in brain development.

A large variety of imaging findings have been reported in BHC, but in general, brain structure appears normal.[18] In some individuals, mild atrophy, empty sella, agenesis of corpus callosum, and signal change in striatum and cerebellum are reported.[27-29] Postmortem studies show no major abnormalities; however, loss of a subset of striatal interneurons[30] and mild degeneration of white matter and striatum[31] were reported. As in structural imaging, functional/metabolic imaging can be normal or can show many alterations.[18] For example, one study utilizing technetium single-photon emission computed tomography (SPECT) showed decreased uptake in the striatum and thalamus[25] and another utilizing 18-fluoro-2-deoxy-glucose positron emission tomography (FDG-PET) demonstrated reduced metabolism in basal ganglia and cortex.[29]

Animal studies to date generate a complex picture of the pathophysiology. Homozygous knockout of the *NKX2* gene in mice results in a very severe phenotype and still birth. Prenatally, mice develop severe lung, thyroid, and pituitary deficits, with abnormal development of the striatum, basal forebrain, and cerebral cortical GABAergic neurons, which are incompatible with extrauterine life.[32,33] The heterozygous mice, which would be the model for the human disease, do not have readily apparent neurologic deficits.[32] However, conditional removal of TITF1 function at various early stages of embryo- and neurogenesis adversely affects differentiation of interneurons, projections of striatal medium spiny neurons, and formation of globus pallidus.[34,35]

DIAGNOSTIC APPROACH

BHC should be considered in children with relatively isolated chorea in the first 5 years of life and an autosomal dominant family history. Features supporting this diagnosis include the presence of broadly normal intellectual development with no regression or loss of cognitive skills, absence of other significant neurologic problems such as epilepsy, normal general examination with no dysmorphic features, and, with the exception of chorea, a normal neurologic examination. As is often true in movement disorders, it is important to examine other family members in addition to taking a multigeneration history. The presence of mild symptoms in a parent would support the presence of autosomal dominant inheritance in BHC. Elevated blood levels of thyroid-stimulating hormone are also supportive. Neuroimaging should usually be obtained to evaluate for diagnoses with more serious, degenerative prognoses. Brain imaging will often be normal in children with BHC.

The differential diagnosis of chorea is broad due in part to difficulty differentiating chorea from mixed movement disorders involving dystonia, myoclonus, and ataxia. Other diagnoses to consider in a child under age 5 with chorea include ataxia telangiectasia (AT),[36] which is autosomal recessive (see Chapter 14), dyskinetic cerebral palsy (see Chapter 20), myoclonus dystonia (DYT 11) (see Chapter 12), and various metabolic disorders (see Chapter 17). Past medical history and family history can assist in prioritizing the differential diagnosis. With regard to AT, a mixed movement disorder occurs prior to development of telangiectasias. Testing for elevated serum alpha fetoprotein is inexpensive and vital in clarifying whether AT may be the diagnosis.[37] With regard to myoclonus dystonia, which has autosomal dominant transmission, there can be substantial overlap in phenotypes in later childhood and early adulthood. BHC should have a more significant effect on gait. Myoclonus dystonia (DYT11), usually caused by mutations in the gene coding for epsilon-sarcoglycan, is manifested by jerk-like movement and dystonia, exacerbated by action, associated with a variety of behavioral comorbidities including obsessive compulsive behavior[38] and substance abuse.[39] Adult family members with myoclonus dystonia may have noticed improved symptoms with alcohol.

TREATMENT

There are no disease-modifying treatments. No symptomatic treatment has been shown in clinical trials to be beneficial in genetically confirmed BHC; however, good treatment results have been described in individuals. In general, dopamine receptor blocking and dopamine depleting agents can be expected to reduce chorea and may be considered when chorea interferes with function and quality of life.[23,29] Response to low dose levodopa has also been described.[40,41]

Secondary (Acquired) Choreas

The majority of childhood-onset diseases where chorea is the predominant movement disorder are acquired, with acute or subacute onset. SC is the most commonly acquired chorea in children aged between 5 and 15 years, and chorea associated with SLE and APS manifest similarly. The majority of acquired chorea in childhood is self-limited.

Choreas Occurring in Immunologic/Autoimmune Disease

SYDENHAM CHOREA (SC)

CLINICAL FEATURES   SC is considered a manifestation of rheumatic disease, a group of sequelae of group A β-hemolytic streptococci (GABHS) infections. GABHS are gram-positive bacteria that colonize or invade the upper respiratory tract. Two surface antigens, surface M proteins and N-acetyl-glucosamine have been implicated as important for virulence and generating antibodies playing a role in pathophysiology of the movement disorder.[42] (see also Chapter 18 on autoimmune diseases). Elevated measurements of both antistreptolysin O (ASO) and anti-DNAse B (ADB) titers in blood are markers of prior infections.[43]

The relationship of GABHS to SC is supported by epidemiologic observations, including the reduction in cases in the postantibiotic era and common co-occurrence of chorea and other manifestations of rheumatic disease, particularly carditis and arthritis.[8] The chorea appears the same whether or not carditis and arthritis occur. In the proper setting, chorea only following GABHS is also classified as rheumatic disease. That is, children manifest with subacute chorea, with or without carditis or arthritis/arthralgia, weeks or months after GABHS infections, and meet the Jones Criteria for Rheumatic Disease.[44] In addition to GABHS, other subtypes of streptococci can cause "strep throat," a highly prevalent bacterial infection that occurs one or more times in many children. Most infections are uncomplicated, responding readily to penicillin or other appropriate antibiotics with few sequelae, and many infections are self-limited, resolving without antibiotics. Infections may also be minor, so that affected individuals do not seek medical attention.

SC is rare in the United States. In three regions with relatively higher prevalence, Utah,[2] Western Pennsylvania,[8] and Southwest Ohio,[45] academic centers report evaluating just 3–10 children with this diagnosis per year. The presence of markers of streptococcal infection is nonspecific due to the high prevalence of these infections.[46] Further, single antibody titer measures can be misleading, as these may remain elevated for months to years after infections.[43] Therefore, in atypical or recurrent cases or those with chorea but no cardiac or joint symptoms, the possibility of SLE and APS should be considered, as discussed later in this chapter. Consultation with rheumatology may be considered in cases involving joints or multiple body systems, or when antibody testing results do not confirm SC.

Chorea in SC develops over hours to days (Videos 10.5 and 10.6). Parents and children can often identify the day or week and sometimes may remember the hour of onset. Symptom severity varies widely. Difficulty with activities of daily living and fine motor tasks such as dressing or writing is common. Patients may describe that they are clumsy or weak, often dropping items in their hands. Abnormal movements diminish or cease during sleep.

In addition to abnormal involuntary movements, cognitive and emotional symptoms, including inattention, anxiety, obsessive compulsiveness, paranoia, and reluctance to speak, may occur.[45,47–50] Interestingly, children with rheumatic fever not only commonly develop obsessive-compulsive symptoms, but they also have a higher than expected prevalence of these symptoms in first-degree relatives.[51]

On examination, affected children appear restless or fidgety while sitting. There may be a paucity of speech[52] and facial movements, combined with inappropriate adventitious facial expressions or facial tics. Speech articulation may be slurred. Coordination is often poor with erratic performance of finger-to-nose testing and intermittent lurching while walking. Falls are not common. Delirium is rare.

There are four classic neurologic signs. These are nonspecific and may be present in chorea due to other causes, but they nearly always occur together and support the diagnosis of SC:

1. *Spooning sign.* The examiner asks the child to extend both arms straight forward, horizontally from the shoulders, with hands pronated (palms down) and fingers spread wide. Children with SC tend to hyperextend at the metacarpophalangeal joint. This "spooning" is dystonic posturing. This maneuver also tends to induce more chorea in proximal and distal arm muscles. Often, the movements are asymmetric. These movements may worsen further if an additional task is added, such as protruding the tongue.
2. *Touchdown (or three-point shot) sign.* The examiner asks the child to extend both arms up vertically from the shoulders with palms facing each other. This induces choreiform movements and results in hand pronation and elbow flexion, again often asymmetric.
3. *Milkmaid's grip.* The examiner offers her or his index and middle fingers together, both hands, for the child to squeeze. The child attempts to squeeze both hands and typically is unable to persist in squeezing. This is *motor impersistence.* The cooperative child, each time the grip releases, tries to squeeze again. As this happens repeatedly, this resembles "milking" the examiner's fingers. Even in cases where hand and arm signs 1 and 2 are highly asymmetric, in SC there is usually some degree of grip impersistence in the less involved hand.
4. *Darting tongue.* The examiner asks the child to stick out his or her tongue. The child attempts to cooperate but the tongue protrusion cannot be maintained, resulting in a "darting tongue."

Because SC is a form of rheumatic disease, it is critical to assess the child carefully for the presence of a systolic heart murmur, or of arthritis or arthralgia.[8] The presence of a systolic murmur in this setting, particularly if the parents believe a murmur was not previously reported to them by their primary physician, is virtually pathognomonic for rheumatic chorea. Carditis is typically mild.[53]

Long-term prognosis of SC is generally good, with resolution of symptoms in most cases in less than 1 year.[45,54,55] In some cases, chorea may persist chronically.[56] Chorea may also recur in up to 20% of children, despite secondary prevention with penicillin.[53] Recurrence appears to be more common, at least in Brazil, in women at the time of pregnancy. A long-term follow-up case-series reported a *chorea gravidarum* rate of 75%, with a higher than expected rate of miscarriages. Oral contraceptives also induced recurrent chorea in these women.[57] In addition, a high proportion of adults who had SC in childhood appear to have a mild degree of bradykinesia[58] and executive dysfunction[59] in adulthood.

The high prevalence of psychiatric symptoms, as well as tics, in SC has led to a great deal of important clinical, epidemiological, and immunological research devoted to determining whether there is a parallel but distinct acquired condition in which GABHS induces tics and obsessive-compulsive disorder symptoms but no (or minimal) chorea.[60] This entity has been called *pediatric autoimmune neuropsychiatric disorders associated with streptococcal infections* (PANDAS). Based on the original operational definition of PANDAS, which emphasized tics and required observation of temporal association between GABHS and neuropsychiatric symptoms on two or more occasions, prospective studies were undertaken. These failed to support PANDAS as a discrete diagnostic entity.[61–63] Identification of overlapping antibodies between SC and explosive tic/OCD cases remains an area of active investigation.[64,65] The use of serum from children diagnosed with PANDAS has been used to generate animal models,[66–68] with interesting but not always consistently replicated results.[69,70]

Recently, the relationship between GABHS and non-SC neuropsychiatric symptoms was reconceptualized and renamed.[71] The new diagnostic criteria de-emphasize tics. The cardinal symptoms are now psychiatric and include other symptoms such as eating disorders.[72]

The relationship between GABHS infection and tics is addressed in greater detail in Chapter 7. The terms "PANDAS" and "SC" should *not* be used interchangeably (See Chapter 18).

PATHOPHYSIOLOGY Although the clinical phenomenology of SC has been recognized for centuries, a causal relationship with GABHS infection was not established until the 1950s.[73] Antibodies to the caudate and subthalamic nucleus have been identified in children with SC.[74] Preliminary studies of antibodies administered via passive transfer to rodents appear to support an effect of SC antibodies on dopaminergic activity.[75] It is important to point out that some antibasal ganglia antibodies were found elevated in HD and Parkinson's disease, as well as in lower proportions of healthy people,[76] so these findings are not specific and may in some cases be epiphenomena or effects, rather than causes. In addition, some studies find high titers of antibrain antibodies in healthy control groups.[77] This suggests that circulating antibodies may not always have sufficient access to the brain required to produce symptoms. The identification of M proteins on streptococci that can evoke antibodies that cross-react with human brain[78] suggested that molecular mimicry may play a role. The relative rarity of SC and other rheumatic complications suggests that some important bacterial or host factors or susceptibility may be required.

Another recent series of studies found elevated immunoglobulin G (IgG) antibodies to neuronal tubulin in blood and cerebrospinal fluid (CSF) in SC. These antibodies cross-react with GABHS epitopes. *In vitro*, binding to caudate and putamen brain sections was blocked by both lysoganglioside GM1 and by an antitubulin antibody. Functionally, in a neuronal cell line, the acute chorea sera induced calcium/calmodulin-dependent protein kinase II activity in human neuronal cells.[49] This same laboratory reported that an antibody and immunoglobulin from SC sera binds to D2 receptors *in vivo* in a mouse model.

DIAGNOSTIC APPROACH The differential diagnosis of chorea is large. Fortunately, only a few categories of disease need to be considered in a school-age, previously healthy, child when chorea develops over a period of hours to days. Most such children will have SC. After careful history, family history, and examination, diagnostic evaluation can therefore often focus on GABHS and rheumatic disease.

A number of other etiologies may in certain settings trigger subacute or acute chorea. Drug-induced choreic movements may be considered (see also Chapter 22 on drug-induced movement disorders). In toddlers, this may result from accidental ingestions. Common offenders are stimulants used to treat ADHD. In older children and teens, stimulant overdose, cocaine, or abrupt withdrawal of high-potency dopamine receptor blocking agents such as risperidone or aripiprazole should also be considered. In one case, azithromycin was reported to induce agitation and chorea.[79] Chorea caused by endocrine disorders such as hyperthyroidism, hyperparathyroidism, and hyperglycemia may also be considered in the appropriate clinical setting and ruled out with laboratory testing. Hyperthyroidism can cause chorea, but usually tachycardia, diarrhea, and skin changes should also be present.[80] Vascular diseases are unlikely in childhood to produce solely chorea because of the low prevalence of small vessel intracranial disease. Vascular causes may be considered in cases of acute, thunderclap onset of unilateral chorea or ballism, or when careful neurologic examination suggests a constellation of symptoms in a distribution supporting vascular disease (see Figure 10.4). Mitochondrial diseases may selectively affect basal ganglia and produce chorea (see Figure 10.5) (Video 10.3).[81] These should be accompanied by characteristic findings of signal change on MRI or basal ganglia lactate elevation on magnetic resonance spectroscopy. Psychogenic movement disorders may have a choreic phenomenology.[3,82]

LABORATORY TESTING Chorea with a subacute course, with gradual evolution of symptoms over minutes to hours or days, is typical of an inflammatory disease and thus these should be the focus of laboratory investigation. GABHS is the most common etiology of subacute chorea in otherwise healthy children. Obtaining a history of infection during the prior 6 months with headache, fever, and sore throat is important. Documenting a prior positive throat culture is also helpful. Even in the absence of this information, with the proper time course, physical, and neurological examination, SC is the most likely diagnosis.

This high pretest probability is important for interpreting the results of confirmatory SC testing. In the presence of a typical history and examination, if there is no documented antecedent GABHS infection, blood testing for both streptococcal antibodies—ASO and ADB—should be obtained. It is important that these studies be run in an experienced laboratory and compared against childhood normative levels for that laboratory. Case series in the United States, 40 years apart, found the sensitivity when both ASO and ADB were tested was 87%[83] and 90%.[45] Thus, the absence of elevations and either titer should prompt consideration of other diagnoses such as lupus (SLE) or APS. Note the presence of a positive throat culture at the time of chorea presentation is not needed for the diagnosis of SC.

If the history and examination are not typical for SC, such that the pretest probability is lower, then interpreting the significance of elevated ASO or ADB titers requires caution. Because GABHS infections are so common, and antibody titers may remain elevated for months,[43] the specificity is lower and, in the setting of clinical uncertainty, the positive predictive value is therefore lower. Moreover, in some developing countries, the background rate of elevated antibody titers is higher,[84] reducing the specificity of this testing in the setting of chorea even further.

Chorea caused by other infections, such as Lyme disease, human immunodeficiency virus, mycoplasma pneumonia, or Legionnaire's disease, parvovirus B19 may be considered, in the appropriate clinical setting, if no history, clinical, or laboratory evidence of GABHS infection, SLE, or APS can be identified.

NEUROIMAGING   Obtaining a brain MRI scan to rule out brain structural causes should be considered as part of the evaluation of any child with subacute chorea. A number of studies have reported subtle signal change or volume increase in basal ganglia nuclei.[8,10,85] However, in most cases where the clinical diagnosis is SC, neuroimaging does not guide further management.[8] MRI findings would also point toward diagnoses of mitochondrial/metabolic diseases, degenerative, neoplastic, vascular,[86] and other inflammatory diseases targeting the basal ganglia. However, experienced clinicians, in the presence of a classic, unambiguous case of SC, may elect not to obtain neuroimaging, because of the expense, the common need for sedation to allow for high-quality images in the presence of hyperkinetic chorea, and the low clinical utility. Subsequently, if the patient's clinical course diverges from what is expected for SC, neuroimaging can be reconsidered and, after the acute period, some striatal changes may be present (see Figure 10.3). SPECT scans show striatal hyperperfusion,[87–89] and PET scans show hypermetabolism[90] in basal ganglia during the acute phase of the illness. Volumetric MRI scans show increases in basal ganglia size which are statistically, though not clinically, apparent.[10] Similarly, diffusion weighted imaging shows apparent diffusion coefficients which are lower in striatum and which increase after steroid treatment.[91] Although informative regarding pathophysiology, these MRI, SPECT, and PET findings are not specific and do not guide clinical management.

OTHER TESTING AND SPECIALTY CONSULTATION   Echocardiography or cardiology consultation is recommended in the presence of a new murmur. If no murmur is heard, an echocardiogram need not be obtained at the time of chorea presentation because identification of a trivial murmur will not change management. However, careful surveillance with a thorough cardiac examination should be emphasized at regular, early follow-up visits. In general, carditis in children with SC is mild and may resolve completely.[92]

TREATMENT   There are three treatment issues to be considered: secondary prevention, chorea symptom suppression, and immune modulation.

Secondary Prevention of GABHS Infections   The standard of care for all children diagnosed with SC, even in cases of isolated chorea, is secondary prevention with penicillin.[44] The purpose is to reduce the risk of recurrences of chorea but especially to reduce the likelihood that future GABHS infections could cause carditis and permanent valvular damage.[93] An appropriate alternative may be selected for children with penicillin allergies. Current recommendations in the United States are for treatment until age 21 years with either monthly intramuscular (IM) penicillin or daily oral penicillin. Some physicians favor monthly IM penicillin to ascertain compliance. Infectious disease consultation may be considered if GABHS recurs despite prophylaxis, which is rare, or if there is concern that the individual or family members are asymptomatic GABHS carriers. Some otolaryngologists will operate to remove adenoids and tonsils in children with SC who have moderate or large tonsils, but this has not been systematically studied.

Chorea Symptom Suppression   A more general discussion of pharmacologic treatment of chorea appears at the end of this chapter in the treatment section. Symptom-suppressing medication is not needed in mild cases. However, treatment is reasonable for children for whom important daily activities are impaired by chorea. As is the case for many movement disorders, there are many small, uncontrolled case series reporting benefit of many medications. These include benzodiazepines and several anticonvulsants, most commonly valproic acid.[94,95] Because chorea in SC is self-limited, it is difficult to interpret these positive reports. Many experts consider dopamine receptor blocking agents, typical neuroleptics, and the dopamine depleting agent, tetrabenazine, to be the most effective chorea-suppressing agents.[45,96,97] Although parents and some physicians may be understandably reluctant to use these medications because of concerns about side effects, it is helpful to emphasize that the expected course of treatment will be brief, usually less than 1 year, and that often low doses are sufficient. These factors reduce the risk of neurologic side effects of dopamine receptor blockers.

Anticholinergic agents such as benztropine or trihexyphenidyl should not be used to treat chorea. These agents, although helpful in some primary, lesional, and drug-induced dystonias, can make chorea worse.

Immune Modulation   Based on the pathophysiology of SC, it is reasonable to consider immune-modulating therapies to shorten the course of illness. By analogy with other subacute neurologic and medical conditions, including acute inflammatory demyelinating polyneuropathy, Kawasaki's disease, and idiopathic thrombocytopenic purpura, treatment with steroids, intravenous immune globulin, or plasmapheresis is also worth investigation in severe cases.

A number of case reports, series, and small trials report benefit with immune-modulating treatment. These are summarized in Table 10.2. The most compelling evidence for benefit from steroids comes from a randomized, blinded, placebo-controlled study by Paz and colleagues.[55] Relative to placebo, a 4-week 2 mg/kg daily oral dose of prednisone, followed by a taper, reduced duration of chorea and accelerated the reduction in symptoms. Weight gain was substantial by the end of 2 months, and long-term results including recurrence rates were similar in both groups. More supportive evidence comes from a clinical trial by Garvey and colleagues,[98] comparing a lower dose of prednisone to intravenous immunoglobulin (IVIG) and plasmapheresis. This study was not blinded, and the 4-week response to prednisone appeared to be less robust. Additional suggestive evidence comes from both small case series[99,100] and a large retrospective observational study. Treatment allocation was nonrandom, and follow-up was nonstandardized and nonblinded.[101] The estimate of treatment effects is likely imprecise because of low follow-up ascertainment. In addition, because there were substantially fewer untreated patients who were followed up, bias due to case mix (untreated patients with persistent chorea were more likely to be followed up) makes interpretation of treatment versus no-treatment effects difficult. Case reports, small case series, and small clinical trials report benefits in use of immunoglobulins,[102,103] and use of anti-TNF alpha therapy.[104]

TABLE 10.2   Immune-Modulating Treatment for Sydenham Chorea

Sample size	Treatment details	Study design	Outcome reported	Result	Citation
102 SC cases over 18 years (48 PRED; 54 NO PRED)	No protocol for treatment	Retrospective, nonrandom treatment allocation, nonblinded and nonstandardized follow-up	Median time to chorea resolution	No data available for 1/2 cases PRED ($n = 32$): 4 weeks NO PRED ($n = 17$): 9 weeks	[101]
18 SC cases over 9 years	PRED PO 1 mg/kg 10 days, 10 day taper IVIG 2 g/kg; PEX 5–6 courses	Randomized controlled, active comparator, no placebo, standard but nonblinded assessment at 1 month, 12 months	Mean chorea scale severity reduction at 4 weeks	PRED ($n = 6$): 29% IVIG ($n = 4$) 72% PEX ($n = 8$) 50%	[98]
37 SC cases over 3 years	PRED PO 2 mg/kg (max 60 mg) × 4 weeks, then 3-week taper; PLACEBO	Randomized, placebo-controlled, double-blinded, standardized longitudinal assessments	Mean time to chorea resolution (mean chorea scale reduction severity)	PRED ($n = 22$): 54 days (85% reduction at 4 weeks); PLACEBO ($n = 15$): 120 days (33% reduction at 4 weeks)	[55]

IVIG, intravenous immune globulin; PEX, plasmapheresis; PO, by mouth; PRED, prednisone; SC, Sydenham's chorea.

Chorea in Primary Anti-Phospholipid Antibody Syndrome (APS) and Systemic Lupus Erythematosus (SLE)

CLINICAL FEATURES

The clinical features of APS and SLE manifesting with chorea overlap with those of SC and cannot be reliably differentiated solely based on the neurological examination (Videos 10.2 and 10.9).[105] APS can manifest with other neurologic signs and symptoms, such as epilepsy, which are rare in SC. Cerebrovascular disease, cognitive impairment, and transverse myelopathy can also be symptoms of APS, and SLE may have multiorgan disease. Arthralgia, arthritis, and mitral valve carditis are characteristic of SC.

PATHOPHYSIOLOGY (SEE ALSO CHAPTER 18)

As for SC, the pathophysiology of APS is believed to be the generation of antibodies, although the trigger is unknown. These are believed to enter the brain, cross-reacting with striatal epitopes due to a process of molecular mimicry, resulting in altered striatal function. A biologically relevant animal model has been developed. In this model, mice are immunized with β_2-glycoprotein I, which induces both persistent high levels of antiphospholipid antibodies and motoric (hyperactive) and adverse cognitive changes.[106]

DIAGNOSTIC APPROACH

SC is a much more prevalent cause of acute/subacute chorea in childhood, but both APS and SLE can manifest initially with isolated chorea and associated neuropsychiatric symptoms, particularly in children.[107] Because of the long-term implications of these diagnoses, and differences in management, it is important to carefully consider the possibility of APS and SLE in children with new chorea.[108] If there is clinical or laboratory evidence of prior GABHS infection and if the chorea is classic for SC, as described previously, the likelihood of SLE or APS is very low. Some authors advocate obtaining testing for lupus anticoagulant and/or anticardiolipin antibodies in all children in this clinical setting.[108] However, as discussed previously, it may be reasonable to consider APS or SLE in some previously healthy, school-age children with acute/subacute chorea in the presence of negative antistreptococcal antibody tests.[11,109] The diagnosis of APS should also be considered in apparent SC cases which recur.

As discussed in more detail in the diagnostic approach to SC, several caveats regarding laboratory testing are needed. First, because of the high prevalence of GABHS infections, elevated antistreptococcal antibody titers are common, and these may persist for months or years in some children. Thus, a child with APS or SLE may have elevated streptococcal antibodies. Second, antibodies elevated in APS may also be elevated in SC, including anticardiolipin β_2-microglobulin antibodies.[85]

TREATMENT

Treatment of SLE, a systemic, multiorgan disease, lies outside the scope of this chapter. However, in general, immune-suppressive therapies will reduce chorea associated with SLE or APS. Prednisone has been reported to reduce chorea in a case where neuroleptic medication was not helpful.[11]

Anti-NMDA Receptor Encephalitis with Chorea and Psychiatric Changes

This entity was only recently described.[110] Case series are emerging in children.[111,112]

CLINICAL FEATURES

Anti-NMDA receptor encephalitis presents as a subacute encephalitis with a multistage course. The initial features may be psychiatric, followed by an acute or subacute emergence of a characteristic movement disorder, orofacial and other stereotypies, chorea, dystonia, and myorhythmia (slow tremor), or seizures.[111] In a case series of 571 patients with IgG antibodies against the NR1 subunit of the NMDA receptor, 23 (4%) had isolated psychiatric episodes as the only manifestation of anti-NMDA receptor encephalitis.[113] Predominant symptoms included delusional thinking (74%), mood disturbances (70%, usually manic), and aggression (57%). Brain MRI findings were abnormal in 10 of 22 patients (45%) and CSF showed pleocytosis in 17 of 22 patients (77%). Eighty-three percent of the patients had full or substantial recovery after immunotherapy and tumor resection when appropriate.

PATHOPHYSIOLOGY

Antibodies to NMDA receptors are implicated. These antibodies may be triggered by the presence of a teratoma or other neoplasm, or triggered by other infections. Antibody binding to NMDA receptors is thought to interfere with glutamatergic transmission as a basis for the symptoms.

DIAGNOSTIC APPROACH

As our understanding of the clinical features of this diagnosis are still evolving, it is important to consider this diagnosis in all children and young adults presenting with an unexplained subacute encephalopathy and movement disorder. The movement disorder in adults usually includes orofacial dyskinesias and this is described in children as well.[114] Psychiatric symptoms may be prominent but there should also be a delirium present.

In adult females, the trigger is often an ovarian teratoma. As in the case of opsoclonus myoclonus syndrome, it is important to be thorough in searching for a tumor. Contrast MRI of the chest, abdomen, and pelvis should be obtained. Blood and CSF should be sent to an appropriate laboratory for anti-NMDA receptor antibody testing. As these results take time, imaging and immune-modulating treatments should be undertaken, in the appropriate clinical setting, prior to receiving the antibody testing results.

TREATMENT

Treatment should be aggressive. If identified, a tumor should be surgically removed. Immunotherapy is standard, including steroid, IVIG, plasmapheresis, and if need be other immunosuppressive agents such as rituximab or cyclophosphamide. Most patients will respond to treatment although the course of the illness may be protracted, lasting months.

Vascular/Hypoxic Ischemia

CHOREA IN MOYAMOYA

Reversible chorea has been described in 3% of children with moyamoya disease or progressive occlusive disease of the intracranial branches of the internal carotid arteries. Angiography showed hypertrophied perforating, collateral lenticulostriate vessels. In general, chorea was resolved after surgical revascularization using pial synangiosis from the external carotid arteries. However, resolution took months, and relapses occurred years later in one case.[115]

"POSTPUMP CHOREA"—CHOREA AFTER NEONATAL AND INFANT CARDIAC SURGERY

CLINICAL FEATURES   Chorea has long been described as a neurologic complication of cardiac surgery in neonates and infants.[116] Dyskinetic movements may be very dramatic, and may be transient or prolonged. Long-term outcomes in these children include persistent chorea in some cases and significant cognitive problems in all cases.[117,118] The incidence of this problem has markedly diminished in the past two decades due to improved surgical techniques.

PATHOPHYSIOLOGY   This occurs because of injury to striatum, likely selectively vulnerable at this age. Postmortem studies in two children showed reactive gliosis, neuronal loss, and degeneration of myelinated fibers, relatively selectively localized to the external globus pallidus.[119]

TREATMENT   The best treatment is prevention and, fortunately, with careful attention to the clinical features of this complication and improvement of surgical technique, there are far fewer cases. Only anecdotal descriptions of treatment are available with little success.[118,120]

Dyskinetic/Choreoathetoid Cerebral Palsy

The basal ganglia appear to be selectively vulnerable to hypoxic/ischemic or metabolic injury in term infants, possibly because of developmental features of neurophysiologic activity and neurotransmitter expression (Videos 10.7 and 10.8).[121,122] This can result in athetoid cerebral palsy[123] (see Chapter 20 on cerebral palsy for further discussion). A small number of cases of patients with dyskinetic cerebral palsy, some idiopathic, have been described where movements worsen markedly to the point of severe, life-threatening ballism with rhabdomyolysis, during febrile illnesses.[4–6,124]

Kernicterus/Chronic Bilirubin Encephalopathy

CLINICAL FEATURES

The three classic neurologic sequelae in children with chronic bilirubin encephalopathy are hearing loss, hyperkinetic movement disorder, and impaired upgaze.[125–127] Dystonia, athetosis, or choreic movements may be prominent in severe cases in both term and preterm infants,[128] with higher total bilirubin levels overall.[129] Symptoms are chronic. Cognitive impairment is variable. Brain MRI may appear normal in the first year or may have subtle T1 signal hyperintensity in the GPi.[130] Subsequently, damage in the GPi is more obvious, with increased T2 signal.

PATHOPHYSIOLOGY

Damage to selective brain cell populations occurs in the neonatal period. Unconjugated bilirubin elevations occur as part of physiologic jaundice in healthy newborns. Excessive bilirubin elevations may occur because of other factors, including hemolytic diseases of the newborn and excessive bruising during delivery. In most cases, there is a history of markedly elevated serum unconjugated bilirubin in the early postnatal period. However, in some sick infants, chronic sequelae have occurred in the absence of marked hyperbilirubinemia.[128,130] Parameters for neonatal intervention with phototherapy and exchange transfusion have traditionally been based on total bilirubin levels, postconceptual age, and illness in the child. A more relevant laboratory finding may be the molar ratio of bilirubin to albumin (bound bilirubin remains in the blood). Ratios exceeding 0.5 may be a more reliable indicator of risk, as recent case series have emphasized.[128,130] Postmortem studies show bilirubin staining and neuronal damage in globus pallidus, subthalamic nucleus, hippocampus, substantia nigra pars reticulata, and brainstem and cerebellar nuclei.[126,131]

Hyperglycemia/Diabetes–Associated Subacute Hemichorea or Hemiballism

CLINICAL FEATURES

Subacute-onset chorea, hemiballism, or hemichorea have been described in adults, typically elderly adults with chronic hyperglycemia. Women and Asians are more commonly affected, and patients usually present with chorea during an episode of nonketotic hyperglycemia. The chorea is usually transient, although symptoms can persist or relapse. Computed tomography (CT) scans show bright signal in contralateral putamen. MRI shows increased signal in putamen on T1 imaging[132–134] and may show signs of hemorrhage.[135] Uncontrolled diabetes appears to be the main risk factor; however, this clinical and imaging syndrome has been described in diabetic adolescent twins with a polyendocrine deficiency syndrome and a polymerase gamma I (*POLG1*) mutation.[136]

PATHOPHYSIOLOGY

A spectrum of focal striatal pathology may be responsible, as there are reports of focal microhemorrhage and of striatal gliosis.[137,138] A biopsy in an adult patient showed necrosis with thickening and hyaline degeneration of all layers of arteriolar wall.[139] Acute/subacute disruption of function of fronto-striatal pallido-thalamic circuits, particularly because of putamenal pathology, appears to be likely. The hyperglycemic hemichorea–hemiballism syndrome is one manifestation of a movement disorder associated with cerebrovascular disease.[140]

DIAGNOSTIC APPROACH

Laboratory testing should include basic serum chemistries, thyroid studies, lactate, and pyruvate for metabolic disorders. In the case of known or suspected diabetes, appropriate studies including hemoglobin A_{1c} are indicated. Tests for chronic neurodegenerative disorders such as Wilson's disease or pantothenate kinase–associated neurodegeneration would typically not be appropriate in this setting. Neuroimaging should be obtained in cases of acute and subacute hemichorea or hemiballism, particularly if there is no history supportive of SC.

TREATMENT

Acute treatment of hyperglycemia may improve the chorea. In some cases, symptomatic treatment with dopamine receptor blocking or dopamine depleting agents (e.g., tetrabenazine) is needed.[141,142]

Multisystem and Genetic Diseases Where Chorea is Prominent

In most diseases in which heredodegenerative or symptomatic chorea occur, encephalopathy symptoms dominate the movement disorder (Video 10.4). Choreas that occur as part of the ataxias are discussed in Chapter 14. A vast number of genetic diseases (see Table 10.3) and acquired brain insults can preferentially affect the basal ganglia and may result in chorea, athetosis, or ballism. These include hypoxic ischemic injury, viral encephalitides, metabolic insults, hypoxia/anoxic insults, and exposure to heavy metals and other toxins that can produce chorea.

Huntington Disease (HD) with onset in Late Teens

CLINICAL FEATURES

HD (see Figure 10.1) is a neurodegenerative disease that produces chorea, cognitive decline, and psychiatric disturbances in adults. Juvenile/childhood-onset HD typically produces parkinsonism (see Chapter 15) and dystonia, but may also present as chorea (Video 10.1). Onset of HD in late teens may yield motor symptoms more similar to adult cases, including chorea, clumsiness, and speech and gait difficulties, as well as cognitive and emotional disturbances.

DIAGNOSTIC APPROACH

The diagnosis of HD is based on characteristic clinical features, autosomal dominant family history, and detection in the *HTT* gene of an expansion to 36 or more CAG trinucleotide repeats. For a variety of psychological and economic reasons, as well as to respect the autonomy of the individual in adulthood, presymptomatic testing in children is strongly discouraged (Huntington's Disease Society of America, www.hdsa.org). Neurologists familiar with HD in children should be consulted, and, in the presence of characteristic symptoms and family history, diagnostic genetic testing may be performed at an HD center or clinic where psychological and genetic counseling services are available.

TREATMENT

At present, there is no therapy available to prevent neurodegeneration in persons genetically at risk for HD. If future treatments are shown to slow the progression of HD, these recommendations may change. Candidates include coenzyme Q (ubiquinone), a component of the electron transport chain in mitochondria and an antioxidant, which is being tested for several neurodegenerative diseases. In addition, both lithium[143] and the mammalian target of rapamycin inhibitors[144] have shown promise in animal models of HD as they may reduce the toxicity of protein aggregates in HD by upregulating autophagy. In 2008 tetrabenazine was approved by the Food and Drug Administration as treatment for chorea associated with HD.[141,145] Tetrabenazine and other dopamine-depleting drugs currently in development provide only symptomatic relief but do not slow disease progression.[146]

Infantile Bilateral Striatal Necrosis

Choreoathetosis, along with developmental regression, mental retardation, pendular nystagmus, optic atrophy, dysphagia, dystonia, spasticity, and severe bilateral striatal atrophy, is a feature of familial infantile bilateral striatal necrosis (IBSN). IBSN, an extremely rare autosomal recessive neurodegenerative disease, is associated with mutation of nup62 on chromosome 19q13.32-13.41.[147] Biotin may slow disease progression.[148] A summary of other genetic diseases which may have childhood onset and in which chorea may be a feature is shown in Table 10.3.

SUMMARY OF DIAGNOSTIC AND THERAPEUTIC APPROACH

Chorea as an isolated symptom is rare in children but asymptomatic chorea minima is quite common and probably under-recognized. In otherwise healthy children who acquire chorea, poststreptococcal SC is most common, but chorea associated with SLE, APS, hyperthyroidism, toxins, and acute metabolic and vascular injuries may need to be considered. In chronic encephalopathies, chorea may also occur. The presence of acute or chronic chorea suggests disordered neural transmission or structural pathology in the basal ganglia or occasionally in other structures. Athetosis and ballism have similar etiologies. Athetosis is more likely to occur in chronic neurologic conditions, and ballism may occur in SC or as hemiballism in acute basal ganglia injury.

Therapeutics

Etiology-specific treatment is the goal, but is not available in most cases. For autoimmune-mediated forms of chorea, prednisone or other immune-modulating treatments may be helpful.

TABLE 10.3 Genetic Diseases in Which Chorea may be a Feature, Arranged by Disease Category

Disease	Inheritance	Gene	Protein	Clinical features	Age of onset
3-methylglutaconic aciduria type III[149]	AR	OPA3	Optic Atrophy 3 protein (OPA3A and OPA3B)	Early onset optic atrophy and choreiform movement, later spasticity, ataxia, dementia	Infants
Ataxia telangiectasia[36]	AR	ATM	ATM protein	Initial movement disorder may present as predominantly chorea between ages 18 months and 5 years. Movement disorder precedes skin findings	Childhood
Congenital Cataracts, facial dysmorphism, and neuropathy[150]	AR	CTDP1	c-terminal domain of the phosphatase of RNA polymerase II	Multisystem disease with skeletal abnormalities, cataracts and microcornea, progressive neuropathy, hypomyelination, developmental cognitive impairment, hearing loss, mild chorea	Infancy or childhood
Dentatorubral-pallidoluysian atrophy[151]	AD	CAGn in atrophin-1	Atrophin-1	Multisystem neurodegenerative disorder with chorea, tics, dementia, seizures	Has been described in a few children, mainly in adults
Huntington's Chorea / Disease HD[152]	AD	CAGn in HTT	Huntingtin	Juvenile/childhood HD presents with hypokinetic/rigid symptoms, dystonia, and psychiatric problems; early/adolescent onset HD may present with chorea and psychiatric symptoms	Mode is 30–40's, childhood onset cases associated with greater repeat length, paternal inheritance
Huntington's Disease Like - 3 HDL3[153]	AR	Linked to chromosome 4p15.3	N/A	Multisystem neurodegenerative disorder with dystonia, chorea, ataxia, dementia, seizures.	Childhood
Idiopathic basal ganglia calcification (IBGC), childhood onset, aka bilateral striopallidodentate calcinosis[154-156]	AR or AD (adult form)	SLC20A2 or PDGFRB	Sodium-dependent phosphate transporter 2 or platelet-derived growth factor receptor-beta	Infantile onset tetraplegia, chorea, severe cognitive impairment, with basal ganglia calcification. Microcephaly. Early death.	Infancy

Disease	Inheritance	Gene	Protein	Clinical features	Onset
Choreoacanthocytosis[157,158]	AR	VPS13A	Chorein	Multisystem neurodegenerative disorder with chorea, tics, dementia, seizures	Has been described in a few children, mainly in adults
Pontocerebellar hypoplasia type II[159]	AR	TSEN54	tRNA-splicing endonuclease subunit Sen54	Microcephaly, severe cognitive impairment, seizures, poor feeding, severe choreiform dyskinesias, brainstem and cerebellar hypoplasia, early death	Infancy
Spinocerebellar ataxia 1[160]	AD	CAGn in ATXN1	Ataxin 1	Neurodegenerative disease with progressive ataxia, mild cognitive impairment, dysarthria, ophthalmoplegia, spasticity, dystonia, chorea	Childhood
Spinocerebellar ataxia 17[161,162]	AD	CAGn or CAAn in TBP	TATA-Box binding protein	Multisystem neurodegenerative disorder with psychiatric symptoms, nystagmus, ataxia, seizures, cerebral and cerebellar atrophy, dementia. Dystonia, chorea occasionally present	Early adults, adolescents have been reported
Spinocerebellar ataxia 7[163]	AD	CAGn in ATXN7	Ataxin 7	Neurodegenerative disease with progressive ataxia, dysarthria, retinal degeneration, optic atrophy, ophthalmoplegia, spasticity, dystonia, chorea	Childhood
Leigh Syndrome, X-linked[164,165]	X-linked	PDHA1	E1 alpha polypeptide-1 of the pyruvate dehydrogenase complex 1	Multisystem disease with hypotonia, chorea, basal ganglia / cerebral / cerebellar / spinal cord lesions, lactic acidemia, respiratory failure	Infancy or childhood
Nonketotic hyperglycinemia (aka Glycine Encephalopathy)[166,167]	AR	GLDC (P protein) GCST (T protein) GCSH (H protein)	'P', 'T', and 'H' proteins in mitochondrial glycine cleavage system	Neonatal classic: hypotonia, severe myoclonic epilepsy, profound cognitive impairment; restlessness	Infancy or childhood

(*Continued*)

TABLE 10.3 Continued

Disease	Inheritance	Gene	Protein	Clinical features	Age of onset
Paroxysmal Nonkinesogenic Dyskinesia 1[168]	AD	MR1	Myofibrillogenesis regulator-1	Episodic, with choreoathetoid or dystonic movement lasting minutes to hours, usually several times per week, precipitated by stress, caffeine, alcohol	Infancy or childhood
Benign Hereditary Chorea BHC[21,22]	AD	NKX2-1	Thyroid transcription factor TITF1	Non progressive or minimally progressive, normal to slightly subnormal intelligence	Childhood or adolescence
Choreoathetosis, hypothyroidism, neonatal respiratory distress[169,170]	AD	Allelic to BHC	Thyroid transcription factor TITF1	Hypotonia, choreoathetosis, hypothyroidism	Neonatal

It is helpful in considering pharmacologic, symptom-suppressing treatment for chorea to consider the following possible alterations in neurotransmission: (1) relatively increased transmission of dopamine into striatum, particularly into the indirect pathway (see Chapter 1); (2) relatively decreased GABAergic projection from striatum, particularly to the globus pallidus externa; and (3) relative preservation of cholinergic transmission within striatum.

On this basis, chorea suppression with typical, high-potency dopamine receptor blocking agents has been used for many years and is reasonable in cases where chorea causes significant functional interference, particularly in autoimmune conditions where the disease process is likely to be self-limited. Anticonvulsants such as valproic acid, perhaps through increasing striatal gamma-aminobutyric acid, may also be helpful. Anticholinergics should not be used. Similarly, dopaminergic agents—psychostimulants, levodopa–carbidopa, or dopamine agonists—should not be used or should be used in low doses, with caution. Tetrabenazine, a monoamine depleting medication, has been used for years in a variety of hyperkinetic movement disorders, including in children, and has the advantage over dopamine blocking drugs in that it does not cause tardive dyskinesia.[146,171,172]

References

1. Wijemanne S, Jankovic J. Hemidystonia-hemiatrophy syndrome. *Mov Disord*. 2009;24(4):583–589.
2. Gowers WR. *General and Functional Diseases of the Nervous System: Chorea. A Manual of Diseases of the Nervous System*. Philadelphia, PA: Blakiston; 1888.
3. Ferrara J, Jankovic J. Psychogenic movement disorders in children. *Mov Disord*. 2008;23(13):1875–1881.
4. Harbord MG, Kobayashi JS. Fever producing ballismus in patients with choreoathetosis. *J Child Neurol*. 1991;6(1):49–52.
5. Kakinuma H, Hori A, Itoh M, Nakamura T, Takahashi H. An inherited disorder characterized by repeated episodes of bilateral ballism: a case report. *Mov Disord*. 2007;22(14):2110–2112.
6. Okun MS, Jummani RR, Carney PR. Antiphospholipid-associated recurrent chorea and ballism in a child with cerebral palsy. *Pediatr Neurol*. 2000;23(1):62–63.
7. PeBenito R, Talamayan RC. Fever-induced protracted ballismus in choreoathetoid cerebral palsy. *Clin Pediatr*. 2001;40(1):49–51.
8. Zomorrodi A, Wald ER. Sydenham's chorea in western Pennsylvania. *Pediatrics*. 2006;117(4):e675–e679.
9. Cardoso F, Eduardo C, Silva AP, Mota CC. Chorea in fifty consecutive patients with rheumatic fever. *Mov Disord*. 1997;12(5):701–703.
10. Giedd JN, Rapoport JL, Kruesi MJ, et al. Sydenham's chorea: magnetic resonance imaging of the basal ganglia. *Neurology*. 1995;45(12):2199–2202.
11. O'Toole O, Lennon VA, Ahlskog JE, et al. Autoimmune chorea in adults. *Neurology*. 2013;80(12):1133–1144.
12. Foroud T, Gray J, Ivashina J, Conneally PM. Differences in duration of Huntington's disease based on age at onset. *J Neurol Neurosurg Psychiatry*. 1999;66(1):52–56.
13. Cloud LJ, Rosenblatt A, Margolis RL, et al. Seizures in juvenile Huntington's disease: frequency and characterization in a multicenter cohort. *Mov Disord*. 2012;27(14):1797–1800.
14. Rossi Sebastiano D, Soliveri P, Panzica F, et al. Cortical myoclonus in childhood and juvenile onset Huntington's disease. *Parkinsonism Relat Disord*. 2012;18(6):794–797.
15. Hallett M, Kaufman C. Physiological observations in Sydenham's chorea. *J Neurol Neurosurg Psychiatry*. 1981;44(9):829–832.
16. Cole WR, Mostofsky SH, Larson JC, Denckla MB, Mahone EM. Age-related changes in motor subtle signs among girls and boys with ADHD. *Neurology*. 2008;71(19):1514–1520.
17. Haerer AF, Currier RD, Jackson JF. Hereditary nonprogressive chorea of early onset. *N Engl J Med*. 1967;276(22):1220–1224.
18. Inzelberg R, Weinberger M, Gak E. Benign hereditary chorea: an update. *Parkinsonism Relat Disord*. 2011;17(5):301–307.

19. Mencacci NE, Erro R, Wiethoff S, et al. *ADCY5* mutations are another cause of benign hereditary chorea. *Neurology.* 2015;85(1):80–88.
20. Gras D, Jonard L, Roze E, et al. Benign hereditary chorea: phenotype, prognosis, therapeutic outcome and long term follow-up in a large series with new mutations in the TITF1/NKX2-1 gene. *J Neurol Neurosurg Psychiatry.* 2012;83(10):956–962.
21. Peall KJ, Lumsden D, Kneen R, et al. Benign hereditary chorea related to NKX2.1: expansion of the genotypic and phenotypic spectrum. *Dev Med Child Neurol.* 2014;56(7):642–648.
22. Breedveld GJ, van Dongen JW, Danesino C, et al. Mutations in TITF-1 are associated with benign hereditary chorea. *Hum Mol Genet.* 2002;11(8):971–979.
23. Patel NJ, Jankovic J. NKX2-1-related disorders. <http://www.ncbi.nlm.nih.gov/books/NBK185066/>; 2014; Accessed 2014.
24. Kleiner-Fisman G, Rogaeva E, Halliday W, et al. Benign hereditary chorea: clinical, genetic, and pathological findings. *Ann Neurol.* 2003;54(2):244–247.
25. Mahajnah M, Inbar D, Steinmetz A, Heutink P, Breedveld GJ, Straussberg R. Benign hereditary chorea: clinical, neuroimaging, and genetic findings. *J Child Neurol.* 2007;22(10):1231–1234.
26. Hageman G, Ippel PF, van Hout MS, Rozeboom AR. A Dutch family with benign hereditary chorea of early onset: differentiation from Huntington's disease. *Clin Neurol Neurosurg.* 1996;98(2):165–170.
27. Carre A, Szinnai G, Castanet M, et al. Five new TTF1/NKX2.1 mutations in brain-lung-thyroid syndrome: rescue by PAX8 synergism in one case. *Hum Mol Genet.* 2009;18(12):2266–2276.
28. Costa MC, Costa C, Silva AP, et al. Nonsense mutation in TITF1 in a Portuguese family with benign hereditary chorea. *Neurogenetics.* 2005;6(4):209–215.
29. Salvatore E, Di Maio L, Filla A, et al. Benign hereditary chorea: clinical and neuroimaging features in an Italian family. *Mov Disord.* 2010;25(10):1491–1496.
30. Kleiner-Fisman G, Calingasan NY, Putt M, Chen J, Beal MF, Lang AE. Alterations of striatal neurons in benign hereditary chorea. *Mov Disord.* 2005;20(10):1353–1357.
31. Yoshida Y, Nunomura J, Shimohata T, Nanjo H, Miyata H. Benign hereditary chorea 2: pathological findings in an autopsy case. *Neuropathology.* 2012;32(5):557–565.
32. Kimura S, Hara Y, Pineau T, et al. The T/ebp null mouse: thyroid-specific enhancer-binding protein is essential for the organogenesis of the thyroid, lung, ventral forebrain, and pituitary. *Genes Dev.* 1996;10(1):60–69.
33. Sussel L, Marin O, Kimura S, Rubenstein JL. Loss of Nkx2.1 homeobox gene function results in a ventral to dorsal molecular respecification within the basal telencephalon: evidence for a transformation of the pallidum into the striatum. *Development.* 1999;126(15):3359–3370.
34. Butt SJ, Sousa VH, Fuccillo MV, et al. The requirement of Nkx2-1 in the temporal specification of cortical interneuron subtypes. *Neuron.* 2008;59(5):722–732.
35. Flandin P, Kimura S, Rubenstein JL. The progenitor zone of the ventral medial ganglionic eminence requires Nkx2-1 to generate most of the globus pallidus but few neocortical interneurons. *J Neurosci.* 2010;30(8):2812–2823.
36. Lavin MF, Gueven N, Bottle S, Gatti RA. Current and potential therapeutic strategies for the treatment of ataxia-telangiectasia. *Br Med Bull.* 2007;81–82:129–147.
37. Cabana MD, Crawford TO, Winkelstein JA, Christensen JR, Lederman HM. Consequences of the delayed diagnosis of ataxia-telangiectasia. *Pediatrics.* 1998;102(1 Pt 1):98–100.
38. Heiman GA, Ottman R, Saunders-Pullman RJ, Ozelius LJ, Risch NJ, Bressman SB. Obsessive-compulsive disorder is not a clinical manifestation of the DYT1 dystonia gene. *Am J Med Genet B Neuropsychiatr Genet.* 2007;144B(3):361–364.
39. Hess CW, Raymond D, Aguiar Pde C, et al. Myoclonus-dystonia, obsessive-compulsive disorder, and alcohol dependence in SGCE mutation carriers. *Neurology.* 2007;68(7):522–524.
40. Asmus F, Horber V, Pohlenz J, et al. A novel TITF-1 mutation causes benign hereditary chorea with response to levodopa. *Neurology.* 2005;64(11):1952–1954.
41. Salvado M, Boronat-Guerrero S, Hernandez-Vara J, Alvarez-Sabin J. Chorea due to TITF1/NKX2-1 mutation: phenotypical description and therapeutic response in a family. *Rev Neurol.* 2013;56(10):515–520.
42. Baizabal-Carvallo JF, Jankovic J. Movement disorders in autoimmune diseases. *Mov Disord.* 2012;27(8):935–946.
43. Johnson DR, Kurlan R, Leckman J, Kaplan EL. The human immune response to streptococcal extracellular antigens: clinical, diagnostic, and potential pathogenetic implications. *Clin Infect Dis.* 2010;50(4):481–490.
44. Pickering LK, ed. *American Academy of Pediatrics 2006 Group A Streptococcal Infections. Red Book: 2006 Report of the Committee on Infectious Diseases.* Elk Grove, IL: American Academy of Pediatrics; 2006.

45. Ridel KR, Lipps TD, Gilbert DL. The prevalence of neuropsychiatric disorders in Sydenham's chorea. *Pediatr Neurol*. 2010;42(4):243–248.

46. Murphy TK, Snider LA, Mutch PJ, et al. Relationship of movements and behaviors to Group A Streptococcus infections in elementary school children. *Biol Psychiatry*. 2007;61(3):279–284.

47. Asbahr FR, Garvey MA, Snider LA, Zanetta DM, Elkis H, Swedo SE. Obsessive-compulsive symptoms among patients with Sydenham chorea. *Biol Psychiatry*. 2005;57(9):1073–1076.

48. Freeman JM, Aron AM, Collard JE, Mackay MC. The emotional correlates of Sydenham's chorea. *Pediatrics*. 1965;35:42–49.

49. Kirvan CA, Cox CJ, Swedo SE, Cunningham MW. Tubulin is a neuronal target of autoantibodies in Sydenham's chorea. *J Immunol*. 2007;178(11):7412–7421.

50. Maia DP, Teixeira Jr. AL, Quintao Cunningham MC, Cardoso F. Obsessive compulsive behavior, hyperactivity, and attention deficit disorder in Sydenham chorea. *Neurology*. 2005;64(10):1799–1801.

51. Hounie AG, Pauls DL, do Rosario-Campos MC, et al. Obsessive-compulsive spectrum disorders and rheumatic fever: a family study. *Biol Psychiatry*. 2007;61(3):266–272.

52. Bye AM, Cunningham CA, Chee KY, Flanagan D. Outcome of neonates with electrographically identified seizures, or at risk of seizures. *Pediatr Neurol*. 1997;16(3):225–231.

53. Ekici F, Cetin II, Cevik BS, et al. What is the outcome of rheumatic carditis in children with Sydenham's chorea? *Turk J Pediatr*. 2012;54(2):159–167.

54. Aron AM, Freeman JM, Carter S. The natural history of Sydenham's chorea. Review of the literature and long-term evaluation with emphasis on cardiac sequelae. *Am J Med*. 1965;38:83–95.

55. Paz JA, Silva CA, Marques-Dias MJ. Randomized double-blind study with prednisone in Sydenham's chorea. *Pediatr Neurol*. 2006;34(4):264–269.

56. Cardoso F, Vargas AP, Oliveira LD, Guerra AA, Amaral SV. Persistent Sydenham's chorea. *Mov Disord*. 1999;14(5):805–807.

57. Maia DP, Fonseca PG, Camargos ST, Pfannes C, Cunningham MC, Cardoso F. Pregnancy in patients with Sydenham's Chorea. *Parkinsonism Relat Disord*. 2012;18(5):458–461.

58. Barreto LB, Maciel ROH, Maia DP, Teixeira AL, Cardoso F. Parkinsonian signs and symptoms in adults with a history of Sydenham's chorea. *Parkinsonism Relat Disord*. 2012;18(5):595–597.

59. Beato R, Maia DP, Teixeira Jr. AL, Cardoso F. Executive functioning in adult patients with Sydenham's chorea. *Mov Disord*. 2010;25(7):853–857.

60. Swedo SE, Leonard HL, Garvey M, et al. Pediatric autoimmune neuropsychiatric disorders associated with streptococcal infections: clinical description of the first 50 cases. *Am J Psychiatry*. 1998;155(2):264–271.

61. Kurlan R, Johnson D, Kaplan EL. Streptococcal infection and exacerbations of childhood tics and obsessive-compulsive symptoms: a prospective blinded cohort study. *Pediatrics*. 2008;121(6):1188–1197.

62. Leckman JF, King RA, Gilbert DL, et al. Streptococcal upper respiratory tract infections and exacerbations of tic and obsessive-compulsive symptoms: a prospective longitudinal study. *J Am Acad Child Adolesc Psychiatry*. 2011;50(2):108–118. e103.

63. Gilbert DL. The relationship between group A streptococcal infections and Tourette syndrome. *Dev Med Child Neurol*. 2011;53(10):883–884.

64. Dale RC, Merheb V, Pillai S, et al. Antibodies to surface dopamine-2 receptor in autoimmune movement and psychiatric disorders. *Brain*. 2012;135(Pt 11):3453–3468.

65. Singer HS, Mascaro-Blanco A, Alvarez K, et al. Neuronal antibody biomarkers for sydenham's chorea identify a new group of children with chronic recurrent episodic acute exacerbations of tic and obsessive compulsive symptoms following a streptococcal infection. *PLOS ONE*. 2015;10(3):e0120499.

66. Hallett JJ, Harling-Berg CJ, Knopf PM, Stopa EG, Kiessling LS. Anti-striatal antibodies in Tourette syndrome cause neuronal dysfunction. *J Neuroimmunol*. 2000;111(1–2):195–202.

67. Brimberg L, Benhar I, Mascaro-Blanco A, et al. Behavioral, pharmacological, and immunological abnormalities after streptococcal exposure: a novel rat model of Sydenham chorea and related neuropsychiatric disorders. *Neuropsychopharmacology*. 2012;37(9):2076–2087.

68. Cox CJ, Sharma M, Leckman JF, et al. Brain human monoclonal autoantibody from Sydenham chorea targets dopaminergic neurons in transgenic mice and signals dopamine D2 receptor: implications in human disease. *J Immunol*. 2013;191(11):5524–5541.

69. Singer HS, Mink JW, Loiselle CR, et al. Microinfusion of antineuronal antibodies into rodent striatum: failure to differentiate between elevated and low titers. *J Neuroimmunol*. 2005;163(1–2):8–14.

70. Ben-Pazi H, Sadan O, Offen D. Striatal microinjection of Sydenham chorea antibodies: using a rat model to examine the dopamine hypothesis. *J Mol Neurosci*. 2012;46(1):162–166.
71. Macerollo A, Martino D. Pediatric autoimmune neuropsychiatric disorders associated with streptococcal infections (PANDAS): an evolving concept. *Tremor Other Hyperkinet Mov (N Y)*. 2013:3.
72. Chang K, Frankovich J, Cooperstock M, et al. Clinical evaluation of youth with pediatric acute onset neuropsychiatric syndrome (PANS): recommendations from the 2013 PANS consensus conference. *J Child Adolesc Psychopharmacol*. 2014.
73. Taranta A, Stollerman GH. The relationship of Sydenham's chorea to infection with group A streptococci. *Am J Med*. 1956;20(2):170–175.
74. Husby G, van de Rijn I, Zabriskie JB, Abdin ZH, Williams Jr. RC. Antibodies reacting with cytoplasm of subthalamic and caudate nuclei neurons in chorea and acute rheumatic fever. *J Exp Med*. 1976;144(4):1094–1110.
75. Doyle F, Cardoso F, Lopes L, et al. Infusion of Sydenham's chorea antibodies in striatum with up-regulated dopaminergic receptors: a pilot study to investigate the potential of SC antibodies to increase dopaminergic activity. *Neurosci Lett*. 2012;523(2):186–189.
76. Husby G, Li L, Davis LE, Wedege E, Kokmen E, Williams Jr. RC. Antibodies to human caudate nucleus neurons in Huntington's chorea. *J Clin Invest*. 1977;59(5):922–932.
77. Singer HS, Hong JJ, Yoon DY, Williams PN. Serum autoantibodies do not differentiate PANDAS and Tourette syndrome from controls. *Neurology*. 2005;65(11):1701–1707.
78. Bronze MS, Dale JB. Epitopes of streptococcal M proteins that evoke antibodies that cross-react with human brain. *J Immunol*. 1993;151(5):2820–2828.
79. Farooq O, Memon Z, Stojanovski SD, Faden HS. Azithromycin-induced agitation and choreoathetosis. *Pediatr Neurol*. 2011;44(4):311–313.
80. Seeherunvong T, Diamantopoulos S, Berkovitz GD. A nine year old girl with thyrotoxicosis, ataxia, and chorea. *Brain Dev*. 2007;29(10):660–661.
81. Wong LJ, Naviaux RK, Brunetti-Pierri N, et al. Molecular and clinical genetics of mitochondrial diseases due to POLG mutations. *Hum Mutat*. 2008;29(9):E150–E172.
82. Isaacs KM, Johnson MD, Kao E, Gilbert DL. Childhood disorders: another perspective. In: Hallett M, Lang AE, Jankovic J, Fahn S, Halligan P, Voon V, eds. *Psychogenic Movement Disorders and Other Conversion Disorders*. Cambridge, UK: Cambridge University Press; 2011:56–58.
83. Ayoub EM, Wannamaker LW. Streptococcal antibody titers in Sydenham's chorea. *Pediatrics*. 1966;38(6): 946–956.
84. Ayoub EM, Nelson B, Shulman ST, et al. Group A streptococcal antibodies in subjects with or without rheumatic fever in areas with high or low incidences of rheumatic fever. *Clin Diagn Lab Immunol*. 2003;10(5):886–890.
85. Faustino PC, Terreri MT, da Rocha AJ, Zappitelli MC, Lederman HM, Hilario MO. Clinical, laboratory, psychiatric and magnetic resonance findings in patients with Sydenham chorea. *Neuroradiology*. 2003;45(7):456–462.
86. Cardenas JF, Chapman K. Sydenham's chorea as a presentation of Moyamoya disease. *Semin Pediatr Neurol*. 2010;17(1):30–34.
87. Barsottini OG, Ferraz HB, Seviliano MM, Barbieri A. Brain SPECT imaging in Sydenham's chorea. *Braz J Med Biol Res*. 2002;35(4):431–436.
88. Kabakus N, Balci TA, Kurt A, Kurt AN. Cerebral blood flow abnormalities in children with Sydenham's chorea: a SPECT study [see comment]. *Indian Pediatr*. 2006;43(3):241–246.
89. Lee PH, Nam HS, Lee KY, Lee BI, Lee JD. Serial brain SPECT images in a case of Sydenham chorea. *Arch Neurol*. 1999;56(2):237–240.
90. Aron AM. Sydenham's chorea: positron emission tomographic (PET) scan studies. *J Child Neurol*. 2005;20(10):832–833.
91. Gumus H, Gumus G, Per H, et al. Diffusion-weighted imaging in Sydenham's chorea. *Childs Nerv Syst*. 2013;29(1):125–130.
92. Ekici F, Cetin II, Cevik B-S, et al. What is the outcome of rheumatic carditis in children with Sydenham's chorea? *Turk J Pediatr*. 2012;54(2):159–167.
93. Panamonta M, Chaikitpinyo A, Auvichayapat N, Weraarchakul W, Panamonta O, Pantongwiriyakul A. Evolution of valve damage in Sydenham's chorea during recurrence of rheumatic fever. *Int J Cardiol*. 2007;119(1):73–79.
94. Daoud AS, Zaki M, Shakir R, al-Saleh Q. Effectiveness of sodium valproate in the treatment of Sydenham's chorea. *Neurology*. 1990;40(7):1140–1141.

95. Kulkarni ML. Sodium valproate controls choreoathetoid movements of kernicterus. *Indian Pediatr*. 1992;29(8):1029–1030.

96. Diaz-Grez F, Lay-Son L, del Barrio-Guerrero E, Vidal-Gonzalez P. Sydenham's chorea. A clinical analysis of 55 patients with a prolonged follow-up. *Rev Neurol*. 2004;39(9):810–815.

97. Fahn S, Jankovic J. Chorea, ballism, athetosis: phenomenology and etiology *Principles and Practice of Movement Disorders*. Philadelphia, PA: Churchill Livingstone/Elsevier; 2007: 393–407.

98. Garvey MA, Snider LA, Leitman SF, Werden R, Swedo SE. Treatment of Sydenham's chorea with intravenous immunoglobulin, plasma exchange, or prednisone. *J Child Neurol*. 2005;20(5):424–429.

99. El Otmani H, Moutaouakil F, Fadel H, Slassi I. Chorea paralytica: a videotape case with rapid recovery and good long-term outcome. *Acta Neurol Belg*. 2013;113(4):515–517.

100. Fusco C, Ucchino V, Frattini D, Pisani F, Della Giustina E. Acute and chronic corticosteroid treatment of ten patients with paralytic form of Sydenham's chorea. *Europ J Paediatr Neurol*. 2012;16(4):373–378.

101. Walker AR, Tani LY, Thompson JA, Firth SD, Veasy LG, Bale Jr. JF. Rheumatic chorea: relationship to systemic manifestations and response to corticosteroids. *J Pediatr*. 2007;151(6):679–683.

102. van Immerzeel TD, van Gilst RM, Hartwig NG. Beneficial use of immunoglobulins in the treatment of Sydenham chorea. *Eur J Pediatr*. 2010;169(9):1151–1154.

103. Walker K, Brink A, Lawrenson J, Mathiassen W, Wilmshurst JM. Treatment of Sydenham chorea with intravenous immunoglobulin. *J Child Neurol*. 2012;27(2):147–155.

104. Cimaz R, Gana S, Braccesi G, Guerrini R. Sydenham's chorea in a girl with juvenile idiopathic arthritis treated with anti-TNFalpha therapy. *Mov Disord*. 2010;25(4):511–514.

105. Baizabal-Carvallo JF, Bonnet C, Jankovic J. Movement disorders in systemic lupus erythematosus and the antiphospholipid syndrome. *J Neural Transm*. 2013;120(11):1579–1589.

106. Katzav A, Chapman J, Shoenfeld Y. CNS dysfunction in the antiphospholipid syndrome. *Lupus*. 2003;12(12):903–907.

107. Cervera R, Piette JC, Font J, et al. Antiphospholipid syndrome: clinical and immunologic manifestations and patterns of disease expression in a cohort of 1,000 patients. *Arthritis Rheum*. 2002;46(4):1019–1027.

108. Kiechl-Kohlendorfer U, Ellemunter H, Kiechl S. Chorea as the presenting clinical feature of primary antiphospholipid syndrome in childhood [see comment]. *Neuropediatrics*. 1999;30(2):96–98.

109. Demonty J, Gonce M, Ribai P, Verellen-Dumoulin C, Hustinx R. Chorea associated with anti-phospholipid antibodies: case report. *Acta Clin Belg*. 2010;65(5):350–353.

110. Dalmau J, Gleichman AJ, Hughes EG, et al. Anti-NMDA-receptor encephalitis: case series and analysis of the effects of antibodies. *Lancet Neurol*. 2008;7(12):1091–1098.

111. Baizabal-Carvallo JF, Stocco A, Muscal E, Jankovic J. The spectrum of movement disorders in children with anti-NMDA receptor encephalitis. *Mov Disord*. 2013;28(4):543–547.

112. Mohammad SS, Fung VS, Grattan-Smith P, et al. Movement disorders in children with anti-NMDAR encephalitis and other autoimmune encephalopathies. *Mov Disord*. 2014;29(12):1539–1542.

113. Kayser MS, Titulaer MJ, Gresa-Arribas N, Dalmau J. Frequency and characteristics of isolated psychiatric episodes in anti-*N*-methyl-ᴅ-aspartate receptor encephalitis. *JAMA Neurol*. 2013;70(9):1133–1139.

114. Armangue T, Titulaer MJ, Malaga I, et al. Pediatric anti-*N*-methyl-ᴅ-aspartate receptor encephalitis-clinical analysis and novel findings in a series of 20 patients. *J Pediatr*. 2013;162(4):850–856.e852.

115. Ahn ES, Scott RM, Robertson Jr. RL, Smith ER. Chorea in the clinical presentation of Moyamoya disease: results of surgical revascularization and a proposed clinicopathological correlation. *J Neurosurg Pediatr*. 2013;11(3):313–319.

116. du Plessis AJ, Bellinger DC, Gauvreau K, et al. Neurologic outcome of choreoathetoid encephalopathy after cardiac surgery. *Pediatric Neurol*. 2002;27(1):9–17.

117. Holden KR, Sessions JC, Cure J, Whitcomb DS, Sade RM. Neurologic outcomes in children with post-pump choreoathetosis. *J Pediatr*. 1998;132(1):162–164.

118. Medlock MD, Cruse RS, Winek SJ, et al. A 10-year experience with postpump chorea. *Ann Neurol*. 1993;34(6):820–826.

119. Kupsky WJ, Drozd MA, Barlow CF. Selective injury of the globus pallidus in children with post-cardiac surgery choreic syndrome. *Dev Med Child Neurol*. 1995;37(2):135–144.

120. Kirkham FJ. Recognition and prevention of neurological complications in pediatric cardiac surgery. *Pediatr Cardiol*. 1998;19(4):331–345.

121. Calabresi P, Centonze D, Bernardi G. Cellular factors controlling neuronal vulnerability in the brain: a lesson from the striatum. *Neurology*. 2000;55(9):1249–1255.

122. Johnston MV, Hoon Jr. AH. Possible mechanisms in infants for selective basal ganglia damage from asphyxia, kernicterus, or mitochondrial encephalopathies. *J Child Neurol.* 2000;15(9):588–591.

123. Morris JG, Grattan-Smith P, Jankelowitz SK, Fung VS, Clouston PD, Hayes MW. Athetosis II: the syndrome of mild athetoid cerebral palsy. *Mov Disord.* 2002;17(6):1281–1287.

124. Beran-Koehn MA, Zupanc ML, Patterson MC, Olk DG, Ahlskog JE. Violent recurrent ballism associated with infections in two children with static encephalopathy. *Mov Disord.* 2000;15(3):570–574.

125. Connolly AM, Volpe JJ. Clinical features of bilirubin encephalopathy. *Clin Perinatol.* 1990;17(2):371–379.

126. Shapiro SM. Chronic bilirubin encephalopathy: diagnosis and outcome. *Semin Fetal Neonatal Med.* 2010;15(3):157–163.

127. Watchko JF, Tiribelli C. Bilirubin-induced neurologic damage—mechanisms and management approaches. *N Engl J Med.* 2013;369(21):2021–2030.

128. Merhar SL, Gilbert DL. Clinical (video) findings and cerebrospinal fluid neurotransmitters in 2 children with severe chronic bilirubin encephalopathy, including a former preterm infant without marked hyperbilirubinemia [video]. *Pediatrics.* 2005;116(5):1226–1230.

129. Powers KM, Miller SJ, Shapiro SM. Exposure to excessive hyperbilirubinemia earlier in neurodevelopment is associated with auditory-predominant kernicterus subtype. *Ann Neurol.* 2008;64(S12):S105.

130. Govaert P, Lequin M, Swarte R, et al. Changes in globus pallidus with (pre)term kernicterus. *Pediatrics.* 2003;112(6 Pt 1):1256–1263.

131. Ahdab-Barmada M, Moossy J. The neuropathology of kernicterus in the premature neonate: diagnostic problems. *J Neuropathol Exp Neurol.* 1984;43(1):45–56.

132. Ahlskog JE, Nishino H, Evidente VG, et al. Persistent chorea triggered by hyperglycemic crisis in diabetics. *Mov Disord.* 2001;16(5):890–898.

133. Lai PH, Tien RD, Chang MH, et al. Chorea-ballismus with nonketotic hyperglycemia in primary diabetes mellitus. *Am J Neuroradiol.* 1996;17(6):1057–1064.

134. Oh SH, Lee KY, Im JH, Lee MS. Chorea associated with non-ketotic hyperglycemia and hyperintensity basal ganglia lesion on T1-weighted brain MRI study: a meta-analysis of 53 cases including four present cases. *J Neurol Sci.* 2002;200(1–2):57–62.

135. Alves C, Sampaio S, Barbosa V, Machado M. Acute chorea and type 1 diabetes mellitus: clinical and neuroimaging findings. *Pediatr Diabetes.* 2012;13(6):e30–e34.

136. Hopkins SE, Somoza A, Gilbert DL. Rare autosomal dominant POLG1 mutation in a family with metabolic strokes, posterior column spinal degeneration, and multi-endocrine disease. *J Child Neurol.* 2010;25(6):752–756.

137. Mestre TA, Ferreira JJ, Pimentel J. Putamenal petechial haemorrhage as the cause of non-ketotic hyperglycaemic chorea: a neuropathological case correlated with MRI findings. *J Neurol Neurosurg Psychiatry.* 2007;78(5):549–550.

138. Ohara S, Nakagawa S, Tabata K, Hashimoto T. Hemiballism with hyperglycemia and striatal T1-MRI hyperintensity: an autopsy report. *Mov Disord.* 2001;16(3):521–525.

139. Abe Y, Yamamoto T, Soeda T, et al. Diabetic striatal disease: clinical presentation, neuroimaging, and pathology. *Intern Med.* 2009;48(13):1135–1141.

140. Mehanna R, Jankovic J. Movement disorders in cerebrovascular disease. *Lancet Neurol.* 2013;12(6):597–608.

141. Kenney C, Hunter C, Davidson A, Jankovic J. Short-term effects of tetrabenazine on chorea associated with Huntington's disease. *Mov Disord.* 2007;22(1):10–13.

142. Kenney C, Jankovic J. Tetrabenazine in the treatment of hyperkinetic movement disorders. *Expert Rev Neurother.* 2006;6(1):7–17.

143. Sarkar S, Floto RA, Berger Z, et al. Lithium induces autophagy by inhibiting inositol monophosphatase. *J Cell Biol.* 2005;170(7):1101–1111.

144. Ravikumar B, Vacher C, Berger Z, et al. Inhibition of mTOR induces autophagy and reduces toxicity of polyglutamine expansions in fly and mouse models of Huntington disease. *Nat Genet.* 2004;36(6):585–595.

145. Frank S, Ondo W, Fahn S, et al. A study of chorea after tetrabenazine withdrawal in patients with Huntington disease. *Clin Neuropharmacol.* 2008;31(3):127–133.

146. Jankovic J, Roos RA. Chorea associated with Huntington's disease: to treat or not to treat? *Mov Disord.* 2014;29(11):1414–1418.

147. Basel-Vanagaite L, Muncher L, Straussberg R, et al. Mutated nup62 causes autosomal recessive infantile bilateral striatal necrosis. *Ann Neurol.* 2006;60(2):214–222.

148. Straussberg R, Shorer Z, Weitz R, et al. Familial infantile bilateral striatal necrosis: clinical features and response to biotin treatment. *Neurology.* 2002;59(7):983–989.

149. Anikster Y, Kleta R, Shaag A, Gahl WA, Elpeleg O. Type III 3-methylglutaconic aciduria (optic atrophy plus syndrome, or Costeff optic atrophy syndrome): identification of the OPA3 gene and its founder mutation in Iraqi Jews. *Am J Hum Genet*. 2001;69(6):1218–1224.

150. Varon R, Gooding R, Steglich C, et al. Partial deficiency of the C-terminal-domain phosphatase of RNA polymerase II is associated with congenital cataracts facial dysmorphism neuropathy syndrome. *Nat Genet*. 2003;35(2):185–189.

151. Burke JR, Wingfield MS, Lewis KE, et al. The Haw River syndrome: dentatorubropallidoluysian atrophy (DRPLA) in an African-American family. *Nat Genet*. 1994;7(4):521–524.

152. Letort D, Gonzalez-Alegre P. Huntington's disease in children. *Handb Clin Neurol*. 2013;113:1913–1917.

153. Kambouris M, Bohlega S, Al-Tahan A, Meyer BF. Localization of the gene for a novel autosomal recessive neurodegenerative Huntington-like disorder to 4p15.3. *Am J Hum Genet*. 2000;66(2):445–452.

154. Hsu SC, Sears RL, Lemos RR, et al. Mutations in SLC20A2 are a major cause of familial idiopathic basal ganglia calcification. *Neurogenetics*. 2013;14(1):11–22.

155. Nicolas G, Pottier C, Maltete D, et al. Mutation of the PDGFRB gene as a cause of idiopathic basal ganglia calcification. *Neurology*. 2013;80(2):181–187.

156. Wang C, Li Y, Shi L, et al. Mutations in SLC20A2 link familial idiopathic basal ganglia calcification with phosphate homeostasis. *Nat Genet*. 2012;44(3):254–256.

157. Rampoldi L, Dobson-Stone C, Rubio JP, et al. A conserved sorting-associated protein is mutant in chorea-acanthocytosis. *Nat Genet*. 2001;28(2):119–120.

158. Ueno S, Maruki Y, Nakamura M, et al. The gene encoding a newly discovered protein, chorein, is mutated in chorea-acanthocytosis. *Nat Genet*. 2001;28(2):121–122.

159. Budde BS, Namavar Y, Barth PG, et al. tRNA splicing endonuclease mutations cause pontocerebellar hypoplasia. *Nat Genet*. 2008;40(9):1113–1118.

160. Banfi S, Servadio A, Chung MY, et al. Identification and characterization of the gene causing type 1 spinocerebellar ataxia. *Nat Genet*. 1994;7(4):513–520.

161. Koide R, Kobayashi S, Shimohata T, et al. A neurological disease caused by an expanded CAG trinucleotide repeat in the TATA-binding protein gene: a new polyglutamine disease? *Hum Mol Genet*. 1999;8(11):2047–2053.

162. Nakamura K, Jeong SY, Uchihara T, et al. SCA17, a novel autosomal dominant cerebellar ataxia caused by an expanded polyglutamine in TATA-binding protein. *Hum Mol Genet*. 2001;10(14):1441–1448.

163. David S, Kelly C, Poppas DP. Nerve sparing extravesical repair of bilateral vesicoureteral reflux: description of technique and evaluation of urinary retention. *J Urol*. 2004;172(4 Pt 2):1617–1620, discussion 1620.

164. Matthews PM, Marchington DR, Squier M, Land J, Brown RM, Brown GK. Molecular genetic characterization of an X-linked form of Leigh's syndrome. *Ann Neurol*. 1993;33(6):652–655.

165. Naito E, Ito M, Yokota I, et al. Biochemical and molecular analysis of an X-linked case of Leigh syndrome associated with thiamin-responsive pyruvate dehydrogenase deficiency. *J Inherit Metab Dis*. 1997;20(4):539–548.

166. Takayanagi M, Kure S, Sakata Y, et al. Human glycine decarboxylase gene (GLDC) and its highly conserved processed pseudogene (psiGLDC): their structure and expression, and the identification of a large deletion in a family with nonketotic hyperglycinemia. *Hum Genet*. 2000;106(3):298–305.

167. Dinopoulos A, Kure S, Chuck G, et al. Glycine decarboxylase mutations: a distinctive phenotype of nonketotic hyperglycinemia in adults. *Neurology*. 2005;64(7):1255–1257.

168. Rainier S, Thomas D, Tokarz D, et al. Myofibrillogenesis regulator 1 gene mutations cause paroxysmal dystonic choreoathetosis [see comment]. *Arch Neurol*. 2004;61(7):1025–1029.

169. Devriendt K, Vanhole C, Matthijs G, de Zegher F. Deletion of thyroid transcription factor-1 gene in an infant with neonatal thyroid dysfunction and respiratory failure. *N Engl J Med*. 1998;338(18):1317–1318.

170. Krude H, Schutz B, Biebermann H, et al. Choreoathetosis, hypothyroidism, and pulmonary alterations due to human NKX2-1 haploinsufficiency. *J Clin Invest*. 2002;109(4):475–480.

171. Kenney C, Hunter C, Jankovic J. Long-term tolerability of tetrabenazine in the treatment of hyperkinetic movement disorders. *Mov Disord*. 2007;22(2):193–197.

172. Jankovic J, Beach J. Long-term effects of tetrabenazine in hyperkinetic movement disorders. *Neurology*. 1997;48(2):358–362.

Dystonia

*Harvey S. Singer[1], Jonathan W. Mink[2],
Donald L. Gilbert[3] and Joseph Jankovic[4]*

[1]Department of Neurology, Johns Hopkins Hospital, Baltimore, MD, USA;
[2]Division of Child Neurology, University of Rochester Medical Center,
Rochester, NY, USA; [3]Division of Neurology, Cincinnati Children's Hospital
Medical Center, Cincinnati, OH, USA; [4]Department of Neurology, Baylor
College of Medicine, Houston, TX, USA

OUTLINE

Movement Disorders in Childhood, Second Edition.
DOI: http://dx.doi.org/10.1016/B978-0-12-411573-6.00011-5

INTRODUCTION

The use of the term "dystonia" appears to have originated with Oppenheim coining the term "dystonia musculorum deformans" in 1911 to name a progressive childhood-onset syndrome characterized by twisted postures, muscle spasms, bizarre walking with bending and twisting of the trunk, and eventually fixed postural deformities.[1] The hallmark of dystonia for Oppenheim was the apparent unpredictable fluctuation of tone. Wilson argued against the term dystonia, because he viewed the disorder as one of movement and not of tone.[2] Denny-Brown used "dystonia" to refer to any abnormal posture that resists displacement such that a displaced body part tends to return to its initial posture.[3] Over the years, there have been numerous attempts to refine the definition of dystonia. In 1984, the Dystonia Medical Research Foundation provided the first consensus definition of dystonia as a syndrome consisting "of sustained muscle contractions, frequently causing twisting and repetitive movements, or abnormal postures."[4] This was in wide-spread use until recently, when an international consensus committee was established by the Dystonia Medical Research Foundation, the Dystonia Coalition, and the European Dystonia COST Action to review and revise the definition.[5] The revised International Consensus is as follows:

> Dystonia is defined as a movement disorder characterized by sustained or intermittent muscle contractions causing abnormal, often repetitive, movements, postures, or both. Dystonic movements are typically patterned, twisting, and may be tremulous. Dystonia is often initiated or worsened by voluntary action and associated with overflow muscle activation.

Many characteristic clinical features of dystonia are present regardless of age, etiology, or affected body parts. Some of these features are seen in several types of movement disorders, but others are relatively specific to dystonia. These features can aid in the diagnosis of dystonia and in distinguishing organic dystonias from functional dystonia (Chapter 23). Dystonic contractions cannot be suppressed voluntarily. Indeed, the biggest problem in dystonia appears to be the inability to relax unwanted muscle activity. Dystonia may be absent when the patient is at rest, but appear with mental activity or attempted voluntary movement of the affected or distant body parts. Dystonia may fluctuate in presence and severity over time. The "patterned" nature of movements is a characteristic feature of dystonia. Two important characteristic features of dystonia are task-specificity and the so-called "geste antagoniste" or sensory trick. These features are typically not seen in other hyperkinetic movement disorders and may be important clues to understanding the underlying pathophysiology of dystonia.

Task-specificity has been most frequently described in focal dystonias, but patients with segmental and generalized dystonia often have exacerbation of their dystonia when performing a skilled movement. Task-specificity manifests as dystonic posturing occurring only with selected movements and paradoxically not with others that may use the same muscles. For example, a patient with writer's cramp may have dystonia only while writing, but not while knitting, typing, or using a screwdriver. In cranial dystonia, lower facial grimacing may occur only when talking and not when eating. The strained, strangled speech of adductor laryngeal dystonia may only affect talking, but not singing, whispering, or breathing. Walking forward may elicit severe lower extremity and truncal twisting, yet walking backward, running, or swimming may be completely normal in someone with generalized dystonia. Some people with generalized dystonia can dance, but cannot walk. All of these observations suggest that the dysfunctional motor control is at a level higher than the final output for selected muscle contraction.

Many people with dystonia find that lightly touching a part of the body may relieve dystonic spasms in that or adjacent body parts. This phenomenon, called a sensory trick, or *geste antagoniste*, has been described best in isolated or inherited dystonias, but can occur in certain acquired dystonias, too. Examples of *geste antagoniste* include touching near the lateral canthus may relieve the eyelid squeezing of blepharospasm; a straw in the mouth may reduce jaw closing dystonia; touching the side of the chin may decrease cervical dystonia; and rubbing the back of the hand may diminish writer's cramp. Even in generalized dystonia, light touch to the neck or an affected limb may transiently reduce dystonic contractions.

CLASSIFICATION OF DYSTONIAS

The etiologies of dystonia in childhood are numerous. In many disorders, dystonia exists as just one neurological sign or symptoms among others. In other disorders, dystonia is the main or the only manifestation. A common approach to the classification of disorders characterized by dystonia divides them into primary (idiopathic) and secondary etiologies. Primary dystonias lack other neurological deficits and are distinguished further from secondary dystonias by lack of an identifiable etiology such as birth injury, stroke, or drug reaction.[6] Another classification scheme considers "primary dystonias" to be disorders that consist of only dystonia or of dystonia plus tremor. Disorders consisting of dystonia and other movement disorders are referred to as "dystonia-plus."[7,8] As additional specific genetic etiologies have been identified and as the phenotypes of primary dystonias are further clarified and reveal comorbid neurological and psychiatric manifestations, division into primary and secondary categories has proven to be increasingly difficult. In recognition of the changing landscape, an International Consensus Committee has recently recommended abandoning the use of "primary" and "secondary" as a classification scheme.[5]

A recently revised classification scheme identifies two distinct axes: clinical features and etiology. A combination of these two axes provides meaningful information on any dystonia patient that can serve to guide diagnosis and to develop research and treatment strategies (Tables 11.1 and 11.2).[5]

TABLE 11.1   Classification of Dystonia: Clinical Characteristics (Axis I)[5]

CLINICAL CHARACTERISTICS OF DYSTONIA

• Age at onset	• Infancy (birth to 2 years) • Childhood (3–12 years) • Adolescence (13–20 years) • Early adulthood (21–40 years) • Late adulthood (>40 years)
• Body distribution	• Focal • Segmental • Multifocal • Generalized (with or without leg involvement) • Hemidystonia

• Temporal patterns	• Disease course
	  ○ Static
	  ○ Progressive
	• Variability
	  ○ Persistent
	  ○ Action-specific
	  ○ Diurnal
	  ○ Paroxysmal

ASSOCIATED FEATURES

• Isolated dystonia or combined with another movement disorder	• Isolated dystonia • Combined dystonia
• Occurrence of other neurological or systemic manifestations	• List of co-occurring neurological manifestations

TABLE 11.2   Classification of Dystonia: Etiology (Axis II)[5]

• Nervous system pathology	• Evidence of degeneration • Evidence of static lesions • No evidence of degeneration or structural lesion

• Inherited or acquired	• Inherited
	  ○ Autosomal dominant
	  ○ Autosomal recessive
	  ○ X-linked recessive
	  ○ Mitochondrial
	• Acquired
	  ○ Perinatal brain injury
	  ○ Infection
	  ○ Drug
	  ○ Toxic
	  ○ Vascular
	  ○ Neoplastic
	  ○ Brain injury
	  ○ Psychogenic
	• Idiopathic
	  ○ Sporadic
	  ○ Familial

Axis I—Clinical Characteristics

Five elements specify the key clinical characteristics: age at onset, body distribution, temporal pattern, coexistence of other movement disorders, and other neurological manifestations (Table 11.1).

Age at Onset

Classification by age is important for both diagnostic testing and prognostic value. Dystonia that begins in childhood is more likely to have a discoverable cause and more likely to progress from focal to generalized dystonia. Because there is no evidence that a single age cutoff can be applied to all forms of dystonia, age categories have been employed in this element. These age categories include infancy (birth to 2 years), childhood (3–12 years), adolescence (13–20 years), early adulthood (21–40 years), and late adulthood (>40 years). Dystonia that emerges during the first year of life has a very high probability of being due to an inherited metabolic disorder (Chapter 17). Dystonia that emerges between 2–6 years of age may be more consistent with dystonic cerebral palsy, or with dopa-responsive dystonia (DRD). Other dystonia syndromes, such as DYT1 dystonia, tend to emerge between 6 and 14 years of age. Sporadic focal dystonia usually emerges after 40 years of age.[156]

Body Distribution

Classification by body region affected has important implications for diagnosis and therapy. The diagnostic considerations in adult-onset focal dystonia are quite different from those in child- or adolescent-onset generalized dystonia. Describing the body distribution has a relevant clinical value, including the possibility to evaluate spread of motor symptoms over time. *Focal dystonia* involves only one body region, such as the upper face, the neck, the larynx, or the hand. *Segmental dystonia* involves two or more contiguous body regions such as the upper plus lower face, or both upper extremities. *Multifocal* dystonia involves two or more noncontiguous body regions. *Generalized* dystonia involves the trunk and at least two other adjacent sites, i.e., neck, upper extremity, and lower extremity. *Hemidystonia* involves multiple body regions on one side of the body only. The presence of hemidystonia suggests, but does not always mean, that there is an underlying focal brain lesion.

Temporal Patterns

Recognizing the temporal pattern can facilitate diagnosis and treatment choices. Two types of temporal patterns are relevant. The first refers to disease course and the second refers to variability of symptom presence. Disease course can be either static or progressive. Variability occurs over a shorter time frame and can be momentary or daily in relation to voluntary actions, external triggers, compensatory phenomena, *geste antagoniste* or psychological state. Variability is characterized by four different patterns: *persistent dystonia* is present to approximately the same extent throughout the day, *action-specific dystonia* occurs only during a particular activity or task, *dystonia with diurnal fluctuations* changes with recognizable circadian variation in presence and severity, and *paroxysmal dystonia* is characterized by sudden and discrete episodes of dystonia with normal function in between episodes (Chapter 9).

Combination with Another Movement Disorder

Dystonia may occur in isolation or in combination with other movement disorders. The resulting syndromes may give rise to recognizable associations, such as isolated dystonia or dystonia with myoclonus, parkinsonism, spasticity, and ataxia. The presence or absence of these associations may have important diagnostic and treatment implications. *Isolated dystonia* has dystonia as the only motor feature, with the exception of tremor. Tremor is an exception because it is so commonly associated with dystonia. *Combined dystonia* has dystonia in combination with other movement disorders. Isolated dystonia encompasses many forms previously described as "primary" and combined dystonia encompasses forms that would have been described previously "dystonia-plus" or "secondary." It should be noted that the terms "isolated" and "combined" refer to the phenomenology and not to the underlying etiology.

Occurrence of Other Neurological or Systemic Manifestations

The presence or absence of other neurologic or systemic features has substantial impact diagnosis of dystonia syndromes. Many of these syndromes are described in Chapters 17 and 20; others are described in this chapter.

Axis II—Etiology

The second axis addresses etiology under two broad elements: anatomically identifiable nervous system pathology and pattern of inheritance (Table 11.2). Anatomical causes may be identified using brain imaging or by pathology. Inheritance differentiates inherited from acquired conditions by means of metabolic, genetic, or other tests. These two elements, anatomical change and pattern of inheritance, are complementary for the purpose of etiological classification.

Nervous System Pathology

Evidence of degeneration, whether at the imaging, gross anatomic, microscopic, or molecular level, provides a useful means to discriminate subgroups of dystonia into degenerative and nondegenerative forms. For the purposes of classification, specific pathology is grouped under *degeneration* in which there is evidence for progressive structural abnormality, such as neuronal loss, and *static lesions*, which are nonprogressive neurodevelopmental anomalies or acquired lesion. There are many forms of dystonia in which there is no evidence of degeneration or structural lesion.

Pattern of Inheritance

The first level of differentiation in this element is whether the dystonia is inherited, acquired, or idiopathic. *Inherited dystonias* with proven genetic causes can have autosomal dominant, autosomal recessive, x-linked recessive, or mitochondrial patterns of inheritance (Tables 11.3 and 11.4). Other genetic dystonias may not be inherited, but may result from *de novo* mutations. These genetic disorders can result in isolated dystonia, dystonia combined with other movement disorders, or dystonia combined with other neurological or system features. *Acquired dystonia* can result from a large number of causes. These are listed in Table 11.5 and described later in this chapter. *Idiopathic dystonia* refers to those forms for

TABLE 11.3 Genetic Causes of Dystonia (DYT Scheme)

Designation	Dystonia type	Inheritance	Gene locus	Protein
DYT1	Early-onset generalized torsion dystonia (dystonia musculorum deformans, Oppenheim's dystonia)	Autosomal dominant	9q34	TorsinA
DYT2	Autosomal recessive torsion dystonia	Autosomal recessive	1p35	Hippocalcin
DYT3[a]	Dystonia-parkinsonism ("lubag")	X-linked recessive	Xq13.1	TATA-binding protein-associated factor-1 (TAF1)
DYT4	Non-DYT1 dystonia (whispering dysphonia)	Autosomal dominant	19p13.3	β-tubulin 4a
DYT5	Dopa-responsive dystonia (DRD)	Autosomal dominant	14q22.1-2	GTP cyclohydrolase 1
DYT6	Adolescent-onset dystonia of mixed type	Autosomal dominant	8p21-22	THAP1
DYT7[a]	Adult-onset focal dystonia	Autosomal dominant	18p	Unknown
DYT8	Paroxysmal nonkinesigenic dyskinesia	Autosomal dominant	2q33-35	Myofibrillogenesis regulator 1
DYT9	Paroxysmal choreoathetosis with episodic ataxia and spasticity	Autosomal dominant	1p21	GLUT1 (glucose transporter 1)
DYT10	Paroxysmal kinesigenic dyskinesia	Autosomal dominant	16p11.2	PRRT2 (proline-rich transmembrane protein 2)
DYT11	Myoclonus dystonia	Autosomal dominant (maternal imprinting)	7q21	ε-Sarcoglycan
DYT12	Rapid-onset dystonia-parkinsonism	Autosomal dominant	19q	Na^+/K^+ ATPase α3 subunit
DYT13	Multifocal/segmental dystonia	Autosomal dominant	1p	Unknown
DYT14 (DYT5)	DRD	Autosomal dominant	14q22.1-2	GTP cyclohydrolase 1
DYT15	Myoclonus dystonia	Autosomal dominant	18p	Unknown
DYT16	Early-onset dystonia-parkinsonism	Autosomal recessive	2q31.3	Protein kinase activator PRKRA
DYT17[a]	Focal torsion dystonia	Autosomal recessive	20p11.22-q13.12	Unknown
DYT18 (DYT9)	Paroxysmal exertion-induced dystonia	Autosomal dominant	1p35-31.3	GLUT1

(Continued)

TABLE 11.3   (Continued)

Designation	Dystonia type	Inheritance	Gene locus	Protein
DYT19	Paroxysmal kinesigenic dyskinesia 2	Autosomal dominant	16q13-q22.1	Unknown
DYT20	Paroxysmal non kinesigenic dyskinesia 2	Autosomal dominant	2q31	Unknown
DYT21[a]	Generalized torsion dystonia	Autosomal dominant	2q14.3-q21.3	Unknown
DYT22	Reserved but unassigned			
DYT23[a]	Adult-onset cervical dystonia	Autosomal dominant	9q34.3	N-type calcium channel (*CACNA1AB*)
DYT24[a]	Adult-onset cranial-cervical dystonia	Autosomal dominant	11p14.2	Anoctamin 3 (*ANO3*)
DYT25[a]	Adult-onset focal dystonia	Autosomal dominant	18p11.21	G-alpha subunit of the G protein receptor (*GNAL*)

[a]*Adult-onset dystonias that are not discussed in this chapter.*

which a cause has not been identified. Idiopathic dystonias can be inherited or sporadic, and many of the sporadic forms may be due to *de novo* mutations. This is a fluid category as new genes are being discovered at a rapid rate. Most genetic forms of dystonia with onset in infancy, childhood, or adolescence were considered to be idiopathic at one time, but are now classified as inherited.

LOCALIZATION AND PATHOPHYSIOLOGY

Dystonia has been associated with a number of diseases, but there is often no discrete, identifiable pathological abnormality in the brain. Abnormalities at many levels of cellular function have been described in genetic forms of dystonia.[9] Together, many of the physiologic abnormalities in dystonia can be related to one of three major processes.[10] These include (i) loss of inhibition leading to excess movement and to the overflow phenomena seen in dystonia, (ii) sensory dysfunction, which may result from or may drive some of the motor abnormalities, and (iii) abnormal, often enhanced, plasticity.

Most studies of dystonia have revealed abnormal cocontraction of agonist and antagonist muscles at rest that is often exacerbated by movement[11–14]; however, one study in children with primary and secondary dystonia failed to confirm cocontraction as a basis for dystonia.[15] At rest, the abnormal contractions can be sustained or intermittent. The intermittent contractions usually last 1–2 sec, although some are as short as 100 msec. During voluntary movement, excessive voluntary contractions are seen in muscles that would not normally be active in the task. In addition to the excessive activity of nearby muscles, agonist muscle

TABLE 11.4   Other Genetic Disorders in Which Dystonia Is a Prominent Feature

Autosomal recessive	Autosomal dominant	Mitochondrial	X-linked
AADC deficiency	DRPLA	Leber disease	dystonia-deafness
Ataxia telangiectasia	Hereditary spastic paraparesis with dystonia	Leigh syndrome	Lesch–Nyhan
Dopamine transporter deficiency	Huntington's disease	MERRF	Pelizaeus Merzbacher
Gangliosidoses	Spinocerebellar ataxias (SCAs)	MELAS	Rett syndrome
Glutaric aciduria			
Hartnup disease			
Homocystinuria			
Juvenile Parkinson's disease			
Metachromatic leukodystrophy			
Methylmalonic aciduria			
Niemann–Pick type C			
Neuroferritinopathy			
PKAN (Hallervorden–Spatz)			
Sepiapterin reductase deficiency			
TH deficiency			
Thiamine transporter 2 deficiency			
Triose phosphate isomerase deficiency			
Tyrosinemia			
Vitamin E deficiency			
Wilson disease			

TABLE 11.5   Acquired Causes of Dystonia

Autoimmune

Cerebral palsy

Drugs

Functional (psychogenic)

Infection

Kernicterus

Psychogenic

Stroke

Toxins

Trauma

IV. HYPERKINETIC AND HYPOKINETIC MOVEMENT DISORDERS

activity is prolonged[16] and movement-related cortical potentials are reduced just prior to movement.[17] The combination of slight reduction in agonist activity and excessive activity in antagonist muscles causes movement to be slow. Movement sequences are relatively more impaired than are the individual components.[18]

In dystonia, the monosynaptic and long-latency stretch reflexes are normal at rapid rates of stretch, but with slower stretches the long-latency reflex is prolonged compared with normal.[19] Stretch of one muscle group often results in "overflow" activation of other muscle groups,[11] and it has been suggested that people with dystonia have impaired reciprocal inhibition on a supraspinal basis.[20,21] People with dystonia often have a paradoxical activation of a passively shortened muscle (the so-called shortening reaction).[11] Thus, a variety of mechanisms may contribute to the abnormal muscle activity seen in dystonia. What these mechanisms appear to have in common is an inability to inhibit unwanted reflex activity in response to stretch.[22] This view is supported by evidence that focal dystonia can be decreased by blocking γ-motorneuron drive to spindles with lidocaine.[23]

It is apparent that the basal ganglia play a central role in many forms of dystonia, but there is also evidence for participation of cerebellar mechanisms in some forms of dystonia. When dystonia is seen after stroke the most common lesion locations are the putamen (most common), globus pallidus, or thalamus.[24,25] Furthermore, metabolic disorders that have dystonia as a prominent feature are often associated with basal ganglia involvement. Lesions of basal ganglia structures in primates can cause abnormal postures that are characteristic of human dystonia.[22] Dopamine D_2 receptor binding is reduced in the putamen of patients with primary focal dystonia and in an animal model of transient dystonia.[26,27] These observations and other data suggest that dystonia is due to abnormal basal ganglia function, which in turn causes altered regulation of cortical, spinal, and probably brainstem and cerebellar sensorimotor mechanisms. The result is abnormal muscular cocontraction and overflow of activity to muscle adjacent to the prime movers or to the contralateral body part, the so-called "mirror dystonia."[13]

There is a large body of evidence implicating dysfunction of the nigrostriatal dopamine system in the pathophysiology of dystonia. Although much of the evidence is circumstantial, impaired dopamine neurotransmission appears to be the common theme: (i) drugs that block dopamine receptors can produce acute dystonic reactions[28]; (ii) in the syndrome of DRD, there is a remarkable symptomatic response to levodopa (L-dopa).[29] In DRD, there is decreased production of dopamine despite no loss of nigrostriatal neurons; (iii) patients with idiopathic focal dystonia have reduced dopamine D_2 receptor binding in the putamen[30]; (iv) dystonia is an early manifestation of Parkinson's disease in 20–40% of patients[31]; (v) the expression of messenger RNA that encodes torsinA, the protein product of a gene (DYT1) that is responsible for childhood-onset generalized torsion dystonia, is particularly concentrated in nigrostriatal dopamine neurons.[32] There is impaired D_2 receptor function in an animal model of DYT1 dystonia.[33]

There is substantial evidence for abnormal neural plasticity in many forms of dystonia.[10] Most studies of plasticity in dystonia have been performed in adults with idiopathic adult-onset focal dystonia.[34,35] Few studies have been performed in children or even in adults with childhood-onset genetic dystonias. However, there is evidence for impaired motor learning in nonmanifesting carriers of the DYT1 mutation[36] and individuals with DYT11 dystonia.[37] Studies in transgenic mice with the DYT1 mutation knocked in have shown abnormal synaptic plasticity in the striatum.[38]

ETIOLOGIES

The tremendous advance in molecular and genetic research and diagnostic tools has led to the identification of specific etiologies of dystonias that were previously considered to be idiopathic. Many genetic forms of dystonia have assigned genetic loci identified as DYTx (Table 11.3). However, there is a much longer list of genetic disorders in which dystonia is an important feature (Table 11.4). In some of these disorders dystonia is the primary feature, but in other it is just one of several neurologic signs or symptoms. Dystonia can also be a prominent feature in acquired disorders (Table 11.5). In the following sections, specific etiologies of nonparoxysmal childhood-onset dystonia will be discussed. Paroxysmal dystonias are covered in Chapter 9. Management and treatment of dystonia is currently based on general characteristics of the dystonia rather than on specific genetic causes and will be discussed after presentation of the specific etiologies. The following section considers DYTx dystonias with onset in childhood. A more complete list, including adult-onset forms is provided in Table 11.3.

DYT1

Diagnostic Features and Natural History

DYT1 dystonia, also known as early-onset primary torsion dystonia, *dystonia musculorum deformans* or Oppenheim dystonia, is an autosomal dominant condition with incomplete (30–40%) penetrance.[39] Genetic studies have found that a GAG deletion in the *TOR1A* (DYT1) gene at 9q34 produces causes most autosomal dominant, early-onset primary generalized dystonias affecting Ashkenazi Jewish patients (90%)[40] and non-Jews (50–60%).[41] In DYT1 dystonia, symptoms usually begin in a limb with a mean onset age of 12.5 years.[42] Approximately equal numbers have onset in an arm (48%) or a leg (49%), but the arm is more likely to be involved first in Ashkenazi Jews (60%) and the leg is more likely to be involved first in non-Jews (60%).[43] Cervical or laryngeal onset is uncommon. Onset is typically after 5 years and before 26 years of age, but can be earlier or later.[8,43,44] Symptoms typically become generalized within 5 years,[42] but may remain multifocal (10%), segmental (12%), or focal (21%) (Videos 11.1, 11.2 and 11.3).[43] Diagnosis is made by genetic testing for the disease-causing GAG deletion in *TOR1A*.

Genetics and Pathophysiology

The product of the *TOR1A* gene is torsinA. TorsinA is a member of a family of ATPases with a variety of cellular activities (AAA +) and bears substantial homology to heat-shock proteins. TorsinA has been implicated in the regulation of the organization of nuclear envelope and endoplasmic reticulum compartments with respect to the cytoskeleton[45,46] and also in the processing of proteins through the secretory pathway.[9] To date, the only known disease-causing mutation of DYT1 dystonia is a GAG deletion causing the loss of one of a pair of glutamic acids in the C-terminal region.[41] Other rare mutations in *TOR1A* have been reported in individuals with dystonia, but a causal role has not been established.[47,48]

The basis for the incomplete penetrance is not known, but genetic, epigenetic, and environmental factors are considered possible contributors. Because of the homology of *TOR1A* with heat-shock proteins, it is possible that early childhood infection or other stressor may play a role in determining penetrance, but this has not been proven. In a small multi-center European study of 110 individuals from 28 families with DYT1, the possible contribution of perinatal adversity, childhood infections, trauma, and general anesthesia to manifestation of dystonia was assessed by questionnaire and clinical interview.[49] A significant association was found between complications of vaginal delivery and development of dystonia, but no other associations were found. A disease-modifying single nucleotide polymorphism in *TOR1A* has been identified in the coding sequence for amino acid residue 216 in torsinA. In 88% of the population, this amino acid is aspartic acid (D), but in 12% of the population it is histidine (H). Frequency of the 216H allele is increased in GAG deletion carriers that do not manifest dystonia and is decreased in GAG deletion carriers that do manifest dystonia compared to controls.[50,51] Interestingly, the protective effect of the D216H polymorphism is only seen when present on the allele without the GAG deletion (trans allele). Although this association is likely to be an important contributor, the D216H polymorphism only partially accounts for the incomplete penetrance of the DYT1 mutation.

There are no consistent neuropathologic abnormalities in DYT1 dystonia. Although perinuclear inclusions and other neurodegenerative changes have been reported in some cases,[52] this initial observation awaits confirmation from other postmortem studies. TorsinA is expressed in several brain regions including substantia nigra, striatum, hippocampus, and cerebellum.[32] It is especially highly expressed in nigral dopamine neurons. TorsinA is expressed in neurons and not in glia.[53] In transgenic mouse models of DYT1 dystonia, there is evidence for impaired dopamine neurotransmission[33,54] and impaired plasticity that can be reversed by application of muscarinic anti-cholinergic medications that act at M1 receptors.[38,55] There is also evidence for decreased inhibitory output from the basal ganglia in transgenic mice,[56] which is consistent with models of human dystonia.[13,57,58]

PET studies of cerebral glucose metabolism have shown abnormal patterns in individuals with DYT1 dystonia.[59] Although the DYT1 dystonia is only 30–40% penetrant, nonexpressing carriers of the deletion have abnormalities on PET imaging that are identical to expressing individuals.[59] This suggests that the DYT1 mutation conveys a vulnerability to a "second hit" that determines whether dystonia manifests or not. An interesting rodent model of cranial dystonia suggests that mild striatal dopamine deficiency may be a permissive factor that allows a relatively modest weakening of the lid-closing orbicularis muscle to produce bilateral forceful blinking of the eyelids resembling blepharospasm.[60] MRI studies in DYT1 dystonia have shown increased activity in sensorimotor networks[61] and altered connectivity including abnormalities in cerebellar outflow pathways.[62]

Management and Treatment

Management and treatment of DTY1 dystonia are discussed at the end of this chapter under a general discussion of dystonia treatments.

DYT2

DYT2 is a recessive form of primary dystonia that has been reported in several families.[63–65] The onset of symptoms is typically in the first decade of life. The dystonia progresses at a slow rate, and individuals may remain functionally independent as adults.[66]

Some of the reported individual cases had atypical features and evidence for this entity had been considered weak, leading to a question of whether DYT2 is a true specific entity.[8] However, a recent study has revealed homozygous mutations in the *HPCA* gene in a consanguineous kindred, and compound heterozygous mutations in *HPCA* in a second family.[66] *HPCA* codes for a neuronal calcium sensory protein in the brain called Hippocalcin. Functional studies have shown that Hippocalcin may play a role in regulating voltage-dependent calcium channels. Due to the apparent rarity of this condition, it remains unknown to what degree DYT2 dystonia has a characteristic phenotype.

DYT4

DYT4 dystonia, also known as "Australian whispering dysphonia," is an autosomal dominant form of early-onset dystonia that was initially described in a large Australian pedigree in which linkage studies excluded the DYT1 locus.[67] The age at onset of symptoms ranged from 13 to 37 years. Most individuals developed dysphonia as the initial manifestation, but also developed generalized dystonia and were described to have a characteristic "hobby horse ataxic gait." Linkage analysis in a seven-generation family followed by exome sequencing has revealed a causative mutation in the β-tubulin 4a (*TUBB4A*) gene.[68,69] A different mutation in *TUBB4A* has also been reported in unrelated individuals with adult-onset dysphonia and segmental dystonia.[69]

TUBB4A mutations have also been associated with hypomyelination with atrophy of the basal ganglia and cerebellum (H-ABC) syndrome.[70] H-ABC syndrome is a rare and sporadic leukodystrophy with a broad phenotypic spectrum. The age at onset ranges from neonatal to childhood periods. Early development can be normal or delayed and progression can range from slow to more rapid neurological deterioration. The symptomatology ranges can include movement disorders, spasticity, ataxia, cognitive deficit, and epilepsy. Brain MRI reveals progressive putaminal atrophy, variable cerebellar atrophy, and highly variable cerebral atrophy. White matter hypomyelination, myelin loss, or both are present. In most patients, the *TUBB4A* mutations are *de novo*.

DYT5

Clinical Features and Natural History

DYT5 refers to the autosomal dominant form of DRD (Segawa Disease) that is due to mutations in the *GCH1* gene resulting in GTP cyclohydrolase deficiency. It is characterized by childhood onset progressive dystonia with sustained dramatic response to low doses of L-dopa, without development of complications related to long-term treatment.[71,72] DRD was first described by Segawa as progressive dystonia with diurnal fluctuations.[73] It typically presents with gait disturbance from foot dystonia with the age of onset ranging from 1 to 12 years. If untreated, there is development of diurnal fluctuation with worsening of symptoms toward the end of the day and marked improvement in the morning. In late adolescence or early adulthood, parkinsonian features can develop if DRD remains untreated. Even if treatment is instituted late in the course, all features typically improve with low-dose L-dopa.[74]

There can be significant phenotypic variability in the presentation of DRD. As noted, the typical presentation is onset of dystonia in childhood, usually affecting gait first, diurnal fluctuation, subsequent development of parkinsonism, and a dramatic response to L-dopa. However, in some children there is hypotonia in infancy and delayed attainment of motor developmental milestones,[75,76] and DRD can be misdiagnosed as cerebral palsy. DRD has also been reported to present as familial spastic paraparesis.[77] Patients with DRD commonly have brisk reflexes and spontaneously upgoing (striatal) toes, but do not have true spasticity. DRD has not been associated with nonmotor features. Specifically, sleep impairment, depression, and anxiety are not more common in patients with DRD than in healthy controls.[78]

Pathophysiology

GTP-cyclohydrolase-I is the initial, and rate-liming, enzyme involved in the biosynthesis of tetrahydrobiopterin (BH_4) from guanidine triphosphate (GTP).[79] BH_4 is a cofactor for tyrosine hydroxylase (TH), the rate-limiting enzyme in dopamine synthesis. Deficiency of BH_4 leads to decreased efficacy of TH and thus to decreased production of dopamine, but without loss of nigrostriatal dopamine terminals.[80] BH_4 is also a cofactor for phenylalanine hydroxylase (PAH) and tryptophan hydroxylase, but DRD does not have associated symptoms related to decreased function of those enzymes.[78] However, the decreased function of PAH allows the use of a phenylalanine loading test for diagnostic evaluation of GTPCH deficiency.[81] To maximize sensitivity and specificity of the oral phenylalanine loading test in children, pediatric reference values, along with combined analysis of the Phe/Tyr ratio and biopterin concentration, are required.[82] CSF can be tested for levels of tetrahydrobiopterin, neopterin, and metabolites of catecholamines and indolamines. Genetic testing for *CGH1* mutations is also available,[83] but the entire gene must be sequenced.

Management and Treatment

Carbidopa/L-dopa is the mainstay of treatment in DRD and may be diagnostic if there is a complete relief of symptoms. A starting dose is 1 mg/kg/day of L-dopa, which can be increased gradually until there is complete benefit or dose-limiting side effects. Most individuals respond to 4–5 mg/kg/day in divided doses, but some authors have suggested doses up to 10 mg/kg/day. If there is no response to a dose of 600 mg/day, it is highly unlikely that DRD is the correct diagnosis. Carbidopa/L-dopa should be given as 25/100 mg tablets. They can be crushed and dissolved in an ascorbic acid solution or in orange juice and used within 24 hours. The 10/100 tablets contain insufficient carbidopa to prevent nausea in most patients and should be avoided. The most common side effects are somnolence, nausea and vomiting, decreased appetite, dyskinesia, and hallucinations. Nausea and vomiting can be reduced by given additional carbidopa, available in the United States as 25 mg tablets. Dyskinesia may occur upon initiation of treatment or in older individuals who are treated with relatively higher doses of L-dopa. Dyskinesia can be reduced or eliminated by reducing the dose of L-dopa. If dyskinesia is present with the initiation of treatment, reduce the dose. If inadequate benefit at the lower dose, it can usually be increased again slowly without recurrence of dyskinesia. Motor complications of L-dopa therapy that are seen in Parkinson's disease do not occur in DRD.

In rare cases of DRD, L-dopa is not tolerated. In those cases, trihexyphenidyl is a reasonable alternative. The dosing of trihexyphenidyl for treatment of DRD is not well established. Starting dose should be 0.5 mg/day in children <4 years old and 1 mg/day in older children. The dose should be increased by 1 mg every 3–7 days in a t.i.d. schedule until benefit or side effects. In DRD, there is benefit from relatively low doses compared to those used to treat other forms of dystonia. Trihexyphenidyl should be considered second-line treatment in DRD because it does not reverse the biochemical defect of decreased dopamine synthesis in DRD. Side effects are uncommon at low doses.

DYT6

DYT6 is an autosomal dominant dystonia that was initially identified in two large Amish-Mennonite families.[84] In these families, the dystonia has been attributed to a founder mutation in the Thanatos-associated (THAP) domain containing, apoptosis-associated protein 1 (*THAP1*).[85] In a study of 27 Amish-Mennonite individuals with *THAP1* mutations, the mean age at onset was 15.5 years (range 5–38 years).[86] Forty-four percent had onset of dystonia in one arm. The majority progressed to have generalized dystonia, with 90% having arm involvement, 52% having leg involvement, and 33% having jaw/tongue involvement. Some affected individuals had a phenotype indistinguishable from the typical DYT1 phenotype, but 26% of patients had onset in cervical musculature, which is uncommon in DYT1 dystonia.[43,86]

DYT6 dystonia is not limited to individuals with Amish-Mennonite ancestry. In studies screening larger number of individuals with dystonia for *THAP1* mutations, missense mutations have been found at many locations in the gene.[87–89] These studies confirmed an average age at onset in the mid-teens, and more likely onset in cranial or cervical muscles than in DYT1. In one study the neck was the most frequently affected anatomic site.[87]

DYT8 (see Chapter 9—PNKD)
DYT9 (see Chapter 9—PED)
DYT10 (see Chapter 9—PKD)

DYT11

Clinical Features and Natural History

DYT11, also known as myoclonus-dystonia syndrome (MDS), is an autosomal dominant disorder characterized by myoclonus, dystonia, or both.[90,91] The gene responsible for DYT11 is *SCGE*, which codes for the ε-sarcoglycan protein. Onset is typically in childhood or early adolescence, with a mean onset age of 5 years.[92] Myoclonus is usually the initial symptom, but dystonia is the first symptom in about 20%.[92] In rare cases, there is a history of neonatal hypotonia. Myoclonus is usually more severe than the main feature and may be the only manifestation in some affected individuals.[91] The neck and upper limbs are usually more involved than legs and gait. The myoclonus often improves with ingestions of ethanol.[90,92] The dystonia is often mild and usually involves the neck or arms (Video 12.2). Alcohol abuse and psychiatric symptoms (obsessive–compulsive disorders, panic attacks) are common among patients with MDS.[93] In a study of 27 adult individuals with *SCGE* mutations, 77% had psychiatric symptoms, including obsessive–compulsive disorder, generalized anxiety disorder, alcohol dependence, or a combination.[94] However, cognitive function is normal.[95]

The rate of progression and severity are highly variable ranging from mild nonprogressive symptoms to marked disability in adolescence or early adulthood. The course of the myoclonus and the dystonia are often independent. Worsening of myoclonus is not necessarily accompanied by worsening of dystonia.[96] There may be spontaneous improvement of myoclonus[96] or of dystonia.[92] Dystonia may completely resolve in approximately 20% of patients.

Diagnostic criteria for MDS have been proposed.[97] Criteria for definite MDS include (i) onset before 20 years of age; (ii) myoclonus predominating in the upper body, either isolated or associated with dystonia; (iii) positive family history with paternal transmission (paternal transmission is applicable only for MDS due to *SGCE* mutation or deletion—see below); (iv) exclusion of additional neurologic features, such as cerebellar ataxia, spasticity, and dementia; and (v) normal brain MRI. Additional suggestive features include (i) short myoclonic bursts (25–250 ms) without cortical premyoclonic potential; negative C-reflex response and lack of giant somatosensory evoked potentials; (ii) spontaneous remission of limb dystonia during childhood or adolescence; and (iii) alcohol responsiveness.

Another genetic locus for inherited myoclonus-dystonia has been identified on chromosome 18p11 and listed as DYT15.[98] This was defined in a large Canadian family with 13 affected individuals. The inheritance pattern was autosomal dominant and the phenotype was similar to what is seen in MDS with *SGCE* mutations.

Pathophysiology

The commonest genetic cause of MDS is mutation of the *SGCE* gene, which encodes ε-sarcoglycan protein.[97] SGCE mutations account for approximately 40% of cases of MDS. ε-Sarcoglycan is expressed predominantly in the brain, and is related to the sarcoglycans that are mutated in limb girdle muscular dystrophies.[99] Most patients with MDS due to SGCE mutations inherit the disorder from the father, suggesting that there is inactivation of the maternal SGCE allele (genomic imprinting), probably by methylation.[99] Indeed, cases of MDS have been described in patients with Russell–Silver syndrome due to maternal uniparental disomy of chromosome 7.[100] ε-Sarcoglycan is highly expressed during brain development and is highly expressed in dopamine neurons in adults.[9] In one MRI volumetric study, dystonia severity in MDS correlated with gray matter volume in the putamen bilaterally.[101] SGCE knockout mice exhibit myoclonus, impaired motor skills, and anxiety-like behaviors. These mice have abnormally increased striatal dopamine and dopamine metabolites.[102]

Management and Treatment

Treatment for MDS is symptomatic and benefit is usually incomplete. There are many reports of trials of various medications.[97] Some benefit from anticholinergic medications: clonazepam, sodium oxybate, valproate, levetiracetam, L-5-hydroxytryptophan, and L-dopa have been reported.[97,103] Botulinum toxin can be used to treat focal dystonia in MDS. Deep brain stimulation (DBS) of the internal globus pallidus has been reported to provide greater than 50% improvement of both myoclonus and dystonia in adults with MDS.[104,105] DBS has not been reported in children or adolescents with MDS.

DYT12

DYT12, otherwise known as rapid-onset dystonia-parkinsonism (RDP), is an autosomal dominant disorder with variable penetrance.[106] RDP typically presents with abrupt onset and rapid progression over hours to weeks, followed by little further progression.[106,107] Onset is usually dramatic and consists of bulbar and limb dystonia with variable features of parkinsonism.[107] Occasional vague symptoms preceding the more dramatic onset were reported in several patients. Age of onset ranges from 8 to 55 years, but is before 20 years of age in 47% and between 20 and 30 years of age in another 39%. Bulbar symptoms are typically worse than appendicular symptoms. Parkinsonism is less prominent than dystonia and usually consists of bradykinesia, postural instability, and hypophonia. Proposed diagnostic criteria consist of (i) abrupt onset of dystonia with features of parkinsonism over a few minutes to 30 days; (ii) rostrocaudal (face > arm > leg) gradient of involvement; and (iii) prominent bulbar findings.[107] Many individuals with RDP also have psychiatric symptoms including psychosis, mood disorders, and substance abuse.[108] Psychiatric symptoms may precede the onset of dystonia.

RDP is caused by mutations in the Na^+/K^+-ATPase $\alpha 3$ subunit (*ATP1A3* gene).[109] The $\alpha 3$ subunit is only expressed in brain and heart, perhaps indicating a role in electrical excitability. It has been suggested that the reported mutations in RDP impair enzyme activity or stability.[9]

More recently, mutations in *ATP1A3* have been associated with alternating hemiplegia of childhood (AHC).[110,111] AHC tends to be more polyphasic whereas RDP is typically monophasic, but other ways these disorders can be viewed as falling on a spectrum.[112] *ATP1A3* mutations affecting transmembrane and functional domains of the protein tend to be associated with AHC, rather than RDP. Other phenotypes have been described with *ATP1A3* mutations, including motor developmental delay and ataxia.[113]

Patients with RDP do not respond consistently to the usual symptomatic treatments for dystonia including L-dopa.[107]

Early-onset Multifocal/Segmental Dystonia (DYT13)

This form of dystonia was described in a large Italian family with early onset of multifocal or segmental dystonia.[114] The average age of onset is 16 years (range 5–40 years). The upper body is most commonly affected, usually involving cranial musculature. Generalization is uncommon. DYT13 has been linked to chromosome 1p,[115] but no gene has been identified.

DYT14 (identical to DYT5)
DYT15 (discussed under DYT11)

DYT16

DYT16 was initially described in three Brazilian families[116] and was subsequently reported in a German boy.[117] Affected individuals had a mean onset age of 9 years (range 2–18 years). In most patients, onset is in a limb with subsequent generalization, although one patient had onset in cranial musculature.[116] Several affected individuals had parkinsonism, pyramidal tract signs, or both. DYT16 is associated with a mutation in the *PRKRA* gene. At least three distinct phenotypes have been reported in *PRKRA* mutations. These include generalized dystonia, dystonia-parkinsonism that is nonresponsive to L-dopa, and acute infantile onset of hypotonia, bradykinesia, pyramidal signs, and developmental regression.[118,119]

PRKRA encodes an interferon-inducible double-stranded RNA activator of protein kinase PKR. This protein is thought to be involved in signal transduction, cell differentiation, and apoptosis.[8] There have been no reports of treatment response for DYT16.

DYT18 (identical to DYT9)

Combined Dystonias and Dystonias Associated with Other Neurologic Features

There is a long list of dystonias associated with other neurologic features due to genetic (Table 11.4) or nongenetic (Table 11.5) etiologies. Most of the genetic etiologies are discussed with metabolic diseases causing movement disorders, including neurotransmitter disorders, in Chapter 17. The great majority of these diseases have a variety of neurological signs and symptoms in addition to dystonia. However, dystonia can be the presenting feature in some. These include neurotransmitter disorders, glutaric aciduria, juvenile parkinsonism, Wilson disease, and pantothenate kinase-associated neurodegeneration (PKAN) (Videos 11.4 and 11.5).

Of acquired etiologies, perinatal brain injury (cerebral palsy) is the most common cause of dystonia. This is discussed in Chapter 20. Other important nongenetic etiologies include drug ingestion (see Chapter 22) and conversion disorder (functional/psychogenic) (see Chapter 23). Stroke is an uncommon cause of dystonia in children, but can present with pure dystonia. Dystonia due to stroke usually affects limbs in a "hemi" distribution. The most common locations of stroke resulting in dystonia are putamen, globus pallidus, and thalamus.[24,25,120]

Dystonic Storm (Status Dystonicus)

This rare complication of dystonia deserves special mention. Dystonic storm is a life-threatening complication of severe dystonia that is characterized by relentless, sustained, severe dystonic muscle contractions.[121,122] Etiologies vary, but can include DYT1 dystonia,[123] medication withdrawal in a variety of forms of dystonia,[121] PKAN,[124] and baclofen pump failure.[125] Prompt diagnosis of this condition is essential. Patients with dystonic storm should be managed in an intensive care unit. They may develop hyperthermia, metabolic derangements, and rhabdomyolysis with acute renal failure. Treatment with intravenous benzodiazepines or general anesthetic agents may be required.[121,124] In extreme intractable cases, intrathecal baclofen, pallidotomy, or DBS of the internal globus pallidus may be beneficial.[124,126,127]

DIAGNOSTIC APPROACH TO DYSTONIA

General diagnostic considerations for movement disorders are discussed in Chapter 4. However, there are some specific considerations for dystonia. Specific diagnostic criteria are provided above for specific genetic etiologies of dystonia where they exist. As for all movement disorders, it is of utmost importance to see the abnormal movements and to evaluate the patient performing a variety of activities. Distribution of affected body parts, task-dependence, and presence or absence of coexisting neurological signs and symptoms are all factors that can help tailor the diagnostic approach. For most children with dystonia, MRI of the brain is indicated to rule out structural causes and to look for disease-specific findings. In children with limb-onset between age 5 years and adulthood, genetic testing for DYT1 and DYT6 should be performed. A therapeutic (and possibly diagnostic) trial of L-dopa is warranted in all children presenting with dystonia, especially those who begin with leg involvement in the first decade of life. Additional metabolic and genetic testing may be warranted depending on the presentation (see above and Chapter 17 for specific descriptions of typical presentations). Because of the large number of entities that can cause dystonia in childhood, a tiered approach to diagnostic testing is advisable, with frequent re-evaluation of the child to assess for progression and development of new signs or symptoms.

MANAGEMENT AND TREATMENT

The management of dystonia can be challenging. Treatment for most forms of dystonia is symptomatic and benefit may be incomplete or accompanied by intolerable side effects. The treatment approach is largely the same regardless of etiology.[128,129] Few controlled trials have been performed, and most trials have included a heterogeneous sample of children with dystonia due to a variety of causes, and surgical trials have focused on adult patients.[130] Nevertheless, with a systematic approach to treatment, good results can be achieved in many cases.[129]

Carbidopa/L-dopa

As discussed above in detail for DRD, carbidopa/L-dopa is the mainstay of treatment in DRD. However, other forms of dystonia may respond partially to L-dopa. Because of its potential for benefit and because complete response to L-dopa can be diagnostic for DRD, a trial of carbidopa/L-dopa is recommended for all children with dystonia unless there is a family history of non-DRD dystonia. Although some patients with acquired dystonia may have benefit from L-dopa,[131] one short term study of children with dystonic cerebral palsy failed to demonstrate benefit on upper limb function.[132]

Trihexyphenidyl

Anticholinergic medications are the most consistently effective in the treatment of dystonia,[133] although the most dramatic reported responses may have come from patients with DRD.[134] Most available data and experiences are with trihexyphenidyl.[133,135] Recent data have shown that the mechanism of action in DYT1 dystonia is likely related to the restoration of abnormal striatal synaptic plasticity.[38] Children may tolerate higher doses than do adults and may find maximum benefit with doses of 60 mg/day or more. However, children may not complain of cognitive side effects, even when they are significant. To minimize side effects, trihexyphenidyl should be started at 1 mg/day at bedtime and increased by 1 mg each week until the desired benefit is obtained or side effects develop. The usual maintenance dose varies from 6 mg/day to over 60 mg/day divided three times per day. The most common side effects of trihexyphenidyl are sedation, dry mouth, decreased concentration and memory, constipation, and blurred vision. Careful monitoring of cognitive function and school performance is required. Chorea can develop with high doses. Sudden cessation should be avoided because it can precipitate mental status changes.

Baclofen

Baclofen is somewhat less effective than trihexyphenidyl in most children, but can be helpful in diminishing pain due to dystonia. It can provide additional benefit with used in combination with trihexyphenidyl. A typical starting dose is 5 mg at bedtime. The dose should be increased slowly until desired benefit or side effects occur. The usual maintenance dose is 10–60 mg/day in the three divided doses, but some older children obtain maximum benefit at doses as high as 180 mg/day. The most common side effect is sedation. Sudden cessation can precipitate seizures or psychosis and should be avoided.

In patients with good benefit from oral baclofen, but who cannot tolerate the effective dose due to side effects, intrathecal baclofen may be an option. There are few data available on the use of intrathecal baclofen in genetic dystonias and benefit may be limited.[136,137] Intrathecal baclofen is used more widely in children with dystonic cerebral palsy than in other forms of dystonia. It may be beneficial, but there is also a high rate of complications, including a 10% risk of infection.[138] A double-blind, placebo-controlled trial of intrathecal baclofen for children with dystonia CP is currently in progress.[139]

Botulinum Toxin

Botulinum toxin injections are highly effective in focal and segmental dystonias due to the limited number of muscles involved.[140] It plays a smaller role in the treatment of generalized dystonia because of the large number of involved muscles. However, it can be quite helpful in reducing symptoms when isolated problematic muscle groups are targeted.[140,141]

Other Medications

Several other medications may be effective in a minority of children with primary dystonia.[128] These include clonazepam, carbamazepine, dopamine antagonists, and dopamine depletors. However, none of these has been studied formally.

Neurosurgical Treatments

Promising neurosurgical treatments of dystonia include thalamotomy, pallidotomy, and DBS of the globus pallidus pars interna.[142–145] Historically, thalamotomy was the most frequently performed ablative procedure, but in the 1990s, pallidotomy became preferred to thalamotomy because of the lower morbidity. Direct comparison has not been performed, but data suggest that pallidotomy is more effective than thalamotomy in genetic dystonias. However, the benefits may be temporary.

In this century, pallidal DBS has become the surgical treatment of choice for dystonia. The effects of DBS are similar to those of pallidotomy, but DBS is programmable and does not involve a destructive lesion. Most systematic studies of pallidal DBS for childhood-onset dystonia have been performed on patients who had DBS as adults.[143,145,146] Outcomes for patients with genetic forms of isolated or combined dystonia are better than for those with acquired dystonia,[146–148] but patients with acquired dystonia may also benefit.[149,150] Some forms of genetic isolated dystonia (e.g., DYT1) may benefit from DBS more than others (e.g., DYT6).[151] Although most candidates for DBS treatment of childhood dystonia are older children or adolescents, DBS can be effective in younger children.[152,153] There is some evidence that the benefit from DBS in children with dystonia may diminish in relation to time between onset of dystonia and initiation of DBS therapy.[150,154,155] Thus, it is likely that this practice will change to consider DBS earlier in the course of dystonia, even in young children.

PATIENT AND FAMILY RESOURCES

The Dystonia Medical Research Foundation (www.dystonia-foundation.org) is a voluntary health organization that provides education and support for individuals and families with dystonia. They also fund research on dystonia and advocate for development of new treatments.

References

1. Oppenheim H. Uber eine eigenartige Krampfkrankheit des kindlichen und jugendlichen Alters (Dysbasia lordotica progressiva, Dystonia musculorum deformans). *Neurol Centrabl.* 1911;30:1090–1107.
2. Wilson SAK. *Modern Problems in Neurology.* London: Arnold; 1928.
3. Denny-Brown D. *The Basal Ganglia and Their Relation to Disorders of Movement.* London: Oxford University Press; 1962.
4. Fahn S, Marsden CD, Calne DB. Classification and investigtaion of dystonia. In: Marsden CD, Fahn S, eds. *Movement Disorders 2.* London: Butterworth; 1987:332–358.
5. Albanese A, Bhatia K, Bressman SB, et al. Phenomenology and classification of dystonia: a consensus update. *Mov Disord.* 2013;28:863–873.
6. Hartmann A, Pogarell O, Oertel W. Secondary dystonias. *J Neurol.* 1998;245:511–518.
7. Bressman SB. Dystonia genotypes, phenotypes, and classification. *Adv Neurol.* 2004;94:101–107.
8. Zorzi G, Zibordi F, Garavaglia B, Nardocci N. Early onset primary dystonia. *Eur J Paediatr Neurol.* 2009.
9. Breakefield XO, Blood AJ, Li Y, Hallett M, Hanson PI, Standaert DG. The pathophysiological basis of dystonias. *Nat Rev Neurosci.* 2008;9:222–234.
10. Quartarone A, Hallett M. Emerging conceptsin the physiological basis of dystonia. *Mov Disord.* 2013;28(7):958–967.
11. Marsden CD, Rothwell JC. The physiology of idiopathic dystonia. *Can J Neurol Sci.* 1987;14:521–527.
12. Bastian AJ, Martin TA, Keating JG, Thach WT. Cerebellar ataxia: Abnormal control of interaction torques across multiple joints. *J Neurophysiol.* 1996;76:492–509.
13. Berardelli A, Rothwell JC, Hallett M, Thompson PD, Manfredi M, Marsden CD. The pathophysiology of primary dystonia. *Brain.* 1998;121:1195–1212.

14. Hallett M. The neurophysiology of dystonia. *Arch Neurol.* 1998;55(5):601–603.
15. Malfait N, Sanger TD. Does dystonia always include co-contraction? A study of unconstrained reaching in children with primary and secondary dystonia. *Exp Brain Res.* 2007;176(2):206–216.
16. van der Kamp W, Berardelli A, Rothwell JC, Thompson PD, Day BL, Marsden CD. Rapid elbow movements in patients with torsion dystonia. *J Neurol Neurosurg Psychiatry.* 1989;52:1043–1049.
17. Deuschl G, Toro C, Matsumoto J, Hallett M. Movement-related cortical potentials in writer's cramp. *Ann Neurol.* 1995;38:862–868.
18. Agostino R, Berardelli A, Formica A, Accornero N, Manfredi M. Sequential arm movements in patients with Parkinson's disease, Huntington's disease and dystonia. *Brain.* 1992;115:1481–1495.
19. Tatton WG, Redingham W, Verrier MC, Blair RDG. Characteristic alterations in responses to imposed wrist displacements in Parksinonian rigidity and dystonia musculorum deformans. *Can J Neurol Sci.* 1984;11:281–287.
20. Chen R, Wassermann EM, Canos M, Hallett M. Impaired inhibition in writer's cramp during voluntary muscle activation. *Neurology.* 1997;49:1054–1059.
21. Nakashima K, Rothwell JC, Day BL, Thompson PD, Shannon K, Marsden CD. Reciprocal inhibition between forearm muscles in patients with writer's cramp and other occupational cramps, symptomatic hemidystonia and hemiparesis due to stroke. *Brain.* 1989;112:681–697.
22. Mink JW. The basal ganglia: focused selection and inhibition of competing motor programs. *Prog Neurobiol.* 1996;50:381–425.
23. Kaji R, Rothwell JC, Katayama M, et al. Tonic vibration reflex and muscle afferent block in writer's cramp. *Ann Neurol.* 1995;38:155–162.
24. Bhatia KP, Marsden CD. The behavioural and motor consequences of focal lesions of the basal ganglia in man. *Brain.* 1994;117:859–876.
25. Marsden CD, Obeso JA, Zarranz JJ, Lang AE. The anatomical basis of symptomatic hemidystonia. *Brain.* 1985;108:463–483.
26. Perlmutter JS, Tempel LW, Black KJ, Parkinson D, Todd RD. MPTP induces dystonia and parkinsonism. Clues to the pathophysiology of dystonia. *Neurology.* 1997;49:1432–1438.
27. Tabbal SD, Mink JW, Antenor JA, Carl JL, Moerlein SM, Perlmutter JS. 1-Methyl-4-phenyl-1,2,3,6-tetrahydropyridine-induced acute transient dystonia in monkeys associated with low striatal dopamine. *Neuroscience.* 2006;141:1281–1287.
28. Rupniak N, Jenner P, Marsden C. Acute dystonia induced by neuroleptic drugs. *Psychopharm.* 1986;88:403–419.
29. Nygaard T. Dopa-responsive dystonia. *Curr Opin Neurol.* 1995;8:310–313.
30. Perlmutter JS, Stambuk MK, Markham J, et al. Decreased [18F]spiperone binding in putamen in idiopathic focal dystonia. *J Neurosci.* 1997;17(2):843–850.
31. Lucking CB, Durr A, Bonifati V, et al. Association between early-onset Parkinson's disease and mutations in the parkin gene. French Parkinson's Disease Genetics Study Group. *N Engl J Med.* 2000;342(21):1560–1567.
32. Augood S, Martin D, Ozelius L, Breakefield X, Penney JJ, Standaert DG. Distribution of the mRNAs encoding torsinA and torsinB in the normal adult human brain. *Ann Neurol.* 1999;46:761–769.
33. Sciamanna G, Bonsi P, Tassone A, et al. Impaired striatal D2 receptor function leads to enhanced GABA transmission in a mouse model of DYT1 dystonia. *Neurobiol Dis.* 2009.
34. Quartarone A, Bagnato S, Rizzo V, et al. Abnormal associative plasticity of the human motor cortex in writer's cramp. *Brain.* 2003;126(Pt 12):2586–2596.
35. Baumer T, Demiralay C, Hidding U, et al. Abnormal plasticity of the sensorimotor cortex to slow repetitive transcranial magnetic stimulation in patients with writer's cramp. *Mov Disord.* 2007;22(1):81–90.
36. Ghilardi MF, Carbon M, Silvestri G, et al. Impaired sequence learning in carriers of the DYT1 dystonia mutation. *Ann Neurol.* 2003;54(1):102–109.
37. Hubsch C, Vidailhet M, Rivaud-Pechoux S, et al. Impaired saccadic adaptation in DYT11 dystonia. *J Neurol Neurosurg Psychiatry.* 2011;82(10):1103–1106.
38. Maltese M, Martella G, Madeo G, et al. Anticholinergic drugs rescue synaptic plasticity in DYT1 dystonia: role of M1 muscarinic receptors. *Mov Disord.* 2014;29(13):1655–1665.
39. Bressman SB, de Leon D, Brin MF, et al. Idiopathic dystonia among Ashkenazi Jews: evidence for autosomal dominant inheritance. *Ann Neurol.* 1989;26(5):612–620.
40. Ozelius L, Kramer P, de Leon D, et al. Strong allelic association between the torsion dystonia gene (DYT1) and loci on chromosome 9q34 in Ashkenazi Jews. *Am J Hum Genet.* 1992;50:619–628.

41. Ozelius L, Hewett J, Page C, et al. The early-onset torsion dystonia gene (DYT1) encodes an ATP-binding protein. *Nat Genet*. 1997;17:40–48.
42. Bressman SB, de Leon D, Kramer PL, et al. Dystonia in Ashkenazi Jews: clinical characterization of a founder mutation. *Ann Neurol*. 1994;36(5):771–777.
43. Bressman SB, Sabatti C, Raymond D, et al. The DYT1 phenotype and guidelines for diagnostic testing. *Neurology*. 2000;54(9):1746–1752.
44. Yilmaz U, Yuksel D, Atac FB, Yilmaz D, Verdi H, Senbil N. Atypical phenotypes of DYT1 dystonia in three children. *Brain Dev*. 2013;35(4):356–359.
45. Goodchild RE, Dauer WT. Mislocalization to the nuclear envelope: An effect of the dystonia-causing torsinA mutation. *PNAS*. 2004;101(3):847–852.
46. Naismith TV, Heuser JE, Breakefield XO, Hanson PI. TorsinA in the nuclear envelope. *Proc Natl Acad Sci USA*. 2004;101(20):7612–7617.
47. Leung JC, Klein C, Friedman J, et al. Novel mutation in the TOR1A (DYT1) gene in atypical early onset dystonia and polymorphisms in dystonia and early onset parkinsonism. *Neurogenetics*. 2001;3(3):133–143.
48. Zirn B, Grundmann K, Huppke P, et al. Novel TOR1A mutation p.Arg288Gln in early-onset dystonia (DYT1). *J Neurol Neurosurg Psychiatry*. 2008;79(12):1327–1330.
49. Martino D, Gajos A, Gallo V, et al. Extragenetic factors and clinical penetrance of DYT1 dystonia: an exploratory study. *J Neurol*. 2013;260(4):1081–1086.
50. Risch NJ, Bressman SB, Senthil G, Ozelius LJ. Intragenic Cis and Trans modification of genetic susceptibility in DYT1 torsion dystonia. *Am J Hum Genet*. 2007;80(6):1188–1193.
51. Kamm C, Fischer H, Garavaglia B, et al. Susceptibility to DYT1 dystonia in European patients is modified by the D216H polymorphism. *Neurology*. 2008;70(23):2261–2262.
52. McNaught KS, Kapustin A, Jackson T, et al. Brainstem pathology in DYT1 primary torsion dystonia. *Ann Neurol*. 2004;56(4):540–547.
53. Shashidharan P, Kramer B, Walker R, Olanow C, Brin M. Immunohistochemical localization and distribution of torsinA in normal humand and rat brain. *Brain Res*. 2000;853:197–206.
54. Zhao Y, DeCuypere M, LeDoux MS. Abnormal motor function and dopamine neurotransmission in DYT1 DeltaGAG transgenic mice. *Exp Neurol*. 2008;210(2):719–730.
55. Sciamanna G, Tassone A, Mandolesi G, et al. Cholinergic dysfunction alters synaptic integration between thalamostriatal and corticostriatal inputs in DYT1 dystonia. *J Neurosci*. 2012;32(35):11991–12004.
56. Chiken S, Shashidharan P, Nambu A. Cortically evoked long-lasting inhibition of pallidal neurons in a transgenic mouse model of dystonia. *J Neurosci*. 2008;28(51):13967–13977.
57. Hallett M. Dystonia: abnormal movements result from loss of inhibition. *Adv Neurol*. 2004;94:1–9.
58. Mink J. The basal ganglia and involuntary movements: Impaired inhibition of competing motor patterns. *Arch Neurol*. 2003;60:1365–1368.
59. Eidelberg D, Moeller J, Antonini A, et al. Functional brain networks in DYT1 dystonia. *Ann Neurol*. 1998;44:303–312.
60. Schicatano EJ, Basso MA, Evinger C. Animal model explains the origins of the cranial dystonia benign essential blepharospasm. *J Neurophysiol*. 1997;77(5):2842–2846.
61. Carbon M, Argyelan M, Habeck C, et al. Increased sensorimotor network activity in DYT1 dystonia: a functional imaging study. *Brain*. 2010;133(Pt 3):690–700.
62. Ulug AM, Vo A, Argyelan M, et al. Cerebellothalamocortical pathway abnormalities in torsinA DYT1 knock-in mice. *Proc Natl Acad Sci USA*. 2011;108(16):6638–6643.
63. Gimenez-Roldan S, Lopez-Fraile IP, Esteban A. Dystonia in Spain: study of a Gypsy family and general survey. *Adv Neurol*. 1976;14:125–136.
64. Eldridge R. The torsion dystonias: literature review and genetic and clinical studies. *Neurology*. 1970; 20(11):1–78.
65. Khan NL, Wood NW, Bhatia KP. Autosomal recessive, DYT2-like primary torsion dystonia: a new family. *Neurology*. 2003;61(12):1801–1803.
66. Charlesworth G, Angelova PR, Bartolome-Robledo F, et al. Mutations in HPCA cause autosomal-recessive primary isolated dystonia. *Am J Hum Genet*. 2015;96(4):657–665.
67. Ahmad F, Davis MB, Waddy HM, Oley CA, Marsden CD, Harding AE. Evidence for locus heterogeneity in autosomal dominant torsion dystonia. *Genomics*. 1993;15(1):9–12.

68. Hersheson J, Mencacci NE, Davis M, et al. Mutations in the autoregulatory domain of beta-tubulin 4a cause hereditary dystonia. *Ann Neurol.* 2013;73(4):546–553.

69. Lohmann K, Wilcox RA, Winkler S, et al. Whispering dysphonia (DYT4 dystonia) is caused by a mutation in the TUBB4 gene. *Ann Neurol.* 2013;73(4):537–545.

70. Hamilton EM, Polder E, Vanderver A, et al. Hypomyelination with atrophy of the basal ganglia and cerebellum: further delineation of the phenotype and genotype-phenotype correlation. *Brain.* 2014;137(Pt 7):1921–1930.

71. Hwang WJ, Calne DB, Tsui JK, de la Fuente-Fernandez R. The long-term response to levodopa in dopa-responsive dystonia. *Parkinsonism Relat Disord.* 2001;8(1):1–5.

72. Nygaard T, Marsden C, Fahn S. Dopa-responsive dystonia: long-term treatment response and prognosis. *Neurology.* 1992;41:174–181.

73. Segawa M, Hosaka A, Miyagawa F, Nomura Y, Imai H. Hereditary progressive dystonia with marked diurnal fluctuation. *Adv Neurol.* 1976;14:215–233.

74. Chaila EC, McCabe DJ, Delanty N, Costello DJ, Murphy RP. Broadening the phenotype of childhood-onset dopa-responsive dystonia. *Arch Neurol.* 2006;63(8):1185–1188.

75. Furukawa Y, Kish SJ, Bebin EM, et al. Dystonia with motor delay in compound heterozygotes for GTP-cyclohydrolase I gene mutations. *Ann Neurol.* 1998;44(1):10–16.

76. Kong CK, Ko CH, Tong SF, Lam CW. Atypical presentation of dopa-responsive dystonia: generalized hypotonia and proximal weakness. *Neurology.* 2001;57(6):1121–1124.

77. Furukawa Y, Graf W, Wong H, Shimadzu M, Kish S. Dopa-responsive dystonia simulating spastic paraplegia due to tyrosine hydroxylase (TH) gene mutations. *Neurology.* 2001;56:260–263.

78. Bruggemann N, Stiller S, Tadic V, et al. Non-motor phenotype of dopa-responsive dystonia and quality of life assessment. *Parkinsonism Relat Disord.* 2014;20(4):428–431.

79. Furukawa Y, Mizuno Y, Narabayashi H. Early-onset parkinsonism with dystonia. Clinical and biochemical differences from hereditary progressive dystonia or DOPA-responsive dystonia. *Adv Neurol.* 1996;69:327–337.

80. Jeon B, Jeong J-M, Park S-S, et al. Dopamine transporter density meaured by [^{123}I]β-CIT single-photon emission computed tomography is normal in dopa-responsive dystonia. *Neurology.* 1998;43:792–800.

81. Hyland K, Fryburg JS, Wilson WG, et al. Oral phenylalanine loading in dopa-responsive dystonia: a possible diagnostic test. *Neurology.* 1997;48(5):1290–1297.

82. Opladen T, Okun JG, Burgard P, Blau N, Hoffmann GF. Phenylalanine loading in pediatric patients with dopa-responsive dystonia: revised test protocol and pediatric cutoff values. *J Inherit Metab Dis.* 2010;33(6):697–703.

83. Ichinose H, Suzuki T, Inagaki H, Ohye T, Nagatsu T. Molecular genetics of dopa-responsive dystonia. *Biol Chem.* 1999;380:1355–1364.

84. Almasy L, Bressman SB, Raymond D, et al. Idiopathic torsion dystonia linked to chromosome 8 in two Mennonite families. *Ann Neurol.* 1997;42(4):670–673.

85. Fuchs T, Gavarini S, Saunders-Pullman R, et al. Mutations in the THAP1 gene are responsible for DYT6 primary torsion dystonia. *Nat Genet.* 2009;41(3):286–288.

86. Saunders-Pullman R, Fuchs T, San Luciano M, et al. Heterogeneity in primary dystonia: lessons from THAP1, GNAL, and TOR1A in Amish-Mennonites. *Mov Disord.* 2014;29(6):812–818.

87. LeDoux MS, Xiao J, Rudzinska M, et al. Genotype-phenotype correlations in THAP1 dystonia: molecular foundations and description of new cases. *Parkinsonism Relat Disord.* 2012;18(5):414–425.

88. Xiromerisiou G, Houlden H, Scarmeas N, et al. THAP1 mutations and dystonia phenotypes: genotype phenotype correlations. *Mov Disord.* 2012;27(10):1290–1294.

89. Groen JL, Ritz K, Contarino MF, et al. DYT6 dystonia: mutation screening, phenotype, and response to deep brain stimulation. *Mov Disord.* 2010;25(14):2420–2427.

90. Obeso JA, Rothwell JC, Lang AE, Marsden CD. Myoclonic dystonia. *Neurology.* 1983;33:825–830.

91. Quinn NP. Essential myoclonus and myoclonic dystonia. *Mov Disord.* 1996;11:119–124.

92. Roze E, Apartis E, Clot F, et al. Myoclonus-dystonia: Clinical and electrophysiologic pattern related to SGCE mutations. *Neurology.* 2008;70(13):1010–1016.

93. Hess CW, Raymond D, Aguiar Pde C, et al. Myoclonus-dystonia, obsessive-compulsive disorder, and alcohol dependence in SGCE mutation carriers. *Neurology.* 2007;68(7):522–524.

94. Peall KJ, Smith DJ, Kurian MA, et al. SGCE mutations cause psychiatric disorders: clinical and genetic characterization. *Brain.* 2013;136(Pt 1):294–303.

95. van Tricht MJ, Dreissen YE, Cath D, et al. Cognition and psychopathology in myoclonus-dystonia. *J Neurol Neurosurg Psychiatry.* 2012;83(8):814–820.

96. Nardocci N, Zorzi G, Barzaghi C, et al. Myoclonus-dystonia syndrome: clinical presentation, disease course, and genetic features in 11 families. *Mov Disord.* 2008;23(1):28–34.

97. Kinugawa K, Vidailhet M, Clot F, Apartis E, Grabli D, Roze E. Myoclonus-dystonia: an update. *Mov Disord.* Dec 31 2008.

98. Grimes DA, Han F, Lang AE, St George-Hyssop P, Racacho L, Bulman DE. A novel locus for inherited myoclonus-dystonia on 18p11. *Neurology.* 2002;59(8):1183–1186.

99. Asmus F, Salih F, Hjermind LE, et al. Myoclonus-dystonia due to genomic deletions in the epsilon-sarcoglycan gene. *Ann Neurol.* 2005;58(5):792–797.

100. Augustine EF, Blackburn J, Pellegrino JE, Miller R, Mink JW. Myoclonus-dystonia syndrome associated with Russell Silver syndrome. *Mov Disord.* 2013;28(6):841–842.

101. Beukers RJ, van der Meer JN, van der Salm SM, Foncke EM, Veltman DJ, Tijssen MA. Severity of dystonia is correlated with putaminal gray matter changes in myoclonus-dystonia. *Eur J Neurol.* 2011;18(6):906–912.

102. Yokoi F, Dang MT, Li J, Li Y. Myoclonus, motor deficits, alterations in emotional responses and monoamine metabolism in epsilon-sarcoglycan deficient mice. *J Biochem.* 2006;140(1):141–146.

103. Luciano MS, Ozelius L, Sims K, Raymond D, Liu L, Saunders-Pullman R. Responsiveness to levodopa in epsilon-sarcoglycan deletions. *Mov Disord.* Jan 9 2009.

104. Magarinos-Ascone CM, Regidor I, Martinez-Castrillo JC, Gomez-Galan M, Figueiras-Mendez R. Pallidal stimulation relieves myoclonus-dystonia syndrome. *J Neurol Neurosurg Psychiatry.* 2005;76(7):989–991.

105. Liu X, Griffin IC, Parkin SG, et al. Involvement of the medial pallidum in focal myoclonic dystonia: a clinical and neurophysiological case study. *Mov Disord.* 2002;17(2):346–353.

106. Dobyns WB, Ozelius LJ, Kramer PL, et al. Rapid-onset dystonia-parkinsonism. *Neurology.* 1993;43(12):2596–2602.

107. Brashear A, Dobyns WB, de Carvalho Aguiar P, et al. The phenotypic spectrum of rapid-onset dystonia-parkinsonism (RDP) and mutations in the ATP1A3 gene. *Brain.* 2007;130(Pt 3):828–835.

108. Brashear A, Cook JF, Hill DF, et al. Psychiatric disorders in rapid-onset dystonia-parkinsonism. *Neurology.* 2012;79(11):1168–1173.

109. de Carvalho Aguiar P, Sweadner KJ, Penniston JT, et al. Mutations in the Na+/K+ -ATPase alpha3 gene ATP1A3 are associated with rapid-onset dystonia parkinsonism. *Neuron.* 2004;43(2):169–175.

110. Heinzen EL, Swoboda KJ, Hitomi Y, et al. De novo mutations in ATP1A3 cause alternating hemiplegia of childhood. *Nat Genet.* 2012;44(9):1030–1034.

111. Rosewich H, Thiele H, Ohlenbusch A, et al. Heterozygous de-novo mutations in ATP1A3 in patients with alternating hemiplegia of childhood: a whole-exome sequencing gene-identification study. *Lancet Neurol.* 2012;11(9):764–773.

112. Rosewich H, Ohlenbusch A, Huppke P, et al. The expanding clinical and genetic spectrum of ATP1A3-related disorders. *Neurology.* 2014;82(11):945–955.

113. Brashear A, Mink JW, Hill DF, et al. ATP1A3 mutations in infants: a new rapid-onset dystonia-Parkinsonism phenotype characterized by motor delay and ataxia. *Dev Med Child Neurol.* 2012;54(11):1065–1067.

114. Bentivoglio AR, Del Grosso N, Albanese A, Cassetta E, Tonali P, Frontali M. Non-DYT1 dystonia in a large Italian family. *J Neurol Neurosurg Psychiatry.* 1997;62(4):357–360.

115. Valente EM, Bentivoglio AR, Cassetta E, et al. DYT13, a novel primary torsion dystonia locus, maps to chromosome 1p36.13--36.32 in an Italian family with cranial-cervical or upper limb onset. *Ann Neurol.* 2001;49(3):362–366.

116. Camargos S, Scholz S, Simon-Sanchez J, et al. DYT16, a novel young-onset dystonia-parkinsonism disorder: identification of a segregating mutation in the stress-response protein PRKRA. *Lancet Neurol.* 2008;7(3):207–215.

117. Seibler P, Djarmati A, Langpap B, et al. A heterozygous frameshift mutation in PRKRA (DYT16) associated with generalised dystonia in a German patient. *Lancet Neurol.* 2008;7(5):380–381.

118. Lemmon ME, Lavenstein B, Applegate CD, Hamosh A, Tekes A, Singer HS. A novel presentation of DYT 16: acute onset in infancy and association with MRI abnormalities. *Mov Disord.* 2013;28(14):1937–1938.

119. Camargos S, Lees AJ, Singleton A, Cardoso F. DYT16: the original cases. *J Neurol Neurosurg Psychiatry.* 2012;83(10):1012–1014.

120. Bejot Y, Giroud M, Moreau T, Benatru I. Clinical spectrum of movement disorders after stroke in childhood and adulthood. *Eur Neurol.* 2012;68(1):59–64.

121. Manji H, Howard RS, Miller DH, et al. Status dystonicus: the syndrome and its management. *Brain.* 1998;121(Pt 2):243–252.

122. Fasano A, Ricciardi L, Bentivoglio AR, et al. Status dystonicus: predictors of outcome and progression patterns of underlying disease. *Mov Disord*. 2012;27(6):783–788.

123. Opal P, Tintner R, Jankovic J, et al. Intrafamilial phenotypic variability of the DYT1 dystonia: From asymptomatic *TOR1A* gene carrier status to dystonic storm. *Mov Disord*. 2002;17(2):339–345.

124. Mariotti P, Fasano A, Contarino MF, et al. Management of status dystonicus: our experience and review of the literature. *Mov Disord*. 2007;22(7):963–968.

125. Alden TD, Lytle RA, Park TS, Noetzel MJ, Ojemann JG. Intrathecal baclofen withdrawal: a case report and review of the literature. *Childs Nerv Syst*. 2002;18(9–10):522–525.

126. Zorzi G, Marras C, Nardocci N, et al. Stimulation of the globus pallidus internus for childhood-onset dystonia. *Mov Disord*. 2005;20(9):1194–1200.

127. Marras CE, Rizzi M, Cantonetti L, et al. Pallidotomy for medically refractory status dystonicus in childhood. *Dev Med Child Neurol*. 2014;56(7):649–656.

128. Jankovic J. Treatment of dystonia. *Lancet Neurol*. 2006;5(10):864–872.

129. Roubertie A, Mariani LL, Fernandez-Alvarez E, Doummar D, Roze E. Treatment for dystonia in childhood. *Eur J Neurol*. 2012;19(10):1292–1299.

130. Mink JW. Special concerns in defining, studying, and treating dystonia in children. *Mov Disord*. 2013;28(7):921–925.

131. Brunstrom J, Bastian A, Wong M, Mink J. Motor benefit from levodopa in spastic quadriplegic cerebral palsy. *Ann Neurol*. 2000;47:662–665.

132. Pozin I, Bdolah-Abram T, Ben-Pazi H. Levodopa does not improve function in individuals with dystonic cerebral palsy. *J Child Neurol*. 2014;29(4):534–537.

133. Fahn S. High dosage anticholinergic therapy in dystonia. *Neurology*. 1983;33:1255–1261.

134. Jarman P, Bandmann O, Marsden C, Wood N. GTP cyclohydrolase I mutations in patients with dystonia responsive to antcholinergic drugs. *J Neurol Neurosurg Psychiatry*. 1997;63:304–308.

135. Carranza-del Rio J, Clegg NJ, Moore A, Delgado MR. Use of trihexyphenidyl in children with cerebral palsy. *Pediatr Neurol*. 2011;44(3):202–206.

136. Walker RH, Danisi FO, Swope DM, Goodman RR, Germano IM, Brin MF. Intrathecal baclofen for dystonia: benefits and complications during six years of experience. *Mov Disord*. 2000;15(6):1242–1247.

137. Hou JG, Ondo W, Jankovic J. Intrathecal baclofen for dystonia. *Mov Disord*. 2001;16(6):1201–1202.

138. Motta F, Antonello CE. Analysis of complications in 430 consecutive pediatric patients treated with intrathecal baclofen therapy: 14-year experience. *J Neurosurg Pediatr*. 2014;13(3):301–306.

139. Bonouvrie LA, Becher JG, Vles JS, et al. Intrathecal baclofen treatment in dystonic cerebral palsy: a randomized clinical trial: the IDYS trial. *BMC Pediatr*. 2013;13:175.

140. Thenganatt MA, Jankovic J. Treatment of dystonia. *Neurotherapeutics*. 2014;11(1):139–152.

141. Sanger TD, Kukke SN, Sherman-Levine S. Botulinum toxin type B improves the speed of reaching in children with cerebral palsy and arm dystonia: an open-label, dose-escalation pilot study. *J Child Neurol*. 2007;22(1):116–122.

142. Lozano AM, Kumar R, Gross RE, et al. Globus pallidus internus pallidotomy for generalized dystonia. *Mov Disord*. 1997;12(6):865–870.

143. Vidailhet M, Vercueil L, Houeto JL, et al. Bilateral deep-brain stimulation of the globus pallidus in primary generalized dystonia. *N Engl J Med*. 2005;352(5):459–467.

144. Vitek JL, Zhang J, Evatt M, et al. GPi pallidotomy for dystonia: clinical outcome and neuronal activity. *Adv Neurol*. 1998;78:211–219.

145. Kupsch A, Benecke R, Muller J, et al. Pallidal deep-brain stimulation in primary generalized or segmental dystonia. *N Engl J Med*. 2006;355(19):1978–1990.

146. FitzGerald JJ, Rosendal F, de Pennington N, et al. Long-term outcome of deep brain stimulation in generalised dystonia: a series of 60 cases. *J Neurol Neurosurg Psychiatry*. 2014;85(12):1371–1376.

147. Castelnau P, Cif L, Valente EM, et al. Pallidal stimulation improves pantothenate kinase-associated neurodegeneration. *Ann Neurol*. 2005;57(5):738–741.

148. Panov F, Gologorsky Y, Connors G, Tagliati M, Miravite J, Alterman RL. Deep brain stimulation in DYT1 dystonia: a 10-year experience. *Neurosurgery*. 2013;73(1):86–93. discussion 93.

149. Olaya JE, Christian E, Ferman D, et al. Deep brain stimulation in children and young adults with secondary dystonia: the Children's Hospital Los Angeles experience. *Neurosurg Focus*. 2013;35(5):E7.

150. Lumsden DE, Kaminska M, Gimeno H, et al. Proportion of life lived with dystonia inversely correlates with response to pallidal deep brain stimulation in both primary and secondary childhood dystonia. *Dev Med Child Neurol.* 2013;55(6):567–574.

151. Panov F, Tagliati M, Ozelius LJ, et al. Pallidal deep brain stimulation for DYT6 dystonia. *J Neurol Neurosurg Psychiatry.* 2012;83(2):182–187.

152. Miyagi Y, Koike Y. Tolerance of early pallidal stimulation in pediatric generalized dystonia. *J Neurosurg Pediatr.* 2013;12(5):476–482.

153. Gimeno H, Tustin K, Selway R, Lin JP. Beyond the Burke-Fahn-Marsden Dystonia Rating Scale: deep brain stimulation in childhood secondary dystonia. *Eur J Paediatr Neurol.* 2012;16(5):501–508.

154. Markun LC, Starr PA, Air EL, Marks Jr. WJ, Volz MM, Ostrem JL. Shorter disease duration correlates with improved long-term deep brain stimulation outcomes in young-onset DYT1 dystonia. *Neurosurgery.* 2012;71(2):325–330.

155. Isaias IU, Volkmann J, Kupsch A, et al. Factors predicting protracted improvement after pallidal DBS for primary dystonia: the role of age and disease duration. *J Neurol.* 2011;258(8):1469–1476.

156. Wijemanne S, Jankovic J. Dopa-responsive dystonia-clinical and genetic heterogeneity. *Nat Rev Neurol.* 2015;11(7):414–424.

Myoclonus

Harvey S. Singer[1], Jonathan W. Mink[2],
Donald L. Gilbert[3] and Joseph Jankovic[4]

[1]Department of Neurology, Johns Hopkins Hospital, Baltimore, MD, USA;
[2]Division of Child Neurology, University of Rochester Medical Center,
Rochester, NY, USA; [3]Division of Neurology, Cincinnati Children's Hospital
Medical Center, Cincinnati, OH, USA; [4]Department of Neurology, Baylor
College of Medicine, Houston, TX, USA

OUTLINE

Movement Disorders in Childhood, Second Edition.
DOI: http://dx.doi.org/10.1016/B978-0-12-411573-6.00012-7

205

INTRODUCTION AND OVERVIEW

Myoclonus can arise from pathological processes in the cerebral cortex, subcortical regions, cerebellum, brainstem, spinal cord, and sometimes peripheral nerves.[1] Both idiopathic disorders and symptomatic conditions can cause myoclonus. In children, myoclonus most commonly manifests with epilepsy, encephalopathy, or other symptoms. Isolated myoclonus is not a common chief complaint in children treated by pediatric neurologists or movement disorder specialists. Thus, clinicians may use the presence of myoclonus as one of several key factors in diagnostic and therapeutic decision making. This chapter encompasses diseases and disorders resulting in clinical syndromes that include prominent myoclonus.

DEFINITION OF MYOCLONUS

Myoclonus refers to quick, shock-like jerks due to sudden involuntary contraction of one or more muscles.[2] The term is usually applied to describe *positive myoclonus*. *Negative myoclonus* refers to a sudden, brief interruption or relaxation of contraction in active postural muscles.[3] *Asterixis* is a form of negative myoclonus. Both *negative myoclonus* and *positive myoclonus* occur in children, but throughout the chapter, *myoclonus* will mainly refer to *positive myoclonus*.

Startle syndromes will also be discussed.[2,4] Startles are brief, generalized motor responses similar to myoclonus.

CLINICAL CHARACTERISTICS—PHENOMENOLOGY OF MYOCLONUS IN CHILDREN

As with other movement disorders, various forms of categorization of myoclonus are useful in describing the phenomenology and facilitating diagnosis. Levels of categorization in wide use are based on clinical features, neuroanatomy, and etiology.[2,5] Table 12.1 emphasizes observable clinical characteristics used in describing forms of myoclonus.

Myoclonus may manifest as synchronous contraction of several muscles or asynchronous contraction of muscles with unpredictable timing. Sometimes myoclonus spreads across muscles predictably. Involvement of muscles may be focal, multifocal, or generalized. Visually, this

TABLE 12.1   Clinical Features of Myoclonus

Clinical features	Types of myoclonus
Muscle action	Contraction—Positive myoclonus
	Relaxation—Negative myoclonus
State	At rest—Spontaneous
	Active—Action
	Stimulated—Reflex
Location	Focal
	Axial
	Multifocal
	Generalized
Timing	Irregular
	Rhythmic

contraction appears to be lightning quick or shock like. Few studies document electrophysiology in children. Electrophysiology in adults generally shows that individual myoclonic jerks having cortical origin last 10–50 ms but that those with brainstem or spinal origin may last up to 200 ms.[6] The relationship of the jerk to rest, voluntary movement, and external triggers is diagnostically important, as is neuroanatomic and body location. *Axial myoclonus* indicates involvement of the trunk. One form of axial myoclonus referred to as propriospinal myoclonus and linked to spinal cord lesions has more recently been considered to be of psychogenic origin.[7,8] *Multifocal myoclonus* refers to randomly appearing jerks in multiple locations. *Generalized myoclonus* refers to jerking in many muscles simultaneously. *Spontaneous* and *action* denote the state of the muscle at myoclonus onset, and *reflex* indicates a preceding sensory input acting as a trigger. Repetitive, *rhythmic myoclonus* is termed by some as *segmental myoclonus* or *myoclonic tremor*. Another oscillatory movement that resembles both myoclonus and tremor is *myorhythmia*. *Myorhythmia* is defined as repetitive, rhythmic, slow (1–4 Hz) movement affecting chiefly cranial and limb muscles; it may be oscillatory and jerky, thus overlapping phenomenologically between tremor and segmental myoclonus.[9] Unilateral rhythmic myoclonus generated by cerebral cortex may be *epilepsia partialis continua* (EPC).

Clinical Differentiation of Myoclonus from Other Movement Disorders

Myoclonus can resemble or co-occur with other movement disorders, and the distinction can be clinically challenging. In addition to observation of phenomenology, documentation of other features is important. The muscle groups involved in an individual patient are usually stereotyped but otherwise the time course and pattern are not predictable. Myoclonus is generally not distractible or suppressible, although some forms of segmental myoclonus may be position-related.

TABLE 12.2   Clinical Features of Myoclonus versus Tics

Clinical features	Myoclonus	Tics
Subjective sense of volition	Involuntary	When noticed seem semivoluntary or both voluntary and involuntary
Relationship to voluntary movement	May occur at onset or during purposeful movements of same muscles	Purposeful movements of same muscles usually "override" tics, so they tend to occur before or after
Suppressibility	Not suppressible	Often, at least briefly, suppressible
Premonitory urge	None	Often present
Co-occurring problems	Epilepsy, encephalopathy, other movement disorders	Anxiety, obsessive–compulsive disorder, attention-deficit hyperactivity disorder, autism spectrum disorder
Age of onset	Any	Usually between 3 and 10 years

The overlap of slow and fast movements in mixed movement disorders requires careful, detailed clinical assessment. Even expert clinicians may be challenged, as has been shown for diagnosis of myoclonus-dystonia versus benign hereditary chorea,[10] although benign hereditary chorea may have infantile onset with a more stable course.[11]

Chorea involves involuntary, ongoing, random-appearing movements or movement fragments. Quick choreic or ballistic (*ballism*) movements may also be difficult to distinguish from multifocal myoclonus.

Dystonia involves involuntary, sustained or intermittent muscle contractions causing abnormal movements or postures. When a dystonic contraction is quick, visual differentiation from myoclonus or tics may be difficult. Both symptoms may occur together, as in myoclonus-dystonia. The presence of other more sustained dystonic posturing, irregular dystonic tremor, or sensory tricks may be clues that the movement in question is dystonic rather than myoclonic.

Fasciculations are spontaneous muscle fiber contractions in denervated, single motor units. These do not cause movement across a joint.

Myokymia denotes continuous muscle rippling usually resulting from peripheral nerve hyperexcitability which does not cause movement across a joint.

Tics, the most common pediatric movement disorder, resemble myoclonus when the tic movements are very quick and involve a small number of muscle groups.

Titubation, truncal ataxia, and limb ataxia may also result in rapid movements that resemble multifocal myoclonus.

It is usually possible to distinguish myoclonus and tics clinically without further diagnostic testing, based on the key distinguishing features described in Table 12.2.

LOCALIZATION AND PATHOPHYSIOLOGY

Myoclonus can originate at multiple levels of the neuraxis, and therefore comprehensive neurological examination is indicated for the purpose of localization and differential

TABLE 12.3   Type of Myoclonus and Neuroanatomic Location

Neuroanatomic substrate	Type of myoclonus
Cerebral cortex	Focal
	Multifocal
	Generalized
	Reflex/stimulus sensitive
Thalamus, basal ganglia	Focal
	Generalized
	Reflex
Brainstem	Reticular, generalized
	Startle, hyperekplexia
	Palatal, myoclonic tremor
Spinal	Segmental
	Propriospinal, axial
Peripheral	Focal
Unknown	Ballistic movement overflow

diagnosis. Myoclonus can also occur in a vast number of neurological conditions. Anatomic sources of myoclonus and types of observed myoclonus are shown in Table 12.3.

Neurophysiology of Myoclonus

By comparison to other movement disorders, myoclonus probably results from a relatively simpler process. The pathophysiology of myoclonus involves a brief discharge of neurons transmitted, inappropriately, out to the body, resulting in brief jerks. Thus, for example, some pathologic processes that disturb the balance of excitation and inhibition within the motor cortex can produce brief abnormal discharges that are propagated to muscles, producing myoclonus. A cortical source of the myoclonus can sometimes be recorded using scalp electroencephalography (EEG). The small amplitude of these abnormal discharges means that the signal does not reliably exceed the background recorded electrical activity. Simultaneous electromyography (EMG) recording of muscle where myoclonus is present demonstrates the burst of less than 50 ms duration electrical activity during the jerk. The relationship between the premotor EEG discharges and EMG bursts can be assessed by superimposing and averaging repeated EEG/EMG tracings to increase the EEG signal-to-noise ratio, bringing out the premotor potential. This method is referred to as *back-averaging*.[6]

Limitations of EEG for understanding the pathophysiology of myoclonus include lack of specificity, lack of information about cellular pathology underlying the cortical discharge, and lack of availability of techniques like back-averaging in many clinics. In addition, this

TABLE 12.4   Categories of Disease Producing Myoclonus

Etiological category	Clinical features
Physiologic	Myoclonus occurs in certain settings in healthy persons. Examples include sleep (hypnic) jerks, hiccoughs, and benign infantile myoclonus with feeding.[15]
Benign, developmental	Myoclonus as a transient symptom during otherwise normal development. Examples include benign neonatal myoclonus and myoclonus of early infancy. See also Chapter 6.
Startle syndromes	Quick, involuntary, stimulus-evoked reflex movements. An exaggerated startle response that may be further subdivided into hereditary, symptomatic, startle epilepsy, and neuropsychiatric startle syndromes (Latah syndrome, jumping Frenchman of Maine, anxiety-induced startle).[4]
Primary myoclonus disorders	Myoclonus occurs as the primary symptom. The cardinal example is *essential myoclonus*.[16,17]
Epileptic	Myoclonus is associated with clinical seizures and/or epileptiform discharges on EEG, supportive of a cortical origin.
Primary epileptic myoclonus disorders	Myoclonus as a seizure type or fragment, or myoclonus as a symptom in addition to seizures in an epilepsy syndrome without encephalopathy.[18,19]
Progressive myoclonic epilepsies and progressive encephalopathies with myoclonus	Myoclonus occurs as part of a multisymptom, progressive neurologic disease.
Secondary myoclonus disorders	Myoclonus occurs secondary to some other identifiable, nongenetic cause or process. Examples include autoimmune diseases, infections/encephalitides, hypoxic ischemic injury (Lance Adams myoclonus), toxins, metabolic derangements such as uremia, acidosis. Also, secondary to medications, e.g., myoclonus triggered by the use of focal antiepileptic medications in patients with generalized epilepsies.[20–22] See also Chapter 22.
Psychogenic/Functional	Pseudomyoclonus as a symptom of a functional neurological symptom disorder/psychogenic movement disorder.[23–25] See also Chapter 23.

method is not always sensitive for cortical sources of myoclonus and cannot be used for deeper sources.

Other neurophysiologic techniques can provide clues about the pathophysiology of myoclonus. For example, cortical myoclonus may be associated with abnormally large amplitude somatosensory-evoked potentials[6,12] or changes in motor cortex excitability measured using transcranial magnetic stimulation (TMS) over motor cortex.[13,14]

Further information about the pathophysiology of myoclonus is available through laboratory, radiologic, and clinical-pathologic correlations in the case of individual diseases. In addition to anatomic localization, it is helpful to consider etiological categories, as shown in Table 12.4, to develop a differential diagnosis for myoclonus. This section is organized into etiological categories and reviews some of the more common or important diseases causing myoclonus in children. The emphasis is on conditions where myoclonus is prominent. A more comprehensive table of diseases in which myoclonus may occur in children appears in Table 12.5.

TABLE 12.5 Genetic Causes of Diseases with Prominent Myoclonus in Childhood, by Category

Disease	Gene (locus); protein	Inheritance	Clinical features	Age of onset
PRIMARY MYOCLONUS				
Hereditary geniospasm[165]	Possible linkage to 9q13-q21	AD	Chin myoclonus/tremor	Childhood
Myoclonus dystonia syndrome : DYT11, DYT15[55,60,166–168]	SGCE; epsilon sarcoglycan; DRD2 dopamine receptor 2	AD	Bilateral myoclonus, tremor, dystonia, torticollis, depression, anxiety, obsessive–compulsive disorder	5–15 years
EPILEPTIC MYOCLONUS WITHOUT ENCEPHALOPATHY				
Juvenile absence epilepsy (EJA1)[169]	EFHC2; EF-hand domain (C-terminal)-containing protein 2	AD	Absence seizures, generalized tonic-clonic seizures, myoclonic seizures	Childhood, around puberty
Juvenile myoclonic epilepsy (JME)[73,74,170–175]	GABRA1 and GABRD GABA receptors; CACNB4 calcium channels; CLCN2 chloride channels	AD	Morning myoclonic jerks, absence and GTC seizures	Childhood and adolescence
MYOCLONUS PLUS ENCEPHALOPATHY				
Amish infantile epilepsy syndrome[176]	SIAT9; sialytransferase-9	AR	Failure to thrive, visual loss, startle myoclonus, epilepsy, no development, early death	Infancy
Aromatic L-amino acid decarboxylase deficiency[177]	DDC; dopa-decarboxylase	AR	Oculogyric crises, opisthotonus, dystonia, myoclonus, hyperreflexia, chorea, irritability	Infancy
Combined saposin deficiency[178,179]	PSAP; prosaposin	AR	Myoclonus, dyskinesias, seizures, organomegaly, respiratory failure	Infancy
Dentatorubral-pallidoluysian atrophy (DRPLA)[180]	ATN1 expanded trinucleotide repeat; atrophin 1	AD	Seizures, ataxia, choreoathetosis, myoclonus, dementia	Usually 30s, can occur in childhood
Gaucher disease IIIA[181]	GBA; acid beta-glucocerebrosidase	AR	Myoclonus, spastic paraparesis, dementia, seizures, ataxia, organomegaly, abnormal saccades, short stature	Early to late childhood
Hyperornithinemia-hyperammonemia-homocitrullinuria syndrome[182,183]	SCLC25A15; solute carrier family 25, member 15	AR	Myoclonic epilepsy, dementia, pyramidal signs and spasticity, neuropathy, episodic vomiting	Infancy

(Continued)

TABLE 12.5 (Continued)

Disease	Gene (locus); protein	Inheritance	Clinical features	Age of onset
Mitochondrial complex II deficiency[184]	SDHAF1; succinate dehydrogenase complex	AR	Short stature, cardiomyopathy, leukoencephalopathy, spongiform encephalopmyopathy, ataxia, myoclonus, seizures	Childhood
Myoclonic epilepsy associated with ragged red fibers (MERRF)[185,186]	Multiple mitochondrial transfer RNA genes, MTTK, MTTL1, MTTH, MTTS1, MTTS2, MTTF	Mitochondrial	Myoclonus, epilepsy, ataxia, spasticity, weakness, deafness	Childhood or adulthood
Neuronal ceroid lipofuscinosis 1[187]	PPT1; palmitoyl-protein thioesterase-1	AR	Progressive visual loss, dementia, myoclonus, ataxia, epilepsy, early death; variable—later onset with psychiatric symptoms	Early childhood; late childhood or adult
Neuronal ceroid lipofuscinosis 2[188]	TPP1; tripeptidyl peptidase 1	AR	Progressive visual loss, dementia, myoclonus, ataxia, epilepsy, early death	Early childhood
Neuronal ceroid lipofuscinosis 3[189]	CLN3; battenin (CLN3 protein)	AR	Progressive visual loss, dementia, myoclonus, ataxia, epilepsy, early death	Childhood
Neuronal ceroid lipofuscinosis 5[190]	CLN5; CLN5 protein	AR	Progressive visual loss, dementia, myoclonus, ataxia, epilepsy, early death	Childhood
Neuronal ceroid lipofuscinosis 8[191]	CLN8; CLN8 protein	AR	Dementia, myoclonus, epilepsy, ataxia, atrophy	Early childhood
Progressive myoclonic ataxias/ Ramsay Hunt syndrome[192]	None—the literature on this syndrome probably represents a collection of diagnoses, including some that now could have molecular diagnosis	AD/other	Myoclonus, ataxia, tremor, GTCs, degeneration of dentate nucleus, globus pallidus, mitochondrial disease findings	Childhood
Progressive neuronal degeneration of childhood with liver disease (Alpers Huttenlocher)[193]	POLG1; DNA mitochondrial polymerase gamma	AR	Failure to thrive, visual loss, myoclonus, epilepsy, ataxia, early death	Infancy
Pyridoxine 5-prime phosphate oxidase deficiency[194]	PNPO; pyridoxine phosphate oxidase	AR	Myoclonus, neonatal epileptic encephalopathy, partial response to pyridoxine, seizure response to pyridoxal phosphate	Infancy, usually preterm delivery

Disease	Gene; Protein	Inheritance	Clinical features	Age of onset
Rett syndrome in males[195,196]	MECP2; Methyl-CpG-Binding Protein 2	X linked	Severe encephalopathy, myoclonus, rigidity, death in 2 years	Infancy
Schindler disease, infantile type[197]	NAGA; alpha-N-acetylgalactosaminidase	AR	Visual loss, dementia, spasticity, myoclonus, brain atrophy	Early childhood
Sialidosis I and II[79]	NEU1; neuraminidase (sialidase)	AR	Storage phenotype—coarse facies, intellectual disabilities	Can be early childhood
Spinocerebellar ataxia type 19[198]	Linkage 1p21-q23	AD	Ataxia, myoclonus, tremor	Usually adult, some child
Spinocerebellar ataxia type 2[199]	ATXN2; expanded trinucleotide repeat; ataxin 2	AD	Dementia, myoclonus, epilepsy, ataxia, atrophy, abnormal eye movements	Usually adult, some infants

PME

Disease	Gene; Protein	Inheritance	Clinical features	Age of onset
Myoclonic epilepsy—Unverricht and Lundborg EPM1A[200]	CSTB; Cystatin B/Stefin B	AR	Myoclonus, ataxia, GTCs, absence seizures, dysarthria, mental deterioration	Childhood
Epilepsy, progressive myoclonic EPM 1B[201]	PRICKLE1; rest-interacting lim domain protein	AR	Upward gaze palsy, motor delays with ataxia early, seizures later childhood	Early childhood
Myoclonic epilepsy—Lafora EPM2A[147]	EPM2A; laforin	AR	Myoclonus, epilepsy, apraxia, dementia, visual loss, psychosis	Late childhood
Myoclonic epilepsy—Lafora EPM2B[148]	NHLRC1; malin	AR	Myoclonus, epilepsy, apraxia, dementia, visual loss, psychosis	Late childhood
Action myoclonus renal failure syndrome[202]	SCARB2; scavenger receptor, class B, member 2	AR	Progressive action myoclonus, finger tremor, ataxia, GTCs, nephropathy/renal failure	Late teens

DISEASES AND DISORDERS

Physiologic Myoclonus—Myoclonus in Certain Settings, in Otherwise Healthy Individuals

Physiologic and Benign Forms of Myoclonus

CLINICAL FEATURES

A common concern for parents is myoclonus related to their child's sleep. Myoclonus at sleep onset is usually a single, full-body jerk, also known as *hypnagogic myoclonus*. Myoclonus during sleep is focal or multifocal and often occurs during rapid eye movement (REM) sleep. Myoclonus related to sleep, including benign neonatal sleep myoclonus, is covered in detail in Chapter 19. In general, these forms of myoclonus do not require diagnostic evaluation or treatment.

Other forms of physiologic myoclonus include hiccups and exercise- or anxiety-induced myoclonus. Anxiety-induced myoclonus is probably an exaggerated startle response.

PATHOPHYSIOLOGY

The pathophysiology is unknown.

DIAGNOSTIC APPROACH

The diagnostic approach is based on history. Brief startles occurring while the child is falling asleep can be diagnosed clinically, for example. In general, no diagnostic testing or treatment is needed.

Startle Syndromes

A startle response to an unexpected stimulus is physiologic and adaptive. The startle response to auditory stimuli appears in the orbicularis oculi and sternocleidomastoid first,[26] and usually habituates rapidly. The neural substrate of the startle response is in the caudal brainstem. A *startle syndrome* involves an abnormal tendency to exhibit startle reflexes— quick, involuntary jerks in response to a surprising stimulus. Although the duration of a startle response is longer than that of cortical myoclonus, many authors include discussions of startle syndromes in reviews of myoclonus.[27]

Hereditary Hyperekplexias

CLINICAL FEATURES

Hyperekplexias may be considered a form of nonepileptic, stimulus-induced myoclonus, or disorders of exaggerated startle responses. Tactile, auditory, visual, and emotional stimuli provoke an excessive response. The phenomenology involves head flexion and extension and abduction of the arms. This category encompasses a number of conditions. When the onset occurs in infancy, the child may have persistent hypertonia and failure to thrive caused by constant startle and stiffening. This is also referred to as the *stiff baby syndrome*.[4,28] This stiffness may eventually resolve. Another disorder associated with stiffness and myoclonus is the *stiff person syndrome*. An autoimmune disorder, stiff person syndrome

TABLE 12.6   Genetically Defined Hyperekplexias

Hyperekplexia type	Inheritance	Gene	Protein	Associated clinical features
HKPX1	AR or AD	GLRA1[32]	Alpha 1 subunit, glycine receptor chloride channel (GlyR)	Infancy onset generalized skeletal muscle contraction, umbilical or inguinal hernia, hip dislocation, hypertonicity in infancy, nocturnal seizures, anxious affect
HKPX2	AR	GLRB[34]	Beta subunit of GlyR	Infancy onset generalized skeletal muscle contraction; improves by early childhood
HKPX3	AD or AR	GLYT2[35]	Glycine neurotransmitter transporter, solute carrier family 6, member 5	Neonatal hypertonia, apnea, stiffness; may resolve in first year
EIEE8	X linked	ARHGEF9[36]	Collybistin, a rho guanine nucleotide exchange factor 9	Occurs in early infantile epileptic encephalopathy-8 with cognitive impairment

typically presents in adults, but may also occur in children and may be associated with myoclonus[29,30] (see Chapter 18). Older children with hyperekplexia may have the classic phenomenology along with other sleep-related symptoms, including periodic limb movements in sleep and hypnagogic myoclonus. In some cases, frequent falls may occur, leading the child to be fearful of walking in open spaces. Sporadic and familial cases are described.

PATHOPHYSIOLOGY

The pathophysiology of startle disorders involves dysfunction within inhibitory synapses, particularly those in reflex circuits. The most common form of hyperekplexia, HKPX1, results from mutations in the GLRA1 gene,[31,32] which encodes the alpha 1 subunit of the glycine receptor chloride channel (GlyR).[33] Three very rare forms, HKPX2,[34] HKPX3,[35] and a form associated with infantile epilepsy,[36] are listed in Table 12.6.

DIAGNOSTIC APPROACH

Hereditary and sporadic hyperekplexias, with startles in the absence of other neurologic signs, may be diagnosed clinically in the presence of characteristic history and examination findings, including an exaggerated head retraction reflex elicited by tapping the tip of the nose.[4] Home videos may be helpful. If the diagnosis appears likely on clinical grounds and symptomatic treatment with clonazepam or other benzodiazepine is effective, then genetic confirmation is not necessary. In less clear cases, genetic testing can be considered based on cost and availability.

TREATMENT

Treatment is nonspecific but can be very helpful. Hereditary hyperekplexias in infants can cause failure to thrive due to difficulty feeding. In children, there can be substantial physical, emotional, and social morbidity. The treatment of choice initially is clonazepam or other benzodiazepines. If these are ineffective, other anticonvulsant agents such as sodium valproate and levetiracetam may be used.

Symptomatic Startle Disorders

CLINICAL FEATURES, PATHOPHYSIOLOGY

The phenomenology of the startle is similar, but other features of the clinical presentation are clues to the diagnosis. Acquired brainstem pathology may result in exaggerated startle, accompanied by other brainstem findings. Perinatal anoxia may result in spastic quadriplegia, profound cognitive impairment, and an exaggerated startle, which may trigger clonus. Other global hypoxic ischemic injuries may also cause this form of myoclonus.[37] Brainstem inflammatory processes, e.g., some viral encephalitides and inflammatory lesions in acute disseminated encephalomyelitis and multiple sclerosis, and auto-antibodies to gephyrin[38] may result in startle disorders. An exaggerated, nonhabituating startle may also occur in neurodegenerative diseases. Diagnostic approach involves history, examination, neuroimaging, and other studies based on the clinical context. Treatment is symptomatic. In cases of diffuse, severe anoxic injury, treatment of stimulus-evoked myoclonus is not necessary.

Startle Epilepsies

CLINICAL FEATURES

Sudden stimuli, such as a loud sound, or photic stimulation may provoke a startle response and then a seizure in children with startle epilepsies. This represents a small proportion of pediatric epilepsies. The seizure semiology may suggest involvement of motor or supplementary motor areas.[39] Startle epilepsies are probably most common after anoxic or ischemic brain injuries in young children,[40] but may occur with occult cerebral lesions in adolescence.[39] They have also been described in children with Down syndrome.[41] Many young children with startle-provoked epilepsies also have significant intellectual disabilities.[42] Idiopathic, reflex myoclonic epilepsy, with myoclonic attacks occurring after unexpected tactile and auditory stimuli, has been described in otherwise normal young children, with good response to treatment with sodium valproate.[43,44]

Neuropsychiatric Startle Syndromes

CLINICAL FEATURES

This diverse but iconic group of movement disorders is characterized by excessive startle plus behavioral symptoms such as shouting out, echolalia, echopraxia, and jumping.[45] The phenomenology of the behaviors may be culturally mediated. Examples include the jumping Frenchmen of Maine, or Latah in Southeast Asia, in which the individual mimics involuntarily the quick movements and sounds of those nearby. Some include in this category patients who exhibit persistent startles with reduced or impaired habituation.

Primary Myoclonic Disorders

The main primary myoclonus is essential myoclonus (EM). The term *essential* classically designates diseases that have no obvious or known cause and normal neuroimaging, and indicates that the named symptom dominates the clinical presentation. In this sense, *essential* overlaps *idiopathic*. Some ambiguity about "unknown cause" occurs when *idiopathic* or *essential* is applied to diseases with high apparent heritability, since a genetic cause is inferred, or to diseases once a causative gene has been identified. The term *primary* is employed as a classification for the neurologic conditions in this section in which myoclonus dominates and either (1) no proximate cause is known, or (2) genetic causes are suspected or identified.

Essential Myoclonus

CLINICAL FEATURES

The phenomenology of EM is multifocal, arrhythmic myoclonus. Onset in hereditary cases is in the first 20 years, and the long-term course is benign. There should be no epilepsy, dementia, ataxia, or other neurologic defects. Some consider geniospasm, a spontaneous or stress-induced intermittent quivering of the chin, to be a form of tremor, others consider it to be a form of EM.[46]

PATHOPHYSIOLOGY

The pathophysiology of EM is unknown, although it appears to be heritable in some cases. Linkage has not been identified, but multiple pedigrees with familial EM have been described in European and Asian populations.[47,48] It should be noted that in older medical literature there is overlap between EM, essential tremor, and myoclonus-dystonia discussed later in this chapter.

DIAGNOSTIC APPROACH

Family history, phenomenology, and careful distinction of myoclonus from tics or rapid dystonic movements should suggest a diagnosis of EM. In adolescents with predominantly morning myoclonic jerks, a diagnosis of juvenile myoclonic epilepsy (JME) should be considered (see later discussion).

TREATMENT

Treatment of EM is symptomatic and often unsatisfactory. Treatment decisions should be based on degree of social and functional impairment. Pharmacological options include benzodiazepines and anticonvulsants such as sodium valproate, levetiracetam, and piracetam. Risks and potential benefits should be considered on an individual basis. For chin myoclonus, a positive response to botulinum toxin injection has been described.[49]

Myoclonus-Dystonia (DYT11)

CLINICAL FEATURES

Myoclonus-dystonia (see also chapter 11) can have early childhood onset. This disorder is described in this chapter because myoclonus may dominate the phenomenology and physiology[209] such that some cases may be diagnosed clinically as EM. Myoclonus is action induced and occurs predominantly in the head, neck, and proximal arms (Video 12.2). Early falls may occur. There is overlap between clinical features of myoclonus dystonia and benign hereditary chorea.[50] However, adult-onset, distal myoclonus has also been described, so the phenotype varies.[51] Alcohol ingestion may reduce symptoms. Psychiatric symptoms, including obsessive–compulsive disorder and anxiety, alcohol abuse, and executive function deficits, are common.[52–55] The long-term adult course is stable.

PATHOPHYSIOLOGY

Myoclonus-dystonia is caused in most cases by mutations in the epsilon sarcoglycan (SGCE) gene.[55] Penetrance, the probability that the individual carrying the SGCE gene mutation will manifest symptoms of the disease, depends on the parent of origin. This disorder demonstrates maternal imprinting, leading to inactivation of the maternal allele. Therefore, if the mutated epsilon sarcoglycan gene is passed on by the mother, the disease is manifest in only approximately 5–10% of cases. However, if the mutated epsilon sarcoglycan gene is passed on by the father, penetrance is approximately 90% (because the healthy, maternally inherited allele is inactivated and cannot dominate the mutated gene). It is important to note also, however, that individual pediatric cases[56] and pedigrees with autosomal dominant inheritance have been identified that are mutation negative.[57–59] Moreover, not all pedigrees support the presence of maternal imprinting.[51] In rare cases, a heterozygous substitution mutation in the DRD2 gene, encoding the dopamine 2 receptor, has been identified.[60]

DIAGNOSTIC APPROACH

The diagnosis should be suspected in children on clinical grounds in the presence of the characteristic features of chronic, action-induced myoclonus which overflows into and interferes with purposeful actions. Dystonia during at least some activities, such as walking, may be apparent. The phenomenology of proximal, action-induced myoclonus can be diagnostically challenging, because there is overlap with the appearance of fast chorea in disorders such as benign hereditary chorea. The presence of a pedigree consistent with autosomal dominant inheritance with incomplete penetrance is helpful. Affected adults' family members may report symptom improvement with alcohol. A molecular diagnosis of DYT11 is useful for understanding the disease, predicting possible outcomes, ruling out other causes, and counseling family members. Specific genetic testing for SGCE is commercially available. If this condition is strongly suspected but sequence testing is negative, testing for TITF1 or DRD2 mutations may be considered. In addition, particularly if there is microcephaly, short stature, or dysmorphic features, chromosome microarray testing for larger deletions should be considered.[61,62]

TREATMENT

There is no specific treatment for myoclonus. General considerations for symptomatic treatment of myoclonus and dystonia apply. Levodopa treatment may be considered.[63] Beneficial treatment of adult cases with deep brain stimulation placed in globus pallidus interna have been described.[64,65] Treatment of anxiety and depression with selective serotonin reuptake inhibitors or cognitive behavioral therapy should be considered.

Benign Myoclonus of Early Infancy

CLINICAL FEATURES

Benign myoclonus of early infancy (BMEI) is a rare disorder of infancy that may mimic infantile spasms.[66] The phenomenology is jerks of the neck or with extension, or tonic flexion, of upper limbs. These may cluster and may appear daily. They tend to occur during waking or during excitement or frustration. Onset is any time in the first year of life[67] (see also Chapter 6). There is some controversy as to whether this should be termed "benign nonepileptic infantile spasms." In contrast to infantile spasms, this condition is benign, with no altered consciousness and no encephalopathy. Symptoms eventually diminish and resolve, usually in a few months. Long-term developmental outcomes are usually good. Pathophysiology is unknown. Generally, the history and examination are completely reassuring, the jerks or shuddering spells are brief without altered consciousness, and interictal and ictal EEGs are normal.[68] Diagnosis is clinical, with characteristic features and normal EEG. Treatment is generally not needed. Additional details are found in Chapter 6.

Epileptic Myoclonus without Encephalopathy

A complete discussion of epileptic myoclonus lies outside the scope of this text but is reviewed elsewhere.[69,70] Epileptic myoclonus can be a fragment of a partial or generalized seizure or be one of multiple seizure types. However, several key phenomena and conditions, in which myoclonic jerks occur prior to generalized seizures, merit discussion, because these conditions may present special diagnostic or therapeutic challenges.

Myoclonus is common in a number of forms of idiopathic and symptomatic epilepsy. If myoclonus is the predominant seizure type or is a prominent phenomenon, the condition is termed *myoclonic epilepsy*.

Juvenile Myoclonic Epilepsy

CLINICAL FEATURES

Adolescents may be seen by neurologists initially with brief myoclonus involving predominantly the arms, which usually occurs in the morning and may characteristically cause fumbling or dropping handheld items. Consciousness is preserved. JME is a subtype of idiopathic generalized epilepsy. Eventually, in most cases, one or more generalized tonic-clonic seizures occur, sometimes triggered by sleep deprivation. Absence seizures may also occur. The disorder is believed to persist throughout life in most individuals, but generalized tonic-clonic seizures may remit in approximately one third of cases.[71] Long-term, individuals with JME have higher risk of psychiatric diagnosis and adverse psychosocial outcomes.[71]

PATHOPHYSIOLOGY

The myoclonus of JME/EJM may be a thalamo-cortically generated myoclonus, or a form of cortical myoclonus.[72] The epilepsy is generalized. The pathophysiology is genetically heterogeneous, as associations have been found with variations in multiple genes (see Table 12.7).

For the forms EJM2, 3, 4, 9, only chromosomal linkages have been identified.

DIAGNOSTIC APPROACH

JME is diagnosed in the setting of the classic clinical presentation with morning myoclonus plus two or more generalized tonic-clonic seizures. In the presence of morning myoclonus only, it is helpful to confirm the JME diagnosis with interictal EEG, which may show characteristic 3–5 Hz spikes and waves. Many clinicians would then advise treatment on the

TABLE 12.7   Genetic Susceptibilities to Juvenile-Onset Epilepsies with Myoclonus

Type of JME	Gene	Protein
EJM1	EFHC1[73]	EF-hand domain containing protein
EJM5	GABRA1[74]	Alpha 1 polypeptide, GABA-A receptor
EJM6	CACNB4[75]	Beta-4 subunit, voltage-dependent calcium channel
EJM7	GABRD[76]	Delta polypeptide, GABA-A receptor
EJM8	CLCN2[77]	Chloride channel 2

basis of the EEG and myoclonus, particularly in individuals who drive. Sleep-deprived EEG may have higher clinical yield in this clinical setting. Nonetheless, interictal EEG may be normal.

TREATMENT

Myoclonus and generalized tonic-clonic seizures of JME are usually well suppressed by sodium valproate.[78] Lamotrigine may be preferred for females because of reproductive and endocrine risks; however, the efficacy for myoclonus may be lower. Other medications effective for generalized epilepsies may also be considered.

Benign Familial Myoclonic Epilepsy

CLINICAL FEATURES

This is a rare form of epilepsy with generalized myoclonic seizures occurring in otherwise normal children, appearing in the first 2 years of life. Febrile seizures and reflex myoclonus may be present. Intellectual outcome is normal in most cases. Ictal EEG shows generalized poly-spikes and waves; interictal EEG is usually normal.

TREATMENT

Sodium valproate is usually effective.[79]

Myoclonia with Childhood Absence Epilepsies

CLINICAL FEATURES

Absence epilepsies are forms of childhood generalized epilepsies that may be accompanied by myoclonus. The classic absence seizure semiology is a stare lasting a few seconds with interruption of ongoing behavior or speech and loss of awareness, followed by immediate return to normal consciousness and no postictal confusion. Absence seizures may occur many hundreds of times per day. Childhood absence epilepsy (ages 3–10), juvenile absence epilepsy (ages 7–20), and JME (ages 7–20) are idiopathic generalized epilepsies that occur in children whose cognitive and behavioral phenotype have typically been viewed as within the normal range. Recent careful studies in childhood absence epilepsy indicate a higher risk of problems with executive function, learning, and anxiety.[80–82] Repetitive movements, or *automatisms*, such as chewing or lip smacking, occur during the seizures in some cases.

Eyelid myoclonia with (Jeavons syndrome) or without absence seizures is a complex syndrome where children may have brief, generalized absence seizures with prominent bilateral *eyelid myoclonus* (also referred to as *blepharoclonus*), associated with generalized bursts on EEG and photosensitive EEG bursts.[83,84] There are also children with photosensitive generalized epilepsies with brief episodes of eyelid closure and then eyelid flutter at approximately 10 Hz, lasting a few seconds, with no EEG correlate. These movements may be triggered voluntarily in some cases, increase with stress, do not respond to antiseizure medication, and may continue after the epilepsy remits.[85] A subset of these children may have a more significant encephalopathy with intellectual disability.[84,86] L-2-hydroxyglutaric aciduria was recently identified in one child with difficult to control seizures and magnetic resonance imaging (MRI) signal change in subcortical white matter and basal ganglia.[87]

Epilepsy with myoclonic absence, ages 3–10, is a more serious syndrome with absence followed by prominent myoclonic jerks and atonic seizures. Cognitive impairment tends to be more significant.[88]

PHENOMENOLOGY

Phenomenology of eyelid myoclonus is rapid eyelid contraction or flutter with eye deviation or jerk, lasting a few seconds. Eyelids are not fully closed in childhood absence epilepsy but may fully close during other forms. In epilepsies associated with cognitive impairment, massive axial myoclonic jerks may occur.

PATHOPHYSIOLOGY

The myoclonus accompanying absence epilepsy is likely an epileptic phenomenon, but the source is unclear in those without EEG correlate.

TREATMENT

Treatment with ethosuximide is first line for childhood absence epilepsy.[89] Sodium valproate, lamotrigine, levetiracetam, or benzodiazepines may in some cases suppress eyelid myoclonus, as well as the absence seizures.

Secondary Myoclonus

In most diseases in which symptomatic (secondary) myoclonus occurs, encephalopathy dominates. A vast number of genetic diseases and acquired brain insults, including viral encephalitidies, metabolic insults, hypoxia/anoxic insults, and exposure to heavy metals and other toxins, can produce myoclonus. This has been thoroughly reviewed elsewhere.[90] In many cases of secondary myoclonus, there is evidence by history of exposure, illness, or hypoxia. In this section, we discuss three secondary causes of myoclonus.

Opsoclonus Myoclonus (Ataxia) Syndrome

CLINICAL FEATURES

Opsoclonus myoclonus (ataxia) syndrome (OMS/OMAS) typically begins abruptly in early childhood, most often before the age of 5 years. Although symptoms of this disease are unusual and appear in its name, the diagnosis can be difficult in some cases. Myoclonus occurs with action and is multifocal and axial. Opsoclonus, rapid bursts of saccadic eye movements in several directions is pathognomonic in this setting (Video 12.3). The early presence of irritability should also be emphasized. The fulminant onset can lead to emergency room presentations[91] or confusion with status epilepticus.[92] OMAS can also present in older children and adolescents and has been described linked to mycoplasma pneumonia[93] and hepatitis C infections.[94]

A common misdiagnosis is acute cerebellar ataxia (ACA) because both ACA and OMAS have subacute, progressive disturbances in gait, truncal instability, and behavioral irritability and neither has a neuroimaging finding or serum biomarker.[95] Irritable toddlers are difficult to examine thoroughly, adding to the challenge of discerning the presence of multifocal mini-myoclonus and action myoclonus plus ataxia in a toddler with OMAS versus truncal titubation, gait, and limb ataxia in ACA. The presence of end-gaze nystagmus supports the diagnosis of ACA, but nystagmus is not universal.[96] The clinician may miss the diagnosis because opsoclonus in OMAS may be intermittent, subtle, or later-appearing.[97] Gait ataxia, tantrums, hypotonia, and varied other signs including reflex abnormalities and head tilt have been described in OMAS. At its peak, OMAS is severely disabling for the child and extremely stressful for the family. In milder cases, the course of OMAS may be monophasic and nonrelapsing.

The prognosis of OMAS, even with treatment, is guarded, with approximately two thirds of children experiencing adverse motor, speech, cognitive, and behavioral outcomes. The prognosis may or may not differ in children with and without neuroblastomas.[98,99] More severe symptoms and younger age at onset and cases with relapse tend to have worse long-term outcomes.[100]

PATHOPHYSIOLOGY

OMAS is an autoimmune condition in which there is abnormal B cell trafficking in the central nervous system (CNS).[101,102] It may be postviral in many cases. A large proportion, 40% in one recent estimate,[100] of children with OMAS have a neuroblastoma, a potentially fatal neural crest tumor. Only a small proportion, probably less than 5%, of children with neuroblastoma have OMAS.[103] Interestingly, in OMAS the neuroblastomas tend to have low-grade histology and favorable molecular markers such as no amplification of n-myc.[104] In most children with OMAS and neuroblastoma, the neuroblastoma is diagnosed at an early stage and has a good prognosis.[98]

The subacute onset of OMAS and the association with neural crest tumors support an autoimmune pathophysiology. The phenomenology suggests that the disease targets multiple CNS sites, including cerebellum and brainstem gaze centers containing burst cells that control saccades. Because the disease is usually not fatal, pathologic confirmation of specific processes and cell type involvement through autopsy studies is sparse. The relative rarity of the disease, delays in its diagnosis, and heterogeneity of prodromes and clinical features all contribute to difficulties in understanding this disease. Intensive research into multiple circulating autoantibodies including antibodies to Purkinje cell targets has not, to date, identified any unique, consistently present, disease-associated antibody. The role of abnormally recruited or activated B cell lymphocytes has been explored with flow cytometry studies of cerebrospinal fluid (CSF).[97] These studies have supported involvement of abnormal profiles of lymphocytes, including increased CD19+ B cells and HLA-DR+ (activated) T cells, and reduced CD4+ helper/inducer T cells. Pathophysiological clues are emerging from more detailed molecular studies of factors which regulate B cell trafficking such as CSF CXCL13 and BAFF.[105,106] The serum concentration of macrophage inflammatory chemokine CCL21 appears to be elevated, correlates with disease severity, and is reduced after adrenocortico-trophin (ACTH) or corticosteroid treatment.[107]

DIAGNOSTIC APPROACH

OMAS is a clinical diagnosis. In the presence of subacute irritability, tremor, and ataxia, a diagnosis of OMAS must be considered, and children diagnosed with ACA should continue to be monitored for emergence of symptoms characteristic of OMAS.[108,109] The presence of end-gaze nystagmus in this setting has a high positive predictive value for ACA. The presence of opsoclonus has a high positive predictive value for OMAS, but its absence does not have a high negative predictive value. That is, because opsoclonus can be subtle, intermittent, or late, clinicians and parents need to continue to remain vigilant for its emergence. Brain MRI should be obtained, but is most often normal. Routine CSF studies are also non-specific and nondiagnostic. Although studies of immune system biomarkers have helped elucidate pathophysiology, none are clinically established for this diagnosis. The search for a neuroblastoma should be thorough and persistent in this clinical setting. MRI with gado-linium or computed tomography with contrast of the chest and abdomen has the highest yield.[110] Nuclear medicine ^{131}I-MIBG (metaiodobenzylguanidine) or ^{111}In-penetreotide (somatostatin receptor ligand) scans and urine collection for elevated 24-h urine catechola-mines and serum neuron-specific enolase may be considered but have lower yield.[110]

TREATMENT

Multimodal treatment is needed. The treatment for a neuroblastoma may involve sur-gery, chemotherapy, or both depending on factors such as size, location, and indicators of malignant potential. The child will likely need immune modulating treatments even if a tumor is identified and resected. If the child was diagnosed with ACA initially,[95] treatment with steroids or intravenous immune globulin may have been tried to shorten the disease course. In many cases, these treatments will not be successful for OMAS.

ACTH treatment protocols are considered optimal based on expert consensus and clini-cal experience.[108] The high-dose ACTH protocol is $150 \, IU/m^2$ intramuscularly or subcutane-ously for 2 weeks, followed by a very gradual taper. Relapses during the taper are common. Possible treatment complications include weight gain, hypertension, elevated blood glu-cose, ulcers, and infections. Exposure to other ill and febrile children should be avoided if possible.

In addition to ACTH, combination treatment with IVIG, plasmaphoresis, rituximab, or other immune-modulating therapies may be needed.[101] Rituximab, an anti-CD20 monoclo-nal antibody treatment, is considered promising in children with CSF B-cell expansion[111] and appears beneficial in refractory cases.[112] Mycophenylate, a lymphocyte proliferation inhibitor, appears not to be useful in treating or preventing relapses.[102]

Acute symptomatic pharmacological and behavioral therapy for myoclonus, behavioral problems, aggression, and insomnia may also be beneficial. When using steroids or ACTH, ulcer prophylaxis is recommended and short-term antihypertensive treatment may be needed. For any immunosuppressive regimen, some also recommend infection prophylaxis with trimethoprim/sulfamethoxazole.

The loss of motor and language skills during the acute phase of this disease can be profound. Physical therapy, occupational therapy, and speech therapy should be provided and may be needed for years. Educational supports through the school are also indicated. Psychological support for the family and long-term behavioral and/or psychopharmacological therapy may be needed as well. Despite successful tumor treatment and resolution of myoclonus, even with intensive rehabilitative interventions, long-term cognitive impairment occurs in most cases.[100,113]

Subacute Sclerosing Panencephalitis

CLINICAL FEATURES

Measles infection remains a common cause of morbidity and mortality in developing countries. Incidence is also increasing in Europe and the United States as a result of parents refusing to vaccinate their children due to unfounded concerns and deliberately misleading reports about links of the measles vaccine to autism.[114]

Measles infections can result in a number of CNS complications including primary measles encephalitis, measles inclusion body encephalitis, acute postinfectious measles encephalomyelitis, and subacute sclerosing panencephalitis (SSPE).[115]

SSPE is a neurologically devastating, potentially fatal, postviral inflammatory condition resulting from measles infection in early childhood. It occurs 3–20 years after measles infection. It can present with emotional lability and behavioral outbursts, followed by progressive cognitive and behavioral problems and myoclonus. Brain MRI early shows decreased gray matter volume, particularly in frontotemporal cortex, amygdala, and cingulate gyrus. T2 weighted images show signal changes occurring focally or diffusely in cerebral cortex, periventricular white matter, basal ganglia, and brainstem. Magnetic resonance spectroscopy (MRS) demonstrates reduced NAA peaks.[116] EEG shows periodic slow-wave complexes every 4–10 s accompanying axial myoclonus. This can progress to burst suppression and diffuse slow waves. Laboratory testing should demonstrate markedly elevated measles-specific antibodies in serum and CSF.

TREATMENT

SSPE is preventable with population measles vaccination. Once acquired, there is no direct disease-modifying treatment. Standard care is supportive. Results of antiviral and immune-modulatory treatments to date have been mixed.[117]

Postanoxic Myoclonus

CLINICAL FEATURES

After diffuse hypoxic/ischemic insults, particularly cardiac arrest in adults, spontaneous and action myoclonus may occur. This has been less frequently described in children, but is reported after neonatal ischemia.[118,119]

PATHOPHYSIOLOGY

Pathophysiology involves cortical and/or Purkinje cell injury.

TREATMENT

Treatment is symptomatic and likely does not improve long-term outcome. Caregivers may find that reducing myoclonus is helpful. Postanoxic myoclonus may respond to levetiracetam[120] or other antimyoclonic agents such as benzodiazepines or sodium valproate.

Epilepsy Partialis Continua (EPC), Rasmussen's Encephalitis, and Myoclonia Continua

CLINICAL FEATURES

Focal jerking, typically in a distal limb, occurs for hours to weeks in EPC. This is discussed in this chapter because the phenomenology of the jerking may be myoclonus. Rasmussen's syndrome is a cause of this rare condition in children and may manifest with focal myoclonus.

PATHOPHYSIOLOGY

Pathophysiology involves either cortical or subcortical pathology, as established with neurophysiologic and imaging studies. Rasmussen's syndrome is an autoimmune disease involving one hemisphere, with cortical, leptomeningeal, and parenchymal perivascular inflammation and infiltration predominantly of T lymphocytes, mainly cytotoxic CD8 T cells. The triggering event is unknown. Antiglutamate receptor antibodies have been identified in some children. The chemokine pathway of CXCR3 in T lymphocytes and CXCL10 in neurons and astrocytes may play a role, as shown by findings in surgical resection specimens in six affected children.[121] A case has also been described after gliomatosis cerebri in two children.[122] Some authors have suggested that EPC be used to designate cases with cortical origin, and *myoclonia continua* be used for those originating elsewhere in the nervous system.[123]

TREATMENT

For EPC, treatment is with anticonvulsant agents. Botulinum toxin injections into the muscles producing focal myoclonus may provide symptomatic relief.[124] For Rasmussen's encephalitis, short- and long-term outcomes after various hemispherectomy procedures[125–127] versus immune-modulatory therapies[128–130] continue to be investigated.

Progressive Myoclonic Epilepsies

Progressive myoclonic epilepsies (PMEs) are rare genetic conditions clustered on the basis of common clinical features of myoclonus, epilepsy, progressive encephalopathy, and ataxia. Genetic causes are denoted as "Epilepsy, Progressive Myoclonic" (EPM). The five main causes are mitochondrial encephalomyopathies, Unverricht–Lundborg disease (EPM1A), Lafora disease (EPM2A, EPM2B), neuronal ceroid lipofuscinoses (NCLs) (See Chapter 17), and sialidoses. A more recently identified form is "North Sea" PME, and there are a number of other rare genetic causes.[131] Clinically, tonic-clonic, clonic, myoclonic, and absence semiologies may be present. Neurophysiologically, seizure types are more often generalized than partial. Light, sound, touch, emotional stress, movements, or posture may induce reflex myoclonus. Spontaneous myoclonus or disabling action myoclonus also occurs. Localization may be multifocal in the face and distal limbs, or bilateral and massive, resulting in falls. Hyperexcitability in PMEs has been demonstrated with giant somatosensory-evoked potentials and reduced intracortical inhibition measured with TMS.[132] Evidence supports origin of myoclonus in cortical, subcortical, and brainstem-reticular loci, possibly related to the pervasively abnormal neural function in these degenerative diseases.

Cerebellar dysfunction is also common, with hypotonia, dysmetria, intention tremor, speech abnormalities, ocular movement disorders, and ataxia variably present. Neuroimaging may be normal or show cerebellar atrophy. Postmortem studies show loss of Purkinje cells and dentate nucleus.[133] MRS in Lafora (*EPM2A* and *EPM2B*) shows reduction in the NAA/choline ratio in the cerebellum with correlations to severity of both myoclonus and ataxia.[134] This pathology may underlie the presence of action myoclonus in PMEs.[135]

Our understanding of the biochemical and molecular pathophysiology of these diagnoses has expanded rapidly with the discovery of a variety of genes and pathways.[131,136,137] However, no rational, disease-modifying therapies are available.

Mitochondrial Myopathies—Myoclonus Epilepsy and Ragged Red Fibers

As mitochondria are ubiquitous, a multitude of neurologic and systemic abnormalities may occur in diseases involving their structure or function. The most frequent manifestations are short stature, hearing loss, neuropathy, diabetes, cardiomyopathy, strokes, migraines, and renal tubular acidosis. Children with muscle weakness, ataxia, dementia, and eye movement abnormalities may have a lactic acidosis and stroke-like episodes or progressive myoclonic epilepsy with ragged red fibers (MERRF) on muscle biopsy.[138] "Ragged red fibers" refers to the histologic appearance of diseased muscle fibers with abnormal mitochondrial proliferation, identified using Gomori trichrome stain. Diagnostic approaches combine identification of the classic clinical features, biochemical features such as elevated serum lactate and pyruvate which are variably present, radiologic features such as characteristic symmetric signal changes in basal ganglia, elevated lactate peak demonstrated with MRS. Testing for mutations in mitochondrial DNA or nuclear DNA regulating mitochondrial function can be accomplished through a targeted approach or a broader genetic panel test, depending on clinical features and inheritance pattern.[139,140] Muscle biopsies are far less commonly used.

CLINICAL FEATURES

Classic symptoms of MERRF are myoclonus, generalized seizures, ataxia, and myopathy. Age of onset of MERRF varies within families, from early childhood to late adulthood.[141] MRI may show atrophy of cerebellum or superior cerebellar peduncles.[142] Serum lactate and pyruvate are characteristically elevated.

PATHOPHYSIOLOGY

This disease is caused by point mutations in mitochondrial DNA encoding tRNA. It is therefore inherited through the maternal line. The most common mutation occurs at position 8344, an A to G coding mutation leading to adenine/guanine substitution.[143] This mutation results in defective translation of mitochondria-encoded DNA, and ultimately adversely affects function of the mitochondrial respiratory chain.

TREATMENT

Therapies at this time for most diseases affecting mitochondrial function are nonspecific and not very effective. A combination of oxygen radical scavengers, enzyme cofactors, artificial electron acceptors, and/or substances to remove noxious metabolites may be considered. Evidence for benefits of this approach is limited, but given the paucity of other options, families and clinicians may feel comforted that something is being done. For seizures, anticonvulsants may be chosen, as for most epilepsies, based on seizure semiology and EEG findings. Sodium valproate is not a drug of choice, because of concern for liver damage, but is not absolutely contraindicated for treatment of epilepsy in patients with mitochondrial diseases involving disordered electron transport. The probability of liver damage, which can be fatal, is higher in disorders of fatty acid oxidation and for children under age 2 years with epilepsy and developmental delay.

Unverricht–Lundborg Disease

This condition, before clarification of the genetic etiology, was previously known by several names describing overlapping clinical presentations. These names included Mediterranean myoclonus, Baltic myoclonus, and Ramsay Hunt syndrome. It is now designated EPM1.

CLINICAL FEATURES

EPM1 onset occurs classically between 6 and 13 years. Inheritance is autosomal recessive. Early visual symptoms, with abnormal photic response on EEG, are followed by segmental action and stimulus-evoked myoclonus (Video 12.1). As the disease progresses, there is severely disabling generalized myoclonus, ataxia, and cognitive impairment. Seizure semiology may be tonic-clonic or absence.[144] Dysarthria, ataxia, tremor, and minimal cognitive decline occur and progress slowly, over decades in individuals homozygous for mutations described originally. However, other genetically confirmed individuals with EPM1 have a much more severe phenotype with progressive cognitive impairment, psychosis, and difficult to control seizures.[145] Some patients present with frequent blinking, which may be initially wrongly diagnosed as tics or blepharospasm.

PATHOPHYSIOLOGY

EPM1 results from mutations in *CSTB*, which encodes cystatin B,[146] a member of the family of cysteine protease inhibitors whose role is protection against excessive, inappropriate intracellular degradation by proteinases leaking from lysosomes. Mutation location and compound heterozygous status confer a more severe phenotype.[145]

TREATMENT

Sodium valproate appears to be effective.[146] Benefit with levetiracetam and with treatment with *N*-acetyl cysteine has also been described. Phenytoin may exacerbate seizures.

Lafora Disease

CLINICAL FEATURES

Clinical features of this disease include childhood onset, usually between ages 8 and 18. Early symptoms include myoclonic jerks, headaches, and generalized tonic-clonic seizures. Spontaneous and action myoclonus then progress rapidly along with dementia, ataxia, and dystonia, and death within 10 years. Adult-onset cases have a slower course. EEG initially shows generalized epileptiform discharges with exacerbation from photic stimulation.

PATHOPHYSIOLOGY

Lafora disease is caused in most cases by mutations in the *EPM2A* gene.[147] EPM2A encodes a protein tyrosine phosphatase termed *laforin*. Lafora disease is also caused by mutations in *EPM2B* (also known as *NHLRC1*), which encodes malin.[148] Malin regulates laforin protein concentration and degradation through ubiquitination.[149,150] Postmortem studies show polyglucosan inclusions (Lafora bodies) in neurons and multiple organs. Lafora bodies are also identified in sweat glands visible on skin biopsy.

Neuronal Ceroid Lipofuscinoses

There are (at least) 11 types of neuronal ceroid lipofuscinoses (NCLs), which tend to occur at various ages. Older literature designated these with eponyms, based on variation in pathological findings and age of onset. For example, the major adult form of NCL, known also as "Kufs disease" was recently discovered to be caused by mutations in the *CLN6* gene,[151] which was already identified as the cause of variant late-infantile NCL. The current nosology is based on identified molecular defects.

CLINICAL FEATURES

These diseases have in common clinical features of relentlessly progressive dementia and disability, and often macular degeneration.[152,153] Several forms have PME, most notably type 2 (*CLN2*). Other movement disorders such as ataxia and Parkinsonism may occur.

PATHOPHYSIOLOGY

The key feature of these heritable disorders is the presence of intracellular lipopigment. This storage material, seen using electron microscopy, takes several forms: granular osmophilic (CLN1), curvilinear (CLN2), fingerprint (CLN3), and mixed.

DIAGNOSTIC APPROACH

In the presence of characteristic features, supported by EEG findings (e.g., photic response), genetic testing is preferable to biopsies. Based on cost considerations and clinical features, targeted gene testing or a larger gene panel may be appropriate. Biopsies of conjunctiva, rectal mucosa, or muscle may be used to identify inclusions, seen by electron microscopy,[154] but more specific diagnostic, prognostic, and ultimately therapeutic information is available through genetic results.

TREATMENT

Management is supportive and palliative. Multiple possible interventions including enzyme replacement, immune modulation, other medications, gene therapy, and stem cell therapies are under investigation.[155]

North Sea PME with Ataxia

This form of PME, termed EPM6, has recently been identified in a number of unrelated, previously undiagnosed families.[156] It presents in early childhood with ataxia, followed several years later by intractable epilepsy with multiple seizure types—generalized tonic-clonic, absence, myoclonic, and atonic/drop attacks. Skeletal deformities, progressive scoliosis, and elevated creatine kinase in blood are additional features.[157] Symptoms progress relentlessly, with loss of ambulation in the second decade and death in early adulthood. The etiology is homozygous mutations in *GOSR2*, the Golgi SNAP receptor complex 2 gene.[156] *GOSR2* encodes a soluble protein important for protein transport through the Golgi apparatus. This transport occurs through formation of pairs of matched vesicle-associated and target membrane-associated proteins which recruit soluble *N*-ethylmaleimide-sensitive factor attachment proteins.[158]

Sialidoses

Two forms of defects in neuraminidase (also known as sialidase) cause PME, as does a related defect causing galactosialidosis.

CLINICAL FEATURES

Sialidosis type I is milder, with later onset. Sialidosis type II is more severe, with more dysmorphic features. Type II is also known as mucolipidosis I. These diseases are characterized by gradual visual failure, myoclonus, tonic-clonic seizures, ataxia, and a cherry-red spot on the macula. Galactosialidosis is characterized by dwarfism, hearing loss, seizures, mental retardation, macular cherry-red spot, and myoclonus.

PATHOPHYSIOLOGY

Sialidosis I and II are allelic, autosomal recessive diseases caused by mutations in the neuraminidase gene,[79] with some correlation between disease severity and residual mutant enzyme activity.[159] Galactosialidosis results from loss of activity of both enzymes beta-galactosidase and alpha-neuraminidase. This has been shown to result from mutations in the gene *CTSA*. *CTSA* encodes the "protective protein"/lysosomal cathepsin A, which stabilizes these enzymes and prevents their degradation. Phenotype severity and age of onset are associated with degree of residual protein activity.[160]

Angelman Syndrome

CLINICAL FEATURES

Clinical features include chronic encephalopathy, with severe mental retardation, absent language, inappropriate paroxysmal laughter, ataxic gait, tremor, myoclonus, and microcephaly with large-appearing mandible.[24] There are multiple seizure types, including absence, myoclonic, and myoclonic status epilepticus.

PATHOPHYSIOLOGY

Angelman syndrome is a sporadic disorder that occurs due to four related genetic mechanisms. The genetic locus is chromosome 15q11-q13. In most cases there is *de novo* deletion at the site of three GABA receptor subunits (GABRB3, GABRA5, and GABRG3) on the maternal chromosome (note that deletion at the same location in the paternal chromosome 15q causes Prader–Willi syndrome).[161] In a small proportion of cases, the cause is (1) disomy of chromosome 15 or (2) chromosomal imprinting defects. Most of the remaining cases are caused by mutations in ubiquitin-protein ligase E3A gene.[162]

TREATMENT

There is no specific treatment. Genetic counseling for the family is recommended, given the complex genetics of this disorder and variable recurrence risk.[163]

AUTOSOMAL DOMINANT, CORTICAL MYOCLONUS WITHOUT EPILEPSY

In a four-generation pedigree, 11 individuals with onset as young as age 18 were characterized as having slowly progressive, multifocal, action-triggered myoclonus in face, arms, and legs leading to falls with injuries. Electrophysiological studies demonstrated giant cortical somatosensory-evoked potentials, consistent with a cortical source for myoclonus. Genetic investigation followed by functional studies supported a mutation in the *NOL3* gene, resulting in a single amino acid substitution in the Nucleolar Protein 3 as the cause.[164]

HEMIFACIAL SPASM

Hemifacial spasm is a rare disorder in children. This topic is addressed in this chapter due to the brief muscle contractions which can be considered peripherally mediated myoclonus. Movements are characterized by involuntary contractions of muscles innervated by the facial nerve. Potential causes include facial nerve compression by vascular or brainstem masses. Hemifacial spasms have also been reported in children with cerebellar astrocytomas[203] and otitis media.[204] Treatment includes carbamazepine and other anticonvulsants, botulinum toxin,[205] and surgical decompression.[206]

SUMMARY OF DIAGNOSTIC AND THERAPEUTIC APPROACH

Myoclonus is highly prevalent but rarely occurs as an isolated finding in children. Nonetheless, some general aid in diagnosis of pediatric neurologic disorders with myoclonus may be gained from the usual principles of neurologic diagnosis.

First, the type of myoclonus may sometimes aid in accurate neuroanatomic localization, as outlined in Table 12.3.

Second, the co-occurring symptoms may provide a critical clue. For example, epilepsy is a clue that the substrate for myoclonus is more likely to be diseased or disordered cerebral cortex. The presence of encephalopathy or a diffuse neurodegenerative disease with dementia makes a cerebral, subcortical, or brainstem source more likely. Secondary epilepsy and PME should be considered, based on clinical features and age of presentation.

The following more specific steps may be helpful:

1. Clarify that myoclonus is the movement disorder. In some cases, this is challenging if there is a mixed phenomenology. In general, dystonia and tics should be distinguishable from myoclonus clinically. Ataxia with titubation versus myoclonus can be more challenging, and these can co-occur. Functional neurological symptom disorder (also known as psychogenic movement disorders) can present with myoclonus-like movements.[25,207,208]
2. Remain vigilant for misdiagnosis and follow up patients carefully. For example, as discussed previously, Opsoclonus Myoclonus Syndrome may be misdiagnosed as Acute Cerebellar Ataxia.
3. Consider a broad differential diagnosis (focal, ictal/ischemic, and toxic/metabolic) for acute myoclonus with encephalopathy if the proximate injury is unknown. Acute

myoclonus is often due to an insult such as an anoxic injury which can be discerned through careful history.

4. Utilize neurophysiological testing appropriately, on a limited basis. Focus on the epilepsy if it is present. Back-averaging, somatosensory-evoked potentials, and other specialized techniques are not critical for diagnosis in most pediatric neurologic diseases with myoclonus.

5. For diseases which seem likely genetic, pursue the diagnosis vigorously. Use the age of onset, inheritance pattern from three-generation family pedigree, and time course (acquired, static, chronic progressive, episodic) to guide diagnostic decisions.

6. For difficult diagnoses, use Web-based resources such as OMIM and Simulconsult (see Appendix B).

7. Referral to a movement disorder specialist for a second opinion for unclear neurological phenotypes may be a more cost-effective approach than expensive testing.

8. Provide referrals for psychiatric or counseling services, as needed.

9. Provide referrals for physical, occupational, and speech therapies as needed.

10. Educate families and encourage them to join advocacy and research support groups.

Treatment in most cases is symptomatic and may not be highly successful. In cases with where myoclonus is part of a global encephalopathy, treating myoclonus may not enhance quality of life. The mainstay symptomatic treatments are antiepileptics (sodium valproate, levetiracetam, and piracetam) as well as benzodiazepines.

References

1. Tyvaert L, Krystkowiak P, Cassim F, et al. Myoclonus of peripheral origin: two case reports. *Mov Disord.* 2009;24(2):274–277.
2. Sanger TD, Chen D, Fehlings DL, et al. Definition and classification of hyperkinetic movements in childhood. *Mov Disord.* 2010;25(11):1538–1549.
3. Shibasaki H. Pathophysiology of negative myoclonus and asterixis. *Adv Neurol.* 1995;67:199–209.
4. Bakker MJ, van Dijk JG, van den Maagdenberg AM, Tijssen MA. Startle syndromes. *Lancet Neurol.* 2006;5(6):513–524.
5. Fahn S, Marsden CD, Van Woert MH. Definition and classification of myoclonus. *Adv Neurol.* 1986;43:1–5.
6. Shibasaki H, Hallett M. Electrophysiological studies of myoclonus. *Muscle Nerve.* 2005;31(2):157–174.
7. Esposito M, Erro R, Edwards MJ, et al. The pathophysiology of symptomatic propriospinal myoclonus. *Mov Disord.* 2014;29(9):1097–1099.
8. Brown P. Propriospinal myoclonus: where do we go from here? *Mov Disord.* 2014;29(9):1092–1093.
9. Baizabal-Carvallo JF, Cardoso F, Jankovic J. Myorhythmia: phenomenology, etiology, and treatment. *Mov Disord.* 2015;30(2):171–179.
10. Schrag A, Quinn NP, Bhatia KP, Marsden CD. Benign hereditary chorea—entity or syndrome? *Mov Disord.* 2000;15(2):280–288.
11. Asmus F, Devlin A, Munz M, Zimprich A, Gasser T, Chinnery PF. Clinical differentiation of genetically proven benign hereditary chorea and myoclonus-dystonia. *Mov Disord.* 2007;22(14):2104–2109.
12. Rothwell JC, Obeso JA, Marsden CD. On the significance of giant somatosensory evoked potentials in cortical myoclonus. *J Neurol Neurosurg Psychiatry.* 1984;47(1):33–42.
13. Manganotti P, Bortolomasi M, Zanette G, Pawelzik T, Giacopuzzi M, Fiaschi A. Intravenous clomipramine decreases excitability of human motor cortex. A study with paired magnetic stimulation. *J Neurol Sci.* 2001;184(1):27–32.
14. Rossi Sebastiano D, Soliveri P, Panzica F, et al. Cortical myoclonus in childhood and juvenile onset Huntington's disease. *Parkinsonism Relat Disord.* 2012;18(6):794–797.

15. Auvin S, Pandit F, De Bellecize J, et al. Benign myoclonic epilepsy in infants: electroclinical features and long-term follow-up of 34 patients. *Epilepsia*. 2006;47(2):387–393.
16. Fahn S, Sjaastad O. Hereditary essential myoclonus in a large Norwegian family. *Mov Disord*. 1991;6(3):237–247.
17. Mahloudji M, Pikielny RT. Hereditary essential myoclonus. *Brain*. 1967;90(3):669–674.
18. Jain S, Padma MV, Maheshwari MC. Occurrence of only myoclonic jerks in juvenile myoclonic epilepsy. *Acta Neurol Scand*. 1997;95(5):263–267.
19. Panayiotopoulos CP, Tahan R, Obeid T. Juvenile myoclonic epilepsy: factors of error involved in the diagnosis and treatment. *Epilepsia*. 1991;32(5):672–676.
20. Huppertz HJ, Feuerstein TJ, Schulze-Bonhage A. Myoclonus in epilepsy patients with anticonvulsive add-on therapy with pregabalin. *Epilepsia*. 2001;42(6):790–792.
21. Perucca E, Gram L, Avanzini G, Dulac O. Antiepileptic drugs as a cause of worsening seizures. *Epilepsia*. 1998;39(1):5–17.
22. Boyer EW, Shannon M. The serotonin syndrome. *N Engl J Med*. 2005;352(11):1112–1120.
23. Brown P, Thompson PD. Electrophysiological aids to the diagnosis of psychogenic jerks, spasms, and tremor. *Mov Disord*. 2001;16(4):595–599.
24. George MS, Wassermann EM, Williams WA, et al. Daily repetitive transcranial magnetic stimulation (rTMS) improves mood in depression. *Neuroreport*. 1995;6(14):1853–1856.
25. Ferrara J, Jankovic J. Psychogenic movement disorders in children. *Mov Disord*. 2008;23(13):1875–1881.
26. Brown P, Rothwell JC, Thompson PD, Britton TC, Day BL, Marsden CD. New observations on the normal auditory startle reflex in man. *Brain*. 1991;114(Pt 4):1891–1902.
27. Espay AJ, Chen R. Myoclonus. *Continuum*. 2013;19(5 Movement Disorders):1264–1286.
28. Thiagalingam S, Flaherty M, Billson F, North K. Neurofibromatosis type 1 and optic pathway gliomas: follow-up of 54 patients. *Ophthalmology*. 2004;111(3):568–577.
29. Fekete R, Jankovic J. Childhood stiff-person syndrome improved with rituximab. *Case Rep Neurol*. 2012;4(2):92–96.
30. Baizabal-Carvallo JF, Jankovic J. Stiff-person syndrome: insights into a complex autoimmune disorder. *J Neurol Neurosurg Psychiatry*. 2015 [in Press]. <http://dx.doi.org/10.1136/jnnp-2014-309201>.
31. Ryan SG, Sherman SL, Terry JC, Sparkes RS, Torres MC, Mackey RW. Startle disease, or hyperekplexia: response to clonazepam and assignment of the gene (STHE) to chromosome 5q by linkage analysis. *Ann Neurol*. 1992;31(6):663–668.
32. Shiang R, Ryan SG, Zhu YZ, Hahn AF, O'Connell P, Wasmuth JJ. Mutations in the alpha 1 subunit of the inhibitory glycine receptor cause the dominant neurologic disorder, hyperekplexia. *Nat Genet*. 1993;5(4):351–358.
33. Lynch JW. Molecular structure and function of the glycine receptor chloride channel. *Physiol Rev*. 2004;84(4):1051–1095.
34. Rees MI, Lewis TM, Kwok JB, et al. Hyperekplexia associated with compound heterozygote mutations in the beta-subunit of the human inhibitory glycine receptor (GLRB). *Hum Mol Genet*. 2002;11(7):853–860.
35. Rees MI, Harvey K, Pearce BR, et al. Mutations in the gene encoding GlyT2 (SLC6A5) define a presynaptic component of human startle disease. *Nat Genet*. 2006;38(7):801–806.
36. Harvey K, Duguid IC, Alldred MJ, et al. The GDP-GTP exchange factor collybistin: an essential determinant of neuronal gephyrin clustering. *J Neurosci*. 2004;24(25):5816–5826.
37. Obeso JA, Lang AE, Rothwell JC, Marsden CD. Postanoxic symptomatic oscillatory myoclonus. *Neurology*. 1983;33(2):240–243.
38. Butler MH, Hayashi A, Ohkoshi N, et al. Autoimmunity to gephyrin in Stiff-Man syndrome. *Neuron*. 2000;26(2):307–312.
39. Manford MR, Fish DR, Shorvon SD. Startle provoked epileptic seizures: features in 19 patients. *J Neurol Neurosurg Psychiatry*. 1996;61(2):151–156.
40. Saenz-Lope E, Herranz FJ, Masdeu JC. Startle epilepsy: a clinical study. *Ann Neurol*. 1984;16(1):78–81.
41. Guerrini R, Genton P, Bureau M, Dravet C, Roger J. Reflex seizures are frequent in patients with Down syndrome and epilepsy. *Epilepsia*. 1990;31(4):406–417.
42. Tibussek D, Wohlrab G, Boltshauser E, Schmitt B. Proven startle-provoked epileptic seizures in childhood: semiologic and electrophysiologic variability. *Epilepsia*. 2006;47(6):1050–1058.
43. Ricci S, Cusmai R, Fusco L, Vigevano F. Reflex myoclonic epilepsy in infancy: a new age-dependent idiopathic epileptic syndrome related to startle reaction. *Epilepsia*. 1995;36(4):342–348.

44. Zafeiriou D, Vargiami E, Kontopoulos E. Reflex myoclonic epilepsy in infancy: a benign age-dependent idiopathic startle epilepsy. *Epileptic Disord.* 2003;5(2):121–122.

45. Brown P. The startle syndrome. *Mov Disord.* 2002;17(suppl 2):S79–S82.

46. Devetag Chalaupka F, Bartholini F, Mandich G, Turro M. Two new families with hereditary essential chin myoclonus: clinical features, neurophysiological findings and treatment. *Neurol Sci.* 2006;27(2):97–103.

47. Lundemo G, Persson HE. Hereditary essential myoclonus. *Acta Neurol Scand.* 1985;72(2):176–179.

48. Phanthumchinda K. Hereditary essential myoclonus. *J Med Assoc Thai.* 1991;74(9):424–427.

49. Gonzalez-Alegre P, Kelkar P, Rodnitzky RL. Isolated high-frequency jaw tremor relieved by botulinum toxin injections. *Mov Disord.* 2006;21(7):1049–1050.

50. Asmus F, Langseth A, Doherty E, et al. "Jerky" dystonia in children: spectrum of phenotypes and genetic testing. *Mov Disord.* 2009;24(5):702–709.

51. Foncke EM, Gerrits MC, van Ruissen F, et al. Distal myoclonus and late onset in a large Dutch family with myoclonus-dystonia. *Neurology.* 2006;67(9):1677–1680.

52. Peall KJ, Smith DJ, Kurian MA, et al. SGCE mutations cause psychiatric disorders: clinical and genetic characterization. *Brain.* 2013;136(Pt 1):294–303.

53. van Tricht MJ, Dreissen YEM, Cath D, et al. Cognition and psychopathology in myoclonus-dystonia. *J Neurol Neurosurg Psychiatry.* 2012;83(8):814–820.

54. Asmus F, Zimprich A, Tezenas Du Montcel S, et al. Myoclonus-dystonia syndrome: epsilon-sarcoglycan mutations and phenotype. *Ann Neurol.* 2002;52(4):489–492.

55. Zimprich A, Grabowski M, Asmus F, et al. Mutations in the gene encoding epsilon-sarcoglycan cause myoclonus-dystonia syndrome. *Nat Genet.* 2001;29(1):66–69.

56. Kock N, Kasten M, Schule B, et al. Clinical and genetic features of myoclonus-dystonia in 3 cases: a video presentation. *Mov Disord.* 2004;19(2):231–234.

57. Orth M, Djarmati A, Baumer T, et al. Autosomal dominant myoclonus-dystonia and Tourette syndrome in a family without linkage to the SGCE gene. *Mov Disord.* 2007;22(14):2090–2096.

58. Fregni F, Thome-Souza S, Bermpohl F, et al. Antiepileptic effects of repetitive transcranial magnetic stimulation in patients with cortical malformations: an EEG and clinical study. *Stereotact Funct Neurosurg.* 2005;83(2–3):57–62.

59. Gerrits M.C., Foncke E.M., de Haan R., et al. Phenotype-genotype correlation in Dutch patients with myoclonus-dystonia [erratum appears in *Neurology.* 2007;68(11):879]. *Neurology.* 2006;66(5):759–761.

60. Klein C, Brin MF, Kramer P, et al. Association of a missense change in the D2 dopamine receptor with myoclonus dystonia. *Proc Natl Acad Sci USA.* 1999;96(9):5173–5176.

61. Saugier-Veber P, Doummar D, Barthez M-A, et al. Myoclonus dystonia plus syndrome due to a novel 7q21 microdeletion. *Am J Med Genet A.* 2010;152A(5):1244–1249.

62. Stark Z, Ryan MM, Bruno DL, Burgess T, Savarirayan R. Atypical Silver–Russell phenotype resulting from maternal uniparental disomy of chromosome 7. *Am J Med Genet A.* 2010;152A(9):2342–2345.

63. Luciano MS, Ozelius L, Sims K, Raymond D, Liu L, Saunders-Pullman R. Responsiveness to levodopa in epsilon-sarcoglycan deletions. *Mov Disord.* 2009;24(3):425–428.

64. Kurtis MM, San Luciano M, Yu Q, et al. Clinical and neurophysiological improvement of SGCE myoclonus-dystonia with GPi deep brain stimulation. *Clin Neurol Neurosurg.* 2010;112(2):149–152.

65. Cantello R, Rossi S, Varrasi C, et al. Slow repetitive TMS for drug-resistant epilepsy: clinical and EEG findings of a placebo-controlled trial. *Epilepsia.* 2007;48(2):366–374.

66. Lombroso CT, Fejerman N. Benign myoclonus of early infancy. *Ann Neurol.* 1977;1(2):138–143.

67. Caraballo RH, Capovilla G, Vigevano F, Beccaria F, Specchio N, Fejerman N. The spectrum of benign myoclonus of early infancy: clinical and neurophysiologic features in 102 patients. *Epilepsia.* 2009;50(5):1176–1183.

68. Pachatz C, Fusco L, Vigevano F. Benign myoclonus of early infancy. *Epileptic Disord.* 1999;1(1):57–61.

69. Guerrini R, Takahashi T. Myoclonus and epilepsy. *Handb Clin Neurol.* 2013;111:667–679.

70. Malek N, Stewart W, Greene J. The progressive myoclonic epilepsies. *Pract Neurol.* 2015;15(3):164–171.

71. Camfield C.S., Camfield P.R. Juvenile myoclonic epilepsy 25 years after seizure onset: a population-based study [summary for patients in *Neurology.* 2009;73(13):e64–e67; PMID: 19786691]. *Neurology.* 2009;73(13):1041–1045.

72. Panzica F, Rubboli G, Franceschetti S, et al. Cortical myoclonus in Janz syndrome. *Clin Neurophysiol.* 2001;112(10):1803–1809.

73. Suzuki T, Delgado-Escueta AV, Aguan K, et al. Mutations in EFHC1 cause juvenile myoclonic epilepsy. *Nat Genet.* 2004;36(8):842–849.

74. Cossette P, Liu L, Brisebois K, et al. Mutation of GABRA1 in an autosomal dominant form of juvenile myoclonic epilepsy. *Nat Genet.* 2002;31(2):184–189.

75. Escayg A, De Waard M, Lee DD, et al. Coding and noncoding variation of the human calcium-channel beta4-subunit gene CACNB4 in patients with idiopathic generalized epilepsy and episodic ataxia. *Am J Hum Genet.* 2000;66(5):1531–1539.

76. Dibbens LM, Feng HJ, Richards MC, et al. GABRD encoding a protein for extra- or peri-synaptic GABAA receptors is a susceptibility locus for generalized epilepsies. *Hum Mol Genet.* 2004;13(13):1315–1319.

77. Saint-Martin C, Gauvain G, Teodorescu G, et al. Two novel CLCN2 mutations accelerating chloride channel deactivation are associated with idiopathic generalized epilepsy. *Hum Mutat.* 2009;30(3):397–405.

78. Glauser T, Ben-Menachem E, Bourgeois B, et al. ILAE treatment guidelines: evidence-based analysis of antiepileptic drug efficacy and effectiveness as initial monotherapy for epileptic seizures and syndromes. *Epilepsia.* 2006;47(7):1094–1120.

79. Bonten E, van der Spoel A, Fornerod M, Grosveld G, d'Azzo A. Characterization of human lysosomal neuraminidase defines the molecular basis of the metabolic storage disorder sialidosis. *Genes Dev.* 1996;10(24):3156–3169.

80. Levav M, Mirsky AF, Herault J, Xiong L, Amir N, Andermann E. Familial association of neuropsychological traits in patients with generalized and partial seizure disorders. *J Clin Exp Neuropsychol.* 2002;24(3):311–326.

81. Barnes GN, Paolicchi JM. Neuropsychiatric comorbidities in childhood absence epilepsy. *Nat Clin Pract Neurol.* 2008;4(12):650–651.

82. Masur D, Shinnar S, Cnaan A, et al. Pretreatment cognitive deficits and treatment effects on attention in childhood absence epilepsy. *Neurology.* 2013;81(18):1572–1580.

83. Panayiotopoulos CP. Fixation-off-sensitive epilepsy in eyelid myoclonia with absence seizures. *Ann Neurol.* 1987;22(1):87–89.

84. Caraballo RH, Fontana E, Darra F, et al. A study of 63 cases with eyelid myoclonia with or without absences: type of seizure or an epileptic syndrome? *Seizure.* 2009;18(6):440–445.

85. Camfield CS, Camfield PR, Sadler M, et al. Paroxysmal eyelid movements: a confusing feature of generalized photosensitive epilepsy. *Neurology.* 2004;63(1):40–42.

86. Capovilla G, Striano P, Gambardella A, et al. Eyelid fluttering, typical EEG pattern, and impaired intellectual function: a homogeneous epileptic condition among the patients presenting with eyelid myoclonia. *Epilepsia.* 2009;50(6):1536–1541.

87. Mete A, Isikay S, Sirikci A, Ozkur A, Bayram M. Eyelid myoclonia with absence seizures in a child with L-2 hydroxyglutaric aciduria: findings of magnetic resonance imaging. *Pediatr Neurol.* 2012;46(3):195–197.

88. Caraballo RH, Chamorro N, Darra F, Fortini S, Arroyo H. Epilepsy with myoclonic atonic seizures: an electroclinical study of 69 patients. *Pediatr Neurol.* 2013;48(5):355–362.

89. Glauser TA, Cnaan A, Shinnar S, et al. Ethosuximide, valproic acid, and lamotrigine in childhood absence epilepsy. *N Engl J Med.* 2010;362(9):790–799.

90. Borg M. Symptomatic myoclonus. *Neurophysiol Clin.* 2006;36(5–6):309–318.

91. Dale RC, Singh H, Troedson C, Pillai S, Gaikiwari S, Kozlowska K. A prospective study of acute movement disorders in children. *Dev Med Child Neurol.* 2010;52(8):739–748.

92. Haden SV, McShane MA, Holt CM. Opsoclonus myoclonus: a non-epileptic movement disorder that may present as status epilepticus. *Arch Dis Child.* 2009;94(11):897–899.

93. Huber BM, Strozzi S, Steinlin M, Aebi C, Fluri S. Mycoplasma pneumoniae associated opsoclonus-myoclonus syndrome in three cases. *Eur J Pediatr.* 2010;169(4):441–445.

94. Ertekin V, Tan H. Opsoclonus-myoclonus syndrome attributable to hepatitis C infection. *Pediatr Neurol.* 2010;42(6):441–442.

95. Desai J, Mitchell WG. Acute cerebellar ataxia, acute cerebellitis, and opsoclonus-myoclonus syndrome. *J Child Neurol.* 2012;27(11):1482–1488.

96. Connolly AM, Dodson WE, Prensky AL, Rust RS. Course and outcome of acute cerebellar ataxia. *Ann Neurol.* 1994;35(6):673–679.

97. Toro C, Pascual-Leone A, Deuschl G, Tate E, Pranzatelli MR, Hallett M. Cortical tremor. A common manifestation of cortical myoclonus. *Neurology.* 1993;43(11):2346–2353.

98. Krug P, Schleiermacher G, Michon J, et al. Opsoclonus-myoclonus in children associated or not with neuroblastoma. *Europ J Paediatr Neurol.* 2010;14(5):400–409.

99. Singhi P, Sahu JK, Sarkar J, Bansal D. Clinical profile and outcome of children with opsoclonus-myoclonus syndrome. *J Child Neurol.* 2014;29(1):58–61.

100. Brunklaus A, Pohl K, Zuberi SM, de Sousa C. Outcome and prognostic features in opsoclonus-myoclonus syndrome from infancy to adult life. *Pediatrics.* 2011;128(2):e388–394.

101. Tate ED, Pranzatelli MR, Verhulst SJ, et al. Active comparator-controlled, rater-blinded study of corticotropin-based immunotherapies for opsoclonus-myoclonus syndrome. *J Child Neurol.* 2012;27(7):875–884.

102. Pranzatelli MR, Tate ED, Travelstead AL, et al. Insights on chronic-relapsing opsoclonus-myoclonus from a pilot study of mycophenolate mofetil. *J Child Neurol.* 2009;24(3):316–322.

103. Aydin GB, Kutluk MT, Buyukpamukcu M, Akyuz C, Yalcin B, Varan A. Neurological complications of neuroblastic tumors: experience of a single center. *Childs Nerv Syst.* 2010;26(3):359–365.

104. Cooper AC, Humphreys GW, Hulleman J, Praamstra P, Georgeson M. Transcranial magnetic stimulation to right parietal cortex modifies the attentional blink. *Exp Brain Res.* 2004;155(1):24–29.

105. Fuhlhuber V, Bick S, Kirsten A, et al. Elevated B-cell activating factor BAFF, but not APRIL, correlates with CSF cerebellar autoantibodies in pediatric opsoclonus-myoclonus syndrome. *J Neuroimmunol.* 2009;210(1–2):87–91.

106. Pranzatelli MR, Tate ED, McGee NR, et al. Key role of CXCL13/CXCR5 axis for cerebrospinal fluid B cell recruitment in pediatric OMS. *J Neuroimmunol.* 2012;243(1–2):81–88.

107. Pranzatelli MR, Tate ED, McGee NR, Ransohoff RM. CCR7 signaling in pediatric opsoclonus-myoclonus: upregulated serum CCL21 expression is steroid-responsive. *Cytokine.* 2013;64(1):331–336.

108. Pranzatelli MR. Opsoclonus-myoclonus-ataxia syndrome. In: Fernandez-Alvarez E, Arzimanoglou A, Tolosa E, eds. *Paediatric Movement Disorders: Progress in Understanding.* Esher, Surrey, UK: John Libbey Eurotext; 2005:121–136.

109. Tate ED, Allison TJ, Pranzatelli MR, Verhulst SJ. Neuroepidemiologic trends in 105 US cases of pediatric opsoclonus-myoclonus syndrome. *J Pediatr Oncol Nurs.* 2005;22(1):8–19.

110. Brunklaus A, Pohl K, Zuberi SM, de Sousa C. Investigating neuroblastoma in childhood opsoclonus-myoclonus syndrome. *Arch Dis Child.* 2012;97(5):461–463.

111. Pranzatelli MR, Tate ED, Travelstead AL, et al. Rituximab (anti-CD20) adjunctive therapy for opsoclonus-myoclonus syndrome. *J Pediatr Hematol Oncol.* 2006;28(9):585–593.

112. Battaglia T, De Grandis E, Mirabelli-Badenier M, et al. Response to rituximab in 3 children with opsoclonus-myoclonus syndrome resistant to conventional treatments. *Europ J Paediatr Neurol.* 2012;16(2):192–195.

113. De Grandis E, Parodi S, Conte M, et al. Long-term follow-up of neuroblastoma-associated opsoclonus-myoclonus-ataxia syndrome. *Neuropediatrics.* 2009;40(3):103–111.

114. Offit PA. *Autism's False Prophets: Bad Science, Risky Medicine, and the Search for a Cure.* New York, NY: Columbia University Press; 2008.

115. Buchanan R, Bonthius DJ. Measles virus and associated central nervous system sequelae. *Semin Pediatr Neurol.* 2012;19(3):107–114.

116. Yuksel D, Diren B, Ulubay H, Altunbasak S, Anlar B. Neuronal loss is an early component of subacute sclerosing panencephalitis. *Neurology.* 2014;83(10):938–944.

117. Tatli B, Ekici B, Ozmen M. Current therapies and future perspectives in subacute sclerosing panencephalitis. *Expert Rev.* 2012;12(4):485–492.

118. Gonzalez de Dios J, Moya M. Asfixia perinatal, encefalopatia hipoxico-isquemica y secuelas neurologicas en recien nacidos a termino. II. Descripcion e interrelaciones. *Revista de Neurologia.* 1996;24(132):969–976.

119. Sarnat HB, Sarnat MS. Neonatal encephalopathy following fetal distress. A clinical and electroencephalographic study. *Arch Neurol.* 1976;33(10):696–705.

120. Genton P, Gelisse P. Antimyoclonic effect of levetiracetam. *Epileptic Disord.* 2000;2(4):209–212.

121. Mirones I, de Prada I, Gomez AM, et al. A role for the CXCR3/CXCL10 axis in Rasmussen encephalitis. *Pediatr Neurol.* 2013;49(6):451–457.

122. Shahar E, Kramer U, Nass D, Savitzki D. Epilepsia partialis continua associated with widespread gliomatosis cerebri. *Pediatr Neurol.* 2002;27(5):392–396.

123. Cockerell OC, Rothwell J, Thompson PD, Marsden CD, Shorvon SD. Clinical and physiological features of epilepsia partialis continua. Cases ascertained in the UK. *Brain.* 1996;119(Pt 2):393–407.

124. Browner N, Azher SN, Jankovic J. Botulinum toxin treatment of facial myoclonus in suspected Rasmussen encephalitis. *Mov Disord.* 2006;21(9):1500–1502.

125. Freeman JM. Rasmussen's syndrome: progressive autoimmune multi-focal encephalopathy. *Pediatr Neurol.* 2005;32(5):295–299.

126. Moosa AN, Gupta A, Jehi L, et al. Longitudinal seizure outcome and prognostic predictors after hemispherectomy in 170 children. *Neurology.* 2013;80(3):253–260.

127. Moosa AN, Jehi L, Marashly A, et al. Long-term functional outcomes and their predictors after hemispherectomy in 115 children. *Epilepsia.* 2013;54(10):1771–1779.

128. Bien CG, Tiemeier H, Sassen R, et al. Rasmussen encephalitis: incidence and course under randomized therapy with tacrolimus or intravenous immunoglobulins. *Epilepsia.* 2013;54(3):543–550.

129. Takahashi Y, Yamazaki E, Mine J, et al. Immunomodulatory therapy versus surgery for Rasmussen syndrome in early childhood. *Brain Dev.* 2013;35(8):778–785.

130. Bittner S, Simon OJ, Gobel K, Bien CG, Meuth SG, Wiendl H. Rasmussen encephalitis treated with natalizumab. *Neurology.* 2013;81(4):395–397.

131. de Siqueira LF. Progressive myoclonic epilepsies: review of clinical, molecular and therapeutic aspects. *J Neurol.* 2010;257(10):1612–1619.

132. Manganotti P, Tamburin S, Zanette G, Fiaschi A. Hyperexcitable cortical responses in progressive myoclonic epilepsy: a TMS study. *Neurology.* 2001;57(10):1793–1799.

133. Lance JW. Action myoclonus, Ramsay Hunt syndrome, and other cerebellar myoclonic syndromes. *Adv Neurol.* 1986;43:33–55.

134. Altindag E, Kara B, Baykan B, et al. MR spectroscopy findings in Lafora disease. *J Neuroimaging.* 2009;19(4):359–365.

135. Mannonen L, Herrgard E, Valmari P, et al. Primary human herpesvirus-6 infection in the central nervous system can cause severe disease. *Pediatr Neurol.* 2007;37(3):186–191.

136. Karkheiran S, Krebs CE, Makarov V, et al. Identification of COL6A2 mutations in progressive myoclonus epilepsy syndrome. *Hum Genet.* 2013;132(3):275–283.

137. Krabichler B, Rostasy K, Baumann M, et al. Novel mutation in potassium channel related gene KCTD7 and progressive myoclonic epilepsy. *Ann Hum Genet.* 2012;76(4):326–331.

138. Hoffman RE, Cavus I. Slow transcranial magnetic stimulation, long-term depotentiation, and brain hyperexcitability disorders. *Am J Psychiatry.* 2002;159(7):1093–1102.

139. Wong LJ, Naviaux RK, Brunetti-Pierri N, et al. Molecular and clinical genetics of mitochondrial diseases due to POLG mutations. *Hum Mutat.* 2008;29(9):E150–172.

140. Rahman S. Mitochondrial disease and epilepsy. *Dev Med Child Neurol.* 2012;54(5):397–406.

141. Fukuhara T, Gotoh M, Asari S, Ohmoto T. Magnetic resonance imaging of patients with intention tremor. *Comput Med Imaging Graph.* 1994;18(1):45–51.

142. Ito S, Shirai W, Asahina M, Hattori T. Clinical and brain MR imaging features focusing on the brain stem and cerebellum in patients with myoclonic epilepsy with ragged-red fibers due to mitochondrial A8344G mutation. *AJNR Am J Neuroradiol.* 2008;29(2):392–395.

143. Shoffner JM, Lott MT, Lezza AM, Seibel P, Ballinger SW, Wallace DC. Myoclonic epilepsy and ragged-red fiber disease (MERRF) is associated with a mitochondrial DNA tRNA(Lys) mutation. *Cell.* 1990;61(6):931–937.

144. Tassinari CA, Bureau-Paillas M, Grasso E, Roger J. [Electroencephalographic study of myoclonic cerebellar dyssynergia with epilepsy (Ramsay Hunt syndrome)]. *Rev Electroencephalogr Neurophysiol Clin.* 1974;4(3):407–428.

145. Canafoglia L, Gennaro E, Capovilla G, et al. Electroclinical presentation and genotype-phenotype relationships in patients with Unverricht–Lundborg disease carrying compound heterozygous CSTB point and indel mutations. *Epilepsia.* 2012;53(12):2120–2127.

146. Pennacchio LA, Lehesjoki AE, Stone NE, et al. Mutations in the gene encoding cystatin B in progressive myoclonus epilepsy (EPM1). *Science.* 1996;271(5256):1731–1734.

147. Minassian BA, Lee JR, Herbrick JA, et al. Mutations in a gene encoding a novel protein tyrosine phosphatase cause progressive myoclonus epilepsy. *Nat Genet.* 1998;20(2):171–174.

148. Chan EM, Young EJ, Ianzano L, et al. Mutations in NHLRC1 cause progressive myoclonus epilepsy. *Nat Genet.* 2003;35(2):125–127.

149. Gentry MS, Worby CA, Dixon JE. Insights into Lafora disease: malin is an E3 ubiquitin ligase that ubiquitinates and promotes the degradation of laforin. *Proc Natl Acad Sci USA.* 2005;102(24):8501–8506.

150. Lohi H, Ianzano L, Zhao XC, et al. Novel glycogen synthase kinase 3 and ubiquitination pathways in progressive myoclonus epilepsy. *Hum Mol Genet.* 2005;14(18):2727–2736.

151. Arsov T, Smith KR, Damiano J, et al. Kufs disease, the major adult form of neuronal ceroid lipofuscinosis, caused by mutations in CLN6. *Am J Hum Genet*. 2011;88(5):566–573.

152. Kousi M, Lehesjoki AE, Mole SE. Update of the mutation spectrum and clinical correlations of over 360 mutations in eight genes that underlie the neuronal ceroid lipofuscinoses. *Hum Mutat*. 2012;33(1):42–63.

153. Mink JW, Augustine EF, Adams HR, Marshall FJ, Kwon JM. Classification and natural history of the neuronal ceroid lipofuscinoses. *J Child Neurol*. 2013;28(9):1101–1105.

154. Tauscher J, Kufferle B, Asenbaum S, Tauscher-Wisniewski S, Kasper S. Striatal dopamine-2 receptor occupancy as measured with [123I]iodobenzamide and SPECT predicted the occurrence of EPS in patients treated with atypical antipsychotics and haloperidol. *Psychopharmacology*. 2002;162(1):42–49.

155. Kohan R, Cismondi IA, Oller-Ramirez AM, et al. Therapeutic approaches to the challenge of neuronal ceroid lipofuscinoses. *Curr Pharm Biotechnol*. 2011;12(6):867–883.

156. Corbett MA, Schwake M, Bahlo M, et al. A mutation in the Golgi Qb-SNARE gene GOSR2 causes progressive myoclonus epilepsy with early ataxia. *Am J Hum Genet*. 2011;88(5):657–663.

157. Boisse Lomax L, Bayly MA, Hjalgrim H, et al. "North Sea" progressive myoclonus epilepsy: phenotype of subjects with GOSR2 mutation. *Brain*. 2013;136(Pt 4):1146–1154.

158. Hay JC, Chao DS, Kuo CS, Scheller RH. Protein interactions regulating vesicle transport between the endoplasmic reticulum and Golgi apparatus in mammalian cells. *Cell*. 1997;89(1):149–158.

159. Bonten EJ, Arts WF, Beck M, et al. Novel mutations in lysosomal neuraminidase identify functional domains and determine clinical severity in sialidosis. *Hum Mol Genet*. 2000;9(18):2715–2725.

160. Zhou X.Y., van der Spoel A., Rottier R., et al. Molecular and biochemical analysis of protective protein/cathepsin A mutations: correlation with clinical severity in galactosialidosis [erratum appears in *Hum Mol Genet*. 1997;6(1):146]. *Hum Mol Genet*. 1996;5(12):1977–1987.

161. Magenis RE, Toth-Fejel S, Allen LJ, et al. Comparison of the 15q deletions in Prader–Willi and Angelman syndromes: specific regions, extent of deletions, parental origin, and clinical consequences. *Am J Med Genet*. 1990;35(3):333–349.

162. Kishino T, Lalande M, Wagstaff J. UBE3A/E6-AP mutations cause Angelman syndrome. *Nat Genet*. 1997;15(1):70–73.

163. American Society of Human Genetics. Diagnostic testing for Prader–Willi and Angleman syndromes: Report of the ASHG/ACMG Test and Technology Transfer Committee. *Am J Hum Genet*. 1996;58(5): 1085–1088.

164. Russell JF, Steckley JL, Coppola G, et al. Familial cortical myoclonus with a mutation in NOL3. *Ann Neurol*. 2012;72(2):175–183.

165. Jarman PR, Wood NW, Davis MT, et al. Hereditary geniospasm: linkage to chromosome 9q13-q21 and evidence for genetic heterogeneity. *Am J Hum Genet*. 1997;61(4):928–933.

166. Marechal L, Raux G, Dumanchin C, et al. Severe myoclonus-dystonia syndrome associated with a novel epsilon-sarcoglycan gene truncating mutation. *Am J Med Genet B Neuropsychiatr Genet*. 2003;119(1):114–117.

167. Kabakci K, Hedrich K, Leung JC, et al. Mutations in DYT1: extension of the phenotypic and mutational spectrum. *Neurology*. 2004;62(3):395–400.

168. Grimes DA, Han F, Lang AE, St George-Hyssop P, Racacho L, Bulman DE. A novel locus for inherited myoclonus-dystonia on 18p11. *Neurology*. 2002;59(8):1183–1186.

169. Gu W, Sander T, Heils A, Lenzen KP, Steinlein OK. A new EF-hand containing gene EFHC2 on Xp11.4: tentative evidence for association with juvenile myoclonic epilepsy. *Epilepsy Res*. 2005;66(1–3):91–98.

170. Medina MT, Suzuki T, Alonso ME, et al. Novel mutations in myoclonin1/EFHC1 in sporadic and familial juvenile myoclonic epilepsy. *Neurology*. 2008;70(22 Pt 2):2137–2144.

171. Ma S, Blair MA, Abou-Khalil B, Lagrange AH, Gurnett CA, Hedera P. Mutations in the GABRA1 and EFHC1 genes are rare in familial juvenile myoclonic epilepsy. *Epilepsy Res*. 2006;71(2–3):129–134.

172. Kapoor A, Vijai J, Ravishankar HM, Satishchandra P, Radhakrishnan K, Anand A. Absence of GABRA1 Ala322Asp mutation in juvenile myoclonic epilepsy families from India. *J Genet*. 2003;82(1–2):17–21.

173. Iannetti P, Parisi P, Spalice A, Ruggieri M, Zara F. Addition of verapamil in the treatment of severe myoclonic epilepsy in infancy. *Epilepsy Res*. 2009;85(1):89–95.

174. Singh B, Monteil A, Bidaud I, et al. Mutational analysis of CACNA1G in idiopathic generalized epilepsy. Mutation in brief #962 [online]. *Hum Mutat*. 2007;28(5):524–525.

175. Haug K, Warnstedt M, Alekov AK, et al. Mutations in CLCN2 encoding a voltage-gated chloride channel are associated with idiopathic generalized epilepsies. *Nat Genet*. 2003;33(4):527–532.

176. Simpson MA, Cross H, Proukakis C, et al. Infantile-onset symptomatic epilepsy syndrome caused by a homozygous loss-of-function mutation of GM3 synthase. *Nat Genet.* 2004;36(11):1225–1229.

177. Hyland K, Surtees RA, Rodeck C, Clayton PT. Aromatic L-amino acid decarboxylase deficiency: clinical features, diagnosis, and treatment of a new inborn error of neurotransmitter amine synthesis. *Neurology.* 1992;42(10):1980–1988.

178. Kuchar L, Ledvinova J, Hrebicek M, et al. Prosaposin deficiency and saposin B deficiency (activator-deficient metachromatic leukodystrophy): report on two patients detected by analysis of urinary sphingolipids and carrying novel PSAP gene mutations. *Am J Med Genet A.* 2009;149A(4):613–621.

179. Harzer K, Paton BC, Poulos A, et al. Sphingolipid activator protein deficiency in a 16-week-old atypical Gaucher disease patient and his fetal sibling: biochemical signs of combined sphingolipidoses. *Eur J Pediatr.* 1989;149(1):31–39.

180. Burke JR, Wingfield MS, Lewis KE, et al. The Haw River syndrome: dentatorubropallidoluysian atrophy (DRPLA) in an African-American family. *Nat Genet.* 1994;7(4):521–524.

181. Patterson MC, Horowitz M, Abel RB, et al. Isolated horizontal supranuclear gaze palsy as a marker of severe systemic involvement in Gaucher's disease. *Neurology.* 1993;43(10):1993–1997.

182. Shih VE, Efron ML, Moser HW. Hyperornithinemia, hyperammonemia, and homocitrullinuria. A new disorder of amino acid metabolism associated with myoclonic seizures and mental retardation. *Am J Dis Child.* 1969;117(1):83–92.

183. Tessa A, Fiermonte G, Dionisi-Vici C, et al. Identification of novel mutations in the SLC25A15 gene in hyperornithinemia-hyperammonemia-homocitrullinuria (HHH) syndrome: a clinical, molecular, and functional study. *Hum Mutat.* 2009;30(5):741–748.

184. Riggs JE, Schochet Jr. SS, Fakadej AV, et al. Mitochondrial encephalomyopathy with decreased succinate-cytochrome c reductase activity. *Neurology.* 1984;34(1):48–53.

185. Fukuhara N, Tokiguchi S, Shirakawa K, Tsubaki T. Myoclonus epilepsy associated with ragged-red fibres (mitochondrial abnormalities): disease entity or a syndrome? Light-and electron-microscopic studies of two cases and review of literature. *J Neurol Sci.* 1980;47(1):117–133.

186. Bindoff LA, Desnuelle C, Birch-Machin MA, et al. Multiple defects of the mitochondrial respiratory chain in a mitochondrial encephalopathy (MERRF): a clinical, biochemical and molecular study. *J Neurol Sci.* 1991;102(1):17–24.

187. Vesa J, Hellsten E, Verkruyse LA, et al. Mutations in the palmitoyl protein thioesterase gene causing infantile neuronal ceroid lipofuscinosis. *Nature.* 1995;376(6541):584–587.

188. Sleat DE, Donnelly RJ, Lackland H, et al. Association of mutations in a lysosomal protein with classical late-infantile neuronal ceroid lipofuscinosis. *Science.* 1997;277(5333):1802–1805.

189. Isolation of a novel gene underlying Batten disease, CLN3. The International Batten Disease Consortium. *Cell.* 1995;82(6):949–957.

190. Savukoski M, Klockars T, Holmberg V, Santavuori P, Lander ES, Peltonen L. CLN5, a novel gene encoding a putative transmembrane protein mutated in Finnish variant late infantile neuronal ceroid lipofuscinosis. *Nat Genet.* 1998;19(3):286–288.

191. Ranta S, Zhang Y, Ross B, et al. The neuronal ceroid lipofuscinoses in human EPMR and mnd mutant mice are associated with mutations in CLN8. *Nat Genet.* 1999;23(2):233–236.

192. Andermann F, Berkovic S, Carpenter S, Andermann E. The Ramsay Hunt syndrome is no longer a useful diagnostic category. *Mov Disord.* 1989;4(1):13–17.

193. Davidzon G, Mancuso M, Ferraris S, et al. POLG mutations and Alpers syndrome. *Ann Neurol.* 2005;57(6):921–923.

194. Mills PB, Surtees RA, Champion MP, et al. Neonatal epileptic encephalopathy caused by mutations in the PNPO gene encoding pyridox(am)ine 5'-phosphate oxidase. *Hum Mol Genet.* 2005;14(8):1077–1086.

195. Philippart M. The Rett syndrome in males. *Brain Dev.* 1990;12(1):33–36.

196. Clayton-Smith J, Watson P, Ramsden S, Black GC. Somatic mutation in MECP2 as a non-fatal neurodevelopmental disorder in males. *Lancet.* 2000;356(9232):830–832.

197. Schindler D, Bishop DF, Wolfe DE, et al. Neuroaxonal dystrophy due to lysosomal alpha-N-acetylgalactosaminidase deficiency. *N Engl J Med.* 1989;320(26):1735–1740.

198. Schelhaas HJ, Ippel PF, Hageman G, Sinke RJ, van der Laan EN, Beemer FA. Clinical and genetic analysis of a four-generation family with a distinct autosomal dominant cerebellar ataxia. *J Neurol.* 2001;248(2):113–120.

199. Pulst SM, Nechiporuk A, Nechiporuk T, et al. Moderate expansion of a normally biallelic trinucleotide repeat in spinocerebellar ataxia type 2. *Nat Genet*. 1996;14(3):269–276.

200. Lalioti MD, Mirotsou M, Buresi C, et al. Identification of mutations in cystatin B, the gene responsible for the Unverricht–Lundborg type of progressive myoclonus epilepsy (EPM1). *Am J Hum Genet*. 1997;60(2):342–351.

201. Bassuk AG, Wallace RH, Buhr A, et al. A homozygous mutation in human PRICKLE1 causes an autosomal-recessive progressive myoclonus epilepsy-ataxia syndrome. *Am J Hum Genet*. 2008;83(5):572–581.

202. Balreira A, Gaspar P, Caiola D, et al. A nonsense mutation in the LIMP-2 gene associated with progressive myoclonic epilepsy and nephrotic syndrome. *Hum Mol Genet*. 2008;17(14):2238–2243.

203. Mezer E, Nischal KK, Nahjawan N, MacKeen LD, Buncic JR. Hemifacial spasm as the initial manifestation of childhood cerebellar astrocytoma. *J AAPOS*. 2006;10(5):489–490.

204. Lavon H, Cohen-Kerem R, Uri N. Hemifacial spasm associated with otitis media with effusion: a first reported case. *Int J Pediatr Otorhinolaryngol*. 2006;70(5):947–950.

205. Ababneh OH, Cetinkaya A, Kulwin DR. Long-term efficacy and safety of botulinum toxin A injections to treat blepharospasm and hemifacial spasm. *Clin Experiment Ophthalmol*. 2014;42(3):254–261.

206. Sandel T, Eide PK. Long-term results of microvascular decompression for trigeminal neuralgia and hemifacial spasms according to preoperative symptomatology. *Acta Neurochir (Wien)*. 2013;155(9):1681–1692. [discussion 1692].

207. Canavese C, Ciano C, Zibordi F, Zorzi G, Cavallera V, Nardocci N. Phenomenology of psychogenic movement disorders in children. *Mov Disord*. 2012;27(9):1153–1157.

208. Thenganatt MA, Jankovic J. Psychogenic movement disorders. *Neurol Clin*. 2015;33(1):205–224.

209. Roze E, Apartis E, Clot F, et al. Myoclonus-dystonia: clinical and electrophysiologic pattern related to SGCE mutations. *Neurology*. 2008;70(13):1010–1016.

Tremor

Harvey S. Singer[1], Jonathan W. Mink[2],
Donald L. Gilbert[3] and Joseph Jankovic[4]

[1]Department of Neurology, Johns Hopkins Hospital, Baltimore, MD, USA; [2]Division of
Child Neurology, University of Rochester Medical Center, Rochester, NY, USA; [3]Division of
Neurology, Cincinnati Children's Hospital Medical Center, Cincinnati, OH, USA; [4]Department
of Neurology, Baylor College of Medicine, Houston, TX, USA

OUTLINE

INTRODUCTION AND OVERVIEW

Tremor is common in children and adults. Prevalence of common forms, such as essential tremor (ET), has been well-studied in adults,[1] but in childhood this has been less well characterized.[2,3] Tremor may be localized to hands-only, or to other locations. Tremor may be *primary*, or *idiopathic*, meaning that pathophysiology is related to relatively isolated dysfunction within tremor-related nodes or networks in the motor system. In children, this designation is typically appropriate when the predominant movement disorder is tremor manifest during action, the remainder of the examination is normal or nearly so, and the results of medical diagnostic testing, if obtained, are also normal. Tremor may also be *secondary*, or symptomatic, resulting from a known cause. The time course can be acute, transient/intermittent, subacute, chronic and stable, or chronic and progressive.

In children, tremor may manifest from infancy through adolescence.[4] Although tremor at any age may distress parents, tremor tends to be brought to medical attention either early in childhood or much later, in adolescence. This is due to both the epidemiology of the more common etiologies and to the age-related impairment. In young children, tremor may interfere with acquiring fine motor skills. Therefore, functional impairment with fine motor tasks often becomes apparent during preschool or early elementary school, with referrals generated by concerns of parents, teachers, or therapists. The differential diagnosis is large, but often a mild static encephalopathy is the cause of tremor at this age. In adolescents, social embarrassment as well as engagement in more complex activities drives more referrals for tremor. At this age, prominent etiologies include enhanced physiologic tremor due to stress or anxiety, medication-induced or substance abuse–induced tremors,[5] ET,[2,6] and functional (psychogenic) tremors.[7]

Finally, a large variety of other neurologic conditions can manifest with tremor. Although most children with tremor do not have a serious, progressive neurologic condition, as is often the case in pediatrics, vigilance and clinical acumen is needed to detect low prevalence, serious illnesses. It is important to have a systematic approach to diagnosis, based on childhood development, epidemiology, primary features, associated symptoms, and understanding of neuroanatomy and pathophysiology. This chapter encompasses diseases and disorders resulting in clinical syndromes that may manifest with prominent tremor in childhood. The many diseases where tremor is a part of a mixed movement disorder or other encephalopathy and not the prominent symptom are covered in more detail in other chapters, indicated in the text.

DEFINITION OF TREMOR

Tremor refers to a rhythmic, relatively symmetric oscillatory involuntary movement about a joint axis.[8] Usually, this involves rhythmic alternating contraction of agonist and antagonist muscles and produces a visible, sinusoidal-appearing movement. Several alternating phenomena are not tremor. Nystagmus is not considered tremor, although it may be oscillatory or pendular. Repetitive contractions that do not move a muscle across a joint, such as myokymia (within a muscle bundle) or fasciculation (within a small number of fibers), are not included within *tremor* nosology. Myoclonus involves jerk-and-release and is therefore distinguished from tremor in part by its lack of both symmetry and midpoint. Continuous palatal myoclonus is considered by some authors to be a form of tremor, but, since it involves contractions of agonists only, "rhythmic myoclonus" is a better description. Athetosis or athetoid movements may be distal and accompany dystonia, as can tremor, but the athetotic movements are generally more complex and less regular in their timing than tremor.

CLINICAL CHARACTERISTICS—PHENOMENOLOGY OF TREMOR IN CHILDREN

Evaluation of tremor involves considering body distribution (distal/proximal limbs, trunk, etc.), the relationship to rest versus action, and frequency. Various forms of categorization of tremor are employed. The most useful, primary distinction is based on the relation to voluntary movement, as described in Table 13.1. Nosology is not always consistent. In Table 13.1, the primary distinction employed is whether the motor system involved is at rest or not.

Rest tremor is most common in hypokinetic syndromes (see Chapter 15) although it can also be drug-induced or functional. Rest tremor generally indicates a serious neurologic illness, often accompanied by other neurological symptoms and signs and therefore often part of diseases discussed in other chapters. The emphasis in this chapter will be on action tremors, which are much more common in children, particularly the postural and kinetic tremors.

Because tremor is continuous and regular around a fixed location, two key features set it apart from other movement disorders: amplitude and frequency. Electromyography (EMG), accelerometers, and other instruments are sometimes used to quantitate tremors, but the *clinical* utility of this information, i.e., its ability to improve diagnostic and/or therapeutic medical decision making, has not been demonstrated in children.[9] There have been many attempts to quantitate tremor,[10] but in practice, instrumentation is seldom used in child neurology for clinical classification of tremor. Systematic clinical assessment by an experienced neurologist, in some cases employing tremor rating scales, is usually adequate for evaluation of tremors and their response to therapy.[11]

TABLE 13.1   Summary of Clinical Features and Classification of Tremor

Type of tremor	Relationship to action or muscle state
Rest	When limbs are fully supported against gravity
Action	During movement of various types
Postural	While holding a limb or body part in a position, against gravity
Kinetic	With directed voluntary movement
Intention/Terminal	While moving the limb toward a target. This is not synonymous with dysmetria but, like dysmetria, is characteristic of cerebellar origin
Isometric	While contracting muscle without an observable movement
Task-specific tremor	During performance of skilled tasks such as writing or playing a musical instrument

Clinical Differentiation from Other Movement Disorders, and Some Special Types of Tremor

Tremor can co-occur with other movement disorders, and the distinction can be clinically challenging, particularly when movement disorders are mixed.[4,8,12] Tremors can be classified according to their phenomenology, distribution, frequency, or etiology.[13] Phenomenologically, tremors are divided into two major categories: rest tremors and action tremors. Rest tremor is present when the affected body part is fully supported against gravity and not actively contracting; rest tremor is diminished or absent during voluntary muscle contraction and during movement. Action tremors occur with voluntary contraction of muscles, and they can be subdivided into postural, kinetic, task-specific or position-specific, and isometric tremors. Postural tremor is evident during maintenance of an antigravity posture, such as holding the arms in an outstretched horizontal position in front of the body. Kinetic tremor can be seen when the voluntary movement starts (initial tremor), during the course of the movement (dynamic tremor), and as the affected body part approaches the target, such as while performing the finger-to-nose or the toe-to-finger maneuver (*terminal tremor*, also called *intention tremor*). Task-specific tremors occur only during, or are markedly exacerbated by, a certain task, such as while writing (primary handwriting tremor), while speaking or singing (voice tremor) or while smiling. Position-specific tremors occur while holding a certain posture (e.g., the "wing-beating" position or holding a spoon or a cup close to the mouth). *Dystonic tremor* is an irregular tremor in the presence of underlying dystonia.[14] The tremor is most prominent when the patient resists and attempts to correct the abnormal dystonic posture and it diminishes or can be completely abolished when the affected body part is allowed to assume the dystonic posture (the so-called null point).

Dentate-Rubral (Holmes) tremor, also known as midbrain tremor, is a large-amplitude, slow tremor present at rest and increasing with posture and movement (Video 13.2). Pathophysiology may involve disruption of the Guillain-Mollaret Triangle, comprised of tracts between the red nucleus, the ipsilateral inferior olivary nucleus, and the contralateral cerebellar dentate nucleus.[15] The lesion may lie nearby in the superior cerebellar peduncle or in the thalamus.[16]

Myorhythmia is a slow (1–3 Hz), continuous or intermittent, relatively rhythmic movement sometimes associated with palatal or ocular myoclonus, usually related to brainstem or diencephalic pathology.[17] Facial myorhythmia, along with vertical ophthalmoparesis or ocular myoclonus, is a characteristic movement disorder in Whipple disease. Myorhythmia may also occur in children with anti-*N*-methyl-D-aspartate receptor encephalitis.[18] *Orthostatic tremor* is an isometric tremor that occurs in the legs and trunk during standing, usually occurring a few minutes after assuming erect posture. This occurs rarely in children.

Trembling usually refers to the chin, as in isolated hereditary chin tremor (Video 13.1).[19-21]

Jitters/jitteriness is a transient high-frequency tremor in neonates (see Chapter 6).

Shuddering is brief episodes of shaking with no electroencephalogram correlate, usually occurring in infancy (see Chapter 6). Although some have suggested that "shuddering attacks" of infancy might be the initial manifestation of ET, this observation has not been validated.[22]

LOCALIZATION AND PATHOPHYSIOLOGY

Tremor involves alternating, relatively symmetric contractions of agonist and antagonist muscles leading to movement around a fixed point, axis, or plane. Visually, the movements are oscillatory. The mathematical regularity of these oscillations is demonstrable with instrumentation such as accelerometers, which allow for quantification of the frequency and amplitude of the tremor, and can also be seen when asking the patient to draw a freehand spiral.

Tremor can be conceptualized as abnormal movement resulting from the insufficient inhibition of or excessive facilitation of oscillatory activity in the central nervous system, transmitted out to muscles. This central oscillatory activity is localized in part in the cortical-striatal-pallidal-thalamocortical circuits (see Chapter 1) and the cortical-cerebellar-thalamocortical circuits (see Chapter 2). These circuits subserve movement and contain nodes in which there is physiological oscillatory or cycling electrical activity. These nodes are sometimes called "central oscillators," and information about them has been gained through direct cell recording in mammals and in cell culture and slice preparations and from human neurophysiology data obtained during functional neurosurgery, particularly deep brain stimulation (DBS) surgery.[23] These central oscillators probably include the ventral thalamus,[24-26] the inferior olive,[27,28] and the subthalamic nucleus.[29-31]

Physiologic oscillating electrical activity in brain circuits usually does not lead directly to observable, oscillating motor activity, i.e., tremor, unless one of several types of processes occurs.

Central and Peripheral Processes Which May Result in Tremor

1. Abnormal function of inhibitory or "damping" systems. Acute, chronic, or progressive processes may cause inefficient neural transmission within inhibitory systems. For example, damage to cerebral cortical inhibitory systems may allow transmission of subcortical oscillatory neural activity to propagate to the motor system.
2. Changes within or among central oscillators. Enhanced activity or pathologic synchronization of oscillatory activity can overload inhibitory systems and lead to propagation of the inappropriate activity out to the motor system. Selective damage to certain critical cell types, e.g., cerebellar Purkinje cells, due to hypoxia or toxins, affects central oscillation patterns.
3. Changes in afferent neural activity to central oscillators. An example would be changes in pallido-thalamic transmission caused by upstream nigrostriatal dopaminergic dysregulation. Another example would be altered peripheral input through muscle spindle feedback, related to stiffness or external mass load on the limbs. This affects central oscillatory activity and alters components of tremor frequency. This mechanical input dysregulation may influence the presentation of tremor in children with spastic cerebral palsy, hypotonia, or neuropathies.

The frequency of the spontaneous activity in these nodes has been shown in some cases to correspond to the tremor frequency recorded with EMG. Tremors of various frequencies appear, based on lesioning studies and clinical–pathologic correlations, to have characteristic anatomic locations. For example, cerebellar hemispheric lesion tremors vary from

5 to 11 Hz, and dentate nucleus lesion results in slower, 6–8 Hz tremor. Midbrain tremors are slower at 2–3 Hz, high brainstem lesions have 5–7 Hz tremor, and low brainstem lesions have 8–11 Hz tremor.[32,33] In addition to anatomic location, the type of lesion may also be important, with destructive or multifocal processes causing lower frequency tremors than compressive lesions.[34] A population of neurons in ventral thalamus in Parkinson's disease (PD) was demonstrated to have rates of firing that correlated with tremor in the contralateral hand,[35] and, similarly, thalamic neural activity has been shown to correlate with EMG recording of ET.[36] The frequency of tremor may be age-dependent. ET frequency is higher in children than adults but generally slower than physiological tremor. Neuroanatomic localization based on frequency has scientific interest but lesser clinical utility or verifiability without instrumentation.

At the cellular and molecular level, there is growing scientific interest in ion channels and cyclic firing patterns, because they seem to play an important role in the neuronal substrate of tremor. In olivary neurons, there is a cycle of autorhythmic depolarization, hyperpolarization, and recurrent depolarization related to Ca^{2+} conductance.[31] It is thought that one mechanism of antitremorigenic action of thalamic DBS is desynchronization of pathologically synchronous oscillating systems.

Thus three main etiologic categories of tremor can be partially understood in terms of effects on central oscillatory activity:

1. *Enhanced physiologic tremor*—physiologic tremor that is normally measurable but not visible becomes more apparent when stressors on the system allow for increased amplitude. Acute emotional stressors, fatigue, and stimulating substances such as caffeine, amphetamines, and thyroid hormones may transiently perturb the inhibitory systems that dampen normal oscillatory activity.
2. *Essential tremor* (ET)—primary tremor that occurs in the absence of other prominent neurologic symptoms. The source of this tremor may be abnormal activity in central oscillators in the cerebellar-thalamocortical loop. This is supported by the observation that adults with ET commonly have some cerebellar symptoms (e.g., abnormal tandem gait). ET case control studies demonstrate increased cerebellar and red nucleus activity during tremor, measured using positron emission tomography (PET).[37–39] Alcohol use, which clinical observation has shown improves ET symptoms, acts in the anterior cerebellum to impair gait coordination. Alcohol also suppresses this cerebellar overactivity as quantified using PET,[40] which may account for its ability to improve ET. ET phenomenology has also been reported ipsilateral to affected unilateral cerebellar hemispheres in congenital as well as postoperative[26] cases in childhood. This suggests ET phenomenology may emerge from aberrant structure or function in multiple locations within cerebellar-thalamic loops. Cerebellar pathology, including loss of Purkinje cells, has been described in some brains of patients with ET, but there is no consensus whether ET-specific pathology is present in the cerebellum of patients with ET.[41,42] Recent findings suggest that more subtle pathology may play a role, e.g., changes in subcellular and gross distributions of climbing fiber/Purkinje cell synapses.[42]
3. *Symptomatic tremor*—secondary tremor due to injuries of central oscillators or proximate afferent or efferent motor circuit nodes or pathways. Examples of anatomical processes include the following: toxins (carbon monoxide—globi pallidi), medications (dopamine

receptor blocking agents—striatum; anticonvulsants—cerebellum), structural lesions (infarctions, tumors, cysts), and genetic and metabolic diseases (Wilson's disease—striatum, globi pallidi, midbrain; galactosemia—Purkinje cells, cerebral/cerebellar white matter).

DISEASES AND DISORDERS

This section reviews some of the more common or important diseases causing tremor in children. Note that many secondary tremors present with mixed movement disorders, and are covered in other chapters. For example, tremor associated with dystonia is covered in greater detail in chapters on dystonia (see Chapter 11) and Parkinsonism (see Chapter 15). Secondary tremor may also occur in the presence of metabolic disorders (see Chapter 17) and static encephalopathies/cerebral palsy (see Chapter 20). Tremors as part of a constellation of significant, nonprogressive ataxia or developmental motor difficulties with clumsiness are discussed in the chapter on ataxia (see Chapter 14). The important features of and etiologies of drug-induced tremor (see Chapter 22) and psychogenic tremor (see Chapter 23) are covered briefly here and in more detail in the dedicated chapters.

Primary Tremors

Enhanced Physiologic Tremor

CLINICAL FEATURES

Physiologic tremor occurs in healthy individuals and is not apparent visually. The tremor frequency increases through childhood, related to normal brain maturation. Certain environmental factors result in enhancement of the tremor, such that it becomes apparent to the child or parent. These factors are usually transient in children. The tremor may have been witnessed repeatedly by the parents but may not be present during the clinic visit. Parents of young children and adolescents typically describe symmetric hand tremor, although other body areas may also be involved. Typically this is faster and has lower amplitude than Essential Tremor.

PATHOPHYSIOLOGY

Common factors that seem to trigger enhancement include stressors such as increased emotion (anxiety, anger, sadness, and frustration), fatigue, fever, hunger, and waking from sleep. Because all children experience these stressors, but not all children develop visible tremors, there are probably some innate factors that predispose certain children to develop a more robust, enhanced physiologic tremor. These factors are unknown. Commonly used medications such as decongestants and bronchodilators[43] and substances such as caffeine may also enhance tremor. More serious endocrinological conditions such as thyrotoxicosis and pheochromocytoma may present with tremor. Typically, the tremor is not isolated, e.g., in childhood thyrotoxicosis there is usually some combination of weight loss, fatigue/tiredness, behavioral changes, and heat intolerance.[44] The history and presence of other characteristic symptoms guide diagnostic evaluation toward these conditions.

DIAGNOSTIC APPROACH AND TREATMENT

The diagnostic approach is guided by the history and physical examination findings. Often just reassurance but no additional diagnostic testing, no pharmacological or habilitative therapy, and no medication are needed. To the extent that the origin of a physiological tremor involves peripheral oscillators and mechanical stretch reflexes, inertial loading testing may demonstrate reduced frequency.

Intermittent Tremor or Persistent Tremor in the Otherwise Healthy Young Child

In the vast majority of cases where there are brief episodes of tremor described by parents, there is no underlying neurologic disease of any consequence. However, diligence is still necessary, for several reasons, depending on the child's age.

If the child is young and the parents are highly anxious about episodes of tremor, it is important to make the parents feel that their concerns have been validated. If this is not accomplished, parents may continue to "shop around" for other opinions or seek out complementary medicine practitioners who prescribe expensive, nonvalidated, and possibly unsafe treatments. A careful history followed by a detailed neurologic examination is therapeutic in this way, and adds credibility when explaining the benign nature of the tremor to the parents. The careful history often reveals the trigger and this can be addressed if necessary. Parents often describe excessive tremulousness on awakening in the morning or after naps. In addition, intermittent tremor in the young child is often increased by frustration. The clinician should note that if the frustration consistently occurs around performance of fine motor tasks, this child may have a mild static encephalopathy (see also Chapter 14, discussion of clumsy children with nonprogressive ataxia). In these children, there is usually some other evidence on examination of subnormal motor function. Asking the child to reach for or manipulate small toys, write, or color a picture in clinic may demonstrate the tremor. These tremors may also be brought out during a detailed motor examination that fatigues the child. It is helpful in order to induce mild fatigue to examine for postural tremor, for terminal/intention tremor with finger-to-nose testing, and for rate and rhythm of fine rapid and sequential finger movements without pausing or allowing the child to rest his or her arms.

There is no evidence-based treatment. Referral to occupational therapy is sometimes warranted to find strategies to improve coordination or accommodate tremor.

A follow-up neurologic examination in 12 months is recommended. Comparison at 12 months of the writing and drawing samples, along with other recorded details of the examination, is critical for distinguishing the rare child with progressive neurologic disease from the majority of children with nonprogressive problems.

Intermittent Tremor in the Adolescent

Adolescents often have bilateral hand tremor. In some cases, they have ET (see later discussion) and describe tremor that is continuously present. In many cases, however, the tremor is intermittent and probably represents stress-induced, enhanced physiologic tremor or functional/psychogenic tremor. For many reasons, adolescence is a stressful time of life. At inopportune moments, physical symptoms may ensue—headaches, irritable or irregular bowel function, enhanced physiologic tremor, or functional neurological disorders. Tremor may embarrass a self-conscious adolescent. As described earlier for the parents of a young child, a careful history and detailed neurological and physical examination in an adolescent can be therapeutic in reassuring both the adolescent and parent. The adolescent can answer questions about functional interference from tremor and can give a writing sample and perform a freehand spiral. Even if the tremor is intermittent, it is important to take a family history and briefly examine both parents, if possible, for resting and action tremor. This is because sometimes the adolescent's subtle, intermittent tremor reflects the onset of ET. Parents may not acknowledge their own ET by history, yet it is readily apparent on postural and finger-to-nose testing.

A review of systems, a medication and substance abuse history, and a brief screen for signs of a mood disorder are also important. Anxiety and other mood disorders often begin in adolescence, and the episodes of tremor may be physical manifestations of these emotional problems. In the presence of isolated, intermittent tremor, without dysarthria or other neurological or general medical symptoms, a thorough diagnostic evaluation involving laboratory tests and neuroimaging is rarely needed. Laboratory testing (for anemia, endocrine disorders, Magnesium, B12, rheumatologic disorders, or rare diseases such as Wilson's disease) can often be deferred and reassurance provided. Referral for psychological consultation is sometimes needed. As for the younger child, a 1-year follow-up examination is recommended. If symptoms clearly progress over 6–12 months, neuroimaging and other diagnostic studies are needed. Some screening labs may reassure anxious families.

Essential Tremor

CLINICAL FEATURES

The term *essential tremor* (ET) denotes relatively isolated tremor, normal brain imaging, and the absence of other etiologies. ET lacks any specific biologic marker, but it is not solely a diagnosis of exclusion. The phenomenology of ET is typically a bilateral postural or intention hand tremor, although it may be asymmetric (Videos 13.3 and 13.4).[45] Sometimes hand tremor is accompanied by head and voice tremor. The prevalence of other cerebellar[46] as well as nonmotor psychiatric symptoms may also be increased.[47]

ET diagnostic thinking differs in adult patients, because tremor is also a cardinal symptom of PD, which is highly prevalent in adult neurology and movement disorder clinics. The phenomenologies of PD, usually a unilateral, resting tremor with bradykinesia and/or rigidity, and ET differ. However, the presence of some clinical overlap, and the observation that some adults with ET later develop clinical features of PD,[48] means that follow-up examinations are important for adults. The diagnosis of ET must also be approached carefully and longitudinally in children, because tremor is a nonspecific symptom of many genetic and acquired neurologic diseases. Therefore, for both patient care and research, it has been important to designate consensus criteria for this diagnosis. Although no specific criteria have been established for diagnosis of ET in children, there has been a general consensus on the diagnosis of ET in adults (Table 13.2).

The *duration* criterion of 5 years for definite ET for adults allows time for the diagnosis to solidify with an absence of progression to PD. Since PD is extremely rare in children, the duration criterion for ET can be relaxed. A follow-up examination 1 year after initial clinic presentation to document persistence without progression of symptoms is generally adequate.

TABLE 13.2   Consensus Criteria for ET in Adults[49,50]

Inclusion—required	Permitted	Exclusion
DEFINITE		
Bilateral postural hands	Intention/Terminal tremor	Other abnormalities on examination (except Froment Sign[a])
Visible tremor	Involvement of other body parts, e.g., head, voice	Causes of enhanced physiological tremor
Continuously present >5 years	Asymmetry	Concurrent exposure to tremorigenic medication
	Amplitude fluctuation	Direct or indirect CNS or PNS trauma
	Lack of functional impairment	Psychogenic tremor
		Time course: sudden onset; stepwise deterioration
PROBABLE		
Bilateral postural hand tremor with duration greater than 3 years	Involvement of other body parts, e.g., head	Primary orthostatic
	Lack of hand involvement, e.g., head only	Isolated voice, tongue, chin tremor
		Position or task-specific tremor
POSSIBLE		
Criteria met for *Definite* or *Probable*, but – Other neurologic signs present – Or instead of both hands, body location is isolated voice, chin, tongue, one-hand only		

[a]*Froment sign is cogwheeling elicited by passively moving one limb while the patient voluntarily moves the other limb. The utility of this sign is not established in children, particularly in young children in whom there is commonly contralateral motor overflow.*
CNS = central nervous system. PNS = peripheral nervous system.

The epidemiology of ET in adults worldwide, including in developing countries, has become better characterized with more community-based studies.[51–53] The adult prevalence appears to be about 2% overall, with peak onset in decades two and six,[54] and higher prevalence in the elderly.[1] The prevalence in children remains less characterized but is likely lower. Current estimates based on small, clinic-referred samples[2,6,55,56] likely contain a number of biases related to referral patterns and higher prevalence of specific comorbidities.

PATHOPHYSIOLOGY

The pathophysiology of ET is probably related to considerations described previously for central oscillators. Indirect evidence comes from clinical observations as well, such as abolition of ET symptoms after a cerebellar stroke[57] and reduction in symptoms with alcohol or centrally acting medications. Despite high heritability of ET, no unique causative gene has been identified.[12,58] However, with careful neurological phenotyping combined with genomewide scans and exome sequencing, much progress has been made. Although all discovered findings only account for a small fraction of ET cases, recent findings are instructive with regard to pathophysiology of tremor as well as genetics of other common neurological conditions with varying degrees of heritability.

The nomenclature for inherited forms of ET is "ETMn." Forms of ETM are currently designated as follows: ETM1 (chromosome 3q13/Ser9Gly polymorphisms in dopamine receptor DRD3[59]); ETM2 (chromosome locus 2p24.1[60]); ETM3 (chromosome locus 6p23[61]); and ETM4 (chromosome 16p11.2; heterozygous mutation in the *FUS* gene,[62] which encodes the FUS nucleoprotein that functions in DNA and RNA metabolism[63]). ETM4 may be due to loss of FUS function. Mutations in FUS are also a cause of amyotrophic lateral sclerosis, possibly due to toxic gain-of-function effects.[63]

Several other genes and polymorphisms have been implicated in the pathophysiology of ET. Possibly the most robust is polymorphisms in the gene *LINGO1*,[12] also called *LRRN6A*, which encodes neuronal Leucine-Rich Repeat Protein 6A and is involved in myelination[64] and neuroprotection[65] pathways. Studies in several distinct ethnic populations support a link between *LINGO1* polymorphisms and ET.[66] Intriguing new findings in a *TENM4*,[67] a gene regulating axon guidance and myelination, and in an intronic variant in *SLC1A2*, which encodes the major glial high-affinity glutamate reuptake transporter, provide new insights into mechanisms and risk factors for ET.[12,68]

There has been increased research into postmortem pathology, in histological studies of brains from elderly adults diagnosed with ET. Postmortem findings of Purkinje cells with axonal swelling, termed "torpedoes," have been identified in some studies.[69] Dendritic swelling in Purkinje cells has also been identified.[70] Case mix in recruitment as well as different pathological staining techniques may play a role in the diverging findings of various studies.[41] The clinical relevance of these findings for children meeting clinical criteria for ET is unknown.

DIAGNOSTIC APPROACH

In the presence of an insidious onset of bilateral, regular postural hand tremor, continually present for longer than 1 year, a stable to gradually progressive severity over time, and a normal detailed neurologic examination otherwise, the diagnosis of ET is likely. The diagnosis of ET would be less likely if tremor is intermittent. Because a diagnosis of ET in a family member is helpful, it is reasonable to briefly examine one or both parents and use family history data. More significant neurologic symptoms in the child or parent, such as gait problems, spasticity, ataxia, dysarthria, or dystonia, should prompt a more careful assessment of the child for other causes. Of course, a positive parental history of a common diagnosis like ET does not exclude the presence of another diagnosis in the child.[71] It is helpful, in addition, to document the detailed neurologic examination, to obtain a writing sample and freehand spiral with both hands, and to videotape the key portions of the tremor examination (full rest, postures with arms fully extended/palms flat/fingers spread in cardinal supination/pronation positions, finger-to-nose testing). These can be used for comparison at a follow-up visit, at a reasonable interval of 12 months. If these findings are all stable over a 12-month period, follow-up thereafter may be "as needed."

TABLE 13.3   Brief Tremor Rating Scale

Score	Detail
0	Absent (no tremor or writing impairment)
1	Slight and infrequently present (mild tremor, writing, and drawing of spiral minimally impaired)
2	Moderate; bothersome to most patients (writing and drawing of spiral moderately impaired)
3	Severe tremor (writing and drawing severely impaired; interferes with many activities such as drinking liquids)
4	Marked tremor (interferes with most activities)

TREATMENT OF ET

Many children and adolescents with ET can be diagnosed and observed without a specific treatment intervention. The decision to treat is based on interference with activities important to the child's quality of life. These may include activities of daily living, academic tasks such as writing, or participation in music or sports-related tasks. Social embarrassment may also contribute to treatment decisions; however, it is important that expectations for tremor reduction should not be overly optimistic.

The clinician and family should also agree on a method for assessing benefit prior to initiating treatment. One helpful, easy-to-use scale for assessing tremor severity is the Brief Tremor Rating Scale (BTRS), shown in Table 13.3. It is generally prudent to defer treatment if the BTRS score is 0 or 1. For higher scores, it is reasonable to advise families that treatment will be at best partially effective, and that possible side effects need to be weighed against benefits. A reasonable goal is symptom reduction, not elimination, with reduction of tremor-related impairment. The clinician, parent, and patient may find it helpful to identify a specific task that the child currently struggles with specifically due to tremor, and then to target improvement in performance of that task, rather than using a rating scale.

For clinical trials or genetic study phenotyping, more detailed, well-standardized scales are recommended. The Tremor Research Group (TRG) Essential Tremor Rating Scale (TETRAS)[72-73] or the Fahn-Tolosa Marin Tremor Rating Scales (TRS)[74] may be used.

With regard to pharmacologic treatment, expert consensus and clinical observation favor use of primidone or propranolol.

For primidone, the dosing regimen is starting at 25 mg at night and increasing weekly as needed to 125–250 mg at night (it is not known whether primidone or its metabolite PEMA is the more effective component).

For propranolol (or other beta-blocker) the dosing regimen starts at 1–2 mg/kg/day up to 30–120 mg per day (twice a day), consistent with the practice guideline for treatment in adults.[13,75]

Other possibilities include gabapentin, pregabalin, and topiramate,[76] starting with low doses and titrating gradually. These recommendations are based on small case series in adults. Botulinum toxin injections in the forearms, posterior neck muscles, or the vocalis muscle are often used before recommending surgical treatment, namely DBS.[77] Botulinum toxin is considered the treatment of choice for dystonic tremor, discussed in Chapter 11. However, ET is rarely sufficiently severe in children or adolescents to consider botulinum toxin or DBS.

Tremor in Functional (Psychogenic) Illness

Tremor is a common phenomenology in children and adolescents with functional (psychogenic) movement disorders.[7,78] In severe, acute-onset cases, parents often bring their child to the emergency room.[79,80] The history generally involves rapid onset and offset of symptoms, often on multiple occasions without any proximate trigger that is apparent to the parent or acknowledged by the child or adolescent. Features of the phenomenology include variable rate, amplitude, and direction. One or multiple limbs may be involved. The clinician should review videos, often brought in by the family.

On examination of an individual suspected of having functional tremor, it is important for the clinician to document the presence of one or more of three positive symptoms, ideally on video. For functional tremor, three key positive findings are *variability, distractability,* and *entrainability*:

1. *Variability* is based on the idea that tremors occurring in neurological conditions have a consistent, characteristic amplitude, direction, and frequency (or rate), but that in patients with functional tremor these all tend instead to vary.

   Maneuver: Perform the routine examination for resting and postural tremor. Observe the tremor's amplitude, direction, and frequency for characteristics that do or do not fit with known phenomenologies of neurological diseases.

2. *Distractibility* is based on the idea that in neurological conditions, a tremoring body part will maintain its basic, pathologic features (amplitude, direction, and frequency) and not be abruptly attenuated by thoughts or actions in uninvolved body parts. In contrast, in functional tremors, cognitive input briefly attenuates or stops the tremor. The examiner can demonstrate this through ambiguous or complex commands during the neurological examination.

   Maneuver: Instruct the child or adolescent to perform a complex finger sequence with the uninvolved hand or perform a sequence of right/left commands. Observe whether this task interrupts the tremor, which supports a functional tremor diagnosis. It is possible that as the patient devotes cognitive resources to deciding how to execute the command, the higher level neural substrate of the functional tremor is thereby diverted, resulting in a pause in the functional tremor.

3. *Entrainability* is also based on the idea that in pathological neurological conditions there is a high degree of consistency of amplitude, direction, and frequency of tremor. In contrast, in functional disorders, the patient's tremor is not fixed within the parameters dictated by underlying pathology. Rather, it is inherently more variable and therefore can be synchronized with either the examiner's movements or movements of another of the patient's body parts.

   Maneuver: Instruct the patient to mimic the examiner in repetitively tapping a finger to thumb, flexing at a joint, or rotating a joint at different rates. As the examiner changes his rate of movement, the patient's functional tremor changes or "entrains" to the examiner's rate. This maneuver should be repeated on both sides of the body, individually and together. *Positive entrainability* means that functional tremors will tend to synchronize their rate and sometimes amplitude and direction with another perceived oscillation (of self or of another person).

These examinations can be challenging and there are pitfalls. For example, a dystonic or Parkinsonian tremor may sometimes appear to be distractible or entrainable on examination. The asymmetric tremor in dystonia may be diminished by action in the less-involved or uninvolved hand in a way that mimics distraction, for example. Second opinions, follow-up visits, and viewing videotaped examinations with movement disorder colleagues can be helpful in such cases. When in doubt, it is not incorrect to list a series of possible diagnoses for the patient and include functional tremors as one among several.

Often, however, for neurologist experienced with movement disorders, after a thorough history and systematic physical and neurological examination, the positive clinical features of functional or psychogenic tremor[81] often suffice for clinical diagnosis without further medical testing or neuroimaging.[82,83] The neurologist then should discuss these positive findings, as well as other negative findings, at the end of the encounter. The neurologist can play a vital role in improving the outcome of these patients. It is helpful to emphasize that functional tremor is common, that the diagnosis is made based on positive findings[84] and not merely as a diagnosis of exclusion, and that many acute and chronic neurological and medical diagnoses, including migraine and irritable bowel, are made primarily on the basis of presenting symptoms and physical examination findings. Depending on clinical circumstances, the neurologist may recommend occupational or physical therapy or psychological therapy. As is the case for other forms of tremor and other forms of functional or psychogenic illness, interval follow-up with the neurologist is advised.

Additional clinical details and treatment strategies for functional/psychogenic tremor are discussed in Chapter 23.

Symptomatic Tremors

A list of diseases and conditions causing tremor in children is given in Table 13.4.

Tremor Due to Structural Abnormalities or Space-Occupying Lesions

Symptomatic or secondary tremors can be caused by a vast number of conditions (Video 13.5).[4] Many of these processes affect nodes or pathways in cortical-striatal-pallidal-thalamic circuits or cortical-ponto-cerebellar-thalamic pathways, as described earlier in this chapter. In addition, most of these secondary conditions manifest with multiple types of abnormal movements and/or additional neurologic symptoms, not merely isolated tremor.

Tremor may be caused by cerebellar malformations and cysts (see also Chapters 2 and 14). Examples include hydrocephalus, e.g., due to aqueductal stenosis.[112,113] Acquired space-occupying lesions may also cause tremor, particularly when the lesions are found in cerebellum.[114] Examples include tuberculomas.[115,116] Various congenital malformations involving the posterior cerebellar hemispheres and deep cerebellar nuclei may result in tremor.[117] Malformations, neoplasms, autoimmune processes, and infarctions in thalamus can also result in tremor.

Tremor Due to Medications or Toxins

Tremor due to use of medications is a common cause of referral (see Chapter 22). Stimulants,[118] dopamine receptor blocking agents,[119,120] and antiseizure medications such as valproate[121] and phenytoin[122] are common causes. Use of immunosuppressive drugs, particularly tacrolimus, for organ transplant or other inflammatory conditions such as ulcerative

TABLE 13.4   Diseases and Conditions Causing Tremor in Children

	References
STRUCTURAL/CONGENITAL	
Bobble-headed doll—third ventricular dilatation in infancy	[85]
Thalamic cyst	[86]
Pineal cyst, resolved with surgery	[87]
Thalamic infarction	[16]
Rhombencephalosynapsis	[88]
ENDOCRINE/METABOLIC	
Hyperthyroidism	[89]
Hyperadrenaline state	[90]
Low magnesium	[91]
Hepatic encephalopathy	[92]
METABOLIC	
Galactosemia	[93]
Phenylketonuria	[94]
Biopterin synthesis defect	[95]
DEGENERATIVE DISEASES	
Wilson's disease	[96]
Leukodystrophy	[97]
Ataxia with oculomotor apraxia	[98]
Rett syndrome/MECP2 mutations	[99,100]
Mitochondrial diseases	[101]
CHROMOSOMAL	
Aneuploidy extra X or Y chromosome syndromes	[102] (Video 13.6)
TOXIC	
Gas sniffing	[103]
Lead, mercury	[104,105]
NUTRITIONAL	
B12 (Cobalamin) deficiency	[106]
Kwashiorkor (protein deficiency)	[107]
Tetrahydrobiopterin deficiency	[108]
Indian infantile tremor syndrome (zinc, B12, vitamin C—multifactorial nutritional deficiency)	[106,109–111]
IATROGENIC	
Anticonvulsants, stimulants, tricyclic antidepressants, neuroleptics, selective serotonin reuptake inhibitors, synthroid, cyclosporine, bronchodilators	See Chapter 22

colitis can also induce tremor.[123–127] Similarly, a large number of toxins exert tremorigenic effects along with other neurologic symptoms. These include acute and chronic exposure to heavy metals such as lead or manganese.[128,129]

Tremor in Glucose Transporter (Glut-1) Deficiency

Movement disorders are a common part of the clinical presentation of children with Glut-1 deficiency as well as other metabolic conditions (see Chapter 17). Tremor may occur at rest with Parkinsonism or with action, in a cerebellar phenomenology. Ketogenic diet treatment may improve paroxysmal events and gait but not other movement disorders.[130]

Tremor in Neurodegenerative Diseases

Neurodegenerative diseases may cause tremor, but tremor is rarely the dominant feature. Table 13.4 lists a number of these diseases (see also Chapters 11—dystonia; 14—ataxia; 15—Parkinsonism; and 17—metabolic movement disorders).

Tremor in Vitamin or Mineral Deficiencies

Zinc deficiency[109] and vitamin B12 deficiency can cause tremor in infants. The syndrome of B12 deficiency usually occurs in developing countries where nursing mothers are B12 deficient related to low protein intake. It presents with hypotonia, anemia, developmental delay, and sometimes seizures.[131] Tremor and myoclonus may appear during B12 treatment.[132]

Clinicians in developed countries should also be aware of another common scenario, where families present with a false belief that their child has a vitamin or mineral excess or deficiency producing tremor or other neurological or behavioral symptoms. The family's beliefs are often promoted by quack physicians or other deceptive practitioners who have a financial conflict of interest. For example, the practitioner may own laboratories that perform and charge families for nonvalidated tests of hair or body fluids for vitamin or mineral levels. They may then subsequently prescribe and profit from mineral chelators or vitamin preparations. Helping families avoid these needless expenses and potentially harmful interventions is important, but can be challenging and time-consuming.

TREATMENT OF SYMPTOMATIC TREMOR

Treatment of clinically significant symptomatic tremor is directed, when possible, toward the underlying etiology. Otherwise, nonspecific tremor-suppressing medications such as primidone or propranolol, as used for ET, may be employed, although benefit tends to be less.

APPROACH TO DIAGNOSIS AND MANAGEMENT

To summarize, when a child with tremor is seen for initial evaluation, a stepwise approach is helpful. Usually, the tremor is not an emergency, but it can cause substantial disability. A thoughtful assessment based on the history, examination findings, and common epidemiology can guide a cost-effective diagnostic evaluation.

1. Clarify that tremor is the movement disorder.
2. Categorize the tremor: Resting, action? Unilateral, bilateral?

3. Stratify into a time-course group—acute, static, chronic progressive, episodic.
4. Consider carefully the findings from the detailed neurologic and general examination. The presence of other motor findings attributable to cortical spinal tract, peripheral neuromotor system, basal ganglia, or cerebellum, or other general findings such as hepatomegaly, may provide the key to the differential diagnosis and decisions about medical diagnostic testing.
5. For idiopathic, isolated, action tremor, clinical monitoring without further testing may be adequate.
6. For tremor that could be inherited, take a careful family history and examine parents and siblings, if possible.
7. Unilateral or predominantly midline cerebellar signs may indicate focal cerebellar pathology.
8. Consider all possible treatable or curable causes of tremors.
9. Rate the severity of the tremor on a clinical scale, and document the tremor via a video recording, to characterize the tremor and document its severity.
10. Consider medical treatment or occupational therapy if tremor causes functional disability.
11. Even if not treating, always reassess the child's tremor in 6–12 months. If a child's tremor has clearly worsened during that time, an aggressive diagnostic evaluation is needed, including in most cases brain magnetic resonance imaging.
12. Genetic testing is not routinely indicated but may be helpful in selected cases. Collaboration with colleagues in Genetics and/or Genetic Counseling may facilitate addressing issues of test cost, emotional issues, confidentiality, and testing other family members.
13. Educate the family about the disease.
14. Provide referrals for supportive services, as needed, and encourage families to read about the disease and join advocacy and research groups.

References

1. Louis ED, Ferreira JJ. How common is the most common adult movement disorder? Update on the worldwide prevalence of essential tremor. *Mov Disord.* 2010;25(5):534–541.
2. Ferrara J, Jankovic J. Epidemiology and management of essential tremor in children. *Paediatr Drugs.* 2009;11(5):293–307.
3. Louis ED, Cubo E, Trejo-Gabriel-Galan JM, et al. Tremor in school-aged children: a cross-sectional study of tremor in 819 boys and girls in Burgos, Spain. *Neuroepidemiology.* 2011;37(2):90–95.
4. Keller S, Dure LS. Tremor in childhood. *Semin Pediatr Neurol.* 2009;16(2):60–70.
5. Gilbert DL. Drug-induced movement disorders in children. *Ann NY Acad Sci.* 2008;1142:72–84.
6. Tan EK, Lum SY, Prakash KM. Clinical features of childhood onset essential tremor. *Eur J Neurol.* 2006;13(12):1302–1305.
7. Thenganatt MA, Jankovic J. Psychogenic tremor: a video guide to its distinguishing features. *Tremor Other Hyperkinet Mov.* 2014;4:253.
8. Sanger TD, Chen D, Fehlings DL, et al. Definition and classification of hyperkinetic movements in childhood. *Mov Disord.* 2010;25(11):1538–1549.
9. Fusco C, Valls-Sole J, Iturriaga C, Colomer J, Fernandez-Alvarez E. Electrophysiological approach to the study of essential tremor in children and adolescents. *Dev Med Child Neurol.* 2003;45(9):624–627.
10. Pulliam CL, Eichenseer SR, Goetz CG, et al. Continuous in-home monitoring of essential tremor. *Parkinsonism Relat Disord.* 2014;20(1):37–40.

11. Elble R, Bain P, Forjaz MJ, et al. Task force report: scales for screening and evaluating tremor: critique and recommendations. *Mov Disord.* 2013;28(13):1793–1800.

12. Kuhlenbaumer G, Hopfner F, Deuschl G. Genetics of essential tremor: meta-analysis and review. *Neurology.* 2014;82(11):1000–1007.

13. Elias WJ, Shah BB. Tremor. *JAMA.* 2014;311(9):948–954.

14. Cardoso F. Difficult diagnoses in hyperkinetic disorders—a focused review. *Front Neurol.* 2012;3:151.

15. Tartaglione T, Izzo G, Alexandre A, et al. MRI findings of olivary degeneration after surgery for posterior fossa tumours in children: incidence, time course, and correlation with tumour grading. *Radiol Med.* 2015;120(5):474–482.

16. Tan H, Turanli G, Ay H, Saatci I. Rubral tremor after thalamic infarction in childhood. *Pediatr Neurol.* 2001;25(5):409–412.

17. Baizabal-Carvallo JF, Cardoso F, Jankovic J. Myorhythmia: phenomenology, etiology, and treatment. *Mov Disord.* 2015;30(2):171–179.

18. Baizabal-Carvallo JF, Stocco A, Muscal E, Jankovic J. The spectrum of movement disorders in children with anti-NMDA receptor encephalitis. *Mov Disord.* 2013;28(4):543–547.

19. Erer S, Jankovic J. Hereditary chin tremor in Parkinson's disease. *Clin Neurol Neurosurg.* 2007;109(9):784–785.

20. Goraya JS, Virdi V, Parmar V. Recurrent nocturnal tongue biting in a child with hereditary chin trembling. *J Child Neurol.* 2006;21(11):985–987.

21. Johnson LF, Kinsbourne M, Renuart AW. Hereditary chin-trembling with nocturnal myoclonus and tongue-biting in dizygous twins. *Dev Med Child Neurol.* 1971;13(6):726–729.

22. Kanazawa O. Shuddering attacks-report of four children. *Pediatr Neurol.* 2000;23(5):421–424.

23. Raethjen J, Deuschl G. The oscillating central network of Essential tremor. *Clin Neurophysiol.* 2012;123(1):61–64.

24. Lamarre Y. Tremorgenic mechanisms in primates. *Adv Neurol.* 1975;10:23–34.

25. Lamarre Y, Filion M, Cordeau JP. Neuronal discharges of the ventrolateral nucleus of the thalamus during sleep and wakefulness in the cat. I. Spontaneous activity. *Exp Brain Res.* 1971;12(5):480–498.

26. Chahine LM, Ghosh D. Essential tremor after ipsilateral cerebellar hemispherectomy: support for the thalamus as the central oscillator. *J Child Neurol.* 2009;24(7):861–864.

27. Llinas R, Muhlethaler M. Electrophysiology of guinea-pig cerebellar nuclear cells in the in vitro brain stem-cerebellar preparation. *J Physiol.* 1988;404:241–258.

28. Kazantsev VB, Nekorkin VI, Makarenko VI, Llinas R. Self-referential phase reset based on inferior olive oscillator dynamics. *Proc Natl Acad Sci USA.* 2004;101(52):18183–18188.

29. Hadipour Niktarash A. Transmission of the subthalamic nucleus oscillatory activity to the cortex: a computational approach. *J Comput Neurosci.* 2003;15(2):223–232.

30. Bevan MD, Magill PJ, Hallworth NE, Bolam JP, Wilson CJ. Regulation of the timing and pattern of action potential generation in rat subthalamic neurons in vitro by GABA-A IPSPs. *J Neurophysiol.* 2002;87(3):1348–1362.

31. Bevan MD, Magill PJ, Terman D, Bolam JP, Wilson CJ. Move to the rhythm: oscillations in the subthalamic nucleus-external globus pallidus network. *Trends Neurosci.* 2002;25(10):525–531.

32. Cole JD, Philip HI, Sedgwick EM. Stability and tremor in the fingers associated with cerebellar hemisphere and cerebellar tract lesions in man. *J Neurol Neurosurg Psychiatry.* 1988;51(12):1558–1568.

33. Hallett M. Overview of human tremor physiology. *Mov Disord.* 1998;13(suppl 3):43–48.

34. Netravathi M, Pal PK, Ravishankar S, Indira Devi B. Electrophysiological evaluation of tremors secondary to space occupying lesions and trauma: correlation with nature and sites of lesions. *Parkinsonism Relat Disord.* 2010;16(1):36–41.

35. Lenz FA, Tasker RR, Kwan HC, et al. Single unit analysis of the human ventral thalamic nuclear group: correlation of thalamic "tremor cells" with the 3–6 Hz component of Parkinsonian tremor. *J Neurosci.* 1988;8(3):754–764.

36. Hua SE, Lenz FA, Zirh TA, Reich SG, Dougherty PM. Thalamic neuronal activity correlated with essential tremor. *J Neurol Neurosurg Psychiatry.* 1998;64(2):273–276.

37. Jenkins IH, Bain PG, Colebatch JG, et al. A positron emission tomography study of essential tremor: evidence for overactivity of cerebellar connections. *Ann Neurol.* 1993;34(1):82–90.

38. Wills AJ, Jenkins IH, Thompson PD, Findley LJ, Brooks DJ. Red nuclear and cerebellar but no olivary activation associated with essential tremor: a positron emission tomographic study. *Ann Neurol.* 1994;36(4):636–642.

39. Wills AJ, Jenkins IH, Thompson PD, Findley LJ, Brooks DJ. A positron emission tomography study of cerebral activation associated with essential and writing tremor. *Arch Neurol.* 1995;52(3):299–305.

40. Boecker H, Wills AJ, Ceballos-Baumann A, et al. The effect of ethanol on alcohol-responsive essential tremor: a positron emission tomography study. *Ann Neurol.* 1996;39(5):650–658.

41. Jellinger KA. Is there cerebellar pathology in essential tremor? *Mov Disord.* 2014;29(4):435–436.

42. Lin CY, Louis ED, Faust PL, Koeppen AH, Vonsattel JP, Kuo SH. Abnormal climbing fibre-Purkinje cell synaptic connections in the essential tremor cerebellum. *Brain.* 2014;137(Pt 12):3149–3159.

43. Saito T, Hasunuma T. Safety and tolerability of high-dose budesonide/formoterol via Turbuhaler in Japanese patients with asthma: a randomized, double-blind, crossover, active comparator-controlled, phase III study. *Clin Drug Invest.* 2012;32(1):51–61.

44. Williamson S, Greene SA. Incidence of thyrotoxicosis in childhood: a national population based study in the UK and Ireland. *Clin Endocrinol (Oxf).* 2010;72(3):358–363.

45. Phibbs F, Fang JY, Cooper MK, Charles DP, Davis TL, Hedera P. Prevalence of unilateral tremor in autosomal dominant essential tremor. *Mov Disord.* 2009;24(1):108–111.

46. Deuschl G, Wenzelburger R, Loffler K, Raethjen J, Stolze H. Essential tremor and cerebellar dysfunction clinical and kinematic analysis of intention tremor. *Brain.* 2000;123(Pt 8):1568–1580.

47. Chandran V, Pal PK, Reddy JYC, Thennarasu K, Yadav R, Shivashankar N. Non-motor features in essential tremor. *Acta Neurol Scand.* 2012;125(5):332–337.

48. Shahed J, Jankovic J. Exploring the relationship between essential tremor and Parkinson's disease. *Parkinsonism Relat Disord.* 2007;13(2):67–76.

49. Deuschl G, Bain P, Brin M. Consensus statement of the Movement Disorder Society on Tremor. Ad Hoc Scientific Committee. *Mov Disord.* 1998;13(suppl 3):2–23.

50. Elble RJ. Diagnostic criteria for essential tremor and differential diagnosis. *Neurology.* 2000;54(11 suppl 4):S2–S6.

51. Das SK, Banerjee TK, Roy T, Raut DK, Chaudhuri A, Hazra A. Prevalence of essential tremor in the city of Kolkata, India: a house-to-house survey. *Eur J Neurol.* 2009;16(7):801–807.

52. Okubadejo NU, Bankole IA, Ojo OO, Ojini FI, Danesi MA. Prevalence of essential tremor in urban Lagos, Nigeria: a door-to-door community-based study. *BMC Neurol.* 2012;12:110.

53. Sur H, Ilhan S, Erdogan H, Ozturk E, Tasdemir M, Boru UT. Prevalence of essential tremor: a door-to-door survey in Sile, Istanbul, Turkey. *Parkinsonism Relat Disord.* 2009;15(2):101–104.

54. Lou JS, Jankovic J. Essential tremor clinical correlates in 350 patients. *Neurology.* 1991;41(2):234.

55. Jankovic J, Madisetty J, Vuong KD. Essential tremor among children. *Pediatrics.* 2004;114(5):1203–1205.

56. Louis ED, Dure LS, Pullman S. Essential tremor in childhood: a series of nineteen cases. *Mov Disord.* 2001;16(5):921–923.

57. Dupuis MJ, Delwaide PJ, Boucquey D, Gonsette RE. Homolateral disappearance of essential tremor after cerebellar stroke. *Mov Disord.* 1989;4(2):183–187.

58. Deng H, Le W, Jankovic J. Genetics of essential tremor. *Brain.* 2007;130(Pt 6):1456–1464.

59. Lucotte G, Lagarde JP, Funalot B, Sokoloff P. Linkage with the Ser9Gly DRD3 polymorphism in essential tremor families. *Clin Genet.* 2006;69(5):437–440.

60. Higgins JJ, Jankovic J, Lombardi RQ, et al. Haplotype analysis of the ETM2 locus in familial essential tremor. *Neurogenetics.* 2003;4(4):185–189.

61. Shatunov A, Sambuughin N, Jankovic J, et al. Genomewide scans in North American families reveal genetic linkage of essential tremor to a region on chromosome 6p23. *Brain.* 2006;129(Pt 9):2318–2331.

62. Merner ND, Girard SL, Catoire H, et al. Exome sequencing identifies FUS mutations as a cause of essential tremor. *Am J Hum Genet.* 2012;91(2):313–319.

63. Vance C, Rogelj B, Hortobagyi T, et al. Mutations in FUS, an RNA processing protein, cause familial amyotrophic lateral sclerosis type 6. *Science.* 2009;323(5918):1208–1211.

64. Mi S, Lee X, Shao Z, et al. LINGO-1 is a component of the Nogo-66 receptor/p75 signaling complex. *Nat Neurosci.* 2004;7(3):221–228.

65. Inoue H, Lin L, Lee X, et al. Inhibition of the leucine-rich repeat protein LINGO-1 enhances survival, structure, and function of dopaminergic neurons in Parkinson's disease models. *Proc Natl Acad Sci USA.* 2007;104(36):14430–14435.

66. Stefansson H, Steinberg S, Petursson H, et al. Variant in the sequence of the LINGO1 gene confers risk of essential tremor. *Nat Genet.* 2009;41(3):277–279.

67. Hor H, Francescatto L, Bartesaghi L, et al. Missense mutations in *TENM4*, a regulator of axon guidance and central myelination, cause essential tremor. *Human Molecular Genetics.* 2015; ddv281.

68. Thier S, Lorenz D, Nothnagel M, et al. Polymorphisms in the glial glutamate transporter SLC1A2 are associated with essential tremor. *Neurology*. 2012;79(3):243–248.

69. Louis ED, Faust PL, Vonsattel JP, et al. Torpedoes in Parkinson's disease, Alzheimer's disease, essential tremor, and control brains. *Mov Disord*. 2009;24(11):1600–1605.

70. Yu M, Ma K, Faust PL, et al. Increased number of Purkinje cell dendritic swellings in essential tremor. *Eur J Neurol*. 2012;19(4):625–630.

71. Nicholl DJ, Ferenci P, Polli C, Burdon MB, Pall HS. Wilson's disease presenting in a family with an apparent dominant history of tremor. *J Neurol Neurosurg Psychiatry*. 2001;70(4):514–516.

72. Elble RJ, Comella C, Fahn S, et al. The essential tremor rating assessment scale (TETRAS). *Mov Disord*. 2008;23(suppl 1):S357.

73. Mostile G, Giuffrida JP, Adam OR, Davidson A, Jankovic J. Correlation between kinesia system assessments and clinical tremor scores in patients with essential tremor. *Mov Disord*. 2010;25(12):1938–1943.

74. Stacy MA, Elble RJ, Ondo WG, Wu SC, Hulihan J. Assessment of interrater and intrarater reliability of the Fahn-Tolosa-Marin Tremor Rating Scale in essential tremor. *Mov Disord*. 2007;22(6):833–838.

75. Zesiewicz TA, Elble R, Louis ED, et al. Practice parameter: therapies for essential tremor: report of the Quality Standards Subcommittee of the American Academy of Neurology. *Neurology*. 2005;64(12):2008–2020.

76. Ondo WG, Jankovic J, Connor GS, et al. Topiramate in essential tremor: a double-blind, placebo-controlled trial. *Neurology*. 2006;66(5):672–677.

77. Jankovic J. Disease oriented approach to botulinum toxin use. *Toxicon*. 2009;54(5):614–623.

78. Canavese C, Ciano C, Zibordi F, Zorzi G, Cavallera V, Nardocci N. Phenomenology of psychogenic movement disorders in children. *Mov Disord*. 2012;27(9):1153–1157.

79. Kirkham FJ, Haywood P, Kashyape P, et al. Movement disorder emergencies in childhood. *Eur J Paediatr Neurol*. 2011;15(5):390–404.

80. Dale RC, Singh H, Troedson C, Pillai S, Gaikiwari S, Kozlowska K. A prospective study of acute movement disorders in children. *Dev Med Child Neurol*. 2010;52(8):739–748.

81. Stone J. Functional neurological symptoms. *J R Coll Physicians Edinb*. 2011;41(1):38–41. [quiz 42].

82. Espay AJ, Goldenhar LM, Voon V, Schrag A, Burton N, Lang AE. Opinions and clinical practices related to diagnosing and managing patients with psychogenic movement disorders: An international survey of movement disorder society members. *Mov Disord*. 2009;24(9):1366–1374.

83. Morgante F, Edwards MJ, Espay AJ, et al. Diagnostic agreement in patients with psychogenic movement disorders. *Mov Disord*. 2012;27(4):548–552.

84. Stone J, Edwards M. Trick or treat? Showing patients with functional (psychogenic) motor symptoms their physical signs. *Neurology*. 2012;79(3):282–284.

85. Mussell HG, Dure LS, Percy AK, Grabb PS. Bobble-head doll syndrome: report of a case and review of the literature. *Mov Disord*. 1997;12(5):810–814.

86. Colnat-Coulbois S, Marchal JC. Thalamic ependymal cyst presenting with tremor. *Childs Nerv Syst*. 2005;21(10):933–935.

87. Morgan JT, Scumpia AJ, Webster TM, Mittler MA, Edelman M, Schneider SJ. Resting tremor secondary to a pineal cyst: case report and review of the literature. *Pediatr Neurosurg*. 2008;44(3):234–238.

88. Canturk S, Oto S, Kizilkilic O, Karaca S, Akova YA. Rhombencephalosynapsis associated with infantile strabismus. *Strabismus*. 2008;16(1):23–27.

89. Sherman J, Thompson GB, Lteif A, et al. Surgical management of Graves disease in childhood and adolescence: an institutional experience. *Surgery*. 2006;140(6):1056–1061. [discussion 1061–1052].

90. Brouwers FM, Eisenhofer G, Lenders JW, Pacak K. Emergencies caused by pheochromocytoma, neuroblastoma, or ganglioneuroma. *Endocrinol Metab Clin North Am*. 2006;35(4):699–724.

91. Flink EB. Magnesium deficiency. Etiology and clinical spectrum. *Acta Med Scand Suppl*. 1981;647:125–137.

92. Wakamoto H, Manabe K, Kobayashi H, Hayashi M. Subclinical portal-systemic encephalopathy in a child with congenital absence of the portal vein. *Brain Dev*. 1999;21(6):425–428.

93. Ridel KR, Leslie ND, Gilbert DL. An updated review of the long-term neurological effects of galactosemia. *Pediatr Neurol*. 2005;33(3):153–161.

94. Perez-Duenas B, Valls-Sole J, Fernandez-Alvarez E, et al. Characterization of tremor in phenylketonuric patients. *J Neurol*. 2005;252(11):1328–1334.

95. Factor SA, Coni RJ, Cowger M, Rosenblum EL. Paroxysmal tremor and orofacial dyskinesia secondary to a biopterin synthesis defect. *Neurology*. 1991;41(6):930–932.

96. Machado A, Chien HF, Deguti MM, et al. Neurological manifestations in Wilson's disease: report of 119 cases. *Mov Disord*. 2006;21(12):2192–2196.

97. Linnankivi T, Lundbom N, Autti T, et al. Five new cases of a recently described leukoencephalopathy with high brain lactate. *Neurology*. 2004;63(4):688–692.

98. Mahajnah M, Basel-Vanagaite L, Inbar D, Kornreich L, Weitz R, Straussberg R. Familial cognitive impairment with ataxia with oculomotor apraxia. *J Child Neurol*. 2005;20(6):523–525.

99. Lundvall M, Samuelsson L, Kyllerman M. Male Rett phenotypes in T158M and R294X MeCP2-mutations. *Neuropediatrics*. 2006;37(5):296–301.

100. Einspieler C, Kerr AM, Prechtl HF. Is the early development of girls with Rett disorder really normal? *Pediatr Res*. 2005;57(5 Pt 1):696–700.

101. Lee HF, Lee HJ, Chi CS, Tsai CR, Chang TK, Wang CJ. The neurological evolution of Pearson syndrome: case report and literature review. *Eur J Paediatr Neurol*. 2007;11(4):208–214.

102. Tartaglia N, Davis S, Hench A, et al. A new look at XXYY syndrome: medical and psychological features. *Am J Med Genet A*. 2008;146A(12):1509–1522.

103. Remington G, Hoffman BF. Gas sniffing as a form of substance abuse. *Can J Psychiatry*. 1984;29(1):31–35.

104. Despres C, Beuter A, Richer F, et al. Neuromotor functions in Inuit preschool children exposed to Pb, PCBs, and Hg. *Neurotoxicol Teratol*. 2005;27(2):245–257.

105. Yorifuji T, Tsuda T, Takao S, Harada M. Long-term exposure to methylmercury and neurologic signs in Minamata and neighboring communities. *Epidemiology*. 2008;19(1):3–9.

106. Garg BK, Srivastava JR. Infantile tremor syndrome. *Indian J Pediatr*. 1969;36(257):213–218.

107. Thame M, Gray R, Forrester T. Parkinsonian-like tremors in the recovery phase of kwashiorkor. *West Indian Med J*. 1994;43(3):102–103.

108. Neville BG, Parascandalo R, Farrugia R, Felice A. Sepiapterin reductase deficiency: a congenital dopa-responsive motor and cognitive disorder. *Brain*. 2005;128(Pt 10):2291–2296.

109. Vora RM, Tullu MS, Bartakke SP, Kamat JR. Infantile tremor syndrome and zinc deficiency. *Indian J Med Sci*. 2002;56(2):69–72.

110. Thora S, Mehta N. Cranial neuroimaging in infantile tremor syndrome (ITS). *Indian Pediatr*. 2007;44(3):218–220.

111. Ratageri VH, Shepur TA, Patil MM, Hakeem MA. Scurvy in infantile tremor syndrome. *Indian J Pediatr*. 2005;72(10):883–884.

112. Seiler FA, Lew SM. Aqueductal stenosis presenting as isolated tremor: case report and review of the literature. *Pediatr Neurosurg*. 2010;46(5):392–395.

113. Yang S-H, Kulkarni AV. Successful treatment of tremor by endoscopic third ventriculostomy in an adolescent with obstructive hydrocephalus due to tectal glioma: case report. *Childs Nerv Syst*. 2011;27(6):1007–1010.

114. Netravathi M, Pal PK, Indira Devi B. A clinical profile of 103 patients with secondary movement disorders: correlation of etiology with phenomenology. *Eur J Neurol*. 2012;19(2):226–233.

115. Alarcon F, Maldonado JC, Rivera JW. Movement disorders identified in patients with intracranial tuberculomas. *Neurologia*. 2011;26(6):343–350.

116. Krygowski JD, Brennen DFP, Counselman FL. Intracranial tuberculomas: an unusual cause of altered mental status in a pediatric patient. *J Emerg Med*. 2010;38(3):323–327.

117. Wassmer E, Davies P, Whitehouse WP, Green SH. Clinical spectrum associated with cerebellar hypoplasia. *Pediatr Neurol*. 2003;28(5):347–351.

118. Pataki CS, Carlson GA, Kelly KL, Rapport MD, Biancaniello TM. Side effects of methylphenidate and desipramine alone and in combination in children. *J Am Acad Child Adolesc Psychiatry*. 1993;32(5):1065–1072.

119. Pringsheim T, Lam D, Ching H, Patten S. Metabolic and neurological complications of second-generation antipsychotic use in children: a systematic review and meta-analysis of randomized controlled trials. *Drug Saf*. 2011;34(8):651–668.

120. Ardizzone I, Nardecchia F, Marconi A, Carratelli TI, Ferrara M. Antipsychotic medication in adolescents suffering from schizophrenia: a meta-analysis of randomized controlled trials. *Psychopharmacol Bull*. 2010;43(2):45–66.

121. Mehndiratta MM, Satyawani M, Gupta S, Khwaja GA. Clinical and surface EMG characteristics of valproate induced tremors. *Electromyogr Clin Neurophysiol*. 2005;45(3):177–182.

122. Holcomb R, Lynn R, Harvey Jr. B, Sweetman BJ, Gerber N. Intoxication with 5,5-diphenylhydantoin (Dilantin): clinical features, blood levels, urinary metabolites, and metabolic changes in a child. *J Pediatr*. 1972;80(4):627–632.

123. Yilmaz M, Cengiz M, Sanli S, et al. Neurological complications after liver transplantation. *J Int Med Res*. 2011;39(4):1483–1489.

124. Bulatova N, Yousef A-M, Al-Khayyat G, Qosa H. Adverse effects of tacrolimus in renal transplant patients from living donors. *Curr Drug Saf*. 2011;6(1):3–11.

125. Fernandez D, El-Azzabi TI, Jain V, et al. Neurologic problems after pediatric liver transplantation and combined liver and bowel transplantations: a single tertiary centre experience. *Transplantation*. 2010;90(3):319–324.

126. Munhoz RP, Teive HAG, Germiniani FMB, et al. Movement disorders secondary to long-term treatment with cyclosporine A. *Arq Neuropsiquiatr*. 2005;63(3A):592–596.

127. Watson S, Pensabene L, Mitchell P, Bousvaros A. Outcomes and adverse events in children and young adults undergoing tacrolimus therapy for steroid-refractory colitis. *Inflamm Bowel Dis*. 2011;17(1):22–29.

128. Lucchini RG, Guazzetti S, Zoni S, et al. Tremor, olfactory and motor changes in Italian adolescents exposed to historical ferro-manganese emission. *Neurotoxicology*. 2012;33(4):687–696.

129. Wills BK, Christensen J, Mazzoncini J, Miller M. Severe neurotoxicity following ingestion of tetraethyl lead. *J Med Toxicol*. 2010;6(1):31–34.

130. Pons R, Collins A, Rotstein M, Engelstad K, De Vivo DC. The spectrum of movement disorders in Glut-1 deficiency. *Mov Disord*. 2010;25(3):275–281.

131. Incecik F, Herguner MO, Altunbasak S, Leblebisatan G. Neurologic findings of nutritional vitamin B12 deficiency in children. *Turk J Pediatr*. 2010;52(1):17–21.

132. Ozdemir O, Baytan B, Gunes AM, Okan M. Involuntary movements during vitamin B12 treatment. *J Child Neurol*. 2010;25(2):227–230.

Ataxia

Harvey S. Singer[1], Jonathan W. Mink[2],
Donald L. Gilbert[3] and Joseph Jankovic[4]

[1]Department of Neurology, Johns Hopkins Hospital, Baltimore, MD, USA;
[2]Division of Child Neurology, University of Rochester Medical Center,
Rochester, NY, USA; [3]Division of Neurology, Cincinnati Children's Hospital
Medical Center, Cincinnati, OH, USA; [4]Department of Neurology, Baylor
College of Medicine, Houston, TX, USA

OUTLINE

INTRODUCTION AND OVERVIEW

This chapter encompasses diseases and disorders of the cerebellum and its connections.

A vast number of conditions adversely affect cerebellar function in children. The most common of these problems are static and nonspecific, leading to children who, relative to peers, are clumsy. A second common category, acute/subacute ataxias, may result from intoxications, infections, inflammatory processes, or trauma. Many other low prevalence and rare neurological conditions present with signs and symptoms of cerebellar dysfunction. Of particular importance are neoplasms, because early detection is important. Genetic nonprogressive and degenerative ataxias are far rarer, but nonetheless will be seen by child neurologists in practice. Diagnosis is difficult and treatment very limited, but arriving at the most precise diagnosis possible has value for families. Quantitative rating scales have been developed to follow the natural progression of ataxia and response to therapy. One of the most widely used instruments is the assessment and rating of cerebellar ataxia (SARA).[1] A systematic approach is needed for diagnosis of both acquired and genetic ataxias.[2]

DEFINITION OF ATAXIA

Ataxia is defined as an inability to generate a normal or expected voluntary movement trajectory that cannot be attributed to weakness or involuntary muscle activity (chorea, dystonia, myoclonus, tremor) about the affected joints. Ataxia can result from impairment of spatial pattern of muscle activity or from the impairment of the timing of that activity, or both.[3]

CLINICAL CHARACTERISTICS—PHENOMENOLOGY OF ATAXIA IN CHILDREN

The ataxic child may have generalized or localized motor coordination problems. Abnormal eye movements of several kinds, notably nystagmus or oculomotor apraxia, may occur. Speech may be slow and/or slurred. Reaching out of hands to a target or to perform a task may demonstrate significant tremor and clumsiness. Stability of the head and trunk may be poor and there may be consistent bobbing movements. Walking or running may be clumsy, broad based, and lurching or staggering.

Ataxia, or cerebellar disorders and diseases more generally, can adversely affect motor control of eyes, speech, trunk, and limbs in characteristic ways. Complex, multijoint movements are more impaired than single joint movements, with compensatory responses contributing to some aspects of observed movement abnormalities. Inaccuracy is greater at high speed than slow speed.[4] Hallmark findings in patients with cerebellar ataxias are presented in Table 14.1.

LOCALIZATION AND PATHOPHYSIOLOGY

Understanding a simplified model of cerebellar anatomy and neurotransmission is helpful and is addressed in greater detail in Chapter 2. Figures 14.1–14.8 provide an overview of some types of cerebellar pathology in children and link these to symptoms in Table 14.1.

DISEASES AND DISORDERS

This section reviews some of the more common or important diseases causing ataxia in children.

TABLE 14.1   Hallmark Findings in Patients with Cerebellar Diseases

Eye movements	*Nystagmus*—oscillatory, rhythmical movements of the eyes
	Impairment with maintaining gaze
	Difficulties initiating rapid saccades—rapid eye movements to a target
	Difficulties with smooth visual pursuit
	Undershooting (hypometria) or overshooting (hypermetria) of saccades
Speech	*Dysarthria*, imprecise production of consonant sounds
	Dysrhythmia of speech production
	Poor regulation of prosody or volume
	Slow, irregularly emphasized, i.e., *scanning*, speech
Trunk movements	Unsteadiness while standing or sitting, such that the person may have to use visual input or hands for stabilization
	Titubation—characteristic bobbing of the head and trunk
Limb movements	*Hypotonia*—diminished resistance to passive limb displacement
	Pendular reflexes
	Rebound—delay in response to rapid imposed movements and then overshoot of the target
	Imprecise targeting of rapid distal limb movements
	Intention/terminal tremor—more noticeable tremor at the end of movement seen on finger-to-nose and heel-to-shin or toe-to-finger testing
	Delays in initiating movement
	Dysynergia/asynergia—decomposition of normal, coordinated execution of movement—errors in the relative timing of components of complex multijoint movements
	Difficulties with spatial coordination of hand and fine fractionated finger movements
	Dysdiadochokinesia—errors in rate and regularity of movements, including alternating movements
Gait	Broad-based, staggering gait

Nonprogressive Ataxia I: The Clumsy Child

Clinical Features

One of the most common referrals to child neurology is for a child with developmental delay. Often such children have problems with movement and coordination that become apparent between the ages of 3 and 7 years. Parents, teachers, and primary physicians may be concerned about subnormal fine or gross motor skills. Usually, these children do not have progressive disease. More often it is because the child's limited abilities are encountering more complex tasks and expectations in school.

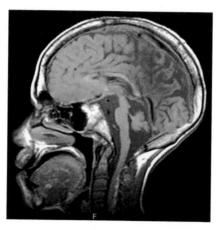

FIGURE 14.1   Diffuse cerebellar and brainstem volume loss in a child with congenital pontocerebellar hypoplasia. In addition to severely abnormal cognition and involuntary movements, the child had intractable epilepsy and apnea, with progressive central nervous system (CNS) volume loss and death before age 10 years.

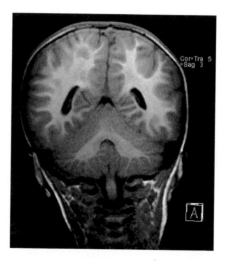

FIGURE 14.2   Coronal T1 magnetic resonance imaging (MRI) of child with partial fusion of the anterior cerebellar lobes, a partial rhombencephalosynapsis. This child had predominantly nonprogressive gait ataxia with significant decompensation during periods of illness. A full syndrome includes cerebellar fusion and absence of vermis. Cerebral abnormalities and epilepsy may also occur.[5]

Typically, there is a nonspecific constellation of motor symptoms. Parents may report tremor of hands and sometimes trunk noted upon awakening, with fatigue or stress, and particularly during fine motor tasks such as drawing, using scissors, or playing with small toys. The child may lag behind typically developing peers in fine and/or gross motor skills and speech articulation. Problems with learning and behavioral regulation may become apparent.

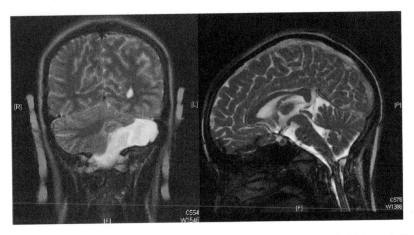

FIGURE 14.3   Coronal and midline sagittal T2 MRI of an adolescent with congenital left cerebellar hemisphere hypoplasia, likely secondary to remote insult. The child had normal intelligence and normal gait, with clumsiness, intention tremor, and postural tremor in the left hand.

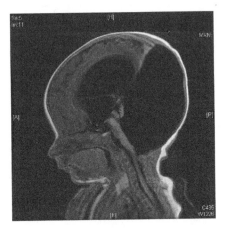

FIGURE 14.4   Dandy–Walker syndrome—enlarged fourth ventricle, absence of cerebellar vermis. This infant has a chromosome 3 deletion. Her lateral ventricles were shunted. She has global developmental delay but can walk with assistance. Developmental disabilities are common but not universal in children with Dandy–Walker syndrome.[6,7]

On general physical examination, special note should be made of any dysmorphic features and skin and cardiac findings. Neurological examination should typically reveal normal mental status and cranial nerves, with no nystagmus or oculomotor apraxia. Strength and bulk should be normal, tone may be normal, low, or high, and reflexes symmetric. Finger tapping and particularly sequential finger tapping may be slow and/or excessively variable in rate and amplitude. Fine regular or irregular postural or intention tremor may be noted. Sensory examination should be grossly normal. Walking and running may be clumsy.

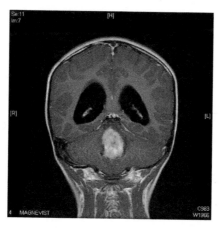

FIGURE 14.5 Coronal Flair MRI of 7-year-old girl with midline cerebellar ependymoma. The child had 2 months of escalating headaches, nocturnal vomiting, fatigue, and finally double vision. Ataxia was not noted, but after tumor resection the child developed cerebellar mutism. This can occur after posterior fossa surgery and may be due to injury to vermis or dentate nucleus.[8,9] Splitting the posterior, inferior vermis can result in predominantly tandem gait difficulty.[10]

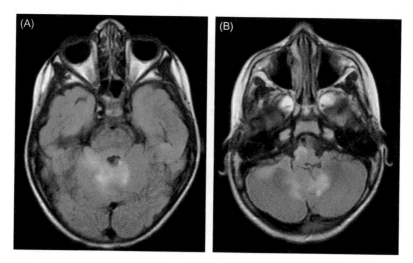

FIGURE 14.6 (A) and (B) Axial Flair images of a 4-year-old girl who presented with subacute progressive vomiting, double vision with right 6th nerve palsy, gait ataxia, and bilateral intention tremor. Over the course of 1 month, clinical symptoms fluctuated and serial images showed migrating, patchy, enhancing lesions in both cerebellar hemispheres as well as midbrain. Etiology was not determined. Within 3 months, both the ataxia and the lesions had largely resolved, although the child had ADHD symptoms long term.

Romberg test typically is normal. A writing sample, drawing sample using the simple Gesell Figures (circle, square, triangle, cross), and bilateral free hand spirals may show tremor, and may be obtained for current assessment. A digital photo pasted into an electronic medical record is useful for comparison at follow-up.

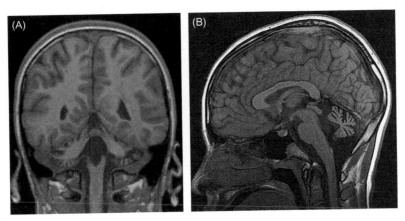

FIGURE 14.7   Coronal (A) and midline sagittal (B) T1 MRI of a 13-year-old boy with 10-year history of progressive gait ataxia, vertigo, nystagmus, intention tremor, and epilepsy. Father and grandfather also have ataxia. Genetic testing revealed heterozygous mutation in the beta-3 spectrin, *SPTBN2* gene, cause of SCA5.

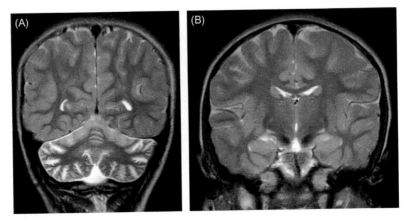

FIGURE 14.8   (A) Coronal T2-weighted MRI showing pan-cerebellar volume loss in 7-year-old girl who presented with 4-year history of progressive spastic paraplegia, gait and limb ataxia, ADHD, OCD, and loss of speech prosody. (B) T2-weighted imaging showing prominent hypointense signal in substantia nigra, consistent with iron deposition. Genetic testing identified mutations in the PLA2G6 gene, consistent with a diagnosis of neurodegeneration with iron accumulation type 2B, also known as atypical neuroaxonal dystrophy (atypical INAD) or PLA2G6-associated neurodegeneration (PLAN).

Pathophysiology

The pathophysiology of routine clumsiness and difficulties with fine motor, gross motor, or speech articulation is variable and nonspecific. Sometimes a history of pre- or perinatal injury is present. A variety of poorly understood genetic and environmental factors may contribute. This heterogeneity is similar to most developmental and behavioral diagnoses, like attention-deficit hyperactivity disorder (ADHD).

Diagnostic Approach—When to Image

In many cases where the problem appears to be static but is relatively mild, and no skills have been lost, a detailed diagnostic evaluation with laboratory testing and neuroimaging will not produce actionable data. A follow-up examination in 6–12 months to ensure there is no skill regression or no new neurological signs is recommended. Although recommendations vary with regard to the yield and utility of neuroimaging in the child with global developmental delay/intellectual disability alone,[11] a number of examination findings increase the yield of imaging. These include (1) abnormalities identified on general examination, suggesting the presence of a syndrome; (2) microcephaly; (3) clearly asymmetric motor findings, or more severe motor problems consistent with a diagnosis of cerebral palsy or "ataxic cerebral palsy."[12] Neuroimaging should definitely be obtained when the following are present: (1) acquired nystagmus and/or acquired ocular mal-alignment; (2) headaches with suspected raised intracranial pressure. The imaging modality of choice is magnetic resonance imaging (MRI). In one study, cerebral palsy was found to be a major contributor to the prevalence of ataxia in childhood.[13]

Treatment

Referral for occupational/physical/speech therapy or special education evaluation may be helpful. In terms of anticipatory guidance for parents of young children, it should be pointed out that when motor problems are present, there is a higher risk for development of cognitive and emotional problems as well. Encouragement of nonfrustrating motor activities that enhance coordination, such as participation in performing or visual arts or sports, may produce positive changes that could be beneficial to motor control over time. There are no strong data on this point; however, a number of studies show structural differences related to music training that might be compensatory for clumsy children.[14–17]

Outcomes

Outcomes are highly variable and likely explained largely by etiology, by nonmedical therapies, and by other positive environmental factors.

Nonprogressive Ataxia II: Ataxia Associated with Congenital Cerebellar Malformations with or without Intellectual Disability

A large number of congenital malformation syndromes as well as prenatal insults may be associated with developmental delay, hypotonia, tremor, and ataxia.[6,13,18,19] Clinical features may relate to the anatomic distribution of the malformation. Congenital ataxias are rare and generally present with hypotonia, developmental delay, and then ataxia, sometimes mild, may be noted. The use of fetal MRI allows increasingly for accurate identification prenatally.[20] Unilateral cerebellar malformations (see Figure 14.3) are generally acquired due to prenatal, perinatal, or postnatal insults. Symptoms vary, with the involvement of the vermis linked to worsen intellectual outcomes.[21] Multiple syndromes are associated with dysgenesis of the midline cerebellar structures. *Dandy–Walker malformations*, characterized by large posterior fossa cystic dilation, upward displacement of the tentorium, midline communication with the fourth ventricle, and complete or partial agenesis of the vermis, can present with early hydrocephalus and later cranial nerve palsies, nystagmus, truncal ataxia, seizures, or cognitive impairments. Dandy–Walker malformations have been associated with numerous chromosomal disorders, gene mutations, inborn errors of metabolism, and teratogens.[7] There is no specific medical therapy for these patients, but neurosurgical consultation for shunting or fenestration of the ventricles or posterior fossa cysts may be needed. *Joubert's syndrome* is an autosomal recessive (AR) syndrome characterized by agenesis of the vermis, dysplasia and heterotopias of cerebellar nuclei, elongation of the superior cerebellar peduncles with deepened interpeduncular fossa (the classic "molar tooth sign" seen on axial MRI), and other brainstem anomalies. Clinically, patients have episodic hyperpnea and apnea, abnormal eye movements, mental retardation, and ataxia.[22–24] *Cerebellar hypoplasia*, which may be global or vermian, and *pontocerebellar hypoplasia* may be part of multiple syndromes that clinically include ataxia as well as other neurologic or organ system dysfunction. Examples include several familial AR or X-linked syndromes, multiple chromosomal trisomies, Smith–Lemli–Opitz syndrome, bilateral periventricular nodular heterotopia/mental retardation syndrome, pontocerebellar hypoplasias types I and II, congenital disorders of glycosylation syndromes types I and II. No specific medical therapies are available for the ataxia symptoms. Outcome varies with etiology.

Recent investigations are expanding the number of genetic causes. For example, a form of autosomal dominant (AD) congenital ataxia with or without intellectual disability has been linked to loss-of-function mutations in the gene *CAMTA1*, a calcium responsive, calmodulin-binding transcription factor expressed in cerebellum.[25] Genetic testing has also resulted in identification of milder phenotypes in cases where biochemical test results are inconsistent, as in a recently described case of congenital disorder of glycosylation 1a.[26]

Acute/Subacute Acquired Ataxias

Overview of Clinical Features

In a previously healthy child, acute ataxia usually presents with gait impairment. A large number of acute processes (partial list in Table 14.2) can affect cerebellar function in an acute or subacute manner. These include intoxications and accidental ingestions, seizures with postictal ataxia, trauma, and autoimmune conditions. A thorough history and examination is essential to identify serious causes. Pathophysiology, treatment, and outcomes are discussed by disease or category.

Intoxications may cause ataxia, sometimes in conjunction with an acute confusional state. Anticonvulsant medications, alcohol, stimulants, and other exposures can often be identified by history, and urine/serum drug screening.[27] Pathophysiology relates to disruption of neural signaling in cerebellum or damage to cerebellar pathways. Illicit sniffing or huffing of toluene-containing solvents can produce diffuse white matter injury and signal change in cerebellar peduncles, resulting in ataxia, kinetic tremor, titubation, and visual loss.[28,29] Acute ataxia and headache evolving to cerebellar stroke after marijuana exposure was reported in three cases, two of which were fatal.[30] Treatment for intoxications is mainly supportive, and outcomes in children are usually excellent.

Acute cerebellar ataxia may occur after a clinical or subclinical infection, particularly with varicella zoster virus,[31] or vaccination.[32,33] After vaccinations in teenagers, functional (psychogenic) illness may also occur, so caution must be taken in verifying the history, time course, and especially the phenomenology. A variety of other preceding infections,

TABLE 14.2   Differential Diagnosis of Acute Ataxia in Childhood

Category	Examples	Clinical features, diagnostic essentials
ACUTE		
Toxic acute ingestion	Alcohol, anticonvulsants, antihistamines, benzodiazepines	Toddlers—accidental ingestion; Adolescents—substance abuse.
		Mental status changes common, urine/serum toxicology screen in Emergency Department may detect unsuspected ingestions.
Trauma/Vascular	Stroke, vertebrobasilar dissection	Consider after neck trauma or if hypercoagulable.
RECURRING		
Metabolic	Many inborn errors of metabolism may occur intermittently	Can be triggered by intercurrent illness.
		Consider if child has preexisting intellectual disabilities, positive family history, consanguinity; or presents with encephalopathy and vomiting.
Migrainous	Basilar migraine, benign paroxysmal vertigo	In the young child, headache may not be prominent. Initial episode consider focal pathology and need for imaging.
Episodic ataxias	Episodic ataxia 1, 2	Bouts of dysarthria, gait ataxia, sometimes with characteristic provoking factors.
Functional	Psychogenic/Functional neurologic symptom disorders	Gait disturbance or abnormal tremor-like movements which have fluctuating, on-off time course, variable direction, amplitude, and frequency, and otherwise do not conform to usual pattern of disease.
		Uneconomical gait, excessive sway without falling may be seen.
SUBACUTE		
Inflammatory	Acute cerebellar ataxia	Symmetric cerebellar findings, gait impairment, truncal ataxia, titubation, nystagmus. Mental status normal. Usually postinfectious. Consider opsoclonus myoclonus ataxia syndrome.
	Acute disseminated encephalomyelitis (ADEM)	Mental status changes; and multifocal neurologic deficits. MRI shows multiple discrete lesions involving white and gray matter.
	Guillain–Barre syndrome, including Miller Fischer variant	Oculomotor paresis, bulbar weakness, hyporeflexia, radicular pain. Risk for respiratory/autonomic failure. Note—weakness localizing peripherally may masquerade as ataxia due to problems with limb control and gait.
	Opsoclonus myoclonus ataxia syndrome	Truncal ataxia, multifocal myoclonus, opsoclonus (may be transient), behavioral irritability. Paraneoplastic (neuroblastoma) or postinfectious.
Mass lesions	Posterior fossa neoplasms	Headaches, vomiting, papilledema, cranial nerve palsies.

including enterovirus, parvovirus, and malaria have been described. Symptoms of gait ataxia occur almost universally, with truncal ataxia less common and nystagmus in fewer than 25%.[34] CSF abnormalities, if present, are nonspecific: elevated WBC in 30–50%, elevated protein in 6–27%. The pathophysiology is unclear but may be similar to paraneoplastic ataxia in adults. Antibodies to multiple glutamate receptors, expressed in Purkinje and other cells, have been described.[35] Recovery is complete in approximately 90%, with mean time to normal gait of 2–3 months.[34] Treatment is not currently recommended although steroids, intravenous immunoglobulin (IVIG), or plasmapheresis should be considered.[36]

Opsoclonus myoclonus ataxia syndrome should be considered carefully in the differential diagnosis of the young child presenting with subacute ataxia.[37] The clinical features are contained in the name of the syndrome, but it is noteworthy that the classic eye movement abnormality, opsoclonus (saccadomania), may be missed due to its transient nature. In addition, truncal myoclonus and multifocal myoclonus may be difficult to distinguish from truncal ataxia, titubation, and action tremor in a toddler. Opsoclonus myoclonus may be postviral or paraneoplastic, related to the solid tumor neuroblastoma. Additional details on the diagnostic testing process and management are found in Chapter 12.

ADEM is an immune-mediated condition that can present in childhood with ataxia[38] or movement disorders, although usually weakness and somnolence are also prominent.[38–40] Clinical features correlate somewhat to the number and localization of central nervous system (CNS) discrete lesions seen on MRI. Time course is usually monophasic, lasting for weeks, with recurrence rate estimates variable.[40,41] The pathophysiology is presumed autoimmune, triggered by infections or in rare cases by vaccinations.[42] The presence of antibodies to myelin oligodendrocyte glycoprotein has been linked to better outcomes.[43] Presentation may overlap with other autoimmune ataxias. The diagnosis should be considered in a child with subacute decline in mental status and motor function, and is generally confirmed through the characteristic MRI. This shows multifocal, multiple sclerosis-like lesions involving both white and gray matter. Many neurologists treat ADEM with immune-modulating therapies such as steroids (IV methylprednisolone at 10–30 mg/kg/day up to a maximum of 1 g/day, followed by a 4–6 week oral taper), or IVIGs (1–2 g/kg dose), and/or plasmapheresis. There are no randomized controlled treatment trials, but reports of treatment outcomes with steroids or IVIG generally show more rapid recovery with treatment.[41] Outcomes are largely good, with more than 80% of children suffering no readily apparent sequelae.

Acute cerebellitis. This term describes a rare acute encephalitis syndrome with altered mental status, dysarthria, mutism, and other cerebellar signs. Brain MRI may show edema with hyperintensity in T2 or Flair images or diffusion restriction.[44,45] Typically, this occurs in young children, usually aged 2–10 years, Many cases are idiopathic, but it has been described with specific infections including varicella,[46] rotavirus,[44,47] and hemolytic streptococcal infection.[45]

Tick paralysis. Children with tick paralysis may present with ascending paralysis, bulbar weakness, and occasionally ataxia,[48] due to a toxin carried in tick saliva.[49] The pathophysiology is believed to involve a failure of neuromuscular transmission.[50] The diagnosis should be considered in the proper clinical context, and the scalp of the child carefully inspected for ticks. Treatment is removal of the tick, and supportive care until symptoms resolve, usually rapidly.

Acute Recurrent Ataxias

This category includes the metabolic diseases causing acute recurrent ataxia as well as other genetic episodic ataxias.

Metabolic Ataxias—Acute Intermittent

A number of metabolic disorders can present with bouts of ataxia (see also Chapter 17). Often, ataxia does not dominate the clinical picture. Specific examples of metabolic diseases which can present as intermittent ataxias include *maple syrup urine disease* (branched chain aminoaciduria), *Hartnup disease*, hyperammonemia, biotinidase deficiency, *mitochondrial disorders*, and pyruvate dehydrogenase (PDH) complex deficiency.

PDH deficiency, resulting from mutations in components of the PDH enzyme complex, can present, sometimes with febrile illness, with intermittent ataxia and weakness that last for days.[51] Supportive laboratory findings include elevated serum pyruvate and alanine, and a CSF lactate level exceeding that in the serum.[52] Administration of 100–200 mg/day of thiamine (B1) and reducing carbohydrate intake may diminish the duration of symptoms and frequency of episodes. Cost/benefit ratio of the ketogenic diet for treatment of patients with the intermittent phenotype is unclear.

Episodic Ataxias

Episodic ataxias may present in childhood or adulthood. They involve bouts (minutes, hours, and sometimes days) of unsteady gait as well as limb, mouth, or eye involvement. Other findings including myokymia, vertigo, hearing loss, tinnitus, or permanent ataxia may develop, and these can be clues to the diagnosis (see Table 14.3). As for the spinocerebellar ataxias (SCAs), the number of associated mutant genes continues to increase including alternate presentations of genetic mutations, for example, in *PRRT2*,[53] known to produce other movement disorders.

EPISODIC ATAXIA TYPE 1 (EA1)

Clinical features of EA1 include childhood onset, brief (minutes) attacks of dysarthria and incoordination. Sudden movement, anxiety, excitement, fevers, and other factors can be triggers. Between attacks, *myokymia*—semirhythmic twitching in hand, the tongue, or the skin around the eyes and mouth—is usually present, although this may be subtle in children. The cause of this disease is a heterozygous mutation in the potassium channel gene *KCNA1*.[54] Penetrance is believed to be complete. Treatment, if desired, is with carbonic anhydrase inhibitors (acetazolamide), up to 375 mg twice per day. This is not always effective chronically, and some patients take small doses intermittently, e.g., before playing sports.

EPISODIC ATAXIA TYPE 2 (EA2)

Clinical features of EA2 include episodes of ataxia lasting hours to days, with gaze-evoked nystagmus between episodes. Triggers for the ataxia episodes include emotional upset, exercise, alcohol, phenytoin, and caffeine. Brief attacks in early childhood, mimicking benign paroxysmal vertigo, have been described.[55] Some children develop chronic, slowly progressive ataxia. Inheritance is AD. The etiology is mutations in the calcium channel subunit gene *CACNA1A*, including both heterozygous point mutations and abnormally

TABLE 14.3   Selected AD Heritable Episodic Ataxias with Childhood Onset

Episodic ataxia type	Classic features, triggers	Interval; duration	Age onset	Gene	Medical treatment
EA1	Gait ataxia, dysarthria, myokymia; Trigger: emotion, postural change	Daily to weekly; seconds to minutes	>2 years	KCNA1 (potassium channel)	Acetazolamide, carbamazepine
EA2	Gait ataxia, nystagmus; Trigger stress (physical, emotional)	Weekly, less; minutes to hours	>2 years	CACNA1A (calcium channel); (migraine)	Acetazolamide, 4-aminopyridine
EA3	Ataxia, vertigo, tinnitus, myokymia Trigger: stress, fatigue, head movement, arousal after sleep	Daily; minutes to sometimes hours	>1 year to adult	Locus 1q42; gene unknown	Acetazolamide
EA5	Ataxia, nystagmus, epilepsy	Hours	>3 years	CACNB4	None
EA6	Severe—episodic and progressive ataxia with seizures, alternating hemiplegia, migraine; milder phenotypes	Hours	13–18 years	SLC1A3 (glutamate transporter EAAT1)	None

AD, autosomal dominant; CACNA/KCNA, calcium and potassium channel subunit genes; EA2 is allelic with spinocerebellar ataxia SCA6 and familial hemiplegic migraine FH1; EAAT1 is Excitatory Amino Acid Transporter 1, also known as Glutamate Aspartate Trasnporter (GLAST).

increased CAG repeats.[56–58] Further increase in CAG repeats cause the allelic disorder SCA6, which usually presents with progressive ataxia and dystonia in adulthood.[59] EA2 and SCA6 are also allelic with familial hemiplegic migraine, caused by a point mutation in this gene. Treatment with acetazolamide 250–750 mg/day can be dramatically effective, although side effects may limit long-term use.[57] A small crossover trial in 10 subjects with EA2 and nystagmus showed short-term benefit from 4-aminopyridine (4-AP) administered 5 mg thrice per day.[60] Aminopyridines inhibit potassium currents, thereby prolonging action potentials.[61]

EPISODIC ATAXIA TYPE 3 (EA3)

Clinical features include episodes generally lasting for minutes, sometimes longer, of ataxia and vertigo severe enough to cause falling. Tinnitus often occurs during episodes. Emotional and physical stress and position can trigger episodes, which may occur daily. This was referred to as EA4 in the initial description in a Menonnite family pedigree,[62] however the nomenclature now is EA3.

EPISODIC ATAXIA 6 (EA6)

More severe clinical features include episodes of ataxia with vertigo, nausea, and vomiting lasting for hours in childhood. Triggers include emotional or physical stress, consuming alcohol or caffeine. The causative gene encodes the glutamate receptor EAAT1[63] and the mutation results in reduced glutamate uptake.[64]

EPISODIC ATAXIA ASSOCIATED WITH SPORADIC SODIUM CHANNEL MUTATION SCN2A

A case report recently described a child with episodic ataxia beginning after the age of 18 months. SCN2A mutations are reported with benign neonatal and intractable infantile seizures as well as with febrile seizures. The child had neonatal seizures followed by episodic ataxia. The authors presented evidence that the missense mutation resulted in a gain of function—increased Na(+) current in cerebellar granule cell axons projecting to Purkinje cells.[65]

Chronic Progressive and Degenerative Ataxias

Overview of Clinical Features and Diagnostic Approach

Chronic progressive ataxias include diseases with primarily ataxia and diseases with ataxia plus other motor, cognitive, and limbic system involvement. In general, any child presenting with chronic progressive cerebellar symptoms and signs (see Tables 14.1 and 14.2) needs a thorough diagnostic investigation.[2] After reviewing all the pertinent findings, including family history and detailed general, ophthalmologic, and neurological examinations, the single most useful initial diagnostic test in virtually all of these cases is a brain MRI scan. IV contrast should be administered in cases with more rapidly progressive symptoms or when neoplasms or inflammatory conditions are suspected.

In some cases, neuroimaging will identify a neoplasm or other space-occupying lesion. A thorough discussion of neoplasms and surgical lesions lies outside the scope of this textbook, but helpful recent reviews may be consulted.[66,67] In general, it should be borne in mind, that the most common pediatric brain tumors—pilocytic astrocytomas, primitive neuroectodermal tumors (PNETS, also known as meduloblastomas), ependymomas (Figure 14.5), and diffuse intrinsic pontine gliomas—are more likely to present in the posterior fossa in children. Thus headache, brainstem findings, and ataxia may develop. Of these tumors, the pilocytic astrocytomas are most amenable to surgery and have the best outcome.[68] Surgical treatment of cerebellar tumors may be curative, but may also induce new neurological problems such as cerebellar mutism. This is most common after resections of midline PNETs with brainstem invasion, and varying degrees of mutism and ataxia may persist for greater than 1 year.[8,69] Cerebellar tumor survivors often have fine motor impairment, ataxia, and cognitive dysfunction, particularly low-performance IQ.[70]

Neuroimaging is vital in evaluation of chronic progressive ataxias. Often, a specific diagnosis will not be made after MRI, but MRI findings in white versus gray matter, and in vermis or cerebellar hemispheres may direct subsequent biochemical, metabolic, or genetic investigations.

If a genetic cause is suspected, the use of updated web-based databases is recommended (see Chapter 4 and Appendix B). For example, the National Center for Biotechnology Information's Online Mendelian Inheritance in Man (OMIM) (www.omim.org/) or the free Simulconsult program (www.simulconsult.com/) allows searches based on several signs and symptoms. Links to GeneReviews or PUBMED can be used to gain additional information about published phenotypes. Laboratory testing options can then be determined at the Genetic Testing Registry Website (www.ncbi.nlm.nih.gov/gtr/) or the Genetests Website (https://www.genetests.org/).

Genetic causes may be productively classified based on certain phenotypic characteristics as well as by mode of inheritance. AR diseases are more likely to present in childhood and will be discussed first, followed by other modes of inheritance such as AD ones.

AR Ataxias

AR ataxias may present more commonly in childhood (see Table 14.4).[71] The most common AR ataxias are Friedreich ataxia (FA) and ataxia telangiectasia (AT). A recently advocated approach is to classify pediatric ataxias broadly into three clinical categories: (1) FA; (2) early-onset ataxia; and (3) adolescent-onset ataxia.[2] Unfortunately, there is no effective treatment for most AR ataxias.[72]

TABLE 14.4   Selected AR Ataxias that May Present with Chronic Progressive Ataxia in Childhood

Disease	Classic features	Age of onset	Inheritance	Diagnostic tests	Medical treatment
Friedreich Ataxia	Gait ataxia, axonal neuropathy, areflexia, extensor plantar response, cardiomyopathy, diabetes	>2 years, mean 15 years	AR	Genetic: >90 GAA expansion in *FRDA*	High-dose idebenone, 45 mg/kg/day with inconclusive benefit (see text)
Ataxia with vitamin E deficiency	Progressive ataxia, retinitis pigmentosa, dystonia	Usually early childhood	AR	Low vitamin E levels	High doses vitamin E, 100 IU/kg/day for life
Ataxia Telangiectasia	Progressive movement disorder—ataxia, chorea, dystonia, athetosis; oculomotor signs, telangiectasias (later) recurrent sinopulmonary infections	Movement disorder at 1–4 years	AR	Elevated serum AFP is usually sufficient to confirm the diagnosis. *ATM* gene sequencing, DNA radiosensitivity testing, may be performed	None for ataxia. Dystonia may improve somewhat with trihexyphenidyl or botulinum toxin. IVIG if immune deficiency/frequent infections
Ataxia with Oculomotor Apraxia 1	Ataxia, choreoathetosis, oculomotor apraxia, sensory neuropathy, hyporeflexia, cognitive impairment	2–18 years	AR	Genetic: *APTX*; low serum albumin, high cholesterol; MRI cerebellar atrophy	None
Ataxia with Oculomotor Apraxia 2	Progressive ataxia, areflexia, oculomotor apraxia less prevalent	13–18 years	AR	Genetic: *SETX*; elevated serum AFP; MRI diffuse cerebellar atrophy	None

AFP, alpha-fetoprotein; AR, autosomal recessive; ATM, ataxia telangiectasia mutation; GAA, trinucleotide repeated sequences; IVIG, intravenous immunoglobulin.

Friedreich Ataxia

CLINICAL FEATURES

Clinical features of FA, which is the most prevalent inherited ataxia in children, include progressive, predominantly sensory cerebellar ataxia, dysarthria, areflexia, pyramidal leg weakness, sensorineural hearing loss, hypertrophic cardiomyopathy, scoliosis, and diabetes (Video 6.1).[73] Ambulation is lost by age 15–20 years. A variety of movement disorders, including tremor, dystonia, and myoclonus, may be associated with FA.[74]

PATHOPHYSIOLOGY

FA results from expanded GAA triplet repeats within the first intron of *FRDA* gene, which encodes frataxin.[75] This expansion impairs exon splicing and reduces frataxin expression. Frataxin deficiency decreases actions of iron–sulfur cluster-containing enzymes, resulting in accumulation of iron in the mitochondrial matrix, increases sensitivity to oxidative stress, and impairs ATP production.

DIAGNOSIS

The diagnosis should be considered in the presence of the characteristic clinical symptoms of ataxic gait with weakness, areflexia, and sensory loss. Milder forms with adult onset have been described.[76]

TREATMENT

A large number of agents to modify disease progression have been studied.[77] These target a broad range of areas related to mitochondrial function including oxidative stress responses, ATP production, iron accumulation, and assembly of iron–sulfur clusters. Antioxidant treatment has been emphasized. Phase II and Phase III studies of the lipid-soluble antioxidant idebenone, a synthetic analog of coenzyme Q10, have had primarily cardiac and not neurological benefits.[78–81] To date there are no proven disease-modifying therapies for the cerebellar aspects of FA, but clinical and translational research continues to be quite active.

Clinicians should carefully manage other FA complications. Referral to cardiology is important. Echocardiography is the main tool for monitoring progressive hypertrophic cardiomyopathy.[82] Heart failure is the main cause of death in FA. Effective management of scoliosis and pes cavus may also be important. If scoliosis surgery is considered, a multispecialist, team approach is advised.

Ataxia Telangiectasia

CLINICAL FEATURES

AT presents in early childhood with dyskinesias but is often misdiagnosed initially. Gait, trunk, and limb movement abnormalities occur and are present even when the child is just standing, although patients may maintain surprisingly good balance for the first 5 years. Early movement problems may be ataxic, dystonic, or choreic, but gait and limb symptoms progress, leading to loss of ambulation in childhood.[83] The movement disorder precedes the onset of the characteristic oculocutaneous telangiectasias. Eye movement problems occur in most patients after the age of 5 years, with difficulty initiating horizontal and vertical saccades.[84,85] Immunologic deficiencies can lead to increased sinopulmonary infections. Risk of lymphoreticular neoplasms is also increased. Median survival is approximately 25 years.[86]

PATHOPHYSIOLOGY

The etiology of AT is mutations in the *ATM* (AT-mutated) gene.[87] The pathophysiology of AT involves disruption of mechanisms of DNA damage surveillance and responses. The *ATM* gene is activated in the presence of DNA damage, signaling cell cycle checkpoints to facilitate DNA repair.[88] Over time, the absence of normal ATM plus the presence of environmental stresses results in damage to cerebellar Purkinje and granular cells, as well as other brain areas including basal ganglia.

DIAGNOSIS

The diagnosis of AT should be considered in children presenting with ataxia, dystonia, or chorea between the ages of 18 months and 3 years, prior to the appearance of the telangiectasias (Video 14.1).[89] The initial diagnostic test is the serum level of alpha-fetoprotein (AFP), which is abnormally and persistently elevated after infancy. This test should be sent routinely in all children presenting with this phenomenology. Genetic testing should not be the initial diagnostic approach after the age of 1 year. Additional diagnostic testing, if necessary, may be obtained through the Ataxia Telangiectasia Children's Project and Clinical Centers in the United States. Genetic testing is reasonable in unclear cases.

TREATMENT

Currently, in patients with recurrent infections, aggressive treatment with IVIG is recommended. There is no curative or preventative treatment for the ataxia and neurologic degeneration. When dystonia occurs, this can be treated medically with trihexyphenidyl or botulinum toxin. An open label study of amantadine in seven children suggested modest symptomatic improvement,[90] although such studies require cautious interpretation. A brief study in four severely affected adult patients suggested that 4-AP, via diminution of the inward rectifying potassium conductance, might have favorable effects on abnormal eye movements.[91] Recent clinical trials involving steroids suggest some opportunity for disease stabilization or modification.[92]

Ataxias with Oculomotor Apraxia

CLINICAL FEATURES AND PATHOPHYSIOLOGY

Clinical features of the ataxias with oculomotor apraxia (AOAs) resemble AT, with slightly later onset and predominantly the neurological (and not the immunologic and dermatologic) phenotype. Key features are oculomotor apraxia, ataxia, and choreoathetosis, distal sensory axonal neuropathy, and marked cerebellar atrophy by brain imaging. Hypoalbuminemia and hypercholesterolemia are also present in AOA1. The etiology of AOA1 is mutations in the *APTX* gene, which codes for the histidine triad superfamily protein aprataxin.[93] Mutant aprataxin appears to affect DNA single strand break repair impair DNA ligation.[94]

AOA2, also referred to as AR spinocerebellar ataxia 1 (SCAR1), has a similar phenotype, although oculomotor apraxia may not be present. As in AT, AFP is elevated. The etiology of AOA2 is mutations in the *SETX* gene, which codes for senataxin,[95] and plays a role in DNA repair and transcriptional regulation.[96] AOA3 was recently identified in a single Saudi Arabian family and linked to homozygous missense mutations in *PIK3R5*.[97] There is no specific medical treatment.

Ataxia with Isolated Vitamin E Deficiency

CLINICAL FEATURES

Ataxia with isolated vitamin E deficiency (AVED) symptoms vary from mild to severe. In severe cases presenting in childhood, initial misdiagnosis as FA has been described. Severe progressive cases develop generalized ataxia, hyporeflexia, weakness, strabismus, dementia, and cardiac arrhythmias. Retinitis pigmentosa[98] and dystonia or myoclonus[99] can also occur.

PATHOPHYSIOLOGY

AVED is caused by mutations in the gene *TTPA*, which codes for the alpha-tocopherol transfer protein.[100] Heterogeneity in phenotypes relates partly to variations in genotype.[100] These patients are unable to incorporate vitamin E efficiently into very low-density lipoproteins, leading to excessive vitamin E elimination. Severe vitamin E malabsorption due to gastrointestinal disease can also cause this clinical picture.[101] Pathologically, findings include degeneration of posterior column axons and dorsal root ganglion cells and mild loss of cerebellar Purkinje cells.[98]

DIAGNOSIS

The diagnosis should be considered in children or adults with progressive sensory ataxia and associated neurological symptoms described earlier. Sporadic or sibling cases as well as ethnicity can also provide clues. Although this is rare, it is important in cases of unexplained ataxia to measure vitamin E levels.

TREATMENT AND OUTCOMES

AVED usually responds to oral Vitamin E supplementation, which must be continued for life. The dose is at least 100IU/kg/day of the most active D-form of alpha-tocopherol. Synthetic, water-soluble forms may be better absorbed, e.g., D-alpha tocopherol succinate. With early treatment, many symptoms may be reversed. Genetic counseling, driving assessments, and occupational therapy may be useful. Despite treatment, progression may still occur, and development of progressive dystonia, despite treatment, has been described.[102]

Infantile Onset Spinocerebellar Ataxia

CLINICAL FEATURES

This severe disease generally has onset at 10–18 months with hearing and visual loss, ophthalmoplegia, ataxia, athetosis, hypotonia and hyporeflexia, sensory neuropathy, and cerebellar atrophy. The etiology is a mutation in the C10 open reading frame gene *C10ORF2* which encodes mitochondrial specific helicase proteins Twinkle and its splice variant Twinky.[103] Pathophysiology of this disease involves mitochondrial DNA depletion. Most *C10ORF* mutations identified result in adult onset progressive external ophthalmoplegia and ptosis.[104]

Posterior Column Ataxia with Retinitis Pigmentosa

CLINICAL FEATURES

This rare AR disease presents in infancy and early childhood with areflexia, progressive sensory ataxia localizable to posterior column dysfunction, and retinitis pigmentosa. There is loss of peripheral vision and subsequent loss of central retinal function. Scoliosis and gastrointestinal dysmotility as well as sensory peripheral neuropathy may occur. Cerebellum appears normal on MRI but high signal will be evident in the posterior columns of the spinal cord.[105] Cause appears to be single-nucleotide coding variant in the transmembrane segment of the *FLVCR1* gene.[106] *FLVCR1* encodes a heme-transporter protein called the feline leukemia virus subgroup C cellular receptor 1. Mutations in *FLVCR1* extracellular loop domains cause the Diamond–Blackfan hematological disorder.

Mitochondrial Recessive Ataxia Syndrome

CLINICAL FEATURES

Clinical features of mitochondrial recessive ataxia syndrome (MIRAS) may include ataxia, involuntary movements, dysarthria, mild cognitive impairment and epilepsy, psychiatric symptoms, and peripheral neuropathy. Etiology may be homozygous or compound heterozygous mutations in polymerase gamma 1 (*POLG1*), resulting in single amino acid substitutions.[107,108]

Childhood Ataxia with Central Hypomyelination/Vanishing White Matter Disease

CLINICAL FEATURES

Childhood ataxia with central hypomyelination (CACH) can occur as a rapidly progressive neurological disease in children, with onset at ages 1–5, or more indolently in adolescents or adults. Diagnostic criteria include: *clinical*—early onset gait ataxia, deterioration with relapsing and remitting course often leading to death by the second decade; *imaging*—symmetric, diffuse white matter changes with CSF-like signal intensity; *neuropathological*—cavitating leukodystrophy with foamy and vacuolated oligodendrocytes and astrocytosis.[109–111] Ataxia dominates the neurological picture, with less prominent cognitive problems and spasticity. A striking feature is the occurrence after minor head trauma or fever of episodes of rapid deterioration in function with hypotonia, seizures, vomiting, and coma, with failure to return to baseline. Epilepsy is also common.[112]

PATHOPHYSIOLOGY

This is a leukodystrophy, caused by mutations in genes encoding any of 5 subunits of the eukaryotic translation initiation factor eIF2B.[113,114] The resulting changes disrupt regulation of protein synthesis during cellular stress in both oligodendrocytes and astrocytes, thereby reducing myelin production and maintenance, but spare of neurons.

DIAGNOSIS

Children with CACH are often diagnosed after neuroimaging, particularly in the context of the striking episodes of deterioration. MRI shows prominent, nonenhancing, diffuse white matter rarefaction or cystic destruction, with signal characteristics close to that of CSF on FLAIR images (Figure 14.6). Additional MRI criteria have been outlined.[112] The differential diagnosis in a child who presents with marked ataxia and mental status changes with fever includes encephalitis and ADEM. ADEM involves multifocal lesions in both white and gray matter. The MRI finding in CACH is readily distinguished from ADEM.

TREATMENT AND OUTCOMES

As no effective treatment is currently available, outcome in childhood onset cases is progressive deterioration and death. Later onset cases may have longer survival but still may have acute deteriorations. Genetic counseling is recommended and prenatal diagnosis is available.

AR Ataxias Identified in Individual Families

Additional AR ataxias have been identified in small families using mapping and next-generation sequencing approaches which should, in the next few years, result in identification of etiologies in more families with unidentified ataxias.[115] For example, in one family, a form of ataxia with epilepsy and mental retardation has been linked to mutations in *KIAA0226* which encodes the protein rundataxin.[116] Mutations in the potassium channel gene *KCNJ10*, which is expressed in brain, inner ear, and kidney, have been found in two consanguineous families where children presented with infantile epilepsy, severe ataxia, deafness, and salt-losing renal tubulopathy with hypokalemic metabolic alkalosis.[117]

X-Linked Ataxia Syndromes

MECP2-Related Syndromes

MECP2 point mutations cause Rett syndrome in girls. Since the recent description of a severe to profound intellectual disability syndrome in boys linked to *MECP2* duplication,[118] case series have identified spastic and ataxic gait as well as later development of epilepsy.[119] Typical severe clinical presentation includes early infantile hypotonia, severe intellectual disability, abnormal gait, lack of speech development, and recurrent infections. Mildly dysmorphic facial features may be present. Gait is ataxic, lumbar lordosis may be noted. Regression may subsequently occur in adolescence with loss of the few acquired skills and more difficult to manage seizures. *MECP2* variant mutations have also been linked to progressive intellectual disability and ataxia in males.[120]

X-Linked Sideroblastic Anemia and Ataxia

Clinical features include ataxia with early childhood ataxia affecting standing, walking, and speech articulation, and mild anemia characterized by hypochromic, microcytic erythrocytes. X-linked sideroblastic anemia and ataxia is caused by mutations in *ABCB7* gene which encodes the ABCB7 protein.[121,122] The ABCB7 protein is a mitochochondrial ATP-binding cassette transporter protein involved in iron homeostasis.

Metabolic Ataxias—Chronic Progressive

A number of metabolic diseases can present with progressive ataxias (see also Chapter 17), some of which have already been discussed. Examples of chronic progressive metabolic ataxias include Refsum disease and cerebrotendinous xanthomatosis. Ataxia occurs as one part of a complex presentation in other neurodegenerative diseases including Niemann Pick type C, gangliosidoses, adrenoleukodystrophy, late-onset Tay–Sachs disease, succinate semialdehyde dehydrogenase deficiency, abetalipoproteinemia, and galactosemia.

Refsum Disease (Heredopathia Atactica Polyneuritiformis)

CLINICAL FEATURES

Clinical features include onset between ages 10 and 20 of impaired night and peripheral vision due to retinitis pigmentosa, and ataxia, polyneuropathy, nystagmus, anosmia, and ichthyosis occurring later. There is also an infantile form with a severe peroxisomal disease phenotype. The etiology of this AR disease is mutations in the *PAHX* gene, which encodes phytanoyl-CoA hydroxylase (PAHX)[123] or the *PEX7* gene, which encodes peroxin-7.[123] Pathophysiology is due to elevated plasma phytanic acid and deposition in brain, spinal cord, and nerves. Reducing dietary intake of phytanic acid containing foods (meats, dairy products) is the typical strategy to slow progression.[124] Beneficial results over a 5- to 13-year period was recently described using lipid apheresis in four severely affected patients.[125]

Polyneuropathy, Hearing Loss, Ataxia, Retinitis Pigmentosa, and Cataract

CLINICAL FEATURES

The phenotype resembles Refsum disease. Key findings include cataracts and early hearing loss, progressive demyelinating polyneuropathy with pes cavus and hammer toes, gait and limb ataxia, and cerebellar atrophy. Onset occurs in childhood or late teens. Causative, null mutations have been identified in the *ABHD12* gene which encodes the microglia-expressed enzyme α/β-hydrolase.[126] This enzyme hydrolyzes 2-arachidonoyl glycerol (2-AG) which in turn acts at presynaptic cannabinoid (CB1) receptors.[127]

Cerebrotendinous Xanthomatosis

CLINICAL FEATURES

Clinical features include progressive ataxia, spasticity, neuropathy, and dementia. Tendon xanthomas and cataracts, associated with elevated serum cholestanol levels, are present. The etiology of this AR disease is point mutations in the *CYP27* gene, which encodes sterol 27-hydroxylase (CYP27), a key enzyme in the bile acid biosynthesis pathway.[128] The pathophysiology is absence of chenodeoxycholic acid, used in bile acid synthesis, resulting in deposits of cholesterol and cholestanol in multiple tissues. Treatment with chenodeoxyholic acid (750 mg/day or 15 mg/kg/day orally divided TID) expands the deficient bile acid pool and reduces elevated plasma cholestanol, partially reversing neurologic symptoms early in the disease course. Later treatment is ineffective.[129] A test for detection in newborns has recently been described.[130] HMG CoA reductase inhibitors, e.g., simvastatin 10–40 mg daily or pravastatin 10 mg daily, may also be useful.[131]

Mitochondrial DNA Ataxias

The neuropathy, ataxia, retinitis pigmentosa (NARP) syndrome[132] may present in childhood.[133] Variants of this syndrome,[134] as well as maternally inherited conditions with unclear pathogenicity, may be identified in mitochondrial DNA (mtDNA) sequencing.[135] A common location for pathogenic point mutations is in the *MTATP6* gene, which encodes a subunit in the F(0) unit of complex V (ATP synthase) in the electron transport chain. Mutations in this gene can also cause Leigh's disease. Ataxia in the presence of neuropathy and characteristic retinal findings, particularly if maternally inherited, supports the utility of obtaining mtDNA sequencing.

The next sections address inherited ataxias, focusing on those that occur in children. The inheritance pattern of a positive family history, when present, assists in narrowing the diagnosis. Therefore, the most common pediatric forms of heritable ataxia will be presented, separated by inheritance pattern.

Autosomal Dominant Spinocerebellar Ataxias

Most AD SCAs present gradually in adulthood.[136] Those which have been reported as having childhood onset will be emphasized in this section. A large proportion of the most common AD SCAs results from extended nucleotide repeats in either coding or noncoding regions. For example, CAG (polyglutamine) repeat expansions within gene reading frames cause SCA1, 2, 3, 7, and 17. Noncoding repeats cause SCA8, 10, and 12. Identification of genetic causes in this setting may involve testing via multigene panels. In children, most may be captured through testing for SCA1, 2, 3, 6, 7, and 17.[137] At present, whole exome sequencing technologies (see Chapter 4) do not detect excess-trinucleotide-repeat mutations.

Subsequent to the initial publications of causative genes, testing in undiagnosed SCA individuals and pedigrees has often broadened and refined our understanding of the phenotypes. For example, diseases once thought to involve certain key features and ages of onset often have a more variable phenotype or earlier onset than was initially appreciated. Thus, while a targeted testing approach based on age of onset and other clinical symptoms remains ideal (see Table 14.5), if these efforts fail then expanding the search and using broad gene panels is rational (Figures 14.7 and 14.8).

The pathophysiology of the SCAs likely involves a variety of mechanisms, including aberrant protein folding, dysregulated transcription, suboptimal bioenergetics, disrupted calcium homeostasis, and ultimately neuronal cell death with apoptotic features.[138]

There are no specific symptom- or disease-modifying treatments shown beneficial in rigorous clinical trials for the SCAs.[139] An open-label, case series study of 5 g/day of the amino acid acetyl-DL-leucine in 13 adults with various degenerative ataxias including SCA1 and 2 suggested broad symptomatic improvement.[140] Coenzyme Q10 may be possibly associated with better clinical outcome in SCA1 and 3, but it is difficult to assess any slowing of progression, especially after 2 years of treatment.[141]

Calcium homeostasis and signaling pathways may be an important target.[142] Various nonpharmacologic therapies have also been recommended and evaluated. Intensive coordinative training (2 weeks in the laboratory, 6 weeks at home) using whole-body controlled video game technology appeared beneficial in an open label study in 10 children with progressive SCA.[143] A recent sham-controlled study of whole body vibration in 32 adults with SCAs 1, 2, 3, and 6 showed improved gait, posture, and speed of speech, but not limb ataxia or speech ataxia.[144]

TABLE 14.5 Selected AD SCAs that May Present with Chronic Progressive Ataxia in Childhood or Early Adulthood, Sorted by Reported Earliest Onset

Spinocerebellar ataxia	Youngest age reported onset in years	Other features in addition to ataxia	MRI findings	Gene	Protein	Mutation type
SCA2	0	Slow saccades and tracking, peripheral sensory loss	Olivopontocerebellar atrophy, posterior column degeneration	ATXN2	Ataxin-2	CAGn
SCA29	0	Congenital nonprogressive, nystagmus, motor delays, mild cognitive impairment	Cerebellar vermis hypotrophy	ITPR1	Inositol 1,4,5-triphosphate receptor, type 1	Various
SCA34	0	Nystagmus; early childhood skin lesions: erythrokeratodermia, papulosquamous erythematous plaques; hyperkeratosis, ataxia, hyporeflexia	Cerebellar atrophy	ELOVL4	Elongation of very long chain fatty acids-like 4	Various
SCA7	1	Pigmentary macular degeneration, ophthalmoplegia, spasticity or Parkinsonism, sensory loss, dementia	Olivopontocerebellar atrophy	ATXN7	Ataxin-7	CAGn
SCA21	1	Oculomotor abnormalities, nystagmus, Parkinsonism, cognitive impairment, hyporeflexia	Cerebellar atrophy	TMEM 240	Transmembrane protein at synapse	Various
SCA25	1	Nystagmus, GI complaints, pes cavus, extensor plantar plus areflexia, sensory neuropathy	Cerebellar atrophy	2p locus	Unknown	Unknown
SCA5 (Video 14.2)	2	Downbeat nystagmus, gaze-evoked nystagmus, facial myokymia, hyperreflexia	Cerebellar atrophy	SPTBN2	Beta III spectrin, associated with glutamate transporter EAAT4	Various
SCA1	3	Oculomotor abnormalities, spasticity/hyperreflexia, EPS, neuropathy	Olivopontocerebellar atrophy, posterior column degeneration	ATXN1	Ataxin-1	CAGn

SCA13	4	Nystagmus, ataxia, hyperreflexia, developmental delay, intellectual disability	Cerebellar atrophy	KCNC3	Voltage-gated potassium channel	Various
SCA14	5	Myokymia, ocular movement abnormality, nystagmus, ataxia, hyperreflexia, dementia, depression, attention deficits, decreased vibratory sense	Cerebellar atrophy	PRKCG	Protein kinase C gamma polypeptide	Various
SCA28	6	Oculomotor abnormalities, ophthalmoparesis, ptosis, rare dystonia/PD, spasticity	Cerebellar atrophy	AFG3L2	ATPase family gene 3-like 2	Various
SCA12	8	Myokymia, ocular movement abnormality, ataxia, tremor, hyperreflexia, dementia, depression, anxiety, delusions	Cortical and cerebellar atrophy	PPP2R-2B	Upstream of coding region for brain-specific regulatory subunit of protein phosphorylase PP2A	CAGn
SCA15	10	Ocular movement abnormalities, nystagmus, ataxia, hyperreflexia, tremor	Cerebellar atrophy	ITPR1	Inositol 1,4,5-triphosphate receptor, type 1	Various
SCA18/SMNA	10	Nystagmus, muscle atrophy and weakness, ataxia, hypo/areflexia, axonal sensory neuropathy	Cerebellar atrophy	IFRD1	Interferon-related developmental regulator gene	Nonsynonymous variant
SCA27	12	Oculomotor abnormalities, nystagmus, pes cavus, intellectual disability, aggression, sensory neuropathy	Cerebellar atrophy; basal ganglia degeneration	FGF14	Fibroblast growth factor 14	Various
SCA3/MJD	13	Parkinsonism, decreased eye movements, loss of reflexes, nystagmus, fasciculations	Cerebellar atrophy, mild	ATXN3	Ataxin-3	CAGn
SCA19	15	Nystagmus, ataxia, hypo- or hyperreflexia, tremor, rigidity, myoclonus, cognitive impairment, reduced vibratory sense	Cerebellar atrophy	KCND3	Voltage-gated potassium channel, SHAL-related subfamily, member 3	Various

(Continued)

TABLE 14.5 (Continued)

Spinocerebellar ataxia	Youngest age reported onset in years	Other features in addition to ataxia	MRI findings	Gene	Protein	Mutation type
SCA4	19	Axonal sensory neuropathy	Cerebellar atrophy	BEAN	Brain-expressed, associated with NEDD4	Insertion within intron
SCA10	19	Seizures, ocular movement abnormalities, mood disorders, polyneuropathy	Cerebellar atrophy	ATXN10	Ataxin-10	ATTCTn
SCA17	19	Ocular movement abnormalities, ataxia, Parkinsonism, dystonia, chorea, dementia, seizures, depression, hallucinations, aggression, frontal release—HD-like or PD-like	Cerebral and cerebellar atrophy, gliosis in stratium, medial thalamic nuclei, inferior olives	TBP	TATA box-binding protein	CAGn
SCA20	19	Dysarthria, dysphonia, nystagmus, tremor, ataxia	Dentate nucleus calcification	11q12.2-11q12.3	Unknown	Contiguous duplication (contains >11 genes)
SCA6	20	Nystagmus, dysarthria, vibratory and proprioceptive loss; some hemiplegic migraine	Cerebellar atrophy	CACNA-1A	Calcium channel, L type, alpha-1A subunit	CAGn
SCA8	20	Spastic dysarthria, spasticity, vibratory loss	Cerebellar atrophy	ATXN8; ATXN8-OS	Ataxin-8	CAGn; CTGn
SCA11	20	Ataxia, dysarthria, hyperreflexia	Cerebellar atrophy	TTBK2	Tau tubulin kinase-2	Indel in coding regions
SCA26	20	Oculomotor abnormalities, nystagmus, ataxia	Cerebellar atrophy	EEF2	Elongation factor 2	Various

SCA		Clinical features		Gene	Protein	Mutation
SCA35	20	Oculomotor abnormalities, torticollis, ataxia, hyperreflexia	Cerebellar atrophy	TGM6	Transglutaminase 6	Various
SCA36	29	Hearing loss, nystagmus, tongue fasciculations/atrophy, skeletal muscle atrophy, denervation, ataxia, hyperrelexia	Cerebellar atrophy	NOP56	Nucleolar ribonucleoprotein complex component of box C/D	GGCCTGn repeat insertion in intron
SCA32	30	Ataxia, azoospermia	Cerebellar atrophy	7q32-q33	Unknown	Unknown
SCA37	38	Oculomotor abnormalities (vertical, horizontal), nystagmus, ataxia	Cerebellar atrophy	1p32	Unknown	Unknown
SCA23	40	Oculomotor abnormalities, ataxia, tremor, mild-cognitive decline, axonal polyneuropathy	Cerebellar atrophy	PDYN	Prodynorphin	Various
SCA30	45	Ataxia, dysarthria, hyperreflexia	Cerebellar atrophy	4q34.3-q35.1	Unknown	Unknown
SCA31	45	Late sensorineural hearing loss, nystagmus, ataxia	Cerebellar atrophy	BEAN	Brain-expressed, associated with NEDD4	TGGAAn repeat insertion in intron

Spinocerebellar Atrophy Type 1 (SCA1)

CLINICAL FEATURES

Clinical features include slow saccades, optic atrophy, nystagmus, amyotrophy, progressive ataxia, dystonia or chorea, and mild cognitive impairment. The disease is caused by a CAG expansion in the gene encoding Ataxin 1.[145] Usually, onset is in adulthood. Genetic testing is available but there is no specific medical treatment. A recent approach in mouse models has involved RNA interference (RNAi). Injection into deep cerebellar nuclei of adeno-associated viruses expressing RNAs targeting ataxin-1 appeared to produce benefits in both cellular pathways and motor function.[146]

Spinocerebellar Atrophy Type 2 (SCA2)

CLINICAL FEATURES

Clinical features are highly variable, with presentation as ataxia or Parkinsonism or both. Other symptoms include slow saccades, nystagmus, retinitis pigmentosa (rare), myoclonus, dementia, posterior spinal cord column degeneration, and peripheral neuropathy. Neuroimaging may show pontocerebellar hypotrophy. The disease is caused by CAG repeat expansion in the gene encoding Ataxin 2.[147] Onset is usually in adulthood, but pediatric cases have been described.[148–150] There is no specific pharmacological treatment. In a mouse model, oral administration of NS13001, a modulator of type 2/3 small conductance calcium-activated potassium channels (SK2), improved neuropathological changes and improved motor function.[151]

Spinocerebellar Atrophy Type 3 (SCA3); Also Known as Machado–Joseph Disease

CLINICAL FEATURES

Clinical features include eye movement abnormalities, ataxia, spasticity, and dystonia. This disease is caused by a trinucleotide CAG repeat expansion in the gene encoding ataxin 3.[152,153] Onset is usually in adulthood, but some cases with rapid progression begin between ages 10 and 30.

Spinocerebellar Atrophy Type 6 (SCA6)

CLINICAL FEATURES

SCA6 is primarily a progressive, adult onset ataxia with nystagmus and dysarthria. This disease is caused by CAG repeat expansion in the CACNA1A gene which encodes the CaV2.1 calcium channel.[154] Mutations in this gene cause EA2 episodic ataxia and familial hemiplegic migraine.

Spinocerebellar Atrophy Type 7 (SCA7)

CLINICAL FEATURES

SCA7 is characterized by progressive ataxia, dysarthria, dysphagia, dysmetria, and slow saccades. Hyperreflexia, chorea, and dystonia also may occur. Visual loss caused by macular and pigmentary retinal generation and optic atrophy set this apart from the other AD SCAs. There is genetic anticipation, particularly with paternal transmission, due to unstable CAG repeat expansion, with age of onset correlating inversely with repeat number.

In early childhood and infantile cases, progression to death is rapid.[155] The pathophysiology of this disease involves expanded CAG repeats in the gene encoding ataxin 7.[156] Postmortem study shows severe neuronal loss and neuronal intranuclear inclusions in the inferior olivary nucleus.[157] The diagnosis should be considered in families with AD ataxia particularly with retinal degeneration. There is no specific treatment available. Outcomes relate to the speed of disease progression, with worse outcomes in children than adults.

Spinocerebellar Atrophy Type 13 (SCA13)

CLINICAL FEATURES

Clinical features of SCA13 are pan-cerebellar. Nystagmus, ataxia of limbs and gait, and dysarthria all occur. Motor development may be delayed and mild intellectual disability may occur. Hyperreflexia and hypotonia are also present, as is cerebellar atrophy. Onset can occur in childhood. Disease progresses slowly.[156,158] The pathophysiology involves mutations in the gene KCNC3, encoding the potassium voltage-gated channel subfamily C member 3.[159] This mutation has a dominant negative effect and slows closing of potassium channels, which prevents fast spiking critical for normal cerebellar function. The diagnosis should be considered in the presence of AD ataxia, but specific features, particularly in adults, do not narrow the differential diagnosis. There is no pharmacological treatment.

Spinocerebellar Atrophy Type 17 (SCA17)

CLINICAL FEATURES

Clinical features of SCA17 are similar to Huntington and Parkinson's diseases. Symptoms may include depression, hallucinations, and frontal release signs, as well as chorea, dystonia, and Parkinsonism. Ocular movement abnormalities may occur. Pathological changes are found diffusely in cerebellum, cerebrum, striatum, and thalami. The disease is caused by CAG repeat expansions in the TBP gene, which encodes the TATA box-binding protein.[160] There is no pharmacological treatment.

Other AD Ataxias

An ataxia presenting in early childhood with gait ataxia, mutism, hypotonia, dysphagia, initially fluctuating, has recently been described associated with mutations in the ATP1A3 gene.[161] Mutations in this gene cause most cases of rapid-onset dystonia-Parkinsonism (RDP, DYT12).

Other Acquired Ataxias

Paraneoplastic, Histiocytosis-Related Cerebellar Leukoencephalopathy

CLINICAL FEATURES

Children may present with progressive cerebellar symptoms affecting gait, coordination, and speech. Spasticity, tremor, dystonia, cognitive decline, and behavioral symptoms may also occur.[162,163] MRI demonstrates symmetric T2 signal change in cerebellar white matter[164] as well as the hilus of the dentate nucleus, pyramidal tracts, basal ganglia, and spinal cord in some cases and calcification of dentate nuclei.[163]

PATHOPHYSIOLOGY

This is believed to be a complication of *histiocytosis*, a disease characterized by abnormally increased numbers of histiocytes, either Langerhans cells (LCH), non-Langerhans cells (nLCH), or malignant cells. A cerebellar leukoencephalopathy may precede or follow the diagnoses of Langerhans or non-Langerhans cell histiocytosis. The cerebellar disease may not respond to treatment of histiocytosis with chemotherapy.

DIAGNOSIS

Characteristic or specific paraneoplastic antibodies have not been identified. The diagnosis should be suspected in children with progressive ataxia and symmetric white matter findings in the clinical context of known or suspected histiocytic disease. Endocrine abnormalities including diabetes and growth failure due to pituitary infiltration may also occur.

TREATMENT

Benefit with chemotherapy and long-term IVIG administration has been described.[165]

Treatment of Degenerative Ataxias

In general, treatment options are quite limited. There are few rational or disease-modifying pharmacological treatments. One recent, small study's approach which appeared beneficial was video-game based. In children with degenerative ataxias, this treatment was followed by improvements in balance and gait.[143]

APPROACH TO DIAGNOSIS AND MANAGEMENT

When presented with a child with ataxia, a flexible, stepwise approach is helpful.

1. Clarify that ataxia is the movement disorder.
2. Localize the lesion. Unilateral or predominantly midline cerebellar signs may indicate focal cerebellar pathology.
3. Stratify into a time-course group—acute/subacute, chronic nonprogressive, chronic progressive, episodic.
4. Identify associated neurological and general medical signs and symptoms outside of the cerebellum and use these to refine the differential diagnosis.
5. For acute/subacute, likely acquired ataxias, assess for intoxications, signs of infection, or inflammation.
6. Obtain a brain MRI for suspected acute or subacute focal cerebellar pathology. Possible causes of focal cerebellar disease include congenital malformation, neoplasm, demyelination, abscess, or vascular event. Treatment of focal neoplasms may be surgical and depends on the cause identified or suspected.
7. For nonprogressive ataxias, monitor clinically, consider brain MRI.
8. For all ataxias that could be inherited, document a three-generation family history and examine parents and siblings, if possible.

9. For early onset, progressive ataxia with no family history or affected siblings only, test for AT with serum AFP level. In the proper settings, consider FA, AVED, AOA types 1 and 2, congenital disorders of glycosylation, and mitochondrial diseases.

10. For children with a family history supportive of AD inheritance, panel test for SCA1, 2, 3, 6, 7, and 17 may capture the majority of likely genetic diagnoses. Targeted testing may be possible depending on other clinical features.

11. For unclear neurologic phenotypes, consider referring for a second opinion.

12. When considering genetic testing, particularly exome sequencing, consider consultation with genetic counselors.

13. Provide general education and referral to general and specific disease Websites.

14. Provide referrals for physical therapy, occupation therapy, and speech therapy as needed.

15. Provide supportive social services as needed.

16. Direct diagnostic and therapeutic efforts outside of the nervous system; e.g., if cardiomyopathy or bone demineralization risks are present, provide appropriate testing or referrals.

17. Consult Clinicaltrials.gov regularly, consider participation in research.

Patient and Family Resources

One advantage of a specific molecular diagnosis is that it helps families network with other affected families and keep track of research. The Clinical Trials Website http:// clinicaltrials.gov/ct2/home lists studies enrolling patients and can be searched by specific disease or disease category.

SUMMARY

A large number of congenital, degenerative, and acquired processes affect cerebellar function, producing ataxia. Diagnosis of inherited, chronic progressive forms is complex, but advancing rapidly. There is hope that rational therapeutic advances may follow.

References

1. du Montcel ST, Charles P, Ribai P, et al. Composite cerebellar functional severity score: validation of a quantitative score of cerebellar impairment. *Brain.* 2008;131(Pt 5):1352–1361.
2. Fogel BL. Childhood cerebellar ataxia. *J Child Neurol.* 2012;27(9):1138–1145.
3. Sanger TD, Chen D, Delgado MR, et al. Definition and classification of negative motor signs in childhood. *Pediatrics.* 2006;118(5):2159–2167.
4. Bastian AJ, Martin TA, Keating JG, Thach WT. Cerebellar ataxia: abnormal control of interaction torques across multiple joints. *J Neurophysiol.* 1996;76(1):492–509.
5. Toelle SP, Yalcinkaya C, Kocer N, et al. Rhombencephalosynapsis: clinical findings and neuroimaging in 9 children. *Neuropediatrics.* 2002;33(4):209–214.
6. Steinlin M. Non-progressive congenital ataxias. *Brain Dev.* 1998;20(4):199–208.
7. Imataka G, Yamanouchi H, Arisaka O. Dandy–Walker syndrome and chromosomal abnormalities. *Congenit Anom (Kyoto).* 2007;47(4):113–118.

8. Robertson PL, Muraszko KM, Holmes EJ, et al. Incidence and severity of postoperative cerebellar mutism syndrome in children with medulloblastoma: a prospective study by the Children's Oncology Group. *J Neurosurg.* 2006;105(6):444–451.

9. Kusano Y, Tanaka Y, Takasuna H, et al. Transient cerebellar mutism caused by bilateral damage to the dentate nuclei after the second posterior fossa surgery. Case report. *J Neurosurg.* 2006;104(2):329–331.

10. Bastian AJ, Mink JW, Kaufman BA, Thach WT. Posterior vermal split syndrome. *Ann Neurol.* 1998;44(4):601–610.

11. Moeschler JB, Shevell M, GENETICS CO Comprehensive evaluation of the child with intellectual disability or global developmental delays. *Pediatrics.* 2014;134(3):e903–e918.

12. Ashwal S, Russman BS, Blasco PA, et al. Practice parameter: diagnostic assessment of the child with cerebral palsy: report of the Quality Standards Subcommittee of the American Academy of Neurology and the Practice Committee of the Child Neurology Society. *Neurology.* 2004;62(6):851–863.

13. Musselman KE, Stoyanov CT, Marasigan R, et al. Prevalence of ataxia in children: a systematic review. *Neurology.* 2014;82(1):80–89.

14. Watanabe D, Savion-Lemieux T, Penhune VB. The effect of early musical training on adult motor performance: evidence for a sensitive period in motor learning. *Exp Brain Res.* 2007;176(2):332–340.

15. Costa-Giomi E. Does music instruction improve fine motor abilities? *Ann NY Acad Sci.* 2005;1060:262–264.

16. Schmithorst VJ, Wilke M. Differences in white matter architecture between musicians and non-musicians: a diffusion tensor imaging study. *Neurosci Lett.* 2002;321(1-2):57–60.

17. Rosenkranz K, Williamon A, Rothwell JC. Motorcortical excitability and synaptic plasticity is enhanced in professional musicians. *J Neurosci.* 2007;27(19):5200–5206.

18. Miller G. Ataxic cerebral palsy and genetic predisposition. *Arch Dis Child.* 1988;63(10):1260–1261.

19. Dyment DA, Sawyer SL, Chardon JW, Boycott KM. Recent advances in the genetic etiology of brain malformations. *Curr Neurol Neurosci Rep.* 2013;13(8):364.

20. Zerem A, Hacohen Y, Ben-Sira L, Lev D, Malinger G, Lerman-Sagie T. Dominantly inherited nonprogressive cerebellar hypoplasia identified in utero. *J Child Neurol.* 2012;27(8):1000–1003.

21. Poretti A, Limperopoulos C, Roulet-Perez E, et al. Outcome of severe unilateral cerebellar hypoplasia. *Dev Med Child Neurol.* 2010;52(8):718–724.

22. Steinlin M, Schmid M, Landau K, Boltshauser E. Follow-up in children with Joubert syndrome. *Neuropediatrics.* 1997;28(4):204–211.

23. Valente EM, Brancati F, Dallapiccola B. Genotypes and phenotypes of Joubert syndrome and related disorders. *Eur J Med Genet.* 2008;51(1):1–23.

24. Choh SA, Choh NA, Bhat SA, Jehangir M. MRI findings in Joubert syndrome. *Indian J Pediatr.* 2009;76(2):231–235.

25. Thevenon J, Lopez E, Keren B, et al. Intragenic CAMTA1 rearrangements cause non-progressive congenital ataxia with or without intellectual disability. *J Med Genet.* 2012;49(6):400–408.

26. Casado M, O'Callaghan MM, Montero R, et al. Mild clinical and biochemical phenotype in two patients with PMM2-CDG (congenital disorder of glycosylation Ia). *Cerebellum.* 2012;11(2):557–563.

27. van Gaalen J, Kerstens F, Maas R, Harmark L, van de Warrenburg B. Drug-induced cerebellar ataxia: a systematic review. *CNC Drugs.* 2014;28(12):1139–1153.

28. Kelly TW. Prolonged cerebellar dysfunction associated with paint-sniffing. *Pediatrics.* 1975;56(4):605–606.

29. Uchino A, Kato A, Yuzuriha T, et al. Comparison between patient characteristics and cranial MR findings in chronic thinner intoxication. *Eur Radiol.* 2002;12(6):1338–1341.

30. Geller T, Loftis L, Brink DS. Cerebellar infarction in adolescent males associated with acute marijuana use. *Pediatrics.* 2004;113(4):e365–e370.

31. Science M, MacGregor D, Richardson SE, Mahant S, Tran D, Bitnun A. Central nervous system complications of varicella-zoster virus. *J Pediatr.* 2014;165(4):779–785.

32. Cutroneo PM, Italiano D, Trifiro G, et al. Acute cerebellar ataxia following meningococcal group C conjugate vaccination. *J Child Neurol.* 2014;29(1):128–130.

33. Yonee C, Toyoshima M, Maegaki Y, et al. Association of acute cerebellar ataxia and human papilloma virus vaccination: a case report. *Neuropediatrics.* 2013;44(5):265–267.

34. Connolly AM, Dodson WE, Prensky AL, Rust RS. Course and outcome of acute cerebellar ataxia. *Ann Neurol.* 1994;35(6):673–679.

35. Levite M. Glutamate receptor antibodies in neurological diseases. *J Neural Transm.* 2014;121(8):1029–1075.

36. Go T. Intravenous immunoglobulin therapy for acute cerebellar ataxia. *Acta Paediatr.* 2003;92(4):504–506.

37. Pranzatelli MR, Tate ED, Wheeler A, et al. Screening for autoantibodies in children with opsoclonus-myoclonus-ataxia. *Pediatr Neurol.* 2002;27(5):384–387.

38. Tenembaum S, Chitnis T, Ness J, Hahn JS. International Pediatric MSSG. Acute disseminated encephalomyelitis. *Neurology.* 2007;68(16 suppl 2):S23–S36.

39. Dale RC, de Sousa C, Chong WK, Cox TC, Harding B, Neville BG. Acute disseminated encephalomyelitis, multiphasic disseminated encephalomyelitis and multiple sclerosis in children. *Brain.* 2000;123(Pt 12): 2407–2422.

40. Javed A, Khan O. Acute disseminated encephalomyelitis. *Handb Clin Neurol.* 2014;123:705–717.

41. Anlar B, Basaran C, Kose G, et al. Acute disseminated encephalomyelitis in children: outcome and prognosis. *Neuropediatrics.* 2003;34(4):194–199.

42. Pellegrino P, Carnovale C, Perrone V, et al. Can HPV immunisation cause ADEM? Two case reports and literature review. *Mult Scler.* 2014;20(6):762–763.

43. Baumann M, Sahin K, Lechner C, et al. Clinical and neuroradiological differences of paediatric acute disseminating encephalomyelitis with and without antibodies to the myelin oligodendrocyte glycoprotein. *J Neurol Neurosurg Psychiatry.* 2014;86(3):265–272.

44. Tang Y, Suddarth B, Du X, Matsumoto JA. Reversible diffusion restriction of the middle cerebellar peduncles and dentate nucleus in acute respiratory syncytial virus cerebellitis: a case report. *Emerg Radiol.* 2014;21(1):89–92.

45. Uchizono H, Iwasa T, Toyoda H, Takahashi Y, Komada Y. Acute cerebellitis following hemolytic streptococcal infection. *Pediatr Neurol.* 2013;49(6):497–500.

46. Bozzola E, Bozzola M, Tozzi AE, et al. Acute cerebellitis in varicella: a ten year case series and systematic review of the literature. *Ital J Pediatr.* 2014;40:57.

47. Zee DS, Chu FC, Leigh RJ, et al. Blink-saccade synkinesis. *Neurology.* 1983;33(9):1233–1236.

48. Li Z, Turner RP. Pediatric tick paralysis: discussion of two cases and literature review. *Pediatr Neurol.* 2004;31(4):304–307.

49. Gorman RJ, Snead OC. Tick paralysis in three children. The diversity of neurologic presentations. *Clin Pediatr.* 1978;17(3):249–251.

50. Vedanarayanan V, Sorey WH, Subramony SH. Tick paralysis. *Semin Neurol.* 2004;24(2):181–184.

51. Kinoshita H, Sakuragawa N, Tada H, Naito E, Kuroda Y, Nonaka I. Recurrent muscle weakness and ataxia in thiamine-responsive pyruvate dehydrogenase complex deficiency. *J Child Neurol.* 1997;12(2):141–144.

52. Uziel G, Bottacchi E, Moschen G, Giovanardi-Rossi P, Cardace G, Di Donato S. Pyruvate-dehydrogenase complex in ataxic patients: enzyme deficiency in ataxic encephalopathy plus lactic acidosis and normal activity in Friedreich ataxia. *Ital J Neurol Sci.* 1982;3(4):317–321.

53. Gardiner AR, Bhatia KP, Stamelou M, et al. PRRT2 gene mutations: from paroxysmal dyskinesia to episodic ataxia and hemiplegic migraine. *Neurology.* 2012;79:2115–2121.

54. Browne DL, Gancher ST, Nutt JG, et al. Episodic ataxia/myokymia syndrome is associated with point mutations in the human potassium channel gene, KCNA1. *Nat Genet.* 1994;8:136–140.

55. Bertholon P, Chabrier S, Riant F, Tournier-Lasserve E, Peyron R. Episodic ataxia type 2: unusual aspects in clinical and genetic presentation. Special emphasis in childhood. *J Neurol Neurosurg Psychiatry.* 2009;80(11):1289–1292.

56. Ophoff RA, Terwindt GM, Vergouwe MN, et al. Familial hemiplegic migraine and episodic ataxia type-2 are caused by mutations in the Ca2+ channel gene CACNL1A4. *Cell.* 1996;87(3):543–552.

57. Wan J, Mamsa H, Johnston JL, et al. Large genomic deletions in CACNA1A cause episodic ataxia type 2. *Front Neurol.* 2011;2:51.

58. Jodice C, Mantuano E, Veneziano L, et al. Episodic ataxia type 2 (EA2) and spinocerebellar ataxia type 6 (SCA6) due to CAG repeat expansion in the CACNA1A gene on chromosome 19p. *Hum Mol Genet.* 1997;6(11):1973–1978.

59. Spacey SD, Materek LA, Szczygielski BI, Bird TD. Two novel CACNA1A gene mutations associated with episodic ataxia type 2 and interictal dystonia. *Arch Neurol.* 2005;62(2):314–316.

60. Strupp M, Kalla R, Claassen J, et al. A randomized trial of 4-aminopyridine in EA2 and related familial episodic ataxias. *Neurology.* 2011;77(3):269–275.

61. Alvina K, Khodakhah K. The therapeutic mode of action of 4-aminopyridine in cerebellar ataxia. *J Neurosci.* 2010;30(21):7258–7268.

62. Steckley JL, Ebers GC, Cader MZ, McLachlan RS. An autosomal dominant disorder with episodic ataxia, vertigo, and tinnitus. *Neurology.* 2001;57(8):1499–1502.

63. Jen JC, Wan J, Palos TP, Howard BD, Baloh RW. Mutation in the glutamate transporter EAAT1 causes episodic ataxia, hemiplegia, and seizures. *Neurology*. 2005;65(4):529–534.

64. de Vries B, Mamsa H, Stam AH, et al. Episodic ataxia associated with EAAT1 mutation C186S affecting glutamate reuptake. *Arch Neurol*. 2009;66(1):97–101.

65. Liao Y, Anttonen AK, Liukkonen E, et al. SCN2A mutation associated with neonatal epilepsy, late-onset episodic ataxia, myoclonus, and pain. *Neurology*. 2010;75(16):1454–1458.

66. Pollack IF. Multidisciplinary management of childhood brain tumors: a review of outcomes, recent advances, and challenges. *J Neurosurg Pediatr*. 2011;8(2):135–148.

67. Khatua S, Sadighi ZS, Pearlman ML, Bochare S, Vats TS. Brain tumors in children—current therapies and newer directions. *Indian J Pediatr*. 2012;79(7):922–927.

68. Fisher PG, Tihan T, Goldthwaite PT, et al. Outcome analysis of childhood low-grade astrocytomas. *Pediatr Blood Cancer*. 2008;51(2):245–250.

69. Gudrunardottir T, Sehested A, Juhler M, Schmiegelow K. Cerebellar mutism: review of the literature. *Childs Nerv Syst*. 2011;27(3):355–363.

70. Rueckriegel SM, Blankenburg F, Henze G, Baque H, Driever PH. Loss of fine motor function correlates with ataxia and decline of cognition in cerebellar tumor survivors. *Pediatr Blood Cancer*. 2009;53(3):424–431.

71. Anheim M, Tranchant C, Koenig M. The autosomal recessive cerebellar ataxias. *N Engl J Med*. 2012;366:636–646.

72. van de Warrenburg BP, van Gaalen J, Boesch S, et al. EFNS/ENS Consensus on the diagnosis and management of chronic ataxias in adulthood. *Eur J Neurol*. 2014;21(4):552–562.

73. Ribai P, Pousset F, Tanguy ML, et al. Neurological, cardiological, and oculomotor progression in 104 patients with Friedreich ataxia during long-term follow-up. *Arch Neurol*. 2007;64(4):558–564.

74. Hou JG, Jankovic J. Movement disorders in Friedreich's ataxia. *J Neurol Sci*. 2003;206(1):59–64.

75. Delatycki MB, Knight M, Koenig M, Cossee M, Williamson R, Forrest SM. G130V, a common FRDA point mutation, appears to have arisen from a common founder. *Hum Genet*. 1999;105(4):343–346.

76. Berciano J, Mateo I, De Pablos C, Polo JM, Combarros O. Friedreich ataxia with minimal GAA expansion presenting as adult-onset spastic ataxia. *J Neurol Sci*. 2002;194(1):75–82.

77. Perlman SL. A review of Friedreich ataxia clinical trial results. *J Child Neurol*. 2012;27(9):1217–1222.

78. Di Prospero NA, Baker A, Jeffries N, Fischbeck KH. Neurological effects of high-dose idebenone in patients with Friedreich's ataxia: a randomised, placebo-controlled trial. *Lancet Neurol*. 2007;6(10):878–886.

79. Lynch DR, Perlman SL, Meier T. A phase 3, double-blind, placebo-controlled trial of idebenone in Friedreich ataxia. *Arch Neurol*. 2010;67(8):941–947.

80. Lagedrost SJ, Sutton MS, Cohen MS, et al. Idebenone in Friedreich ataxia cardiomyopathy—results from a 6-month phase III study (IONIA). *Am Heart J*. 2011;161(3):639–645 e631.

81. Meier T, Perlman SL, Rummey C, Coppard NJ, Lynch DR. Assessment of neurological efficacy of idebenone in pediatric patients with Friedreich's ataxia: data from a 6-month controlled study followed by a 12-month open-label extension study. *J Neurol*. 2012;259(2):284–291.

82. Weidemann F, Rummey C, Bijnens B, et al. The heart in Friedreich ataxia: definition of cardiomyopathy, disease severity, and correlation with neurological symptoms. *Circulation*. 2012;125(13):1626–1634.

83. Crawford TO, Mandir AS, Lefton-Greif MA, et al. Quantitative neurologic assessment of ataxia-telangiectasia. *Neurology*. 2000;54(7):1505–1509.

84. Shaikh AG, Marti S, Tarnutzer AA, et al. Gaze fixation deficits and their implication in ataxia-telangiectasia. *J Neurol Neurosurg Psychiatry*. 2009;80(8):858–864.

85. Lewis RF, Lederman HM, Crawford TO. Ocular motor abnormalities in ataxia telangiectasia. *Ann Neurol*. 1999;46(3):287–295.

86. Crawford TO, Skolasky RL, Fernandez R, Rosquist KJ, Lederman HM. Survival probability in ataxia telangiectasia. *Arch Dis Child*. 2006;91(7):610–611.

87. Savitsky K, Bar-Shira A, Gilad S, et al. A single ataxia telangiectasia gene with a product similar to PI-3 kinase. *Science*. 1995;268(5218):1749–1753.

88. Lavin MF, Gueven N, Bottle S, Gatti RA. Current and potential therapeutic strategies for the treatment of ataxia-telangiectasia. *Br Med Bull*. 2007;81-82:129–147.

89. Cabana MD, Crawford TO, Winkelstein JA, Christensen JR, Lederman HM. Consequences of the delayed diagnosis of ataxia-telangiectasia. *Pediatrics*. 1998;102(1 Pt 1):98–100.

90. Nissenkorn A, Hassin-Baer S, Lerman SF, Levi YB, Tzadok M, Ben-Zeev B. Movement disorder in ataxia-telangiectasia: treatment with amantadine sulfate. *J Child Neurol.* 2013;28(2):155–160.

91. Shaikh AG, Marti S, Tarnutzer AA, et al. Effects of 4-aminopyridine on nystagmus and vestibulo-ocular reflex in ataxia-telangiectasia. *J Neurol.* 2013;260(11):2728–2735.

92. Chessa L, Leuzzi V, Plebani A, et al. Intra-erythrocyte infusion of dexamethasone reduces neurological symptoms in ataxia teleangiectasia patients: results of a phase 2 trial. *Orphanet J Rare Dis.* 2014;9(5).

93. Iwadate Y, Saeki N, Namba H, Odaki M, Oka N, Yamaura A. Post-traumatic intention tremor—clinical features and CT findings. *Neurosurg Rev.* 1989;12(suppl 1):500–507.

94. Reynolds JJ, El-Khamisy SF, Katyal S, Clements P, McKinnon PJ, Caldecott KW. Defective DNA ligation during short-patch single-strand break repair in ataxia oculomotor apraxia 1. *Mol Cell Biol.* 2009;29(5):1354–1362.

95. Gonzalez-Vioque E, Blazquez A, Fernandez-Moreira D, et al. Association of novel POLG mutations and multiple mitochondrial DNA deletions with variable clinical phenotypes in a Spanish population. *Arch Neurol.* 2006;63(1):107–111.

96. Suraweera A, Lim Y, Woods R, et al. Functional role for senataxin, defective in ataxia oculomotor apraxia type 2, in transcriptional regulation. *Hum Mol Genet.* 2009;18(18):3384–3396.

97. Al Tassan N, Khalil D, Shinwari J, et al. A missense mutation in PIK3R5 gene in a family with ataxia and oculomotor apraxia. *Hum Mutat.* 2012;33(2):351–354.

98. Yokota T, Uchihara T, Kumagai J, et al. Postmortem study of ataxia with retinitis pigmentosa by mutation of the alpha-tocopherol transfer protein gene. *J Neurol Neurosurg Psychiatry.* 2000;68(4):521–525.

99. Angelini L, Erba A, Mariotti C, Gellera C, Ciano C, Nardocci N. Myoclonic dystonia as unique presentation of isolated vitamin E deficiency in a young patient. *Mov Disord.* 2002;17(3):612–614.

100. Cavalier L, Ouahchi K, Kayden HJ, et al. Ataxia with isolated vitamin E deficiency: heterogeneity of mutations and phenotypic variability in a large number of families. *Am J Hum Genet.* 1998;62(2):301–310.

101. Sokol RJ, Guggenheim MA, Iannaccone ST, et al. Improved neurologic function after long-term correction of vitamin E deficiency in children with chronic cholestasis. *N Engl J Med.* 1985;313(25):1580–1586.

102. Roubertie A, Biolsi B, Rivier F, Humbertclaude V, Cheminal R, Echenne B. Ataxia with vitamin E deficiency and severe dystonia: report of a case. *Brain Dev.* 2003;25(6):442–445.

103. Nikali K, Suomalainen A, Saharinen J, et al. Infantile onset spinocerebellar ataxia is caused by recessive mutations in mitochondrial proteins Twinkle and Twinky. *Hum Mol Genet.* 2005;14(20):2981–2990.

104. Van Hove JL, Cunningham V, Rice C, et al. Finding twinkle in the eyes of a 71-year-old lady: a case report and review of the genotypic and phenotypic spectrum of TWINKLE-related dominant disease. *Am J Med Genet A.* 2009;149A(5):861–867.

105. Higgins JJ, Morton DH, Patronas N, Nee LE. An autosomal recessive disorder with posterior column ataxia and retinitis pigmentosa. *Neurology.* 1997;49(6):1717–1720.

106. Rajadhyaksha AM, Elemento O, Puffenberger EG, et al. Mutations in FLVCR1 cause posterior column ataxia and retinitis pigmentosa. *Am J Hum Genet.* 2010;87(5):643–654.

107. Hakonen AH, Heiskanen S, Juvonen V, et al. Mitochondrial DNA polymerase W748S mutation: a common cause of autosomal recessive ataxia with ancient European origin. *Am J Hum Genet.* 2005;77(3):430–441.

108. Palin EJ, Hakonen AH, Korpela M, Paetau A, Suomalainen A. Mitochondrial recessive ataxia syndrome mimicking dominant spinocerebellar ataxia. *J Neurol Sci.* 2012;315(1–2):160–163.

109. Fogli A, Schiffmann R, Bertini E, et al. The effect of genotype on the natural history of eIF2B-related leukodystrophies. *Neurology.* 2004;62(9):1509–1517.

110. Schiffmann R, Moller JR, Trapp BD, et al. Childhood ataxia with diffuse central nervous system hypomyelination. *Ann Neurol.* 1994;35(3):331–340.

111. Rodriguez D, Gelot A, Della Gaspera B, et al. Increased density of oligodendrocytes in childhood ataxia with diffuse central hypomyelination (CACH) syndrome: neuropathological and biochemical study of two cases. *Acta Neuropathol.* 1999;97(5):469–480.

112. Mierzewska H, van der Knaap MS, Scheper GC, Jurkiewicz E, Schmidt-Sidor B, Szymanska K. Leukoencephalopathy with vanishing white matter due to homozygous EIF2B2 gene mutation. First Polish cases. *Folia Neuropathol.* 2006;44(2):144–148.

113. van der Knaap MS, Leegwater PAJ, Konst AAM, et al. Mutations in each of the five subunits of translation initiation factor eIF2B can cause leukoencephalopathy with vanishing white matter. *Ann Neurol.* 2002;51(2):264–270.

114. Leegwater PA, Vermeulen G, Konst AA, et al. Subunits of the translation initiation factor eIF2B are mutant in leukoencephalopathy with vanishing white matter. *Nat Genet*. 2001;29(4):383–388.

115. Sailer A, Houlden H. Recent advances in the genetics of cerebellar ataxias. *Curr Neurol Neurosci Rep*. 2012;12(3):227–236.

116. Assoum M, Salih MA, Drouot N, et al. Rundataxin, a novel protein with RUN and diacylglycerol binding domains, is mutant in a new recessive ataxia. *Brain*. 2010;133(Pt 8):2439–2447.

117. Bockenhauer D, Feather S, Stanescu HC, et al. Epilepsy, ataxia, sensorineural deafness, tubulopathy, and KCNJ10 mutations. *N Engl J Med*. 2009;360(19):1960–1970.

118. Van Esch H, Bauters M, Ignatius J, et al. Duplication of the *MECP2* region is a frequent cause of severe mental retardation and progressive neurological symptoms in males. *Am J Hum Genet*. 2005;77(3):442–453.

119. Vignoli A, Borgatti R, Peron A, et al. Electroclinical pattern in MECP2 duplication syndrome: eight new reported cases and review of literature. *Epilepsia*. 2012;53(7):1146–1155.

120. McWilliam C, Cooke A, Lobo D, Warner J, Taylor M, Tolmie J. Semi-dominant X-chromosome linked learning disability with progressive ataxia, spasticity and dystonia associated with the novel *MECP2* variant p. V122A: akin to the new *MECP2* duplication syndrome? *Eur J Paediatr Neurol*. 2010;14(3):267–269.

121. Allikmets R, Raskind WH, Hutchinson A, Schueck ND, Dean M, Koeller DM. Mutation of a putative mitochondrial iron transporter gene (ABC7) in X-linked sideroblastic anemia and ataxia (XLSA/A). *Hum Mol Genet*. 1999;8(5):743–749.

122. Pagon RA, Bird TD, Detter JC, Pierce I. Hereditary sideroblastic anaemia and ataxia: an X linked recessive disorder. *J Med Genet*. 1985;22(4):267–273.

123. Egfjord M, Jansen JA, Flachs H, Schou JS. Combined boric acid and cinchocaine chloride poisoning in a 12-month-old infant: evaluation of haemodialysis. *Hum Toxicol*. 1988;7(2):175–178.

124. Baldwin EJ, Gibberd FB, Harley C, Sidey MC, Feher MD, Wierzbicki AS. The effectiveness of long-term dietary therapy in the treatment of adult Refsum disease. *J Neurol Neurosurg Psychiatry*. 2010;81(9):954–957.

125. Zolotov D, Wagner S, Kalb K, Bunia J, Heibges A, Klingel R. Long-term strategies for the treatment of Refsum's disease using therapeutic apheresis. *J Clin Apher*. 2012;27(2):99–105.

126. Fiskerstrand T, H'Mida-Ben Brahim D, Johansson S, et al. Mutations in ABHD12 cause the neurodegenerative disease PHARC: an inborn error of endocannabinoid metabolism. *Am J Hum Genet*. 2010;87(3):410–417.

127. Savinainen JR, Saario SM, Laitinen JT. The serine hydrolases MAGL, ABHD6 and ABHD12 as guardians of 2-arachidonoylglycerol signalling through cannabinoid receptors. *Acta Physiol (Oxf)*. 2012;204(2):267–276.

128. Cali JJ, Hsieh CL, Francke U, Russell DW. Mutations in the bile acid biosynthetic enzyme sterol 27-hydroxylase underlie cerebrotendinous xanthomatosis. *J Biol Chem*. 1991;266(12):7779–7783.

129. Yahalom G, Tsabari R, Molshatzki N, Ephraty L, Cohen H, Hassin-Baer S. Neurological outcome in cerebrotendinous xanthomatosis treated with chenodeoxycholic acid: early versus late diagnosis. *Clin Neuropharmacol*. 2013;36(3):78–83.

130. DeBarber AE, Luo J, Star-Weinstock M, et al. A blood test for cerebrotendinous xanthomatosis with potential for disease detection in newborns. *J Lipid Res*. 2014;55(1):146–154.

131. Luyckx E, Eyskens F, Simons A, Beckx K, Van West D, Dhar M. Long-term follow-up on the effect of combined therapy of bile acids and statins in the treatment of cerebrotendinous xanthomatosis: a case report. *Clin Neurol Neurosurg*. 2014;118:9–11.

132. Holt IJ, Harding AE, Petty RK, Morgan-Hughes JA. A new mitochondrial disease associated with mitochondrial DNA heteroplasmy. *Am J Hum Genet*. 1990;46(3):428–433.

133. Parfait B, de Lonlay P, von Kleist-Retzow JC, et al. The neurogenic weakness, ataxia and retinitis pigmentosa (NARP) syndrome mtDNA mutation (T8993G) triggers muscle ATPase deficiency and hypocitrullinaemia. *Eur J Pediatr*. 1999;158(1):55–58.

134. Kara B, Arikan M, Maras H, Abaci N, Cakiris A, Ustek D. Whole mitochondrial genome analysis of a family with NARP/MILS caused by m.8993T>C mutation in the MT-ATP6 gene. *Mol Genet Metab*. 2012;107(3):389–393.

135. Sikorska M, Sandhu JK, Simon DK, et al. Identification of ataxia-associated mtDNA mutations (m.4052T>C and m.9035T>C) and evaluation of their pathogenicity in transmitochondrial cybrids. *Muscle Nerve*. 2009;40(3):381–394.

136. Rossi M, Perez-Lloret S, Doldan L, et al. Autosomal dominant cerebellar ataxias: a systematic review of clinical features. *Eur J Neurol*. 2014;21(4):607–615.

137. Gasser T, Finsterer J, Baets J, et al. EFNS guidelines on the molecular diagnosis of ataxias and spastic paraplegias. *Eur J Neurol*. 2010;17(2):179–188.

138. Matilla-Duenas A, Ashizawa T, Brice A, et al. Consensus paper: pathological mechanisms underlying neurodegeneration in spinocerebellar ataxias. *Cerebellum*. 2014;13(2):269–302.

139. Nag N, Tarlac V, Storey E. Assessing the efficacy of specific cerebellomodulatory drugs for use as therapy for spinocerebellar ataxia type 1. *Cerebellum*. 2013;12(1):74–82.

140. Strupp M, Teufel J, Habs M, et al. Effects of acetyl-DL-leucine in patients with cerebellar ataxia: a case series. *J Neurol*. 2013;260(10):2556–2561.

141. Lo RY, Figueroa KP, Pulst SM, et al. Coenzyme Q10 and spinocerebellar ataxias. *Mov Disord*. 2015;30(2):214–220.

142. Bettencourt C, Ryten M, Forabosco P, et al. Insights from cerebellar transcriptomic analysis into the pathogenesis of ataxia. *JAMA Neurol*. 2014;71(7):831–839.

143. Ilg W, Schatton C, Schicks J, Giese MA, Schols L, Synofzik M. Video game-based coordinative training improves ataxia in children with degenerative ataxia. *Neurology*. 2012;79(20):2056–2060.

144. Kaut O, Jacobi H, Coch C, et al. A randomized pilot study of stochastic vibration therapy in spinocerebellar ataxia. *Cerebellum*. 2014;13(2):237–242.

145. Banfi S, Servadio A, Chung MY, et al. Identification and characterization of the gene causing type 1 spinocerebellar ataxia. *Nat Genet*. 1994;7(4):513–520.

146. Keiser MS, Boudreau RL, Davidson BL. Broad therapeutic benefit after RNAi expression vector delivery to deep cerebellar nuclei: implications for spinocerebellar ataxia type 1 therapy. *Mol Ther*. 2014;22(3):588–595.

147. Pulst SM, Nechiporuk A, Nechiporuk T, et al. Moderate expansion of a normally biallelic trinucleotide repeat in spinocerebellar ataxia type 2. *Nat Genet*. 1996;14(3):269–276.

148. Dirik E, Yis U, Basak N, Soydan E, Hudaoglu O, Ozgonul F. Spinocerebellar ataxia type 2 in a Turkish family. *J Child Neurol*. 2007;22(7):891–894.

149. Abdel-Aleem A, Zaki MS. Spinocerebellar ataxia type 2 (SCA2) in an Egyptian family presenting with polyphagia and marked CAG expansion in infancy. *J Neurol*. 2008;255(3):413–419.

150. Ramocki MB, Chapieski L, McDonald RO, Fernandez F, Malphrus AD. Spinocerebellar ataxia type 2 presenting with cognitive regression in childhood. *J Child Neurol*. 2008;23(9):999–1001.

151. Kasumu AW, Hougaard C, Rode F, et al. Selective positive modulator of calcium-activated potassium channels exerts beneficial effects in a mouse model of spinocerebellar ataxia type 2. *Chem Biol*. 2012;19(10):1340–1353.

152. Kawaguchi Y, Okamoto T, Taniwaki M, et al. CAG expansions in a novel gene for Machado–Joseph disease at chromosome 14q32.1. *Nat Genet*. 1994;8(3):221–228.

153. Schols L, Vieira-Saecker AM, Schols S, Przuntek H, Epplen JT, Riess O. Trinucleotide expansion within the MJD1 gene presents clinically as spinocerebellar ataxia and occurs most frequently in German SCA patients. *Hum Mol Genet*. 1995;4(6):1001–1005.

154. Ishikawa K, Fujigasaki H, Saegusa H, et al. Abundant expression and cytoplasmic aggregations of [alpha]1A voltage-dependent calcium channel protein associated with neurodegeneration in spinocerebellar ataxia type 6. *Hum Mol Genet*. 1999;8(7):1185–1193.

155. Enevoldson TP, Sanders MD, Harding AE. Autosomal dominant cerebellar ataxia with pigmentary macular dystrophy. A clinical and genetic study of eight families. *Brain*. 1994;117(Pt 3):445–460.

156. David G, Abbas N, Stevanin G, et al. Cloning of the SCA7 gene reveals a highly unstable CAG repeat expansion. *Nat Genet*. 1997;17(1):65–70.

157. Holmberg M, Duyckaerts C, Durr A, et al. Spinocerebellar ataxia type 7 (SCA7): a neurodegenerative disorder with neuronal intranuclear inclusions. *Hum Mol Genet*. 1998;7(5):913–918.

158. Herman-Bert A, Stevanin G, Netter JC, et al. Mapping of spinocerebellar ataxia 13 to chromosome 19q13.3-q13.4 in a family with autosomal dominant cerebellar ataxia and mental retardation. *Am J Hum Genet*. 2000;67(1):229–235.

159. Wong LJ, Naviaux RK, Brunetti-Pierri N, et al. Molecular and clinical genetics of mitochondrial diseases due to POLG mutations. *Hum Mutat*. 2008;29(9):E150–E172.

160. Nakamura K, Jeong SY, Uchihara T, et al. SCA17, a novel autosomal dominant cerebellar ataxia caused by an expanded polyglutamine in TATA-binding protein. *Hum Mol Genet*. 2001;10(14):1441–1448.

161. Brashear A, Mink JW, Hill DF, et al. ATP1A3 mutations in infants: a new rapid-onset dystonia-Parkinsonism phenotype characterized by motor delay and ataxia. *Dev Med Child Neurol*. 2012;54(11):1065–1067.

162. Goldberg-Stern H, Weitz R, Zaizov R, Gornish M, Gadoth N. Progressive spinocerebellar degeneration "plus" associated with Langerhans cell histiocytosis: a new paraneoplastic syndrome? *J Neurol Neurosurg Psychiatry.* 1995;58(2):180–183.

163. van der Knaap MS, Arts WFM, Garbern JY, et al. Cerebellar leukoencephalopathy: most likely histiocytosis-related. *Neurology.* 2008;71(17):1361–1367.

164. Martin-Duverneuil N, Idbaih A, Hoang-Xuan K, et al. MRI features of neurodegenerative Langerhans cell histiocytosis. *Eur Radiol.* 2006;16(9):2074–2082.

165. Imashuku S, Okazaki NA, Nakayama M, et al. Treatment of neurodegenerative CNS disease in Langerhans cell histiocytosis with a combination of intravenous immunoglobulin and chemotherapy. *Pediatr Blood Cancer.* 2008;50(2):308–311.

166. van der Knaap MS, Pronk JC, Scheper GC. Vanishing white matter disease. *Lancet Neurol.* 2006;5(5):413–423.

Parkinsonism

Harvey S. Singer[1], Jonathan W. Mink[2], Donald L. Gilbert[3] and Joseph Jankovic[4]

[1]Department of Neurology, Johns Hopkins Hospital, Baltimore, MD, USA;
[2]Division of Child Neurology, University of Rochester Medical Center, Rochester, NY, USA; [3]Division of Neurology, Cincinnati Children's Hospital Medical Center, Cincinnati, OH, USA; [4]Department of Neurology, Baylor College of Medicine, Houston, TX, USA

O U T L I N E

Movement Disorders in Childhood, Second Edition.
DOI: http://dx.doi.org/10.1016/B978-0-12-411573-6.00015-2

INTRODUCTION

Parkinsonism is a constellation of signs and symptoms that are characteristically observed in Parkinson's disease (PD), but that are not necessarily due to PD. Parkinsonism is the primary type of hypokinetic movement disorder. It is sometimes referred to as the hypokinetic-rigid syndrome or akinetic-rigid syndrome. As discussed elsewhere in this text, hyperkinetic movement disorders are far more common in children than is parkinsonism. Parkinsonism can arise from many different causes in children, including juvenile-onset PD. However, true juvenile-onset PD is quite rare. Parkinsonism may be seen in isolation or in conjunction with other neurologic signs or symptoms.

CLINICAL FEATURES OF PARKINSONISM

Parkinsonism is usually defined by the presence of two or more of the cardinal signs of PD. These signs are tremor at rest, bradykinesia (or akinesia), rigidity, and postural instability.[1] *Rest tremor* is rare in childhood parkinsonism. It is more likely to be seen in juvenile PD (JPD) or drug-induced parkinsonism than in parkinsonism due to other causes. When present, the tremor is typically in the frequency range of 4–6 Hz, and is most prominent at rest but may reemerge with sustained posture. *Bradykinesia* is slowness of movement that is not due to weakness or ataxia. Parkinsonian bradykinesia is commonly accompanied by progressive reduction of movement amplitude with repeated rhythmic movements, such as finger tapping or pronation and supination of the forearm. There may also be *akinesia*, with paucity of movement, reduced spontaneous movements, in some cases the inability to move at all (freezing). Akinesia commonly manifests as diminished spontaneous facial expression (masking or hypomimia), soft speech (hypophonia), and reduced arm-swing during walking. Parkinsonian *rigidity* is increased muscle tone that is equal in all directions of movement, does not increase with increased velocity of passive movement, and does not have a particular preferred posture.[2] Rigidity may have a "lead pipe" quality, in which the limb can be moved with difficulty into arbitrary postures, but, once placed in a posture, will remain there against gravity. If there is superimposed tremor, the rigidity can feel ratchety, like a cog-wheel. It is important to note that "cog-wheeling" is due to underlying tremor and is not a required feature of parkinsonian rigidity. *Postural instability* manifests as increased likelihood of falling and is due to dysregulation of postural reflexes. Clinically, it is evaluated with the "pull-test" in which the patient stands, facing away from the examiner with feet apart at shoulder width. The examiner gives a gentle pull backward at the shoulders bilaterally. A normal individual may take a step backward, but an individual with parkinsonian postural instability will take many steps backward (retropulsion) or may fall backward with no attempt to compensate.

PATHOPHYSIOLOGY OF PARKINSONISM

Adult-onset idiopathic PD is associated with the loss of nigrostriatal dopamine neurons.[3] However, lesions involving nigrostriatal dopamine neurons, the nigrostriatal pathway, the striatum, or other components of the basal ganglia-thalamocortical circuitry can all result in parkinsonism (Chapter 1).[4–6] It has been suggested that parkinsonism results from excessive or disordered inhibitory output from the internal globus pallidus (GPi) and substantia nigra pars reticulata (SNpr), regardless of cause.[5,7–9] Other conditions that are associated with decreased efficacy of nigrostriatal dopamine neurotransmission, including dopamine depleting or blocking medications and inborn errors of dopamine synthesis, can also cause parkinsonism. The pathogenesis of individual disorders causing parkinsonism will be discussed in the context of those specific disorders later in this chapter. It does appear that there may be a common pathophysiology of the cardinal signs of parkinsonism, regardless of specific cause. Almost all data on the pathophysiology of parkinsonism comes from studies in adult patients or nonhuman primate models, but the principles are likely to apply to parkinsonism in children.

Tremor

The pathophysiology of tremor in PD is poorly understood. It is generally agreed that parkinsonian tremor is largely due to central tremor generators, possibly located in the thalamus.[10,11] There is evidence that peripheral afferent activity can modulate and even entrain tremor in PD.[11] However, parkinsonian tremor persists after deafferentation[12] and has been shown to persist without frequency change in wrist flexors after complete radial nerve palsy.[13] Thus, although there may be some modulation of PD tremor by muscle afferent activity, central mechanisms are critical for its production. It has long been known that thalamotomy, particularly of the ventral intermediate nucleus (VIM) is effective in reducing or eliminating parkinsonian tremor.[14] Abnormal oscillatory neuronal activity has been recorded in VIM, subthalamic nucleus (STN), and GPi of parkinsonian subjects.[14–16] However, the oscillatory rate of STN and GPi neurons is twice that of the tremor and VIM neurons, more reliably correlates with parkinsonian tremor.[16] Interestingly, the VIM nucleus is thought to be the site of cerebellar rather than basal ganglia input to the thalamus. It is not known to what degree cerebellar mechanisms might be involved in PD tremor, but it has been suggested that tremor results from downstream mechanisms that attempt to compensate for basal ganglia dysfunction in PD.[16] The fundamental mechanisms causing tremor in PD continue to be investigated in PD and in primate models.

Bradykinesia

Bradykinesia is a hallmark of parkinsonism. However, it should be noted that voluntary movements are slow in almost any disease that affects the motor system. What distinguishes the different conditions is the quality of the impairment. In PD, there is slowness and reduced amplitude of individual movements that typically worsen as movements proceed. The classic example of this is the micrographia of PD where handwriting can be near normal at the beginning of a line, but the size of letters and velocity of strokes decreases as the writing continues. The slowness of movement in parkinsonism has been associated with reduced magnitude of agonist muscle activity during movement.[17] The reduced agonist amplitude often results in a succession of multiple small amplitude submovements instead of a larger amplitude single movement. In addition to decreased agonist activation, there is often excessive cocontraction of the antagonist during movement[18] and muscular cocontraction at rest.[19] This abnormal cocontraction can combine with the abnormally reduced contraction of the agonist to cause slowing of movement. People with parkinsonism are often more impaired when relaxing muscles to reduce force than when activating muscles to generate force.[20–22] Thus, an inability to "turn off" the antagonist may be more impaired than the ability to "turn on" the agonist.

It has also been suggested that individuals with PD have more difficulty performing sequences of movements than individual movements.[23–25] When subjects with PD disease performed a task involving a grasp and elbow flexion separately, simultaneously, or sequentially, they were slower than normal in all conditions. However, they were slower on simultaneous and sequential movements than they were on the individual components.[23,24] Subjects with PD are equally slow when they draw the sides of a pentagon sequentially as when they repeatedly draw one side five times, suggesting that there is progressive slowing of movement with repetition, but not a specific sequencing deficit.[26] Despite the evidence that sequential movements are more impaired in PD, even single stimulus-triggered movement is slow.[17,27] This suggests that the fundamental deficit in PD is not one of sequencing, but that sequential or repetitive movements may exacerbate the deficit.

Akinesia

The paucity of movement and "freezing" in parkinsonism has been attributed to a defect of movement initiation. Indeed some, but not all, people with PD do have prolonged reaction times in stimulus-triggered movements, suggesting that in some cases there is delayed initiation of movement.[27] However, it is not clear that the delayed initiation is due to basal ganglia dysfunction. Instead, the delayed initiation may be due to the loss of dopamine input to prefrontal, premotor, or motor cortex.[28–30] Animals with a focal lesions of the dopamine input to prefrontal cortex have prolonged reaction times,[31] but animals with lesions of the basal ganglia output (GPi or SNpr) usually do not.[5]

It is also possible that the prolonged reaction time in PD is not due to dysfunction of movement initiatory systems. Muscle activity may begin at the normal time in relation to movement, but the magnitude of the initial muscle activity may not be sufficient to overcome inertial and viscoelastic forces rapidly[27] and the mechanically detected onset of movement is delayed. Alternatively, an inability to inhibit unwanted postural reflexes may delay the onset of movement due to competition of antagonistic motor mechanisms. In either case, the initiatory commands may be normal, but other factors cause the onset of movement to be delayed.

Rigidity

People with PD have increased resistance to passive muscle stretch. It is not known if this clinical sign reflects mechanisms that interfere with movement, since bradykinesia and rigidity can vary independently. However, stiffness and an inability to completely relax are common complaints in PD. The rigidity of PD has been attributed in part to hyperactivity of long-latency (transcortical) stretch reflexes.[19,32,33] The monosynaptic stretch reflex is normal in PD.

Postural Instability

People with PD have an inability to inhibit long-latency reflexes other than the trans-cortical stretch reflex. Although it is often stated that PD is accompanied by a "loss of pos-tural reflexes," it appears that there is inability to *inhibit* long-latency postural reflexes that accounts for the postural instability of PD. When normal subjects are subjected to a per-turbation in the anterior-posterior dimension while standing, they have a stereotyped pat-tern of muscle activity in the legs and trunk that maintains upright stance. If they then sit down and are subjected to the same perturbation, this activity no longer occurs. By contrast, patients with PD have an inappropriate cocontraction of leg and back muscles in response to perturbation from upright stance. When the same subjects are subjected to a perturbation in a sitting position, they continue to have the same pattern of muscle activity. Thus, they are not able to inhibit appropriately the postural reflexes that were active during stance.[34] These data, together with the proposed mechanism of rigidity (see above) and the fact that so-called "primitive reflexes" are abnormally active in PD,[35] suggest that there may be an inability to suppress unwanted reflex activity generally.

ETIOLOGIES OF PARKINSONISM IN CHILDREN

In children, parkinsonism can be a manifestation of many different disorders.[36] It is often associated with a dopaminergic deficit, and since dopaminergic deficits can produce dystonia in children, dystonia may be present as well.[37] Most causes of parkinsonism in children are disorders that cause parkinsonism in addition to other signs and symptoms. Parkinsonism beginning in infancy is usually due to a defect in dopamine production, transport, or metabo-lism.[38] Primary parkinsonism in children is rare, but recognition of these entities is important. In discussion of the etiologies of parkinsonism in children, primary causes or JPD will be con-sidered first followed by important secondary causes of parkinsonism. Treatment of parkin-sonism will be discussed in a section following delineation of the etiologies.

Juvenile Parkinson Disease

JPD typically presents with leg dystonia in younger children and bradykinesia and rigid-ity in older children. Tremor is less common in JPD than in adult PD. It should be noted that disorders causing JPD may not present until adulthood, so unlike many other movement disorders of children, childhood-onset is not defining. Table 15.2 lists genetic loci associated with "young-onset" forms of PD.

PARK2

The most common cause of autosomal recessive young-onset PD is *PARK2*, due to muta-tions in the *parkin* gene, located on chromosome 6q25.2-27.[39,40] In 12 Japanese families, the mean age at onset was 27 years, with a range from 9 to 43.[41] The most prominent symp-toms were retropulsion, dystonia of the feet, and classic parkinsonism. Symptoms of tremor, rigidity, and bradykinesia were mild. There was good symptomatic benefit from levodopa but dopa-induced dyskinesias and wearing-off phenomena occurred relatively early in the disease course. Lohmann et al.[42] compared 146 PD patients with parkin mutations to 250 PD patients without parkin mutations. Patients with parkin mutations had an earlier and more symmetric onset, a slower progression of disease, and had greater response to L-dopa at lower doses. Age at onset in the parkin group was 7–70 years. In families with autosomal recessive parkinsonism, more than 80% of patients with age at onset of 20 years or younger had parkin mutations.[42] Heterozygous mutations in the parkin gene have been identified in some patients with later onset disease, raising the possibility that heterozygous mutations may confer increased susceptibility to the disease.[43]

The pathology of parkin-associated PD does not show Lewy bodies, the pathological hallmark of adult-onset idiopathic PD, although there is neuronal loss and neurofibrillary tangles. Fluorodopa PET scanning shows decreased uptake, indicating a presynaptic abnormality consistent with degeneration of the nigrostriatal pathways.[44,45] It has been hypothesized that parkin interacts with alpha-synuclein such that parkin normally ubiquitinates alpha-synuclein and this process is defective in parkin mutations. This leads to pathologic accumulation of a non-ubiquitinated, glycosylated form of alpha-synuclein.[46] Indeed, it appears that parkin interacts with the other proteins implicated in young-onset PD, *PINK1* and *DJ1* (see below), to form a ubiquitin E3 ligase complex that promotes ubiquitination and degradation of Parkin substrates, including Parkin itself.[47] Thus, mutations in any of these three genes may influence the same biochemical pathway.

PARK6

Mutations in a PTEN-induced kinase (*PINK1; PARK6*) with autosomal-recessive early-onset PD.[48] The age at onset for this disorder is typically young adulthood. To date, no cases have been reported to start during childhood or early adolescence.

PARK7

DJ1 mutations (*PARK7*) are associated with onset of symptoms before age 40 years with rest tremor, postural tremor, bradykinesia, postural instability, and asymmetric onset.[49,50] No cases of childhood or early adolescent onset have been reported to date.

Autosomal recessive PD due to *PARK2* (parkin) mutations is substantially more common than *PARK6* or *PARK7* in several populations.[51,52] PINK1, DJ1, and parkin appear to interact functionally,[47] as noted above.

PARK19

Autosomal recessive juvenile parkinsonism has been described in two families with mutation in *DNAJC6* (*PARK19*), which codes for the auxilin protein which is involved in clatharin-mediated exocytosis. In an Arab Palestinian family, two brothers developed parkinsonism at ages 7 and 11 years.[53] Both had normal development prior to the onset of parkinsonism. The parkinsonism included bradykinesia, rigidity, postural instability, and asymmetric rest tremor. Disease progression led to loss of independent ambulation within 10 years, but cognition remained intact. Treatment with levodopa was ineffective. Four patients were also reported from a Turkish family with onset of parkinsonism around 10 years of age.[54] The parkinsonism was similar to that described in the Palestinian family. However, the affected individuals from the Turkish family had mild to moderate intellectual disability. Three of the four patients had absence and generalize tonic-clonic seizures staring in the first 5 years of life and that were well-controlled with medications. These individuals had benefit from levodopa, but developed severe dose-limited side effects.

SECONDARY PARKINSONISM

Secondary causes of parkinsonism in children include a wide variety of disorders (see Tables 15.1 and 15.2). In most of these disorders, parkinsonism is accompanied by other neurological signs and symptoms and this diagnosis is guided by the constellation of manifestations. However, in some disorders, parkinsonism can be the dominant feature or seen in association only with dystonia, a common accompaniment of parkinsonism. Some of these disorders have been assigned PARK*n* designations, but are discussed in the section due to the presence of other neurologic manifestations in addition to parkinsonism.

Structural Lesions

Parkinsonism can result from infarcts or other structural lesions, primarily those that affect the basal ganglia or their connections.[4] Parkinsonism has been reported in association

TABLE 15.1   Etiologies of Parkinsonism in Children

Structural	Infectious/Parainfectious
Stroke	Encephalitis lethargica
Brain tumor	Viral encephalitis
Hydrocephalus	Mycoplasma
Hereditary/Degenerative (see also Chapter 17)	*Metabolic*
JPD	Dopa-responsive dystonia
HD (Westphal variant)	ALAAD deficiency
PKAN	Rapid-onset dystonia-parkinsonism
Rett syndrome	Primary familial brain calcification
Niemann–Pick Type C	*Drugs/Toxins* (Chapter 22)
Juvenile NCL (*CLN3*)	Antipsychotics
Neuronal intranuclear inclusion disease	Antiemetics
Kufor–Rakeb syndrome (*PARK9*)	Dopamine depletors
Pallido-pyramidal syndrome	Isoniazid
Neurodegeneration with brain iron accumulation (*PLA2G6*; *C19orf12*)	Calcium channel blockers
	Meperidine
	Chemotherapy

TABLE 15.2 Genetic Loci for Juvenile Parkinsonism

Designation	Alternative name	Inheritance	Gene locus	Gene	Protein
PARK2	JPD	Autosomal recessive	6q25.2-27	*PRKN*	Parkin
PARK6	*PINK1* early-onset PD	Autosomal recessive	1p36.12	*PINK1*	PTEN-induced putative kinase 1
PARK7	DJ1 early-onset PD	Autosomal recessive	1p36.23	*DJ1*	DJ1 protein
PARK9	Kufor–Rakeb syndrome	Autosomal recessive	1p36.13	*ATP13A2*	Lysosomal type 5 ATPase
PARK14	Dystonia-parkinsonism; neurodegeneration with brain iron accumulation	Autosomal recessive	22q13.1	*PLA2G6*	Phospholipase A2, calcium-independent, group VI
PARK15	Parkinsonian-pyramidal syndrome	Autosomal recessive	22q12.3	*FBXO7*	F-box protein 7
PARK19	DNAJC6 juvenile-onset PD	Autosomal recessive	1p31.3	*DNAJC6*	Auxilin

with brain tumors,[55,56] including gliomatosis cerebri.[57] Parkinsonism has been reported following cranial radiation treatment of a brain tumor in an adolescent.[58] Parkinsonism has been reported as a presenting sign in hydrocephalus[59] or as a result of shunt malfunction.[60] Parkinsonism due to hydrocephalus can be dopa-responsive.[59,60]

Hereditary/Degenerative Diseases

Many of the hereditary degenerative disorders that produce parkinsonism are discussed in Chapter 17.

Huntington Disease

Huntington disease (HD) is an autosomal dominant, caused by a trinucleotide repeat expansion of the IT-15 gene on chromosome 4.[61] This neurodegenerative disorder is characterized by a combination of dystonia, chorea, myoclonus, behavioral abnormalities, ataxia, and ultimately dementia. When HD begins in childhood, the typical presentation is parkinsonism or dystonia, and not chorea (Video 15.1). This has been referred to as the Westphal variant of HD.[62,63] The age at onset is earlier for children with a higher number of repeats.[64] There tends to be amplification of the number of repeats, particularly when it is transmitted from father to child, and therefore most cases of juvenile HD are inherited from the father and involve repeat lengths that are significantly higher than those seen in adults.

Diagnosis is based upon identification of the trinucleotide repeat sequence. Although at least 38 repeats are usually required for the occurrence of symptoms in adults, a larger number of repeats typically over 60 would be expected when symptoms present in childhood.[62,64] Magnetic resonance imaging (MRI) shows atrophy of the caudate heads and, in later stages, generalized cerebral and cerebellar atrophy.

In teenagers, the initial presentation of HD may be with psychiatric illness, and in particular, major depression may be the presenting symptom.[65] Dystonia, myoclonus, or chorea usually supervenes later (Videos 15.2, 15.3, 15.4). The pathology includes basal ganglia, cerebellar, and cortical degeneration.[66–68] In children, there may be a relatively symmetric loss of both D1-bearing and D2-bearing medium spiny neurons which could account for the primarily dystonic and parkinsonian rather than choreatic presentation.[69,70]

Treatment of parkinsonism due to HD can be difficult. However, in many cases, the parkinsonism responds to levodopa.[71] Prognosis is poor for childhood-onset HD, and the movement disorder is expected to worsen progressively over the years following diagnosis. Life expectancy depends upon the severity of symptoms and the number of repeats, but typically children will survive 10–15 years from the time of diagnosis.

Rett Syndrome

Rett syndrome is discussed in Chapter 8. The characteristic movement disorder of Rett syndrome is stereotypies. However, many girls with Rett develop parkinsonism as the disorder progresses.[72] Imaging studies have shown mild reduction of fluorodopa uptake and of dopamine D2-receptor binding.[73] Parkinsonism associated with Rett syndrome usually does not respond to levodopa or dopamine agonists, suggesting a post-synaptic defect.[72]

Neuronal Intranuclear Inclusion Disease

Neuronal intranuclear inclusion disease (NIID) is a rare neurodegenerative disorder with a heterogeneous clinical picture that variably includes parkinsonism, behavioral changes, abnormal eye movements including oculogyric crises, ataxia, pyramidal tract signs, and motor neuron signs. It can present as juvenile parkinsonism[74] or dopa-responsive dystonia.[75] It is characterized by the presence of eosinophilic intranuclear inclusions in neuronal and glial cells,[76] and is diagnosed during life by demonstrating these in a full thickness rectal biopsy or skin biopsy. The age at onset is between 3 and 12 years. Initial symptoms typically include slow cognitive and behavioral decline with mood alteration.[77] Patients with NIID have benefit from levodopa, but may develop substantial dopa-induced dyskinesia early in the treatment course. Deep brain stimulation of the STN may provide some benefit.[78]

Pallido-Pyramidal Syndrome

This syndrome was initially described by Davison who reported 5 patients with juvenile-onset parkinsonism and pyramidal tract signs. In one case, lesions of the pallidum, ansa lenticularis, substantia nigra, and pyramidal tract were described on neuropathology.[79] The clinical phenotype consists of an autosomal recessive, juvenile-onset, progressive parkinsonism with hyperreflexia, spasticity, Babinski signs, and is slowly progressive. This disorder has been associated with mutations in the FBXO7 gene.[80–82] Some individuals have psychiatric symptoms. Response to levodopa is variable, ranging from marked and sustained to moderate and unpredictable. FBXO7 codes for an F-box protein which is thought to be a component of an E3 ubiquitin ligase.[83] It has been proposed that pallido-pyramidal syndrome is more appropriately called "parkinsonism-pyramidal syndrome"[81]; it has been designated as PARK15.

Another form of pallido-pyramidal syndrome has been associated with mutations in C19orf12.[84,85] This disorder is associated with iron deposition in the brain and has been classified as NBIA4. It has also been called mitochondrial membrane protein-associated neurodegeneration. The age at onset ranges from 4 to 30 years (mean 11 years). Most patients present with gait problems and visual impairment due to optic atrophy. They develop progressive weakness and spasticity, and later in the disease have motor neuron dysfunction. Parkinsonism is prominent in some individuals and has variable response to levodopa.[84] Most patients have prominent behavioral symptoms including inattention, emotional lability, and impulsivity. MRI shows increased iron deposition in the globus pallidus and substantia nigra; many patients have cortical and cerebellar atrophy. Neuropathology on one patient showed widespread Lewy bodies.

C19orf12 is one of growing numbers of syndromes classified as neurodegeneration with brain iron accumulation (NBIA). The first NBIA, previously referred to as Hallervorden-Spatz syndrome is pantothenate kinase associated neurodegeneration (PKAN). Other NBIAs include neuroferritinopathy, infantile neuroaxonal dystrophy, aceruloplasminemia, PLA2G6-associated neurodegeneration (PLAN), and others.[107] In addition to a variety of motor and behavioral features, patients with NBIA have characteristic abnormalities on their brain MRI scans, including the "eye-of-the-tiger" sign and other evidence of iron deposition in the basal ganglia.

Kufor–Rakeb Syndrome

Kufor–Rakeb syndrome (PARK9) was initially described in a consanguineous Jordanian family.[86] The clinical features include autosomal recessive pattern of inheritance, mask-like face, rigidity, and bradykinesia. Tremor was not reported. Spasticity, supranuclear upgaze paresis, and dementia were also reported in most individuals. In addition, facial-faucial-finger mini-myoclonus, visual hallucinations, and oculogyric dystonic spasms have been reported.[87] Age of onset was between 12 and 16 years and symptoms progressed rapidly. MRI scans of the brain showed globus pallidus atrophy and later generalized brain atrophy. In this condition, there is variable but often dramatic improvement, limited to extrapyramidal manifestations, within 48h in all affected subjects in response to levodopa therapy.[86] Over time, the response to L-dopa wanes, with narrowing of the therapeutic window and emergence of peak-dose dyskinesias.[87] Kufor–Rakeb syndrome is caused by loss-of-function mutations in a predominantly neuronal P-type ATPase gene, ATP13A2.[88,89]

PLA2G6-Associated Neurodegeneration with Brain Iron Accumulation

PLA2G6 is the causative gene for infantile neuroaxonal dystrophy and for one form of neurodegeneration associated with brain iron accumulation.[90] More recently, PLA2G6 has been associated with an early-onset dystonia-parkinsonism and has been designated PARK14.[91] Patients with this condition have onset of parkinsonism in adolescence or early adulthood.[91,92] The parkinsonism is accompanied by intellectual or cognitive impairment, psychosis, dystonia, hyperreflexia, or a combination, in most patients. The parkinsonism responds to levodopa, but is rapidly progressive. Brain MRI may show iron deposition. Neuropathology has shown widespread Lewy bodies and tau deposition in both children and adults.[93] In one study of Han Chinese patients from Taiwan, it was found that PLA2G6 mutations were the second most common cause of young-onset parkinsonism, next to *PARK2*.[92]

Infectious and Postinfectious Diseases

Postencephalitic parkinsonism was classically described following the pandemics of encephalitis lethargica in the 1920s.[94] These cases were mostly in adults; the exact cause has not been determined. Parkinsonism has also been described as a consequence of viral encephalitis,[95] mycoplasma pneumonia infection, or following vaccination for measles.[96] In many cases, the parkinsonism responded to levodopa or anticholinergic medications.

Metabolic Diseases

Most metabolic diseases that cause parkinsonism are discussed in Chapter 17. However, Fahr syndrome will be discussed in this chapter.

Fahr Syndrome

Fahr syndrome is characterized by basal ganglia calcification, as well as calcification of other gray matter structures, including cerebellar nuclei and punctate calcifications in thalamus and sometimes cortex.[97,98] This is usually an adult-onset disease, but in some cases can occur in the second decade of life. When it does, it is characterized by microcephaly, hypertonia, and choreoathetosis. However, parkinsonism may be a prominent feature. The etiology is often unknown, but in some cases is due to hypoparathyroidism and therefore parathyroid function should be checked. It is autosomal dominant, with reduced penetrance in most families, and appears to be slowly progressive. Diagnosis is based on evidence of calcification detected by head CT scanning.[97,99,100] Treatment is supportive, unless a specific disorder of parathyroid hormone can be found, in which case specific treatment will be available.

Drug-Induced Parkinsonism

Many medications are known to be able to cause parkinsonism. The most important of these are drugs that block dopamine receptors or impair dopamine synthesis. The most potent dopamine receptor blocking medications are the antipsychotic neuroleptic medications. The older high potency medications such as haloperidol are more likely to cause parkinsonism than the newer atypical antipsychotics. Nonetheless, atypical antipsychotics with even weak dopamine D2 receptor blockade can cause parkinsonism. In addition, some antiemetics can be important causes of parkinsonism with chronic use. Dopamine depletors such as tetrabenazine, reserpine, and alphamethylparatyrosine are not used commonly in children but are well-known to have parkinsonism as a side effect. Chemotherapy agents have been reported to cause parkinsonism in rare cases.[95] Other medication classes that can cause parkinsonism are listed in Table 15.1. Cessation of the medication is usually sufficient to reverse the parkinsonism. A broader discussion of drug-induced movement disorders is contained in Chapter 22.

TREATMENT OF PARKINSONISM

JPD is levodopa-responsive, at least in the early years. It will also respond to anticholinergic medication, dopamine agonists, and inhibitors of dopamine breakdown. However, escalating doses are required, and children typically develop dopa-induced dyskinesia similar to those seen in adults on chronic dopaminergic therapy. It is important to differentiate this disorder from dopa-responsive dystonia as well as other disorders that may respond to dopaminergic medication, since the prognosis is different. Some authors recommend use of dopa-sparing medications, including dopamine agonists or inhibitors of dopamine breakdown, in order to prolong the efficacy and delay in the onset of dyskinesia. However, strong evidence to support this strategy is lacking. No prospective studies of treatment in childhood-onset PD have been reported. Studies in adults have shown that levodopa provides more benefit than dopamine agonists.[6]

Secondary parkinsonisms are variably responsive to medications. Bradykinesia is the primary symptom that is responsive to treatment in childhood parkinsonism. It is usually assumed to be due to dopamine deficiency, and therefore is treated with levodopa or dopamine agonists. Levodopa is combined with a peripheral decarboxylase inhibitor such as carbidopa in order to reduce side effects and increase delivery to the brain. Treatment is often initiated with a single dose of levodopa 1 mg/kg (or 50–100 mg total) given in the morning to evaluate for potential side effects including nausea or postural hypotension. If this dose is tolerated for 3–4 days, then therapeutic treatment can be initiated three times per day. Unless symptoms are present at night the doses are usually given during the daytime to maximize effect. Dosage can be increased to a maximum of 10–15 mg/kg/day depending on effectiveness. In addition to nausea and hypotension, common side effects can include dystonia, agitation, sleeplessness, and behavior changes. The dosage must be adjusted gradually in order to find the optimal dose, and the optimal dose may change as the child grows. Additional carbidopa may be given to decrease nausea.

In adults and children with PD, long-term treatment with dopamine or dopamine agonists will eventually lead to dyskinesias and freezing episodes that can limit its use. Some authors have advocated "dopamine sparing" strategies that involve the early use of dopamine agonists such as pramipexole, ropinirole, or dopamine breakdown inhibitors such as entacapone or selegeline.[101] This approach remains controversial and it has not been studied in children.

Amantadine may be used to treat dyskinesias associated with acute or chronic use of levodopa,[102] and it has some antiparkinsonian effects as well.[103,104] Anticholinergic medication will improve parkinsonism, but it is more commonly used to treat associated dystonia. Deep-brain stimulation in the GPi or STN has met with tremendous success in ameliorating symptoms of adult PD.[105,106] Whether similar neurosurgical procedures would be effective in children is not known.

Failure of dopaminergic transmission can be divided into presynaptic and postsynaptic forms. In presynaptic failure, there is reduced production or release of dopamine at nigrostriatal nerve terminals. This is typical in JPD and dopa-responsive dystonia. In postsynaptic failure, there is injury to the striatal targets. This is typical following encephalitis or hypoxic injury. Treatment with dopaminergic medication is most successful when there is presynaptic failure. If injury is primarily postsynaptic, there may be some mild benefit from dopaminergic medication, but the effect will be limited.

References

1. Jankovic J. Parkinson's disease: clinical features and diagnosis. *J Neurol Neurosurg Psychiatry*. 2008; 79(4):368–376.
2. Sanger TD, Delgado MR, Gaebler-Spira D, Hallett M, Mink JW. Classification and definition of disorders causing hypertonia in childhood. *Pediatrics*. 2003;111(1):e89–e97.
3. Ehringer H, Hornykiewicz O. Verteilung von noradrenalin und dopamin (3-hydroxytyramin) in gehirn des menschen und ihr verhalten bei erkrankungen des extrapyramidalen systems. *Klin Wochsenshr*. 1960;39:1236–1239.
4. Bhatia KP, Marsden CD. The behavioural and motor consequences of focal lesions of the basal ganglia in man. *Brain*. 1994;117:859–876.
5. Mink JW. The basal ganglia: focused selection and inhibition of competing motor programs. *Prog Neurobiol*. 1996;50:381–425.
6. Nutt JG, Wooten GF. Diagnosis and initial management of Parkinson's disease. *N Engl J Med*. 2005;353(10):1021–1027.
7. DeLong MR. Primate models of movement disorders of basal ganglia origin. *Trends Neurosci*. 1990;13:281–285.
8. Wichmann T, DeLong M. Physiology of the basal ganglia and pathophysiology of movement disorders of basal ganglia origin. In: Watts R, Koller W, eds. *Movement Disorders: Neurologic Principles and Practice*. New York, NY: McGraw-Hill; 1997:87–97.
9. Wichmann T, DeLong MR. Functional and pathophysiological models of the basal ganglia. *Curr Opin Neurobiol*. 1996;6:751–758.
10. Pare D, Curro'Dossi R, Steriade M. Neuronal basis of the parkinsonian resting tremor: a hypothesis and its implications for treatment. *Neuroscience*. 1990;35:217–226.
11. Rack PMH, Ross HF. The role of reflexes in the resting tremor of Parkinson's disease. *Brain*. 1986;109:115–141.
12. Foerster O. Resection of the posterior roots of spinal cord. *Lancet*. 1911;2:76–79.
13. Pullman SL, Elibol B, Fahn S. Modulation of parkinsonian tremor by radial nerve palsy. *Neurology*. 1994;44(10):1861–1864.
14. Benabid AL, Pollak P, Gao D, et al. Chronic electrical stimulation of the ventralis intermedius nucleus of the thalamus as a treatment of movement disorders. *J Neurosurg*. 1996;84(2):203–214.
15. Lenz FA, Tasker RR, Kwan HC, et al. Single unit analysis of the human ventral thalamic nuclear group: correlation of thalamic "tremor cells" with the 3–6 Hz component of parkinsonian tremor. *J Neurosci*. 1988;8(3):754–764.
16. Rosin B, Nevet A, Elias S, Rivlin-Etzion M, Israel Z, Bergman H. Physiology and pathophysiology of the basal ganglia-thalamo-cortical networks. *Parkinsonism Relat Disord*. 2007;13(suppl 3):S437–S439.
17. Hallett M, Khoshbin S. A physiological mechanism of bradykinesia. *Brain*. 1980;103:301–314.
18. Hayashi A, Kagamihara Y, Nakajima Y, Narabayashi H, Okuma Y, Tanaka R. Disorder in reciprocal innervation upon initiation of voluntary movement in patients with Parkinson's disease. *Exp Brain Res*. 1988;70:437–440.
19. Berardelli A, Sabra AF, Hallett M. Physiological mechanisms of rigidity in Parkinson's disease. *J Neurol Neurosurg Psychiatr*. 1983;46:45–53.
20. Corcos DM, Chen C-M, Quinn NP, McAuley J, Rothwell JC. Strength in Parkinson's disease: relationship to rate of force generation and clinical status. *Ann Neurol*. 1996;39:79–88.
21. Kunesch E, Schnitzler A, Tyercha C, Knecht S, Stelmach G. Altered force release control in Parkinson's disease. *Behav Brain Res*. 1995;67:43–49.
22. Wing AM. A comparison of the rate of pinch grip force increases and decreases in Parkinsonian bradykinesia. *Neuropsychologia*. 1988;26(3):479–482.
23. Benecke R, Rothwell JC, Dick JPR, Day BL, Marsden CD. Performance of simultaneous movements in patients with Parkinson's disease. *Brain*. 1986;109:739–757.
24. Benecke R, Rothwell JC, Dick JPR, Day BL, Marsden CD. Simple and complex movements off and on treatment in patients with Parkinson's disease. *J Neurol Neurosurg Psychiatr*. 1987;50:296–303.
25. Roy EA, Saint-Cyr J, Taylor A, Lang A. Movement sequencing disorders in Parkinson's disease. *Int J Neurosci*. 1993;73:183–194.
26. Agostino R, Berardelli A, Formica A, Stocchi F, Accornero N, Manfredi M. Analysis of repetitive and nonrepetitive sequential arm movements in patients with Parkinson's disease. *Mov Disord*. 1994;9(3):311–314.
27. Evarts EV, Teravainen H, Calne DB. Reaction time in Parkinson's disease. *Brain*. 1981;104:167–186.

28. Gaspar P, Duyckaerts C, Alvarez C, Javoy-Agid F, Berger B. Alterations of dopaminergic and noradrenergic innervations in motor cortex in Parkinson's disease. *Ann Neurol*. 1991;30:365–374.

29. Gaspar P, Stepniewski I, Kaas JH. Topography and collateralization of the dopaminergic projections to motor and lateral prefrontal cortex in owl monkeys. *J Comp Neurol*. 1992;325:1–21.

30. Sawaguchi T, Goldman-Rakic PS. The role of D1-dopamine receptor in working memory: local injections of dopamine antagonists into the prefrontal cortex of rhesus monkeys performing and oculomotor delayed response task. *J Neurophysiol*. 1994;71(2):515–528.

31. Hauber W, Bubser M, Schmidt WJ. 6-Hydroxydopamine lesion of the rat prefrontal cortex impairs motor initiation but not motor execution. *Exp Brain Res*. 1994;99(3):524–528.

32. Rothwell JC, Obeso JA, Traub MM, Marsden CD. The behavior of the long-latency stretch reflex in patients with Parkinson's disease. *J Neurol Neurosurg Psychiatr*. 1983;46:35–44.

33. Tatton WG, Lee RG. Evidence for abnormal long-loop reflexes in rigid Parkinsonian patients. *Brain Res*. 1975;100:671–676.

34. Horak FB, Nutt JG, Nashner LM. Postural inflexibility in Parkinsonian subjects. *J Neurol Sci*. 1992;111:46–58.

35. Vreeling FW, Verhey FRJ, Houx PJ, Jolles J. Primitive reflexes in Parkinson's disease. *J Neurol Neurosurg Psychiatr*. 1993;56:1323–1326.

36. Riederer P, Foley P. Mini-review: multiple developmental forms of parkinsonism. The basis for further research as to the pathogenesis of parkinsonism. *J Neural Transm*. 2002;109(12):1469–1475.

37. Yokochi M. Development of the nosological analysis of juvenile parkinsonism. *Brain Dev*. 2000;22(suppl 1):S81–S86.

38. Garcia-Cazorla A, Ortez C, Perez-Duenas B, et al. Hypokinetic-rigid syndrome in children and inborn errors of metabolism. *Eur J Paediatr Neurol*. 2011;15(4):295–302.

39. Ruiz-Linares A. Juvenile Parkinson disease and the C212Y mutation of parkin. *Arch Neurol*. 2004;61(3):444. [author reply 444].

40. Huynh DP, Scoles DR, Nguyen D, Pulst SM. The autosomal recessive juvenile Parkinson disease gene product, parkin, interacts with and ubiquitinates synaptotagmin XI. *Hum Mol Genet*. 2003;12(20):2587–2597.

41. Ishikawa A, Tsuji S. Clinical analysis of 17 patients in 12 Japanese families with autosomal-recessive type juvenile parkinsonism. *Neurology*. 1996;47:160–166.

42. Lohmann E, Periquet M, Bonifati V, et al. How much phenotypic variation can be attributed to parkin genotype? *Ann Neurol*. 2003;54(2):176–185.

43. Wang Y, Clark LN, Louis ED, et al. Risk of Parkinson disease in carriers of parkin mutations: estimation using the kin-cohort method. *Arch Neurol*. 2008;65(4):467–474.

44. Khan NL, Valente EM, Bentivoglio AR, et al. Clinical and subclinical dopaminergic dysfunction in PARK6-linked parkinsonism: an 18F-dopa PET study. *Ann Neurol*. 2002;52(6):849–853.

45. Pal PK, Leung J, Hedrich K, et al. [18F]-Dopa positron emission tomography imaging in early-stage, non-parkin juvenile parkinsonism. *Mov Disord*. 2002;17(4):789–794.

46. Shimura H, Schlossmacher MG, Hattori N, et al. Ubiquitination of a new form of alpha-synuclein by parkin from human brain: implications for Parkinson's disease. *Science*. 2001;293(5528):263–269.

47. Xiong H, Wang D, Chen L, et al. Parkin, PINK1, and DJ-1 form a ubiquitin E3 ligase complex promoting unfolded protein degradation. *J Clin Invest*. 2009;119(3):650–660.

48. Albanese A, Valente EM, Romito LM, Bellacchio E, Elia AE, Dallapiccola B. The PINK1 phenotype can be indistinguishable from idiopathic Parkinson disease. *Neurology*. 2005;64(11):1958–1960.

49. Abou-Sleiman PM, Healy DG, Quinn N, Lees AJ, Wood NW. The role of pathogenic DJ-1 mutations in Parkinson's disease. *Ann Neurol*. 2003;54:283–286.

50. van Duijn CM, Dekker MCJ, Bonifati V, et al. PARK7, a novel locus for autosomal recessive early-onset parkinsonism, on chromosome 1p36. *Am J Hum Genet*. 2001;69:629–634.

51. Ghazavi F, Fazlali Z, Banihosseini SS, et al. PRKN, DJ-1, and PINK1 screening identifies novel splice site mutation in PRKN and two novel DJ-1 mutations. *Mov Disord*. 2011;26(1):80–89.

52. Lohmann E, Dursun B, Lesage S, et al. Genetic bases and phenotypes of autosomal recessive Parkinson disease in a Turkish population. *Eur J Neurol*. 2012;19(5):769–775.

53. Edvardson S, Cinnamon Y, Ta-Shma A, et al. A deleterious mutation in DNAJC6 encoding the neuronal-specific clathrin-uncoating co-chaperone auxilin, is associated with juvenile parkinsonism. *PLoS One*. 2012;7(5):e36458.

54. Koroglu C, Baysal L, Cetinkaya M, Karasoy H, Tolun A. DNAJC6 is responsible for juvenile parkinsonism with phenotypic variability. *Parkinsonism Relat Disord*. 2013;19(3):320–324.

55. Krauss JK, Paduch T, Mundinger F, Seeger W. Parkinsonism and rest tremor secondary to supratentorial tumours sparing the basal ganglia. *Acta Neurochir (Wien)*. 1995;133(1–2):22–29.

56. Yoshimura M, Yamamoto T, Iso-o N, et al. Hemiparkinsonism associated with a mesencephalic tumor. *J Neurol Sci*. 2002;197(1–2):89–92.

57. Jang W, Ha SH, Khang SK, Kim J, Kim SH, Kim HJ. Juvenile parkinsonism as an initial manifestation of gliomatosis cerebri. *J Neurol*. 2013;260(12):3161–3163.

58. Voermans NC, Bloem BR, Janssens G, Vogel WV, Sie LT. Secondary parkinsonism in childhood: a rare complication after radiotherapy. *Pediatr Neurol*. 2006;34(6):495–498.

59. Curran T, Lang AE. Parkinsonian syndromes associated with hydrocephalus: case reports, a review of the literature, and pathophysiological hypotheses. *Mov Disord*. 1994;9(5):508–520.

60. Racette BA, Esper GJ, Antenor J, et al. Pathophysiology of parkinsonism due to hydrocephalus. *J Neurol Neurosurg Psychiatry*. 2004;75(11):1617–1619.

61. Li SH, Schilling G, Young 3rd WS, et al. Huntington's disease gene (IT15) is widely expressed in human and rat tissues. *Neuron*. 1993;11(5):985–993.

62. Quinn N, Schrag A. Huntington's disease and other choreas. *J Neurol*. 1998;245(11):709–716.

63. Topper R, Schwarz M, Lange HW, Hefter H, Noth J. Neurophysiological abnormalities in the Westphal variant of Huntington's disease. *Mov Disord*. 1998;13(6):920–928.

64. Langbehn DR, Brinkman RR, Falush D, Paulsen JS, Hayden MR. A new model for prediction of the age of onset and penetrance for Huntington's disease based on CAG length. *Clin Genet*. 2004;65(4):267–277.

65. Tost H, Wendt CS, Schmitt A, Heinz A, Braus DF. Huntington's disease: phenomenological diversity of a neuropsychiatric condition that challenges traditional concepts in neurology and psychiatry. *Am J Psychiatry*. 2004;161(1):28–34.

66. Vonsattel JP, Myers RH, Stevens TJ, Ferrante RJ, Bird ED, Richardson Jr. EP. Neuropathological classification of Huntington's disease. *J Neuropathol Exp Neurol*. 1985;44(6):559–577.

67. de la Monte SM, Vonsattel JP, Richardson Jr. EP. Morphometric demonstration of atrophic changes in the cerebral cortex, white matter, and neostriatum in Huntington's disease. *J Neuropathol Exp Neurol*. 1988;47(5):516–525.

68. Myers RH, Vonsattel JP, Stevens TJ, et al. Clinical and neuropathologic assessment of severity in Huntington's disease. *Neurology*. 1988;38(3):341–347.

69. Augood SJ, Faull RL, Emson PC. Dopamine D1 and D2 receptor gene expression in the striatum in Huntington's disease. *Ann Neurol*. 1997;42(2):215–221.

70. Albin RL, Reiner A, Anderson KD, Penney JB, Young AB. Striatal and nigral neuron subpopulations in rigid Huntington's disease: implications for the functional anatomy of chorea and rigidity-akinesia. *Ann Neurol*. 1990;27(4):357–365.

71. Jongen PJ, Renier WO, Gabreels FJ. Seven cases of Huntington's disease in childhood and levodopa induced improvement in the hypokinetic–rigid form. *Clin Neurol Neurosurg*. 1980;82(4):251–261.

72. FitzGerald PM, Jankovic J, Glaze DG, Schultz R, Percy AK. Extrapyramidal involvement in Rett's syndrome. *Neurology*. 1990;40(2):293–295.

73. Dunn HG, Stoessl AJ, Ho HH, et al. Rett syndrome: investigation of nine patients, including PET scan. *Can J Neurol Sci*. 2002;29(4):345–357.

74. O'Sullivan JD, Hanagasi HA, Daniel SE, Tidswell P, Davies SW, Lees AJ. Neuronal intranuclear inclusion disease and juvenile parkinsonism. *Mov Disord*. 2000;15(5):990–995.

75. Paviour DC, Revesz T, Holton JL, Evans A, Olsson JE, Lees AJ. Neuronal intranuclear inclusion disease: report on a case originally diagnosed as dopa-responsive dystonia with Lewy bodies. *Mov Disord*. 2005;20(10):1345–1349.

76. Lindenberg R, Rubinstein LJ, Herman MM, Haydon GB. A light and electron microscopy study of an unusual widespread nuclear inclusion body disease. A possible residuum of an old herpesvirus infection. *Acta Neuropathol*. 1968;10(1):54–73.

77. Goutieres F, Mikol J, Aicardi J. Neuronal intranuclear inclusion disease in a child: diagnosis by rectal biopsy. *Ann Neurol*. 1990;27(1):103–106.

78. Lai SC, Jung SM, Grattan-Smith P, et al. Neuronal intranuclear inclusion disease: two cases of dopa-responsive juvenile parkinsonism with drug-induced dyskinesia. *Mov Disord*. 2010;25(9):1274–1279.

79. Davison C. Pallido-pyramidal disease. *J Neuropathol Exp Neurol*. 1954;13(1):50–59.

80. Shojaee S, Sina F, Banihosseini SS, et al. Genome-wide linkage analysis of a Parkinsonian-pyramidal syndrome pedigree by 500 K SNP arrays. *Am J Hum Genet*. 2008;82(6):1375–1384.

81. Di Fonzo A, Dekker MC, Montagna P, et al. FBXO7 mutations cause autosomal recessive, early-onset parkinsonian-pyramidal syndrome. *Neurology.* 2009;72(3):240–245.

82. Deng H, Liang H, Jankovic J. F-box only protein 7 gene in parkinsonian-pyramidal disease. *JAMA Neurol.* 2013;70(1):20–24.

83. Winston JT, Koepp DM, Zhu C, Elledge SJ, Harper JW. A family of mammalian F-box proteins. *Curr Biol.* 1999;9(20):1180–1182.

84. Hogarth P, Gregory A, Kruer MC, et al. New NBIA subtype: genetic, clinical, pathologic, and radiographic features of MPAN. *Neurology.* 2013;80(3):268–275.

85. Kruer MC, Salih MA, Mooney C, et al. C19orf12 mutation leads to a pallido-pyramidal syndrome. *Gene.* 2014;537(2):352–356.

86. Najim al-Din AS, Wriekat A, Mubaidin A, Dasouki M, Hiari M. Pallido-pyramidal degeneration, supranuclear upgaze paresis and dementia: Kufor–Rakeb syndrome. *Acta Neurol Scand.* 1994;89(5):347–352.

87. Williams DR, Hadeed A, al-Din AS, Wreikat AL, Lees AJ. Kufor Rakeb disease: autosomal recessive, levodopa-responsive parkinsonism with pyramidal degeneration, supranuclear gaze palsy, and dementia. *Mov Disord.* 2005;20(10):1264–1271.

88. Fong CY, Rolfs A, Schwarzbraun T, Klein C, O'Callaghan FJ. Juvenile parkinsonism associated with heterozygous frameshift ATP13A2 gene mutation. *Eur J Paediatr Neurol.* 2011;15(3):271–275.

89. Ramirez A, Heimbach A, Grundemann J, et al. Hereditary parkinsonism with dementia is caused by mutations in ATP13A2, encoding a lysosomal type 5 P-type ATPase. *Nat Genet.* 2006;38(10):1184–1191.

90. Gregory A, Polster BJ, Hayflick SJ. Clinical and genetic delineation of neurodegeneration with brain iron accumulation. *J Med Genet.* 2009;46(2):73–80.

91. Yoshino H, Tomiyama H, Tachibana N, et al. Phenotypic spectrum of patients with PLA2G6 mutation and PARK14-linked parkinsonism. *Neurology.* 2010;75(15):1356–1361.

92. Lu CS, Lai SC, Wu RM, et al. PLA2G6 mutations in PARK14-linked young-onset parkinsonism and sporadic Parkinson's disease. *Am J Med Genet B Neuropsychiatr Genet.* 2012;159B(2):183–191.

93. Paisan-Ruiz C, Li A, Schneider SA, et al. Widespread Lewy body and tau accumulation in childhood and adult onset dystonia-parkinsonism cases with PLA2G6 mutations. *Neurobiol Aging.* 2012;33(4):814–823.

94. Von Economo C. *Encephalitis Lethargica. Its Sequelae and Treatment.* London: Oxford University Press; 1931.

95. Pranzatelli MR, Mott SH, Pavlakis SG, Conry JA, Tate ED. Clinical spectrum of secondary parkinsonism in childhood: a reversible disorder. *Pediatr Neurol.* 1994;10(2):131–140.

96. Alves RS, Barbosa ER, Scaff M. Postvaccinal parkinsonism. *Mov Disord.* 1992;7(2):178–180.

97. Deng H, Zheng W, Jankovic J. Genetics and molecular biology of brain calcification. *Ageing Res Rev.* 2015;22:20–38.

98. Manyam BV. What is and what is not "Fahr's disease". *Parkinsonism Relat Disord.* 2005;11(2):73–80.

99. Koller WC, Klawans HL. Cerebellar calcification on computerized tomography. *Ann Neurol.* 1980;7(2):193–194.

100. Koller WC, Cochran JW, Klawans HL. Calcification of the basal ganglia: computerized tomography and clinical correlation. *Neurology.* 1979;29(3):328–333.

101. Jenner P. Dopamine agonists, receptor selectivity and dyskinesia induction in Parkinson's disease. *Curr Opin Neurol.* 2003;16(suppl 1):S3–S7.

102. Furukawa Y, Filiano JJ, Kish SJ. Amantadine for levodopa-induced choreic dyskinesia in compound heterozygotes for GCH1 mutations. *Mov Disord.* 2004;19(10):1256–1258.

103. Paci C, Thomas A, Onofrj M. Amantadine for dyskinesia in patients affected by severe Parkinson's disease. *Neurol Sci.* 2001;22(1):75–76.

104. Crosby NJ, Deane KH, Clarke CE. Amantadine for dyskinesia in Parkinson's disease. *Cochrane Database Syst Rev.* 2003(2))CD003467.

105. Peppe A, Pierantozzi M, Bassi A, et al. Stimulation of the subthalamic nucleus compared with the globus pallidus internus in patients with Parkinson disease. *J Neurosurg.* 2004;101(2):195–200.

106. Germano IM, Gracies JM, Weisz DJ, Tse W, Koller WC, Olanow CW. Unilateral stimulation of the subthalamic nucleus in Parkinson disease: a double-blind 12-month evaluation study. *J Neurosurg.* 2004;101(1):36–42.

107. Schneider SA, Dusek P, Hardy J, Westenberger A, Jankovic J, Bhatia KP. Genetics and Pathophysiology of Neurodegeneration with Brain Iron Accumulation (NBIA). *Curr Neuropharmacol.* 2013;11(1):59–79.

Hereditary Spastic Paraplegia

Harvey S. Singer[1], Jonathan W. Mink[2],
Donald L. Gilbert[3] and Joseph Jankovic[4]

[1]Department of Neurology, Johns Hopkins Hospital, Baltimore, MD, USA;
[2]Division of Child Neurology, University of Rochester Medical Center,
Rochester, NY, USA; [3]Division of Neurology, Cincinnati Children's Hospital
Medical Center, Cincinnati, OH, USA; [4]Department of Neurology, Baylor
College of Medicine, Houston, TX, USA

INTRODUCTION AND OVERVIEW

This chapter focuses on the clinically and genetically heterogeneous neurodegenerative disorders known as hereditary spastic paraplegias (HSPs), emphasizing those which may begin in childhood. The primary features of these diseases are weakness and spasticity in the legs.

A vast number of conditions adversely affect motor function and cause hypertonia in the legs in children. Most of these conditions cause spasticity. However, unilateral and bilateral leg dystonia or rigidity can also occur, and diseases in which spastic paraplegia combines with other movement disorders are not unusual. Thus, clinically these can be challenging at times to differentiate from one another. As discussed in Chapter 20 (Cerebral Palsy), chronic hypertonia of the legs beginning in infancy or early childhood most often results from hypoxic ischemic encephalopathy. There are numerous other nonhypoxic etiologies. For example, acute and subacute-onset leg spasticity can result from acquired lesions of the spinal cord. These are not addressed in this chapter.

The HSPs are classified as "pure" or "uncomplicated," based on the involvement of spinal cord tracts only, versus "complicated," "complex," or "syndromic" based on involvement of other parts of the nervous system.[1-3] Most of the types of HSP are extremely rare. Genetic diagnosis based on clinical findings is difficult. Despite substantial advancements in genetics and understanding of pathophysiology, treatments remain nonspecific and supportive. However, arriving at the most precise diagnosis possible has value for families. A systematic approach is needed for diagnosis of both acquired and genetic spastic paraplegias.[3-5]

HSPs of the pure or uncomplicated class involve slowly progressive weakness and spasticity of the legs, but may also include reduced vibratory sense or proprioception in the legs or hypertonic urinary bladder. The more extensive problems in the complex HSPs include cognitive or emotional impairments, epilepsy, dystonia or movement disorders, ataxia, cerebellar or callosal abnormalities, muscle wasting, or polyneuropathy.[2,6]

DEFINITIONS OF SPASTICITY AND HYPERTONIA

Hypertonia designates the observation by an examiner of elevated resistance across a joint, when the patient is examined in the resting state. *Spasticity* is a form of hypertonia where the examiner perceives that the resistance increases at faster speed of stretch and differs depending on the direction of joint movement. There is often a "catch," a point at which the resistance increases rapidly once the joint reaches a certain angle or the passive movement reaches a certain speed.[7]

CLINICAL CHARACTERISTICS—PHENOMENOLOGY OF SPASTIC PARAPLEGIA IN CHILDREN

It is generally straightforward for a clinician to identify that a gait is abnormal. However, characterizing the specific difficulties requires experience and careful observation. Even with experience, based on visual or kinematic features, it can be difficult to distinguish the spastic gait due to cerebral palsy from gait in the HSPs.[8] A helpful approach is to observe the child walking while wearing shorts, and to focus sequentially on joints and alternate legs. For example, observe during a number of strides the position of the hip throughout the gait, then the knee, then the ankle, first on one leg, then the other.

Common features of spastic gaits: The child with spastic paraplegia develops a walking strategy to overcome whatever combination of weakness and spasticity their disease involves. Quantitative analyses of spatiotemporal parameters comparing children with spasticity to healthy, typically developing children demonstrate shorter step length, wider step width, and slower step velocity in children with spasticity.[9]

Hips: At the hips, excessive flexion, or pelvic tilt, is present throughout the gait cycle. While children with spastic diplegia (SD) due to cerebral palsy tend to demonstrate excessive internal rotation at the hip, children with HSP do not.

Knees: Knee positioning is also abnormal, with excessive flexion at the point of foot contact and, often, hyperextension during midstance. There may be reduced flexion during the swing phase of gait. The amount and duration of knee hyperextension during stance tends to be greater in HSP than in SD.

Ankles: At the ankle, in HSP the position is generally normal, whereas in SD there is excess plantar flexion at initial contact and reduced ability to dorsiflex during the stance and swing phases.

EMG studies: In children with SD, there tends to be co-activation of rectus femoris and hamstrings. In contrast, in HSP patients there tends to be less activation of the rectus femoris throughout the gait cycle.[9]

LOCALIZATION AND PATHOPHYSIOLOGY

HSPs result from disease localizing to the longest corticospinal tract axons, predominantly. Pathological studies show degeneration of terminal portions of the long descending corticospinal tracts and ascending dorsal columns. Many mechanisms have been implicated through careful study of the large number of causative genes.[3,10] The most prominent involve disruptions in:

1. Axonal transport of macromolecules and organelles via microtubule tracks powered by distinct "motors"
   a. Anterograde—kinesins transporting short microtubules, neurofilaments, other elements critical for growth, repair, and nerve terminal maintenance.
   b. Retrograde—cytoplasmic dyniens transporting mitochondria, RNA-associated proteins, endosomes, injury-response signaling molecules.
2. Membrane trafficking processes such as vesicle assembly, transport, protein- and receptor-mediated fusion with the target membrane.
3. Mitochondrial function which might reduce efficiency of axonal transport among other processes.
4. Myelin production, which then influences anterograde and retrograde transport, resulting in length-dependent axonal loss.

DISEASES AND DISORDERS

Careful history including age of onset and family history, plus neurological and general examinations should guide the diagnostic evaluation. Many phenotypes overlap, and a common diagnostic strategy involves testing using commercially available diagnostic panels. New mutations and variants which may be benign can pose challenges, so it remains important for clinicians to carefully consider specific features. In this section, the HSPs are presented by type of inheritance. Clinical features, genetics, and pathophysiology are presented in the text for the more common, childhood-onset HSPs. More comprehensive lists are presented in Tables 16.1–16.3, sorted for clinical use by earliest reported age of onset.

AD Pure, Uncomplicated HSPs

This category includes conditions involving spasticity and weakness in the legs, with or without accompanying vibratory and joint position sensory loss, and urinary urgency. The

TABLE 16.1   Selected Autosomal Dominant (AD) HSPs That May Present in Childhood, Sorted by Earliest Reported Age of Onset

Spastic paraplegia	Youngest age reported onset in years	Other features	Gene	Protein
SPG3A[11–13]	1	Uncomplicated	ATL1	Atlastin-1
SPG4[14,15]	0–1	Uncomplicated, or may have cognitive impairment late	SPAST	Spastin
SPG10[16,17]	1	Uncomplicated, or may have upper arm involvement, Parkinsonism, axonal neuropathy	KIF5A	Kinesin family member 5A
SPG42[18]	4	Uncomplicated	SLC33A1	Solute carrier family 33 (acetyl-CoA transporter) member 1
SPG12[19,20]	5	Uncomplicated	RTN2	Reticulon 2
SPG17[21–23]	8	Uncomplicated, but may have upper limb involvement and distal limb atrophy	BSCL2	Seipin
SPG6[24,25]	9	Uncomplicated	NIPA1	Nonimprinted gene in Prader–Willi syndrome/Angelman syndrome region
SPG31[26–28]	15	Uncomplicated, or may have dysphagia/dysarthria, upper limb involvement, amyotrophy	REEP1	Receptor expression-enhancing protein 1
SPG13[29]	17	Uncomplicated	HSPD1	Heat-shock 60-KD protein 1
SPG8[30]	18	Uncomplicated or may have upper limb involvement	KIAA0196	Strumpellin

TABLE 16.2   Selected X-Linked HSPs That May Present in Childhood

Spastic paraplegia	Youngest age reported onset in years	Other features	MRI findings	Gene	Protein
SPG1[31]	1	Intellectual impairment, short stature, micro- or macrocephaly, kyphosis, adducted thumbs, pes cavus/talipes equinovarus	Hydrocephalus, agenesis of the corpus callosum	L1CAM	L1 cell-adhesion molecule
SPG2[32]	1	Intellectual disability, nystagmus, optic atrophy, dysarthria, ataxia, upper limb involvement, joint contractures, limb atrophy, allelic to Pelizaeus–Merzbacher disease	Normal, or white matter hyperintensities	PLP1	Myelin proteolipid protein (lipophilin)
SPG22[33,34]	0	Intellectual disability, irritability, neonatal hypotonia, nystagmus, dystonia, athetosis, muscle atrophy, microcephaly, dysmorphic face/ears	White matter changes	SLC16A2	Monocarboxylate transporter-8
SPG34[35]	10	Uncomplicated	Normal	Unknown	

most common (least rare) forms affecting children are SPG3A, SPG4, and SPG31. Less commonly occurring forms in children are SPG6, SPG10, and SPG12.[4] In this section, details are provided about the more common childhood-onset forms. Additional diagnoses, for which genes have been identified, are listed in Table 16.1.

SPG3A

CLINICAL FEATURES

Presents between infancy and early childhood in most cohorts, with spasticity and weakness in legs, reduced vibratory sense, and urinary bladder hyperactivity. Symptoms may be severe. Infancy onset cases may be misdiagnosed as cerebral palsy. Symptoms may progress slowly or remain static.

PATHOPHYSIOLOGY

The etiology of SPG3A is mutations in the *ATL1* gene,[11] which encodes atlastin-1, a GTPase which participates with dynamin in the formation of endoplasmic reticulum and axon elongation.[66] This disease is allelic to hereditary sensory neuropathy type I.

TABLE 16.3 Selected Autosomal Recessive Spastic Paraplegias That May Present in Childhood

Spastic paraplegia	Youngest age reported onset in years	Other features	MRI findings	Gene	Protein
SPG11[36,37]	1	Dementia, dysarthria, dysphagia, amyotrophy, nystagmus, retinal degeneration	Thin corpus callosum	KIAA1840	Spatacsin
SPG15[38]	5	Dementia, dysarthria, ataxia, hearing loss, pigmentary retinal degeneration, neuropathy	Thin corpus callosum, white matter hyperintensities, atrophy cerebrum, and brainstem	ZFYVE26	Spastizin
SPG7[39–41]	10	None, or dysarthria, dysphagia, axonal neuropathy	Cerebral or cerebellar atrophy	SPG7	Paraplegin
SPG45[42]	0	Intellectual disability	Thin corpus callosum, white matter changes	NT5C2	Nucleotidase, 5-prime, cytosolic II
SPG47[43]	0	Severe intellectual disability, stereotypic laughter, seizures, dystonia, dysarthria, short stature, microcephaly, wide nasal bridge, high-arched palate, genu recurvatum, pes planus	Thin corpus callosum, periventricular white matter abnormalities	AP4B1	Adaptor-related protein complex 4
SPG49[44]	0	Intellectual disability, dysarthria, ataxia, poor respiration, short stature, microcephaly, low anterior hairline, round face, dental crowding	Thin corpus callosum, cerebral atrophy	TECPR2	Tectonin beta-propeller repeat-containing protein 2
SPG50[45]	0	Severe intellectual disability, spastic quadriplegia, microcephaly, adducted thumbs, club feet	Cerebral and cerebellar atrophy, white matter abnormalities; mimics perinatal hypoxic ischemic encephalopathy	AP4M1	Adaptor-related protein complex 4, MU-1 subunit
SPG51[46]	0	Severe intellectual disability, seizures, stereotypic laughter, spastic quadriplegia, short stature, down-slanting palpebral fissures, long narrow face, bitemporal narrowing, short philtrum	Cerebral and cerebellar atrophy, white matter abnormalities	AP4E1	Adaptor-related protein complex 4, epsilon-1 subunit

TABLE 16.3 (Continued)

Spastic paraplegia	Youngest age reported onset in years	Other features	MRI findings	Gene	Protein
SPG52[43]	0	Severe intellectual disability, stereotypic laughter, short stature, severe spasticity, microcephaly, coarse faces, joint contractures	Not described	AP4S1	Adaptor-related protein complex 4, sigma-1 subunit
SPG53[47]	0	Intellectual disability, upper limb hyperreflexia, dystonia, pectus carinatum, kyphosis, hypertrichosis	Normal	VPS37A	Vacuolar protein sorting 37, yeast, homolog of A
SPG56[48]	0	Some cognitive impairment, some dystonia	Normal, or thin corpus callosum, white matter abnormalities, basal ganglia calcifications	CYP2U1	Cytochrome P450, family 2, subfamily U, polypeptide 1
SPG5A[49]	1	Upper limb weakness, dysarthria, ataxia	White matter changes	BYP7B1	Cytochrome P450, family 7, subfamily B
SPG18[50]	1	Oculomotor abnormalities, upper limb spasticity, intellectual disability, seizures, high-arched palate, progressive severe contractures, scoliosis, kyphosis	Normal, or thin corpus callosum	ERLIN2	Endoplasmic reticulum lipid raft-associated protein 2
SPG54[51]	1	Intellectual disability, optic atrophy, dysphagia, dysarthria, short stature, telecanthus, high palate, foot contractures	Thin corpus callosum, periventricular white matter changes, abnormal lipid peak on MRS	DDHD2	DDHD domain containing protein 2
SPG20[52–54]	2	Intellectual disability, dysarthria, ataxia, upper limb spasticity, distal amyotrophy, short stature, hypertelorism, kyphoscoliosis, limb contractures, brachy-clino- or camptodactyly, pes cavus	Periventricular white matter changes, cerebellar atrophy	SPG20	Spartin
SPG46[55,56]	2	Dementia, dysarthria, ataxia, cataracts, testicular hypotrophy, scoliosis, pes cavus	Thin corpus callosum, cerebral and cerebellar atrophy	GBA2	Glucosidase, beta, acid-2

(Continued)

TABLE 16.3   (Continued)

Spastic paraplegia	Youngest age reported onset in years	Other features	MRI findings	Gene	Protein
SPG35[57]	3	Dementia, seizures, dysarthria, upper limb spastic weakness, dystonia, ataxia	Leukodystrophy, globus pallidus iron deposition, thin corpus callosum, brainstem and cerebellar atrophy	FA2H	Fatty acid 2-hydroxylase
SPG39[58]	4	Upper limb weakness, ataxia, axonal neuropathy	Cerebellar atrophy	PNPLA6	Patatin-like phospholipase domain-containing protein 6
SPG44[59]	5	Cognitive impairment, seizures, sensorineural hearing loss, slow saccades, upper limb spasticity, intention tremor, ataxia, scoliosis, pes cavus	Hypomyelinating leukoencephalopathy, thin corpus callosum	GJC2	Gap junction protein, gamma-2
SPG28[48]	6	Axonal neuropathy, scoliosis, pes cavus	Not described	DDHD1	DDHD domain-containing protein 1
SPG43[60]	7	Contractures of fingers, distal amyotrophy	Normal	C19ORF12	Chromosome 19 open reading frame 12
SPG55[61]	7	Intellectual disability, optic atrophy, nystagmus, axonal neuropathy, small joint arthrogryposis, distal amyotrophy	Thin corpus callosum, few white matter lesions	C12ORF65	Chromosome 12 open reading frame 65
SPG30[62,63]	10	Lower limb atrophy cerebellar signs, axonal neuropathy	Cerebellar atrophy	KIF1A	Kinesin family member 1A
SPG21[64,65]	17	Dysphagia/bulbar dysfunction, apraxia, dementia, Parkinsonism, peripheral neuropathy	Fronto-temporal atrophy, thin corpus callosum	ACP33	33-kd acidic cluster protein

SPG4

CLINICAL FEATURES

SPG4 may present in childhood or adulthood, with bimodal peaks at ages 10 and 30 years. While most cases described fit with uncomplicated HSP, some individuals may have ataxia, dementia, or posterior fossa abnormalities. This is the most common form of AD HSP and also accounts for some sporadic cases.

PATHOPHYSIOLOGY

The etiology of SPG4 is mutations in the *SPAST* gene, which encodes spastin.[14] Spastin plays a role in regulation and severing of microtubules important for organelle transport in axons.[67]

SPG31

CLINICAL FEATURES

SPG31 may present in the first or second decade of childhood. Lower limbs are affected by weakness and spasticity. Hyperreflexia with clonus and extensor plantar responses, proximal leg weakness, and distal sensory loss are noted on exam. Less commonly, weakness of upper limbs, dysarthria and dysphagia, and amyotrophy may occur.

PATHOPHYSIOLOGY

The etiology of SPG31 is mutations in the *REEP1* gene,[26] which encodes receptor expression-enhancing protein 1. This protein participates in endoplasmic reticulum formation and may affect lipid droplet size in axons[68] and play a role in resistance to oxidative stress.[69]

SPG6

CLINICAL FEATURES

SPG6 presents as an uncomplicated HSP but with severe and rapidly progressive spasticity. Examination shows weakness of hip flexion and ankle dorsiflexion, spasticity, hyperreflexia and extensor plantar responses, and reduced vibratory sense. Pes cavus usually occurs.

PATHOPHYSIOLOGY

The etiology of SPG6 is mutations in the *NIPA1* gene (nonimprinted gene in the Prader–Willi/Angelman syndrome chromosome region 1).[24] The NIPA1 protein binds with atlastin-1 protein and inhibits bone morphogenic protein (BMP1) signaling.[70] BMP1 signaling is important for axon function distally.[71]

SPG10

CLINICAL FEATURES

SPG10 can present with either uncomplicated or complicated AD HSP. Onset is usually in adulthood, but infant onset has been described. Intrafamilial variability may occur, with an alternate phenotype of peripheral, axonal sensorimotor neuropathy and limb amyotrophy. Parkinsonism and cognitive impairment have also been described.

PATHOPHYSIOLOGY

The etiology of SPG10 is mutations in the *KIF5A* gene,[16] which encodes the heavy chain, neuron-specific kinesin protein. Kinesins are motor proteins which contribute to antero-grade axonal transport.[72]

SPG12

CLINICAL FEATURES

SPG12 can present from the first to third decade with progressive symptoms of an uncomplicated, AD HSP.

PATHOPHYSIOLOGY

The etiology of SPG12 is mutations in the *RTN2* gene,[19] which encodes reticulon 2. RTN2 participates, with REEP1, atlastin-1, and spastin in the formation of the endoplasmic reticulum.[19,73]

X-Linked, Complicated HSP

This category includes two important causes of spastic paraplegias, SPG1 and SPG2, described below. Rarer forms are listed in Table 16.2.

SPG1

CLINICAL FEATURES

SPG1 presents as a complicated HSP. This is also known by various eponyms and acronyms: Gareis–Mason, CRASH, and MASA syndrome. Onset is in early childhood, but spastic paraplegia features may not be clearly evident prior to age 4 years. Features on examination also include short stature, microcephaly, intellectual disability, delayed language, spastic gait, and adducted thumbs. Imaging may show agenesis/hypoplasia of the corpus callosum.

PATHOPHYSIOLOGY

The etiology of SPG1 is mutations in the *L1CAM* gene,[74,75] which encodes the L1 cell-adhesion molecule. This is a membrane glycoprotein found primarily in the nervous system, considered to be a "neural recognition molecule" which guides multiple components of neural development including neuronal migration, neurite outgrowth, myelination, and synaptogenesis.[76] This disease is allelic to the disease X-linked aqueductal stenosis also known as Hydrocephalus due to congenital Stenosis of the Aqueduct of Sylvius (HSAS).[31]

SPG2

CLINICAL FEATURES

SPG2 presents as an early onset, slowly progressive, uncomplicated or complicated HSP. Findings vary and may include early or late onset intellectual disability, nystagmus, optic atrophy, dysarthria, and sensory loss.

PATHOPHYSIOLOGY

The etiology of SPG2 is mutations in the myelin proteolipid protein (*PLP1*) gene, making this disease allelic to the hypomyelinating leukodystrophy Pelizaeus–Merzbacher disease.[32]

The *PLP1* gene is transcribed and its mRNA spliced into two myelin proteolipid proteins, PLP and DM20. While duplication of *PLP1* is responsible for Pelizaeus–Merzbacher in most cases, some cases can be caused by gene deletions or a variety of mutations. SPG2 tends to occur in persons with splice-site mutations or changes in the PLP-specific (i.e., not coding for DM20) exons.[77] Myelin proteolipid protein associates with myelin during its biosynthesis. Overexpression results in accumulation in the endoplasmic reticulum, which may overwhelm degradation machinery. Other mutations likely alter trafficking of myelin in the cell, perturbing healthy myelin formation. Differentiation and survival of oligodendrocytes may also be affected.[78]

AR, Complicated HSP

Autosomal recessive forms often present in early childhood. Most have complicated phenotypes. Many have been described in just a few families. Clinical presentations and pathophysiologies for the more common forms are described below, with a more comprehensive list in Table 16.3.

SPG11

CLINICAL FEATURES

SPG11, also known as autosomal recessive HSP with thin corpus callosum (ARHSP-TCC), presents from childhood through adulthood, with peak onset in early adolescence. It is a progressive, complicated HSP. Dementia, dysarthria, dysphagia, amyotrophy, nystagmus, and retinal degeneration may develop. Dopa-responsive dystonia has been also described in patients with genetically confirmed SPG11.[79] Peripheral neuropathy with loss of myelinated fibers also occurs. A key distinguishing feature is thin or atrophied corpus callosum.

PATHOPHYSIOLOGY

The etiology of SPG11 is homozygous or compound heterozygous mutations in the SPG11/*KIAA1840* gene, which encodes spatacsin.[36] Spatacsin contributes to neurite growth, tubulin stabilization, and anterograde axonal transport to synapses.[80]

SPG15

CLINICAL FEATURES

SPG15 has similar features to SPG11.[81] It is an autosomal recessive, complicated HSP with thin corpus callosum that presents from childhood through adulthood. Intellectual impairment may precede spastic paraplegia and may progress. Pigmented maculopathy, nystagmus, distal amyotrophy, dysarthria, dysphagia, amyotrophy, and peripheral neuropathy may occur.

PATHOPHYSIOLOGY

The etiology of SPG15 is homozygous or compound heterozygous mutations in the SPG15/*ZFYVE26* gene, which encodes spatizin.[38] This zinc finger protein co-localizes in mitochondria and microtubules and forms a core protein complex with spatacsin.[82]

SPG7 with Ataxia

CLINICAL FEATURES

SPG7 can present in childhood but more often presents in adulthood. It can present with uncomplicated spastic paraplegia but can also present with optic atrophy, supranuclear palsy, nystagmus, ataxia, dementia, and cerebral and cerebellar atrophy.

PATHOPHYSIOLOGY

The etiology of SPG7 is homozygous or compound heterozygous mutations in the *SPG7/PGN* gene, which encodes paraplegin.[39] This protein is a subunit in the mitochondrial inner membrane, ATP-dependent m-AAA protease. Mutations alter mitochondrial function affecting axonal transport, resulting in axonal degeneration.[83,84]

AD, Complicated HSP

SPG17 (Silver) with Distal Amyotrophy

CLINICAL FEATURES

SPG17, also known as Silver syndrome, presents in childhood or early adulthood with symptoms of spastic paraplegia. It is distinguished by prominent atrophy and weakness of the hands, which may precede the onset of spastic paraplegia. This disease is allelic with hereditary motor neuropathy Type VA.

PATHOPHYSIOLOGY

The etiology of SPG17 is mutation in the *BSCL2* gene,[21] which encodes seipin, an endoplasmic reticulum protein predicted to influence lipid droplet formation or metabolism. It is expressed in motor neurons in spinal cord as well as in frontal lobe cerebral cortical neurons.[85] Heterozygous mutations result in aggregate formation and activation of the unfolded protein responses, thereby leading to apoptosis through endoplasmic reticulum stress[86] and neurodegeneration. Homozygous or compound heterozygous mutations cause progressive encephalopathy with leukodystrophy.[87]

TREATMENT

To date, treatment is symptomatic and follows the usual treatment approaches for spasticity. Most published data on treatment of spasticity in childhood comes from cerebral palsy, not spastic paraplegia. However, similar treatment principles generally apply. A mainstay of management is physical therapy to maintain strength and range of motion and to reduce the occurrence of joint contractures. Pharmacological interventions may also be used, including baclofen and benzodiazepines.[88] Injection of botulinum toxin is commonly performed,[89–91] although it can be difficult to demonstrate clear, long-term benefit in rigorously performed studies.[92] Baclofen pumps are also used in more severe cases.[93,94]

DIAGNOSTIC AND MANAGEMENT APPROACH

When presented with a child who may have HSP, a systematic, stepwise approach to diagnosis is advised.

1. Clarify that spastic paraplegia is the movement disorder.
2. Document by history and examination presence or absence of features of a primary, uncomplicated spastic paraplegia: spasticity and weakness of the legs, distal sensory loss by modality, disturbances in urinary function.
3. Document carefully the remainder of the history and general or neurological examination to identify any findings supportive of involvement elsewhere in the central or peripheral nervous system or body. These could indicate the presence of a complicated spastic paraplegia.
4. Stratify into an age/time-course group:
   a. Infancy, early childhood onset, static: Consider carefully, based on history and examination, whether the diagnosis is SD due to pre- or perinatal hypoxic ischemic encephalopathy.
   b. Later childhood onset, acute/subacute: Consider secondary, upper motor neuron lesions and image spine or brain based on localization.
   c. Infancy, childhood, adolescent onset, static or chronic progressive: Consider possibility of a heritable spastic paraplegia.
5. For all paraplegias that could be inherited, document a three-generation family history pedigree. Examine parents and siblings, if possible. Determine whether likely inheritance is autosomal dominant, autosomal recessive, X-linked, or mitochondrial.
6. Consider carefully whether to perform neuroimaging of the brain and spine. If the clinical presentation strongly supports an uncomplicated spastic paraplegia, particularly for AD inheritance, and other localization, e.g. parasagittal, not suspected, imaging the spine-only may be appropriate. In suspected AR, X-linked, or mitochondrial cases, imaging the brain provides critical information, such as white matter changes or thin corpus callosum, that narrows the differential diagnosis.
7. For children with a family history supportive of AD inheritance, particularly if uncomplicated, the most efficient strategy is often testing for SPG3A and SPG4 initially. Consider the costs of targeted versus panel commercial genetic testing.
8. For children with a family history supportive of autosomal recessive inheritance, the age of onset and additional neurological and nonneurological signs[4] may be used to generate the differential diagnosis. Depending on costs and differential, consider targeted stepwise approach versus commercial genetic testing panels. SPG 7, 11, 15 may be most likely.
9. For boys with clear X-linked family history or complicated symptoms and onset age consistent with known X-linked disease, consider targeted versus stepwise testing approach.
10. For apparent *de novo* cases in family, the best genetic testing approach is not clear. Phenotype and age of onset may be used to optimize testing approach. AD diagnoses

may occur as spontaneous mutations. Penetrance is not always complete, and intrafamilial variation in severity is common, so a parent with only hyperreflexia may have a more severely affected child.

11. When considering genetic testing, particularly exome sequencing, consider consultation with genetic counselors.
12. Provide general education and referral to general and specific disease Websites.
13. Provide referrals for multidisciplinary management, with physical therapy, pharmacologic therapy, and consideration for botulinum toxin or baclofen pump.
14. Provide supportive social services as needed.
15. Consult Clinicaltrials.gov regularly, consider participation in research.

Patient and Family Resources

One advantage of a specific molecular diagnosis is that it helps families network with other affected families and keep track of research. The Clinical Trials Website http://clinicaltrials.gov/ct2/home lists studies enrolling patients and can be searched by specific disease or disease category.

SUMMARY

A large number of congenital, degenerative, and acquired processes cause spasticity and weakness in the legs. Diagnosis of HSPs is complex, but advancing rapidly. There is hope that rational therapeutic advances may follow.

References

1. Harding AE. Classification of the hereditary ataxias and paraplegias. *Lancet*. 1983;1(8334):1151–1155.
2. Fink JK. Hereditary spastic paraplegia: clinical principles and genetic advances. *Semin Neurol*. 2014;34(3):293–305.
3. Finsterer J, Loscher W, Quasthoff S, Wanschitz J, Auer-Grumbach M, Stevanin G. Hereditary spastic paraplegias with autosomal dominant, recessive, X-linked, or maternal trait of inheritance. *J Neurol Sci*. 2012;318(1–2):1–18.
4. de Bot ST, van de Warrenburg BP, Kremer HP, Willemsen MA. Child neurology: hereditary spastic paraplegia in children. *Neurology*. 2010;75(19):e75–e79.
5. Depienne C, Stevanin G, Brice A, Durr A. Hereditary spastic paraplegias: an update. *Curr Opin Neurol*. 2007;20(6):674–680.
6. Tesson C, Koht J, Stevanin G. Delving into the complexity of hereditary spastic paraplegias: how unexpected phenotypes and inheritance modes are revolutionizing their nosology. *Hum Genet*. 2015:1–28.
7. Sanger TD, Delgado MR, Gaebler-Spira D, Hallett M, Mink JW, Task Force on Childhood Motor Disorders Classification and definition of disorders causing hypertonia in childhood. *Pediatrics*. 2003;111(1):e89–e97.
8. Wolf SI, Braatz F, Metaxiotis D, et al. Gait analysis may help to distinguish hereditary spastic paraplegia from cerebral palsy. *Gait Posture*. 2011;33(4):556–561.
9. Piccinini L, Cimolin V, D'Angelo MG, Turconi AC, Crivellini M, Galli M. 3D gait analysis in patients with hereditary spastic paraparesis and spastic diplegia: a kinematic, kinetic and EMG comparison. *Eur J Paediatr Neurol*. 2011;15(2):138–145.
10. Salinas S, Proukakis C, Crosby A, Warner TT. Hereditary spastic paraplegia: clinical features and pathogenetic mechanisms. *Lancet Neurol*. 2008;7(12):1127–1138.

11. Zhao X, Alvarado D, Rainier S, et al. Mutations in a newly identified GTPase gene cause autosomal dominant hereditary spastic paraplegia. *Nat Genet*. 2001;29(3):326–331.

12. Battini R, Fogli A, Borghetti D, et al. Clinical and genetic findings in a series of Italian children with pure hereditary spastic paraplegia. *Eur J Neurol*. 2011;18(1):150–157.

13. Namekawa M, Ribai P, Nelson I, et al. SPG3A is the most frequent cause of hereditary spastic paraplegia with onset before age 10 years. *Neurology*. 2006;66(1):112–114.

14. Svenson IK, Ashley-Koch AE, Gaskell PC, et al. Identification and expression analysis of spastin gene mutations in hereditary spastic paraplegia. *Am J Hum Genet*. 2001;68(5):1077–1085.

15. de Bot ST, van den Elzen RT, Mensenkamp AR, et al. Hereditary spastic paraplegia due to SPAST mutations in 151 Dutch patients: new clinical aspects and 27 novel mutations. *J Neurol Neurosurg Psychiatry*. 2010;81(10):1073–1078.

16. Reid E, Kloos M, Ashley-Koch A, et al. A kinesin heavy chain (KIF5A) mutation in hereditary spastic paraplegia (SPG10). *Am J Hum Genet*. 2002;71(5):1189–1194.

17. Crimella C, Baschirotto C, Arnoldi A, et al. Mutations in the motor and stalk domains of KIF5A in spastic paraplegia type 10 and in axonal Charcot–Marie–Tooth type 2. *Clin Genet*. 2012;82(2):157–164.

18. Lin P, Li J, Liu Q, et al. A missense mutation in SLC33A1, which encodes the acetyl-CoA transporter, causes autosomal-dominant spastic paraplegia (SPG42). *Am J Hum Genet*. 2008;83(6):752–759.

19. Montenegro G, Rebelo AP, Connell J, et al. Mutations in the ER-shaping protein reticulon 2 cause the axon-degenerative disorder hereditary spastic paraplegia type 12. *J Clin Invest*. 2012;122(2):538–544.

20. Orlacchio A, Kawarai T, Rogaeva E, et al. Clinical and genetic study of a large Italian family linked to SPG12 locus. *Neurology*. 2002;59(9):1395–1401.

21. Windpassinger C, Auer-Grumbach M, Irobi J, et al. Heterozygous missense mutations in BSCL2 are associated with distal hereditary motor neuropathy and Silver syndrome. *Nat Genet*. 2004;36(3):271–276.

22. Cafforio G, Calabrese R, Morelli N, et al. The first Italian family with evidence of pyramidal impairment as phenotypic manifestation of Silver syndrome BSCL2 gene mutation. *Neurol Sci*. 2008;29(3):189–191.

23. Irobi J, Van den Bergh P, Merlini L, et al. The phenotype of motor neuropathies associated with BSCL2 mutations is broader than Silver syndrome and distal HMN type V. *Brain*. 2004;127(Pt 9):2124–2130.

24. Rainier S, Chai JH, Tokarz D, Nicholls RD, Fink JK. NIPA1 gene mutations cause autosomal dominant hereditary spastic paraplegia (SPG6). *Am J Hum Genet*. 2003;73(4):967–971.

25. Du J, Hu YC, Tang BS, et al. Expansion of the phenotypic spectrum of SPG6 caused by mutation in NIPA1. *Clin Neurol Neurosurg*. 2011;113(6):480–482.

26. Zuchner S, Wang G, Tran-Viet KN, et al. Mutations in the novel mitochondrial protein REEP1 cause hereditary spastic paraplegia type 31. *Am J Hum Genet*. 2006;79(2):365–369.

27. Beetz C, Schule R, Deconinck T, et al. REEP1 mutation spectrum and genotype/phenotype correlation in hereditary spastic paraplegia type 31. *Brain*. 2008;131(Pt 4):1078–1086.

28. Goizet C, Depienne C, Benard G, et al. REEP1 mutations in SPG31: frequency, mutational spectrum, and potential association with mitochondrial morpho-functional dysfunction. *Hum Mutat*. 2011;32(10):1118–1127.

29. Hansen JJ, Durr A, Cournu-Rebeix I, et al. Hereditary spastic paraplegia SPG13 is associated with a mutation in the gene encoding the mitochondrial chaperonin HSP60. *Am J Hum Genet*. 2002;70(5):1328–1332.

30. Valdmanis PN, Meijer IA, Reynolds A, et al. Mutations in the KIAA0196 gene at the SPG8 locus cause hereditary spastic paraplegia. *Am J Hum Genet*. 2007;80(1):152–161.

31. Rosenthal A, Jouet M, Kenwrick S. Aberrant splicing of neural cell adhesion molecule L1 mRNA in a family with X-linked hydrocephalus. *Nat Genet*. 1992;2(2):107–112.

32. Saugier-Veber P, Munnich A, Bonneau D, et al. X-linked spastic paraplegia and Pelizaeus–Merzbacher disease are allelic disorders at the proteolipid protein locus. *Nat Genet*. 1994;6(3):257–262.

33. Dumitrescu AM, Liao XH, Best TB, Brockmann K, Refetoff S. A novel syndrome combining thyroid and neurological abnormalities is associated with mutations in a monocarboxylate transporter gene. *Am J Hum Genet*. 2004;74(1):168–175.

34. Schwartz CE, May MM, Carpenter NJ, et al. Allan–Herndon–Dudley syndrome and the monocarboxylate transporter 8 (MCT8) gene. *Am J Hum Genet*. 2005;77(1):41–53.

35. Macedo-Souza LI, Kok F, Santos S, et al. Reevaluation of a large family defines a new locus for X-linked recessive pure spastic paraplegia (SPG34) on chromosome Xq25. *Neurogenetics*. 2008;9(3):225–226.

36. Stevanin G, Santorelli FM, Azzedine H, et al. Mutations in SPG11, encoding spatacsin, are a major cause of spastic paraplegia with thin corpus callosum. *Nat Genet*. 2007;39(3):366–372.

37. Hehr U, Bauer P, Winner B, et al. Long-term course and mutational spectrum of spatacsin-linked spastic paraplegia. *Ann Neurol.* 2007;62(6):656–665.

38. Hanein S, Martin E, Boukhris A, et al. Identification of the SPG15 gene, encoding spastizin, as a frequent cause of complicated autosomal-recessive spastic paraplegia, including Kjellin syndrome. *Am J Hum Genet.* 2008;82(4):992–1002.

39. Casari G, De Fusco M, Ciarmatori S, et al. Spastic paraplegia and OXPHOS impairment caused by mutations in paraplegin, a nuclear-encoded mitochondrial metalloprotease. *Cell.* 1998;93(6):973–983.

40. Arnoldi A, Tonelli A, Crippa F, et al. A clinical, genetic, and biochemical characterization of SPG7 mutations in a large cohort of patients with hereditary spastic paraplegia. *Hum Mutat.* 2008;29(4):522–531.

41. Klebe S, Depienne C, Gerber S, et al. Spastic paraplegia gene 7 in patients with spasticity and/or optic neuropathy. *Brain.* 2012;135(Pt 10):2980–2993.

42. Novarino G, Fenstermaker AG, Zaki MS, et al. Exome sequencing links corticospinal motor neuron disease to common neurodegenerative disorders. *Science.* 2014;343(6170):506–511.

43. Abou Jamra R, Philippe O, Raas-Rothschild A, et al. Adaptor protein complex 4 deficiency causes severe autosomal-recessive intellectual disability, progressive spastic paraplegia, shy character, and short stature. *Am J Hum Genet.* 2011;88(6):788–795.

44. Oz-Levi D, Ben-Zeev B, Ruzzo EK, et al. Mutation in TECPR2 reveals a role for autophagy in hereditary spastic paraparesis. *Am J Hum Genet.* 2012;91(6):1065–1072.

45. Verkerk AJ, Schot R, Dumee B, et al. Mutation in the AP4M1 gene provides a model for neuroaxonal injury in cerebral palsy. *Am J Hum Genet.* 2009;85(1):40–52.

46. Moreno-De-Luca A, Helmers SL, Mao H, et al. Adaptor protein complex-4 (AP-4) deficiency causes a novel autosomal recessive cerebral palsy syndrome with microcephaly and intellectual disability. *J Med Genet.* 2011;48(2):141–144.

47. Zivony-Elboum Y, Westbroek W, Kfir N, et al. A founder mutation in Vps37A causes autosomal recessive complex hereditary spastic paraparesis. *J Med Genet.* 2012;49(7):462–472.

48. Tesson C, Nawara M, Salih MA, et al. Alteration of fatty-acid-metabolizing enzymes affects mitochondrial form and function in hereditary spastic paraplegia. *Am J Hum Genet.* 2012;91(6):1051–1064.

49. Tsaousidou MK, Ouahchi K, Warner TT, et al. Sequence alterations within CYP7B1 implicate defective cholesterol homeostasis in motor-neuron degeneration. *Am J Hum Genet.* 2008;82(2):510–515.

50. Al-Yahyaee S, Al-Gazali LI, De Jonghe P, et al. A novel locus for hereditary spastic paraplegia with thin corpus callosum and epilepsy. *Neurology.* 2006;66(8):1230–1234.

51. Schuurs-Hoeijmakers JH, Geraghty MT, Kamsteeg EJ, et al. Mutations in DDHD2, encoding an intracellular phospholipase A(1), cause a recessive form of complex hereditary spastic paraplegia. *Am J Hum Genet.* 2012;91(6):1073–1081.

52. Patel H, Cross H, Proukakis C, et al. SPG20 is mutated in Troyer syndrome, an hereditary spastic paraplegia. *Nat Genet.* 2002;31(4):347–348.

53. Cross HE, McKusick VA. The Troyer syndrome. A recessive form of spastic paraplegia with distal muscle wasting. *Arch Neurol.* 1967;16(5):473–485.

54. Manzini MC, Rajab A, Maynard TM, et al. Developmental and degenerative features in a complicated spastic paraplegia. *Ann Neurol.* 2010;67(4):516–525.

55. Martin E, Schule R, Smets K, et al. Loss of function of glucocerebrosidase GBA2 is responsible for motor neuron defects in hereditary spastic paraplegia. *Am J Hum Genet.* 2013;92(2):238–244.

56. Boukhris A, Feki I, Elleuch N, et al. A new locus (SPG46) maps to 9p21.2-q21.12 in a Tunisian family with a complicated autosomal recessive hereditary spastic paraplegia with mental impairment and thin corpus callosum. *Neurogenetics.* 2010;11(4):441–448.

57. Edvardson S, Hama H, Shaag A, et al. Mutations in the fatty acid 2-hydroxylase gene are associated with leukodystrophy with spastic paraparesis and dystonia. *Am J Hum Genet.* 2008;83(5):643–648.

58. Synofzik M, Gonzalez MA, Lourenco CM, et al. PNPLA6 mutations cause Boucher–Neuhauser and Gordon Holmes syndromes as part of a broad neurodegenerative spectrum. *Brain.* 2014;137(Pt 1):69–77.

59. Orthmann-Murphy JL, Salsano E, Abrams CK, et al. Hereditary spastic paraplegia is a novel phenotype for GJA12/GJC2 mutations. *Brain.* 2009;132(Pt 2):426–438.

60. Landoure G, Zhu PP, Lourenco CM, et al. Hereditary spastic paraplegia type 43 (SPG43) is caused by mutation in C19orf12. *Hum Mutat.* 2013;34(10):1357–1360.

61. Shimazaki H, Takiyama Y, Ishiura H, et al. A homozygous mutation of C12orf65 causes spastic paraplegia with optic atrophy and neuropathy (SPG55). *J Med Genet*. 2012;49(12):777–784.

62. Erlich Y, Edvardson S, Hodges E, et al. Exome sequencing and disease-network analysis of a single family implicate a mutation in KIF1A in hereditary spastic paraparesis. *Genome Res*. 2011;21(5):658–664.

63. Klebe S, Lossos A, Azzedine H, et al. KIF1A missense mutations in SPG30, an autosomal recessive spastic paraplegia: distinct phenotypes according to the nature of the mutations. *Eur J Hum Genet*. 2012;20(6):645–649.

64. Simpson MA, Cross H, Proukakis C, et al. Maspardin is mutated in mast syndrome, a complicated form of hereditary spastic paraplegia associated with dementia. *Am J Hum Genet*. 2003;73(5):1147–1156.

65. Cross HE, McKusick VA. The mast syndrome. A recessively inherited form of presenile dementia with motor disturbances. *Arch Neurol*. 1967;16(1):1–13.

66. Zhu PP, Soderblom C, Tao-Cheng JH, Stadler J, Blackstone C. SPG3A protein atlastin-1 is enriched in growth cones and promotes axon elongation during neuronal development. *Hum Mol Genet*. 2006;15(8):1343–1353.

67. Errico A, Ballabio A, Rugarli EI. Spastin, the protein mutated in autosomal dominant hereditary spastic paraplegia, is involved in microtubule dynamics. *Hum Mol Genet*. 2002;11(2):153–163.

68. Falk J, Rohde M, Bekhite MM, et al. Functional mutation analysis provides evidence for a role of REEP1 in lipid droplet biology. *Hum Mutat*. 2014;35(4):497–504.

69. Appocher C, Klima R, Feiguin F. Functional screening in *Drosophila* reveals the conserved role of REEP1 in promoting stress resistance and preventing the formation of Tau aggregates. *Hum Mol Genet*. 2014;23(25):6762–6772.

70. Tsang HT, Edwards TL, Wang X, et al. The hereditary spastic paraplegia proteins NIPA1, spastin and spartin are inhibitors of mammalian BMP signalling. *Hum Mol Genet*. 2009;18(20):3805–3821.

71. Charron F, Tessier-Lavigne M. The Hedgehog, TGF-beta/BMP and Wnt families of morphogens in axon guidance. *Adv Exp Med Biol*. 2007;621:116–133.

72. Kanai Y, Dohmae N, Hirokawa N. Kinesin transports RNA: isolation and characterization of an RNA-transporting granule. *Neuron*. 2004;43(4):513–525.

73. Roebroek AJ, Contreras B, Pauli IG, Van de Ven WJ. cDNA cloning, genomic organization, and expression of the human RTN2 gene, a member of a gene family encoding reticulons. *Genomics*. 1998;51(1):98–106.

74. Jouet M, Rosenthal A, Armstrong G, et al. X-linked spastic paraplegia (SPG1), MASA syndrome and X-linked hydrocephalus result from mutations in the L1 gene. *Nat Genet*. 1994;7(3):402–407.

75. Vits L, Van Camp G, Coucke P, et al. MASA syndrome is due to mutations in the neural cell adhesion gene L1CAM. *Nat Genet*. 1994;7(3):408–413.

76. Kenwrick S, Watkins A, De Angelis E. Neural cell recognition molecule L1: relating biological complexity to human disease mutations. *Hum Mol Genet*. 2000;9(6):879–886.

77. Cailloux F, Gauthier-Barichard F, Mimault C, et al. Genotype-phenotype correlation in inherited brain myelination defects due to proteolipid protein gene mutations. Clinical European network on brain dysmyelinating disease. *Eur J Hum Genet*. 2000;8(11):837–845.

78. Kobayashi H, Hoffman EP, Marks HG. The rumpshaker mutation in spastic paraplegia. *Nat Genet*. 1994;7(3):351–352.

79. Wijemanne S, Shulman JM, Jimenez-Shahed J, Curry D, Jankovic J. SPG11 mutations associated with a complex phenotype resembling dopa-responsive dystonia. *Mov Disord Clin Pract*. 2015;2(2):149–154.

80. Perez-Branguli F, Mishra HK, Prots I, et al. Dysfunction of spatacsin leads to axonal pathology in SPG11-linked hereditary spastic paraplegia. *Hum Mol Genet*. 2014;23(18):4859–4874.

81. Pensato V, Castellotti B, Gellera C, et al. Overlapping phenotypes in complex spastic paraplegias SPG11, SPG15, SPG35 and SPG48. *Brain*. 2014;137(Pt 7):1907–1920.

82. Murmu RP, Martin E, Rastetter A, et al. Cellular distribution and subcellular localization of spatacsin and spastizin, two proteins involved in hereditary spastic paraplegia. *Mol Cell Neurosci*. 2011;47(3):191–202.

83. Ferreirinha F, Quattrini A, Pirozzi M, et al. Axonal degeneration in paraplegin-deficient mice is associated with abnormal mitochondria and impairment of axonal transport. *J Clin Invest*. 2004;113(2):231–242.

84. Koppen M, Metodiev MD, Casari G, Rugarli EI, Langer T. Variable and tissue-specific subunit composition of mitochondrial m-AAA protease complexes linked to hereditary spastic paraplegia. *Mol Cell Biol*. 2007;27(2):758–767.

85. Ito D, Fujisawa T, Iida H, Suzuki N. Characterization of seipin/BSCL2, a protein associated with spastic paraplegia 17. *Neurobiol Dis*. 2008;31(2):266–277.

86. Ito D, Suzuki N. Molecular pathogenesis of seipin/BSCL2-related motor neuron diseases. *Ann Neurol*. 2007;61(3):237–250.

87. Guillen-Navarro E, Sanchez-Iglesias S, Domingo-Jimenez R, et al. A new seipin-associated neurodegenerative syndrome. *J Med Genet*. 2013;50(6):401–409.

88. McIntyre A, Lee T, Janzen S, Mays R, Mehta S, Teasell R. Systematic review of the effectiveness of pharmacological interventions in the treatment of spasticity of the hemiparetic lower extremity more than six months post stroke. *Top Stroke Rehabil*. 2012;19(6):479–490.

89. Balbaloglu O, Basaran A, Ayoglu H. Functional outcomes of multilevel botulinum toxin and comprehensive rehabilitation in cerebral palsy. *J Child Neurol*. 2011;26(4):482–487.

90. Dai AI, Wasay M, Awan S. Botulinum toxin type A with oral baclofen versus oral tizanidine: a nonrandomized pilot comparison in patients with cerebral palsy and spastic equinus foot deformity. *J Child Neurol*. 2008;23(12):1464–1466.

91. Tedroff K, Granath F, Forssberg H, Haglund-Akerlind Y. Long-term effects of botulinum toxin A in children with cerebral palsy. *Dev Med Child Neurol*. 2009;51(2):120–127.

92. Lannin N, Scheinberg A, Clark K. AACPDM systematic review of the effectiveness of therapy for children with cerebral palsy after botulinum toxin A injections. *Dev Med Child Neurol*. 2006;48(6):533–539.

93. Brochard S, Remy-Neris O, Filipetti P, Bussel B. Intrathecal baclofen infusion for ambulant children with cerebral palsy. *Pediatr Neurol*. 2009;40(4):265–270.

94. de Lissovoy G, Matza LS, Green H, Werner M, Edgar T. Cost-effectiveness of intrathecal baclofen therapy for the treatment of severe spasticity associated with cerebral palsy. *J Child Neurol*. 2007;22(1):49–59.

SELECTED SECONDARY MOVEMENT DISORDERS

Inherited Metabolic Disorders with Associated Movement Abnormalities

Harvey S. Singer[1], Jonathan W. Mink[2], Donald L. Gilbert[3] and Joseph Jankovic[4]

[1]Department of Neurology, Johns Hopkins Hospital, Baltimore, MD, USA;
[2]Division of Child Neurology, University of Rochester Medical Center,
Rochester, NY, USA; [3]Division of Neurology, Cincinnati Children's Hospital
Medical Center, Cincinnati, OH, USA; [4]Department of Neurology, Baylor
College of Medicine, Houston, TX, USA

Movement Disorders in Childhood, Second Edition.
DOI: http://dx.doi.org/10.1016/B978-0-12-411573-6.00017-6

PEDIATRIC NEUROTRANSMITTER DISORDERS

The term *pediatric neurotransmitter disease* has been applied to a broad spectrum of relatively uncommon genetic disorders that affect the synthesis, metabolism, and catabolism of neurotransmitters. The primary neurotransmitters involved in these diseases are the monoamines, which include serotonin and catecholamines (dopamine and norepinephrine), and gamma-aminobutyric acid (GABA).[1–3]

Monoamine Neurotransmitter Disorders

Monoamine-related neurotransmitter diseases can be divided into separate categories based on the site of abnormality in the metabolic pathway, e.g., those affecting (1) the cofactor tetrahydrobiopterin (BH4), (2) enzymes of monoamine biosynthesis, (3) catabolic enzymes, and (4) transporter defects (Table 17.1; Figure 17.1). Despite their differing etiologies, these disorders have many common symptoms, including developmental delay, axial hypotonia, rigidity, movement abnormalities, speech problems, feeding difficulties, abnormal eye movements, and autonomic symptoms. Diagnostic studies include cerebrospinal fluid (CSF) for analysis of monoamines (dopamine, DA; serotonin, 5HT; norepinephrine,

TABLE 17.1   Pediatric Neurotransmitter Disorders

MONOAMINE NEUROTRANSMITTER DEFICIENCIES

---

1. *Biopterin defects*
   With hyperphenylalaninemia
   - GTPCH-1 deficiency (autosomal recessive)
   - Pyruvoyl-tetrahydropterin synthase (PTPS) deficiency
   - DHPR deficiency

   Without hyperphenylalaninemia
   - Dopa-responsive dystonia (DRD) (autosomal dominant)
   - SPR deficiency
2. *Primary defects of monoamine biosynthesis*
   - TH deficiency
   - AADC or ALAAD deficiency
3. *Catabolic enzyme defects*
   - MAO deficiency
   - DBH deficiency
4. *Transporter defects*
   - Brain dopamine-serotonin vesicular monoamine transporter (VMAT2) disease
   - Dopamine transporter deficiency

GABA-RELATED NEUROTRANSMITTER DISORDERS

Succinic semialdehyde dehydrogenase (SSADH) deficiency

NE), neurotransmitter metabolites (homovanillic acid, HVA; 5-hydroxyindoleacetic acid, 5-HIAA; 3-methoxy-4-hydroxylphenylglycol, MHPG; pterins (biopterin and neopterin)), quantitative plasma and urine catecholamines, and phenylalanine loading profiles with and without BH4. The concentrations of these metabolites and other products, however, can vary markedly from one individual to another and some abnormalities may not be necessarily specific for a particular disorder.

Biopterin Defects

BH4 is an essential cofactor for the neurotransmitter synthesizing enzymes TH (which catalyzes the conversion of tyrosine to L-dopa) and TPH (which catalyzes the conversion of tryptophan to 5-hydroxytryptophan, 5-HTP), as well as for PAH (which converts phenylalanine to tyrosine). BH4 itself is synthesized in a multistep pathway starting from guanosine triphosphate (GTP) and, when formed, requires several enzymes to maintain it in its active state (Figure 17.2).

Several enzymatic defects have been identified in BH4 metabolism, e.g., deficiencies in the first and rate-limiting synthesizing enzyme GTPCH-1, in the second and third enzymatic steps, namely, 6-pyruvoyl-tetrahydropterin synthase (6-PTS) and SPR, respectively, and in the maintenance enzyme DHPR. Although one might expect that a defect in BH4 metabolism would be readily detectable based on the presence of hyperphenylalaninemia, which occurs because of a deficiency of PAH activity, this is not always present. Hence, classifications of BH4 metabolism defects are based on presentations with or without hyperphenylalaninemia.

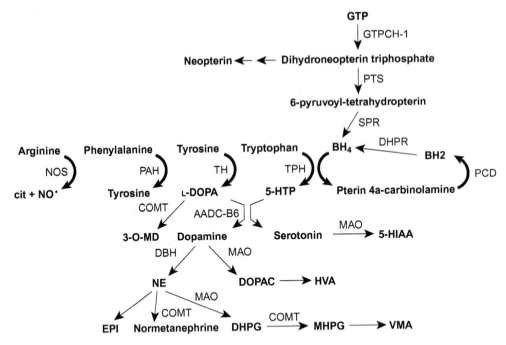

FIGURE 17.1   **Synthesis and catabolism of catecholamine and indoleamine neurotransmitters.** Abbreviations: AADC, aromatic L-amino acid decarboxylase; B6, pyridoxine; COMT, catechol-O-methyltransferase; DBH, dopamine β-hydroxylase; DHPG, dihydrophenyl glycine; DHPR, dihydropteridine reductase; DOPAC, dihydroxphenylacetic acid; EPI, epinephrine; 5-HIAA, 5-hydroxyindoleacetic acid; 5-HTP, 5-hydroxytryptophan; GTPCH, guanosine triphosphate cyclohydrolase; HVA, homovanillic acid; MAO, monoamine oxidase; MHPG, methoxy 4 hydroxphenylglycol; NE, neoepinephrine; NOS, nitric oxide synthase; PAH, phenylalanine hydroxylase; PCD, pterin-4-carbinolamine dehydratase; PTS, 6-pyruvoyl-tetrahydropeterin synthase; qBH2, quinonoid dihydropterin; SPR, sepiapterin reductase; TH, tyrosine hydroxylase; TPH, tryptophan hydroxylase; VMA, vanillylmandelic acid. *Source: Swoboda KJ, Hyland K; Diagnosis and treatment of neurotransmitter related disorders, Neurol Clin 20:1143–1161, 2002.*

BH4 DEFECTS WITH HYPERPHENYLALANINEMIA

Individuals in this group have onset in the neonatal period and include those with autosomal recessively inherited forms of GTPCH-1 deficiency, 6-PTS deficiency, PCD deficiency, and DHPR deficiency.[4–6] Since each produces hyperphenylalaninemia and reduced synthesis of monoamines, clinical signs and symptoms tend to overlap.

CLINICAL PRESENTATION   In the neonatal period, presumably due to hyperphenylalaninemia, hypotonia, poor suck, diminished movements, and microcephaly are usually present. Generally, beginning several months later, more monoaminergic symptoms appear, including autonomic symptoms (hypersalivation, temperature instability, excessive diaphoresis, and blood pressure lability), oculogyric crises, swallowing difficulties, variable hypokinetic and hyperkinetic movements, seizures, and cognitive impairment.[5,7,8] These patients can be detected by neonatal screening for phenylketonuria (PKU). In DHPR deficiency, a secondary reduction in central nervous system (CNS) folate has led to perivascular basal ganglia calcification and multifocal subcortical perivascular demyelination.[9,10]

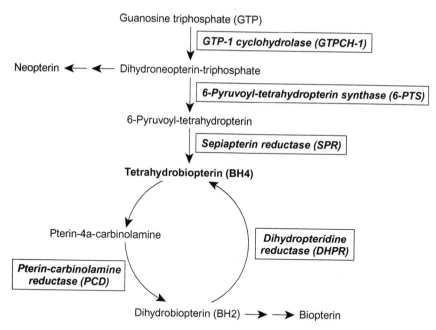

FIGURE 17.2   BH4 synthesis.

Follow-up testing of urine pterins (biopterin and neopterin) and measurement of DHPR activity in blood are necessary to pinpoint the defect.[4]

AUTOSOMAL RECESSIVE INHERITED FORMS OF GTPCH-1 DEFICIENCY (14Q22.1-22.2)

Although one most commonly thinks of the autosomal-dominant form of the disease, i.e., Segawa's disease or DRD, there is an autosomal recessive form of GTPCH deficiency. The autosomal recessive form has hyperphenylalaninemia, due to a deficiency of hepatic PAH activity, and typical symptoms as described previously. Treatment with BH4 is usually insufficient and supplementation with L-dopa and 5-HTP is usually required.[2]

PYRUVOYL-TETRAHYDROPTERIN SYNTHASE (6-PTS) DEFICIENCY (AUTOSOMAL RECESSIVE, LOCUS 11Q22.3-23.3)

This is the most prevalent form of hyperphenylalaninemia not attributed to PAH deficiency. 6-PTS catalyzes dihydroneopterin-triphosphate to form 6-pyruvoyl-tetrahydropterin. Patients have reduced catecholamine and serotonin metabolites and an increased neopterin to biopterin level in the CSF. Two variants have been described, each having elevated levels of phenylalanine in newborn screening tests. The classic severe form shows persistent delays and progressive neurologic deterioration, with truncal hypotonia, subsequent appendicular hypertonia, bradykinesia, extrapyramidal signs (cogwheel rigidity, choreoathetosis, dystonia), and diurnal fluctuation.[1,11] Other features may include swallowing difficulties, oculogyric crises, autonomic symptoms, irritability, and seizures. Patients with milder phenotypes have deteriorated following administration of folate antagonists; the latter interferes with the conversion of BH2 to BH4 (see Figures 17.1 and 17.2), via dihydrofolate reductase.[12] A non-CNS "peripheral form" has been reported that has no biochemical abnormalities in the CSF, mild phenylalaninemia, and the potential for normal neurologic development with appropriate treatment.[13] Treatments include the use of neurotransmitter precursors (L-dopa, 5-HTP), MAO inhibitors, and BH4.[2]

DHPR DEFICIENCY (AUTOSOMAL RECESSIVE, LOCUS 4P15.31)

This disorder results from a defect of BH4 regeneration. The disorder is caused by mutations in the *QDPR* gene. Two forms have been described: the more common neonatal/early infancy form with progressive clinical symptoms similar to 6-PTS deficiency, and a juvenile-onset form with progressive cognitive deterioration, seizures, long-tract signs, extrapyramidal signs, and cerebellar signs.[14,15] CSF shows elevated levels of BH2, raised to normal levels of biopterin, and reduced concentrations of HVA and 5-HIAA. Early recognition and treatment is important. Basal ganglia calcifications may be reversible with folinic acid supplementation.[16] As described in other hyperphenylalaninemia BH4 defects, treatment is designed to replace CSF dopamine and serotonin and to prevent breakdown of the formed neurotransmitter. The use of BH4 supplementation remains controversial whereas oral calcium folinate/folinic acid is routinely used.[2]

BH4 DEFECTS WITHOUT HYPERPHENYLALANINEMIA

Dopa-responsive dystonia: DRD, also known as Segawa's disease, hereditary progressive dystonia, and DYT5, is the hallmark disorder of BH4 metabolism without hyperphenylalaninemia. DRD is an autosomal-dominant disorder caused by heterozygous mutations, spanning a 30kb region with six exons, in the gene for GTPCH-1 located on chromosome 14q22.1-22.2.[17,18] This enzyme is the rate-limiting step in BH4 synthesis. New mutations are frequent, clinical penetrance is incomplete (increased in females), and variable expressivity has occurred in families.[19] Although the spectrum of presentations is wide, patients typically seek treatment in mid-childhood (5–6 years) with dystonic posturing of leg or foot affecting the gait in a child with normal cognition.[20] Symptoms progressively worsen and about one-quarter develop hyperreflexia and spasticity, leading some to be inappropriately labeled with the diagnosis of cerebral palsy. Diurnal variation occurs in all forms with progressive worsening throughout the day and improvement in the morning, after sleep. Cases without diurnal changes, however, have been reported. Investigators have also differentiated differences in clinical presentations at older ages: onset around age 8 years presents with retrocollis, torticollis, and possibly oculogyric crisis; and after age 10, presentation with an asymmetric postural tremor, and a more adult presentation with features of Parkinsonism, i.e., bradykinesia, rigidity, masked facies, hypophonic speech, and postural instability.[4,20,21] An unusual case with myoclonus-dystonia syndrome, i.e., myoclonic jerks beginning in childhood, has been described.[22] Older patients have a greater prevalence of obsessive-compulsive disorder and major depressive disorder.[23]

Patients respond dramatically and in a sustained fashion to low-dose levodopa (or a dopamine agonist), making it important to properly diagnose this disorder. Some DRD patients have also shown a good response to anticholinergics, such as trihexyphenidyl.[24] BH4 may be helpful, but is rarely used. Since dopamine synthesis is more affected than serotonin, serotonin reuptake inhibitors are not typically used.

DIAGNOSIS Diagnosis is typically based on clinical symptoms and response to levodopa. A cardinal feature of this disorder is its responsiveness to a therapeutic trial with L-dopa/carbidopa. In unclear cases or to distinguish DRD from other metabolic diseases or forms of Parkinsonism, genetic testing of GTPCH-1 or CSF testing, as above, may be helpful. CSF analysis shows markedly decreased HVA, normal or low 5-HIAA, reduced BH4 and neopterin levels, with normal plasma phenylalanine levels. CSF findings may not, however, always be classical.[2] The phenylalanine loading test has been advocated for detection of both affected and nonmanifesting GTPCH-1 gene carriers.[25,26] Since individuals with PKU would show similar abnormalities, DRD carriers are distinguished by correction of the loading test after administering biopterin. Nevertheless, in view of limited sensitivity and specificity, the results of phenylalanine loading tests need to be interpreted with caution.[2,27] Genetic testing can be done to identify heterozygous mutations of the *GTPCH1* gene on chromosome 14q, however, over 100 mutations have been identified.[28] If genetic analyses do not demonstrate mutations in GTPCH-1,[29] it is important to ascertain whether analysis included sequencing of the entire gene.

Neuroimaging can occasionally be helpful to distinguish DRD from juvenile Parkinsonism. The density of presynaptic dopamine terminals in striatum should appear normal in DRD but reduced in juvenile Parkinsonism, as demonstrated either by use of fluorodopa positron emission tomography (PET) or by single-photon emission tomography with [^{123}I]beta-CIT. Postsynaptic terminal D2 receptor density, using raclopride PET has been variable, but some PET D2 dopamine receptor studies suggest increased binding in both symptomatic and asymptomatic carriers of GTPCH mutations as well as in some juvenile Parkinsonism cases.[30,31]

DHPR DEFICIENCY WITHOUT HYPERPHENYLALANINEMIA

This disorder has been reported in several cases.[32] Neurologic symptoms include psychomotor retardation, microcephaly, spasticity, dystonia, oculomotor apraxia, and hypersomnolence. The oral phenylalanine loading test in these patients was abnormal, despite the lack of hyperphenylalaninemia. CSF measurements show reduced monoamines and their metabolites, but normal BH4 and neopterin levels. Treatment of this disorder includes the use of levodopa and 5-HTP in combination with carbidopa to correct central monoamine deficits.

SPR DEFICIENCY (AUTOSOMAL RECESSIVE, LOCUS 2P14-P12)

SPR deficiency is another inherited disorder of BH4 metabolism characterized by signs and symptoms related to monoamine neurotransmitter deficiency, but without hyperphenylalaninemia. SPR catalyzes the final two-step reduction of the intermediate 6-pyruvoyltetrahydropterin (PTP) to BH4. Phenylalaninemia is absent, since other reductases in the liver, but not brain, can substitute for this enzyme. SPR deficiency has been reported in the first month of life with progressive psychomotor retardation, axial hypotonia, oculogyric crisis, diurnal fluctuations of dystonia, dyskinesias, athetosis, tremor, behavioral and psychiatric features, and hypersomnolence.[33-35] CSF measurements show low CSF HVA and 5-HIAA and raised levels of total biopterin, dihydrobiopterin (BH2), and sepiapterin.[36] Urine pterins and plasma phenylalanine levels are normal. Several mutations in the SPR gene have been identified.

TREATMENT Nonhyperphenylalaninemia BH4 deficiencies can be treated with dopamine and serotonin precursor supplementation. BH4 has not been beneficial.[34] A low starting dose of L-dopa is recommended.[3]

Primary Defects of Monoamine Biosynthesis

Defects of monoamine biosynthesis have been defined at three sequential enzymatic steps: (1) TH, the rate-limiting step catalyzing the conversion of tyrosine to L-dopa in the formation of dopamine and norepinephrine; (2) ALAAD or AADC, which converts L-dopa to dopamine; and (3) DBH, the enzyme that converts dopamine to norepinephrine (see Figure 17.1).

TH DEFICIENCY (AUTOSOMAL RECESSIVE, LOCUS 11P15.5)

TH, the rate-limiting enzyme in the biosynthesis of dopamine, catalyzes the conversion of L-tyrosine to L-dihydroxyphenylalanine. At least eight different point mutations have been identified in the TH gene, and alternate splicing of TH pre-mRNA can lead to at least four different isoforms.[37] Varying phenotypes have been described including severe early-onset encephalopathy, progressive gait disorder, juvenile Parkinsonism, and hypotonia with ataxia.[38,39] A classification based on phenotype, genotype, and CSF HVA:5-HIAA ratios has been suggested: *Type A* containing an infantile hypokinetic-rigid syndrome with dystonia, promoter mutations, and CSF HVA:5-HIAA ratio <1; and *Type B* with a severe neonatal encephalopathy and CSF ratio <0.7.[40] In cases with a severe reduction of TH activity, onset occurs in infancy with symptoms of psychomotor retardation, rigidity, hypokinesia, axial hypotonia, and oculogyric crises. In other presentations, cases have Parkinsonism, gait disorders, stiffness after exercise, tremor, dystonia, and ataxia. One case had a static encephalopathy with spastic paraplegia and the later development of a progressive dystonic-dyskinetic syndrome.[41] Neuroimaging is normal whereas electroencephalograms (EEGs) may show nonspecific background abnormalities.[42,43] The possibility of an autosomal-dominant presentation has been observed in one family.[44]

DIAGNOSIS Diagnosis is confirmed by genetic analysis and biochemical testing showing reduced CSF levels of dopamine, norepinephrine, HVA, and MHPG with normal 5-HIAA, biopterin, and neopterin levels.[38,40] The CSF HVA:5-HIAA ratio is < 1 (normal 1.0–3.7). Since TH is primarily expressed in the brain and adrenal gland, enzymatic assessment is generally not feasible.

TREATMENT Treatment involves the administration of conservative doses of levodopa/carbidopa in order to minimize L-dopa sensitivity and intolerable dyskinesia.[39] In general, medication responses for motor symptoms and involuntary movements in individuals who tolerate L-dopa are good.[40] Additional therapeutic recommendations include use of a MAO-B inhibitor (selegiline) to prevent breakdown of formed neurotransmitter, dopamine agonists (bromocriptine, pramipexole) and biperiden (a selective central M1 cholinergic receptor blocker).[38,45] Deep brain stimulation was beneficial in a single case.[46]

ALAAD OR AADC DEFICIENCY (AUTOSOMAL RECESSIVE, LOCUS 7P12.1-12.3)

AADC, a pyridoxal-5-phosphate-dependent enzyme, catalyzes both the formation of dopamine from L-dopa and serotonin from 5-HTP. Deficiency of this enzyme leads to a profound reduction of CSF serotonin and catecholamines. AADC deficiency is caused by mutations in the *DDC* gene with a common founder mutation identified in Taiwanese patients.[47] Clinical symptoms usually begin in childhood; although onset and phenotype can be variable. Major presenting problems include developmental delay, hypotonia, and oculogyric crises.[48] About 50% also present with movement disorders including arm and leg extension, dystonia, athetosis, myoclonus, torticollis, and bulbar dysfunction. Autonomic symptoms, associated with monoamine neurotransmitter deficiency, have included ptosis, miosis, sweating, temperature instability, hypotension, gastroesophageal reflux, and sleep disturbances.[48] Milder phenotypes have been reported in siblings with hypersomnolence, fatigability, and dystonia[49] as well as in older individuals.[48,50] Magnetic resonance imaging (MRI) scans may have mild cortical atrophy and EEGs spike or polyspike bursts.[51]

DIAGNOSIS Diagnosis of an AADC deficiency is made by measuring CSF neurotransmitters and metabolites. Classic findings include marked reductions of dopamine, HVA, serotonin, 5-HIAA, norepinephrine, and 3-MHPG. Levels of L-dopa and its metabolite, 3-O-methyldopa, are elevated, since L-dopa cannot be decarboxylated to dopamine. The CSF pterin profile is normal. Plasma and fibroblast AADC is markedly reduced. A secondary deficiency of AADC, caused by a lack of pyridoxal 5-phosphate, has been reported.[52]

TREATMENT Treatments are variable and satisfactory in about 19% of patients.[48] Therapeutic approaches include possibly enhancing enzyme activity by using of high dose cofactor supplementation with pyridoxal phosphate[53]; maintaining any levels of dopamine and serotonin that are produced by use of MAO inhibitors (tranylcypramine, selegiline); stimulating dopaminergic neurotransmission by use of dopamine agonists (bromocriptine, pramipexole, ropinirole); and supplementation with folinic acid, since the folate may be reduced by the excessive metabolism of L-dopa. L-dopa is not expected to be beneficial, although rarely some patients do improve,[54] whereas serotonergic agents have not been of benefit.[8]

Catabolic Enzyme Defects

MAO DEFICIENCY (MAPPED TO THE XP11.23-11.4 REGION)

MAO catalyzes the oxidative deamination of serotonin, epinephrine, and norepinephrine. MAO-A deficiency has been reported in males with mild mental retardation and violent aggressive behavior[55] and MAO-B deficiency has been identified in Norrie disease.

DBH DEFICIENCY

DBH catalyzes the conversion of dopamine to norepinephrine. Deficient individuals have low CSF/plasma/urine levels of norepinephrine, epinephrine, and their metabolites. Typical presenting symptoms are hypotension, hypothermia, and hypoglycemia.[1]

Transporter Defects

BRAIN DOPAMINE-SEROTONIN VESICULAR TRANSPORTER DISEASE (MUTATIONS IN *SLC18A2*)

Mutational defects that alter the VMAT2 result in the defective loading of monoamines into synaptic vesicles and in turn a functional deficiency. A consanguineous family with eight affected children presented with the early onset of delayed milestones, hypotonia, oculogyric crisis, focal dyskinesia, Parkinsonism, tremor, dystonia, sleep disturbance, and autonomic dysfunction.[56] Neuroimaging and CSF neurotransmitter profiles were normal, urine levels of dopamine and norepinephrine were low, and HVA and HIAA were elevated. Treatment with L-dopa caused deterioration in chorea and dystonia, but pramipexole (a dopamine receptor agonist) produced sustained improvement.

DOPAMINE TRANSPORTER DEFICIENCY SYNDROME (MUTATION IN *SLC6A3*)

Defective presynaptic uptake of dopamine from the synaptic cleft results in increased synaptic levels, greater catabolism, and raised CSF HVA levels (HVA:5-HIAA ratio >5). Clinically, this disorder presents in infancy with hypotonia, irritability, and feeding difficulties. Neurological symptoms are progressive with the appearance of Parkinsonian features with bradykinesia, rigidity, and resting tremor.[57,58] Variants have also been reported in older children and adults. The majority of affected patients have been unresponsive to a variety of medications and deep brain stimulation, although some dopamine agonists have produced limited improvement.[59]

GABA-Related Neurotransmitter Disease

SSADH Deficiency (4-Hydroxybutyric Acidurias, Autosomal Recessive, Locus 6p32)

SSADH works in conjunction with GABA transaminase to convert GABA to succinic acid (Figure 17.3). In the absence of SSADH, GABA is converted to 4-hydroxybutyric acid (GHB). Pathophysiologically, despite an excessive concentration of GHB in physiological fluids, it remains unclear whether clinical symptomatology is due to elevated GHB, GABA, or other metabolic alterations. The gene for SSADH, an aldehyde dehydrogenase 5 family member A1 (*ALDH5A1*) is located on chromosome 6p22.

SSADH deficiency has a mean age of onset of about 11 months, but diagnosis is often delayed until a mean of 6.6 years.[60] Clinical phenotype is variable and nonspecific with a variety of neurologic and psychiatric symptoms. Findings include mental retardation, disproportionate language dysfunction, autistic traits, hypotonia, ataxia, aggression, anxiety, hallucinations, hyperactivity, occasionally choreoathetosis, and about half of affected individuals have seizures.[61,62] About 10% have a severe phenotype characterized by

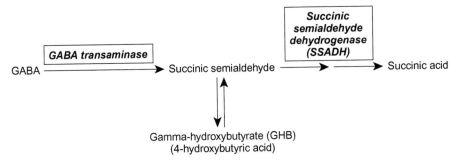

FIGURE 17.3 Succinic acid synthesis.

developmental regression and extrapyramidal manifestations.[63,64] Neuropathological evaluation in a single case showed findings consistent with a chronic excitotoxic injury.[65]

DIAGNOSIS

Neuroimaging has shown cerebral and cerebellar atrophy and T2 hyperintensities in the globus pallidus, cerebellar dentate nucleus, and subthalamic nucleus, although imaging is normal in 40% of cases.[66] EEG may show diffuse background slowing and generalized or multifocal abnormalities, photosensitivity, and sleep spindle asynchrony. Diagnosis is made by detection of massive increases in GHB in urine, plasma, or CSF and confirmed using enzyme analysis in leukocytes and molecular genetic analysis of ALDH5A1. Prenatal diagnosis is possible and prenatal testing/preimplantation testing is available.[67–69]

TREATMENT

Treatment is symptomatic, with anticonvulsants and medication for behavior problems. Valproic acid is contraindicated because it inhibits residual SSADH enzyme activity. Vigabatrin (gamma-vinyl GABA), which blocks GABA transaminase and the conversion of GABA to GHB,[70] has been tried with mixed results.

METABOLIC DISORDERS

Mineral Accumulation

Copper

WILSON'S DISEASE (HEPATOLENTICULAR DEGENERATION) (AUTOSOMAL RECESSIVE, LOCUS 13Q14.3)

PATHOPHYSIOLOGY   The gene for Wilson's disease encodes for a protein (copper-transporting P-type ATPase, ATP7B), localized in the trans-Golgi network, that is responsible for excretion of copper out of the hepatocyte and the incorporation of copper into ceruloplasmin (Figure 17.4).[71] More than 500 *ATP7B* mutations have been described and there is extensive phenotypic:genotypic heterogeneity.[72] Abnormalities lead to failure to excrete copper in the bile and the subsequent accumulation in liver, brain, cornea, kidney, bones, and blood. Intestinal absorption of copper is normal and serum levels of ceruloplasmin, an α-2-globulin that binds and transports copper molecules, are nearly always reduced. Increased excretion of copper in the urine is insufficient to prevent copper accumulation. The accumulation of other metals in the brain, besides copper, has also been speculated to have a contributing pathogenic role, e.g., dysfunction of ceruloplasmin leading to iron accumulation and liver dysfunction.[73] ATP7A, structurally similar to the Wilson's disease ATP7B, affects copper absorption and is responsible for systemic copper deficiency (decreased serum copper and ceruloplasmin) and the X-linked Menkes disease with its clinical symptoms of kinky hair, developmental regression, hypotonia that progresses to spasticity, and paresis.[74]

CLINICAL FEATURES   The typical childhood clinical presentation of Wilson's disease is hepatic dysfunction (asymptomatic hepatomegaly, acute transient or fulminant hepatitis) beginning about age 12 years.[75] An early onset case has been described in 9-month-old child

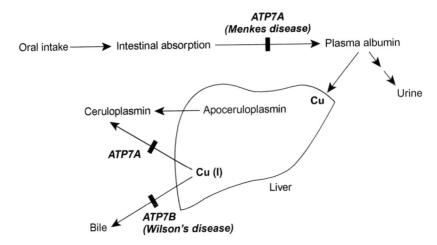

FIGURE 17.4   Copper transport.

and late-onset cases in individuals over age 70 years.[76,77] The mean age for the appearance of neurological symptoms is about 19 years, although symptoms have been reported in a 6-year-old child.[78–80] Clinical presentation tend to be insidious and variable, including alterations in speech, drooling, pharyngeal dysmotility, motor function, and mental changes.[72] Dysarthria described by Wilson[81] as a "trifling indistinctness of speech," clumsiness, tremor, or mental changes may be the initial presentation. In contrast, others have suggested that tremor, chorea, dystonia, and cerebellar impairment are the earliest manifestations.[82,83] Unusual presentations have included spasmodic muscle cramps and myopathy.[84] Several other phenotypes have been described, including an akinetic-rigid (Parkinsonian) form, a generalized dystonic type, and an ataxic phenotype.[85] Psychiatric symptoms precede the neurologic abnormalities in about 20% of cases, ranging from subtle changes in personality and behavior ("a childishness seen in facile laughter, or irritability, or caprice") or decline in school performance, to significant anxiety, depression, and frank psychosis.[86,87] Tremor, although common in Wilson's disease, has variable characteristics and may be unilateral or bilateral; appear at rest or during postural maintenance, with movement, or in any combination of the aforementioned. When presenting as an action tremor, it is typically coarse and irregular and when elicited with arms forward and flexed may have the classical "wing-beating" or proximal quality.[88] Dystonia can be generalized, segmental, focal, or multifocal. With progression of the disease, spasmodic dystonia of the head or body and dyskinesias involving the face (facial grimacing, sardonic smile or risus sardonicus, blepharospasm, and tongue dyskinesia) are common. Abnormal vertical smooth pursuits are frequently observed.[89] A possible association has been identified between genotype and psychopathological symptoms and personality traits.[90] The Kayser–Fleischer (KF) ring, a yellow-brown deposition of copper in the periphery (Descemet's membrane) of the cornea, is characteristic of the disease when it involves the CNS.[91] Although identifiable on examination, especially in individuals with lightly pigmented corneas, KF rings are best observed by slit-lamp examination.

MRI abnormalities include increased signal intensity on T2-weighted images of the tectal plate, basal ganglia, thalamus, and brainstem and central pontine myelinolysis-like changes.[92] Less common findings include the "face of the panda" located in the midbrain. Pathologically, copper accumulates extensively in the basal ganglia, where it can cause necrosis, as well as diffusely in the cortex and adjacent white matter. Although MRI findings can improve with copper chelation therapy,[93] brain content of copper may remain elevated and prominent neuropathological features persist. The severity of neuropathological findings has been correlated with the content of cerebral copper.[94]

DIAGNOSIS Early diagnosis is critical in order to reverse symptoms and prevent further complications. Diagnosis requires consistent clinical findings and supporting laboratory studies that include measurement of serum ceruloplasmin (reduced), quantification of 24-h urine copper (elevated, typically exceeds $100 \mu g/24h$), identification of the Kayser–Fleischer ring on slit-lamp examination, and the most definitive evaluation being a liver biopsy with histologic assessment and determination of copper content. Direct molecular diagnosis can also be a decisive tool, but testing must include screening for the entire ATP7B coding region and adjacent splice sites. In children, ages 6 and above, with neurologic symptoms suggestive of Wilson's disease, the appropriate first test is a serum ceruloplasmin. Detection of ceruloplasmin, an α2-glycoprotein acute-phase reactant, at a level of $20 mg/dL$ or lower has a diagnostic sensitivity of approximately 95%. False positives (low levels) may occur in severe malnutrition, protein losing conditions, acute liver failure, and aceruloplasminemia. False negatives (higher levels) can occur in affected individuals who have hepatitis, other inflammatory disorders, or are using oral contraceptives. In addition, values may differ in local populations.[95]

TREATMENT Treatment for Wilson's disease is divided into an acute de-coppering therapy and lifelong maintenance treatment.[72,96] Existing questions have made it difficult to select the most appropriate de-coppering compound and randomized control trials need to be done. Penicillamine is a powerful copper chelating agent, but because of potential side effects, including sudden and possibly permanent worsening of neurologic symptoms, its use is controversial.[75,97,98] Ammonium tetrathiomolybdate is a newer medication that has four sulfur groups, which allows it to form a tripartite complex with copper and protein.[99] Clinical experience with this drug is limited and its formulation may not be stable. Trientine (triethylene tetramine dihydrochloride) is not beneficial for the acute treatment of patients with neurologic symptoms, because it does not mobilize copper from the brain. It is useful, however, as maintenance therapy and in the treatment of patients with pure hepatic disease. Zinc, which induces the synthesis of metallothionein in the intestine, has a slower onset of action and is only used as maintenance therapy or in case of very early diagnosis. Serum parameters of copper metabolism, urinary copper levels, and liver function tests should be monitored in patients receiving chronic therapy to prevent iatrogenic copper deficiency. Recovery of neurologic problems typically does not begin until after about 6 months of treatment. Although radiographic improvement on brain MRI may be seen for up to 4 years, disabilities that persist for longer than 2 years after initiation of therapy tend to be permanent. Orthotopic liver transplantation may be lifesaving for patients with fulminant liver failure; however, this procedure is controversial for individuals with severe neurological symptoms.[72,100] Deep brain stimulation may be an effective treatment.[101] Gene therapy approaches are potentially effective strategies.[102,103]

HUPPKE–BRENDL SYNDROME (AUTOSOMAL RECESSIVE; MUTATIONS IN *SLC33A1*)

Low ceruloplasmin and copper levels have been identified in children with mutations in SLC33A1, which encodes the acetylcholine transporter AT-1.[104] Clinically this is a lethal autosomal recessive disorder with congenital cataracts, hearing loss, and severe developmental delay. MRI shows cerebellar hypoplasia and hypomyelination.

Manganese

MANGANESE STORAGE DISORDER (AUTOSOMAL RECESSIVE; MUTATIONS IN *SLC30A10*)

A small number of cases with generalized dystonia in childhood and adolescence or Parkinsonism in adulthood have been reported with manganese accumulation secondary to mutations in the manganese transporter gene SLC30A10.[105–107] Laboratory findings include increased serum manganese concentrations, polycythemia, reduced iron stores with low ferritin, and high total iron binding capacity. Similar to Wilson's disease, patients had hepatic cirrhosis and MRI contained hyperintensities in the basal ganglia. Improvement depends on early treatment with repeated intravenous $CaNa_2$-EDTA infusions, which increase urinary excretion of manganese.[105,107]

Neurodegeneration with Brain Iron Accumulation

Neurodegeneration with brain iron accumulation (NBIA) is a group of rare and devastating disorders associated with iron deposition in the brain. Initially labeled Hallervorden–Spatz syndrome (HSS), this heterogeneous group of conditions has been associated with nine different NBIA genes (*PKAN, PLA2G6, C19orf12, WDR45, FTL, CP, ATP13A2, C2orf37,* and *FA2H*).[108–110] Based on their frequency, the two major subtypes are pantothenate kinase–associated neurodegeneration (PKAN) and PLA2G6-associated neurodegeneration (PLAN). Several other phenotypes are listed in Table 17.2.

TABLE 17.2   NBIA Disorders and Gene Abnormality

Pantothenate kinase–associated neurodegeneration (PKAN); *pantothenate kinase 2 (PANK2)*

PLA2G6-associated neurodegeneration (PLAN); *PLA2G6*

Mitochondrial membrane protein-associated neurodegeneration (MPAN); *C19orf12*

Beta-propeller-associated neurodegeneration (BPAN); *WDR45*

Neuroferritinopathy; *FTL*

Aceruloplasminemia; *CP*

Kufor–Rakeb syndrome: *ATP13A2*

Fatty acid hydroxylase-associated neurodegeneration (FAHN); *FA2H*

Woodhouse–Sakati syndrome: *C2orf37* gene

PANTOTHENATE KINASE–ASSOCIATED NEURODEGENERATION

PKAN is a rare autosomal recessive disorder (chromosomal locus 20p12.3-p13) caused by mutations (point mutations, insertions, and deletions in all seven exons) in the gene for pantothenate kinase 2 (PANK2). Pantothenate kinase is an essential regulatory enzyme in the biosynthesis of coenzyme A (CoA) from vitamin B5 (pantothenate) (Figure 17.5). The enzyme is localized to mitochondria and postulated to alter mitochondrial membrane potentials.[111] Pathologically, this disorder is associated with abnormal iron deposition and high concentrations of lipofuscin and neuromelanin in the substantia nigra pars reticulata and the internal segment of the globus pallidus. Patients homozygous for null mutations show typical PKAN phenotypes whereas individuals who are compound heterozygous for null/missense mutations have a more atypical course.[112]

CLINICAL FEATURES   PKAN has variable presentations and has been divided into (a) a classic early-onset form containing 75% of cases with presentation before age 6 years and a rapidly progressive course, and (b) "atypical forms," which present at a mean age of 14 years.[113,114]

In the classical form, onset is in early childhood with progressive motor difficulties, personality changes, cognitive decline, dysarthria, and spasticity. Extrapyramidal dysfunction is typically present, but may be delayed for several years. Dystonia is the most common extrapyramidal feature (orobuccolingual and limb), and rigidity, choreoathetosis, and a resting or action tremor may also be present. Ophthalmologic abnormalities include pigmentary retinal degeneration in about two thirds of patients, alteration of vertical and saccadic pursuits, progressive loss of peripheral visual fields, and blindness. Patients also develop cognitive dysfunction and seizures may be present. Acanthocytosis is the most frequently reported systemic manifestation, occurring in about 8% of classic patients.[114] The course of the early-onset form is variable and is divided into a rapidly and a slowly progressive type. The rapidly progressive early-onset type has a short transition from spasticity to severe movements with opisthotonos, and death within 1–2 years. In contrast, the more prevalent

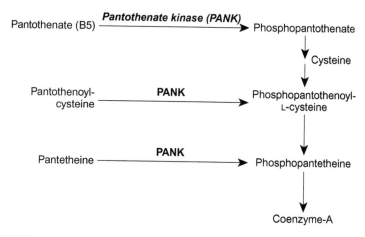

FIGURE 17.5   PANK-mediated reactions.

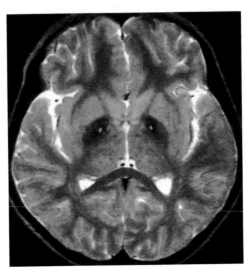

FIGURE 17.6   MRI findings in NBIA type 1 showing decreased T2-weighted and proton density signal in the globus pallidus—the "eye of the tiger" sign.

slowly progressive early-onset type advances at a nonuniform rate and symptoms decline more slowly; dystonia and spasticity leading to being wheelchair-bound by the teens, with death occurring within 20 years.

In the "atypical" late-onset childhood form, patients often have speech defects (palilalia, tachylalia, and dysarthria) as an early sign and develop significant psychiatric symptoms (personality changes, impulsivity, obsessive-compulsive disorder, aggression, episodic outbursts, and depression) and even motor and vocal tics.[108,115,116] Although affected individuals are often described as clumsy, motor involvement (Parkinsonism, akinesia, dystonia, tremor) is a later feature, and spasticity ultimately limits ambulation. Freezing during ambulation, especially when turning or encountering irregular surfaces, has been described.[117] Subclinical retinal changes may be present. In general, the course of atypical PKAN is less severe and more slowly progressive than the early-onset types.

DIAGNOSIS   The diagnosis of PKAN depends on the presence of obligate features: onset in the first two decades, progressive course, extrapyramidal symptoms, and classic MRI findings showing hypointense T2-weighted and proton density signal in the globus pallidus and substantia nigra (Figure 17.6). The presence of a hyperintense area within the hypodense areas, named the "eye of the tiger sign," is thought to be almost pathognomonic for PKAN.[118] Hyperdense lesions may be present in presymptomatic patients, but as the disease progresses hypodensities appear and ultimately predominate.[118–120] In patients with PKAN, 7-Tesla imaging has identified elevated concentrations of iron in the globus pallidus, substantia nigra and internal capsule; not seen in those with heterozygous mutations.[73] Other findings include abnormal cytosomes in lymphocytes and retinal bone spicule pigmentation and accumulation.[113,121] Cultured skin fibroblasts have been reported to accumulate ^{59}Fe-transferrin.

TREATMENT There is no specific treatment for PKAN. Theoretically, in patients with residual PANK2 activity the downstream delivery of phosphopantothenate or products in the coenzyme A pathway might be therapeutic. Iron chelation therapy with desferrioxamine has not been effective, but response was better with deferiprone.[122,123] Therapy for movement disorders and spasticity is symptomatic. Oral baclofen has been helpful in early stages but intrathecal infusion has provided only limited benefit.[124] In 23 PKAN patients, deep brain stimulation improved dystonia and quality of life.[125] Pallidotomy and thalamotomy have produced limited and transient benefit.[126–128]

PLA2G6-ASSOCIATED NEURODEGENERATION; AUTOSOMAL RECESSIVE

The newly termed PLAN represents a second major NBIA phenotype and comprises three previously separate, but overlapping, phenotypes including infantile neuroaxonal dystrophy (INAD), atypical neuroaxonal dystrophy, and PLA2G6-related dystonia Parkinsonism (Video 17.1). The *PLA2G6* gene encodes an 85 kDa calcium-independent phospholipase A_2 enzyme (iPLA$_2$-VIA), which is active in a tetrameric form. Functionally, the enzyme catalyzes the hydrolysis of glycerophospholipids, generates a free fatty acid and lysophospholipid, playing a role in membrane homeostasis through the regulation of phospholipids.[129] MRIs in this group may overlap with that seen in PKAN.

INAD is an autosomal recessive disorder, manifesting between 6 months and 3 years, with a gait disturbance and truncal hypotonia. Onset may occur following an intercurrent infection. Progressive symptoms include motor and sensory impairment, spastic tetraplegia, hyperreflexia, and visual impairment associated with optic atrophy.[130] Seizures are a late manifestation. This is a rapidly progressing disorder with death at the end of the first decade. Electromyography shows denervation and nerve conduction studies a distal axonal sensorimotor neuropathy. MRI demonstrates cerebellar atrophy, "claval hypertrophy,"[131] and brain iron accumulation within the globus pallidus, dentate nucleus, and substantia nigra.[130]

The *atypical form of NAD* has an older age of onset with presenting symptoms including gait impairment, ataxia, speech difficulties, and autistic features.[132,133] The clinical course is relatively stable in early childhood with neurological deterioration in mid-childhood consisting of extrapyramidal manifestations (primarily dystonia), dysarthria, and in later stages spastic tetraplegia. Previously described Karak syndrome[134] is now considered an atypical NAD. MRI shows prominent brain iron accumulation with or without cerebellar atrophy.

PLA2G6-related dystonia Parkinsonism is a rare disorder with a broad range of presentations, mostly occurring in early adulthood. Childhood presentations have initially overlapped with atypical NAD, including development of an extrapyramidal syndrome with dystonia, Parkinsonism, and choreoathetosis. MRIs have shown nonspecific changes including cerebral atrophy. Symptoms may temporarily respond to L-dopa.

MITOCHONDRIAL MEMBRANE PROTEIN-ASSOCIATED NEURODEGENERATION

MPAN is an autosomal recessive disorder caused by mutations in the *C19orf12* gene.[109,135] C19orf12 expression is mainly in the brain, blood cells, and adipocytes with proteins located in the mitochondria. The precise function of C19orf12 proteins remains unclear. The mean age of symptom onset is 10 years, with variability ranging between 3 and 30 years. Frequent symptoms include spasticity, cognitive decline, dysarthria, optic atrophy, dystonia, psychiatric symptoms, dysphagia, and Parkinsonism. About half have a motor axonal neuropathy with muscle atrophy, fasciculations, and EMG changes. Neuroimaging shows brain iron accumulation in the globus pallidus and substantia nigra and generalized cerebral and/or cerebellar atrophy.

BETA-PROPELLER PROTEIN-ASSOCIATED NEURODEGENERATION

BPAN is the only X-linked disorder of NBIA.[136] The disorder is due to X-chromosomal WDR45 *de novo* mutations. WDR45 belongs to a family of WD40 proteins that promote protein–protein interactions with a role in cell cycle control, translational regulation, signal transduction and autophagy. The name beta-propeller is derived from its tertiary structure. Affected children have global developmental delay, epilepsy (multiple seizure types), Rett-like behaviors, stereotypies, dysfunctional sleep, and ocular defects.[137] Regression occurs in adolescence with the appearance of Parkinsonian features (bradykinesia, freezing of gait, rigidity), progressive dyskinesia, and dementia. Early imaging may be normal, but with increasing symptoms shows iron deposition in the globus pallidus and substantia nigra. On T1-weighted imaging, the substantia nigra/cerebral peduncles have a distinctive hyperintense "halo." Parkinsonian symptoms have improved with L-dopa, but medication-induced dyskinesia is common.

NEUROFERRITINOPATHY

Neuroferritinopathy is an autosomal-dominant disorder characterized by mutations in the ferritin light-chain gene (*FTL*), which codes for ferritin light polypeptide, on chromosome 19q13. The mean age of onset is 40 years and presentation includes chorea, dystonia, prominent oromandibular dyskinesias, and Parkinsonism.[138,139] Neurocognitive features include dementia, depression, emotional lability, and acute psychosis.[140] Patients have low serum ferritin levels and MRI is abnormal even early in the disease.[141]

ACERULOPLASMINEMIA (AUTOSOMAL RECESSIVE DISORDER, LOCALIZED TO CHROMOSOME 3)

This disorder is due to mutations altering the function of the ceruloplasmin gene (*CP*) and is often confused with Wilson's disease because of very low levels of ceruloplasmin and overlapping imaging results.[142] In contrast to Wilson's disease, however, aceruloplasminemia is considered to be a disorder of iron metabolism due to its activity as an iron oxidase and its absence resulting in iron accumulation within the brain, liver, and pancreas.[143] Clinical manifestations usually occur in adulthood (fifth–sixth decade) with findings of diabetes mellitus, retinal degeneration, and neurological symptoms. Progressive neurological problems include dystonia, dysarthria, bradykinesia, rigidity, cerebellar ataxia, and dementia.[144,145] Anemia with low serum iron, low transferrin saturation, but elevated serum ferritin is usually present. MRI shows hypointensities in the basal ganglia, dentate, and thalamus. Attempts to treat with iron chelators have been disappointing.[143]

OTHER NBIA DISORDERS

Kufor–Rakeb syndrome (*ATP13A2* gene) is a rare autosomal recessive disorder beginning in adolescence with Parkinsonism, eye movement abnormalities, and possible pyramidal signs. It is also labeled as PARK9.[146,147]

FAHN is associated with mutations in the *FA2H* gene and clinically characterized by the childhood onset of gait abnormalities, spastic quadriparesis, ataxia, and dystonia. Mutations also cause a form of hereditary spastic paraplegia and leukodystrophy.[148,149]

Woodhouse–Sakati syndrome is a rare autosomal recessive disorder associated with mutations in the *C2orf37* gene located on chromosome 2q31.1. Clinically, this syndrome is characterized by hypogonadism, frontotemporal alopecia, hypotrichosis, diabetes, mental retardation, and cervicofacial dystonia.[150,151]

HARP SYNDROME

HARP syndrome has been used to define a phenotype that includes hypoprebetalipoproteinemia, acanthocytosis, retinitis pigmentosa, and pallidal degeneration.[152] This disorder has been shown to be caused by mutations in PANK2, the gene that causes PKAN.[114] A few other patients have been reported with symptoms of acanthocytosis, retinitis pigmentosa, facio-bucco-lingual dyskinesia, and the "eye of the tiger sign" (see Figure 17.6), but with normal serum lipoproteins.[153] Acanthocytes are believed to be caused by lipid peroxidation, a process stimulated by iron.

Lysosomal Storage Disorders

Lysosomes are intracytoplasmic vesicles that contain a variety of degradative enzymes that are used to catabolize complex substrates such as sphingolipids, gangliosides, cerebrosides, sulfatides, mucopolysaccharides, and glycoproteins.[154] The diagnosis of these diseases is based on levels of lysosomal enzyme activity which are readily assayed in serum, white blood cells, or cultured fibroblasts. The inherited absence of a specific enzyme activity, in turn, results in the excessive accumulation of the undegradable substance in the lysosome, with subsequent disruption of either neuronal or myelin function (Figure 17.7).

Neuronal Storage Diseases

Neuronal storage diseases, such as GM1 and GM2 gangliosidosis, Gaucher disease (GD), and Niemann–Pick disease, are typically characterized by the presence in infancy of progressive cognitive and motor deterioration, seizures, retinopathy, and in some cases hepatosplenomegaly. In general, it is the more slowly progressive variants of these disorders, i.e., those that have only partial deficiencies of enzyme activity, which tend to have extrapyramidal signs.

GM1 GANGLIOSIDOSES

GM1 gangliosidoses are caused by a deficiency of β-galactosidase activity resulting in a failure to cleave the terminal β-galactose from the GM1 ganglioside.[155,156] Three types of GM1 gangliosidoses have been defined based on age of onset and the extent of enzyme activity; very low β-galactosidase activity in the infantile form and residual activity in the older forms.[157] At least 102 mutations in the β-galactosidase gene have been described. The infantile form (*Type 1*) is the most common, has its onset between birth and 6 months, and is characterized by coarse facial features, developmental failure, edema, dysostosis multiplex, hepatosplenomegaly, hypotonia, cherry-red macular spot, seizures, vacuolated lymphocytes, and skeletal dysostosis. Progressive spasticity, joint stiffening, vision and hearing

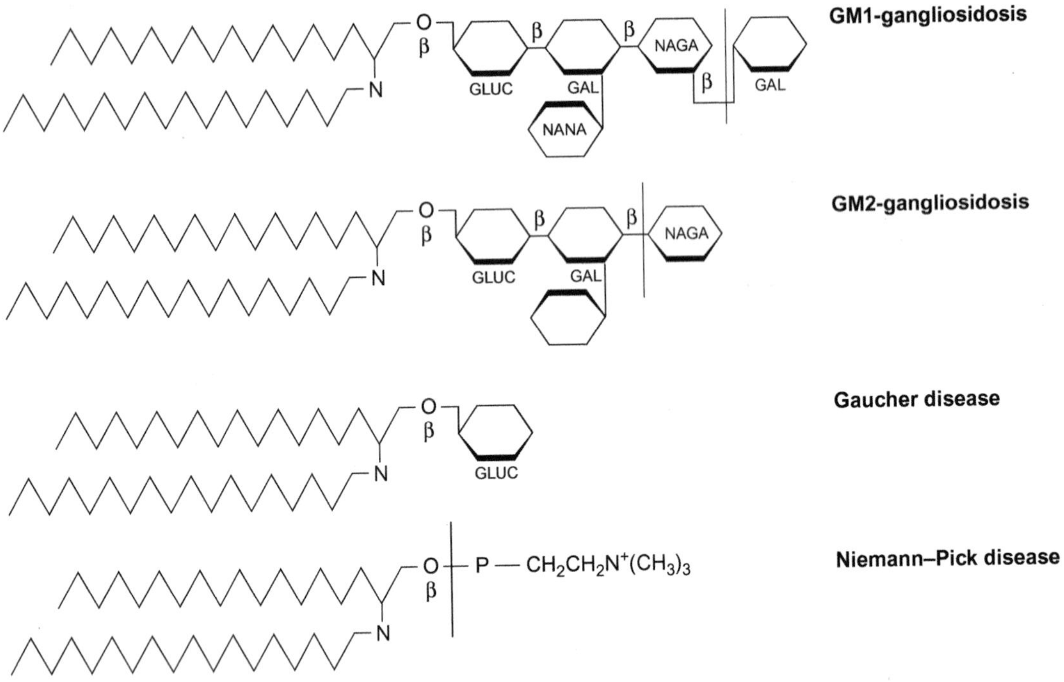

FIGURE 17.7   Neuronal storage diseases.

loss, and seizures are common. Death usually occurs by 1–2 years of age. A single case has been reported with basal ganglia calcifications.[158] *Type 2*, the late-infantile or juvenile form, begins between 1 and 3 years of age with seizures, spasticity, ataxia, extrapyramidal signs, and mental impairment. Dysmorphic features, corneal clouding, and hepatosplenomegaly, a part of the type 1 form, are lacking in types 2 and 3. Cherry-red spots may be present in type 2. *Type 3* GM1 gangliosidosis occurs in children or adults (ages 3–30 years) and is a slowly progressive disorder with dysarthria, dystonia, rigidity, bradykinesia, and gait abnormalities.[159–162] MRI in type 3 shows symmetric hyperintense signal intensities on proton-density and T2-weighted sequences in the caudate and putamen.[159,160,162] Intracytoplasmic storage and cell loss is most prominent in the caudate and putamen, with lesser involvement in the globus pallidus, cerebellar Purkinje cells, and amygdala.[163] The molecular mechanisms leading to disease symptoms are incompletely understood.[164,165]

GM2 GANGLIOSIDOSES

GM2 gangliosidoses are a group of recessively inherited disorders characterized by the accumulation of the GM2 ganglioside within neuronal cells secondary to a deficiency in β-hexosaminidase activity. β-Hexosaminidase has two major isozymes, hexosaminidase A (HEX A), which is composed of α- and β-subunits, and hexosaminidase B (HEX B), containing only β-subunits. The Hex A gene is located at 15q23-24 and encodes the α-subunit and Hex B at 15q13 encodes the β-subunit. Thus a genetic defect encoding α-subunits would affect only HEX A, whereas a defect encoding β-subunits would affect both HEX A and B.

The three major forms of GM2 gangliosidosis include *Tay–Sachs disease* and its variants due to a HEX A deficiency (also known as the B types); *Sandhoff disease* with a deficiency of both HEX A and HEX B (also called the O type); and the *AB variant* caused by an abnormality of the GM2-activator protein. Diagnosis is based on identifying a decreased hexaminidase activity and a change in activity between isoforms. No biochemical test is currently available for the activator deficiency.[166]

The *classic infantile forms* of Tay–Sachs and Sandhoff diseases are characterized by early neurologic deterioration, loss of developmental milestones, exaggerated startle response to auditory stimuli, motor weakness, progressive blindness, cherry-red spots in the macular region, seizures, and early death. Hepatosplenomegaly may be present in Sandhoff disease. MRI findings on T2-weighted images include hyperintensities in both basal ganglia and thalamus.[167] Why specific subpopulations of neurons are targeted remains unclear.

Juvenile GM2 gangliosidosis (deficiency of hexosaminidase A) has an age of onset of 2–6 years and is characterized by combinations of psychomotor deterioration, progressive ataxia, dysarthria, spasticity, dystonic movements, athetoid posturing of the hands and extremities, and seizures, with death by the midteens.[168] Several cases have had progressive proximal muscle weakness and were initially misdiagnosed as having spinal muscular atrophy (SMA) type III (Kugelberg–Welander disease).[169,170]

Adult or chronic GM2 gangliosidosis has a slowly progressive course with neurologic symptoms including cerebellar ataxia, dysarthria, weakness, and atrophy (similar to a motor neuron disease), a combined spinocerebellar ataxia, oculomotor disturbances, and involvement of the peripheral and autonomic nervous system.[171,172] Psychiatric symptoms, including depression, psychosis, and dementia, also occur in this variant and may be a presenting feature.[173]

TREATMENT There is no specific treatment for the gangliosidoses. Several therapies are under investigation in animal models,[174,175] but none have been effective in man.[176]

NIEMANN–PICK DISEASES

The eponym Niemann–Pick disease encompasses a variety of different lysosomal lipid storage diseases. Individuals with type A have an acute neuropathic form with visceromegaly, pulmonary involvement, and death in infancy. Those with type B have chronic visceral disease without neurologic involvement. In both the type A and B autosomal recessive disorders, sphingomyelin accumulates in various tissues and the lysosomal enzyme sphingomyelinase is deficient.

Niemann–Pick type C is an atypical lysosomal storage disease characterized by normal sphingomyelinase levels but the lysosomal accumulation of unesterified cholesterol and glycosphingolipids due to altered lipid trafficking.[177–179] Mutations in the *NPC1* gene on chromosome 18q11-12 (approximately 300) account for about 95% of human cases and the rest are due to *NPC2* gene alterations.[180] Both NPC1, a transmembrane protein, and NPC2, a soluble protein, are involved in lysosomal cholesterol efflux. Loss of function mutations in NPC1 leads to a failure of the calcium-mediated fusion of endosomes with lysosomes.[181] Neuropathological features include neuronal storage, neuronal loss, ectopic dendrites, and neuroaxonal dystrophy. The range of onset has been variable. A juvenile-onset form is characterized by learning difficulties, cognitive deterioration, psychiatric symptoms, supranuclear vertical gaze palsy, cerebellar ataxia, cataplexy, dysarthria, gait problems, seizures, and hepatosplenomegaly. Movement disorders, including dystonia (begins in the extremities and gradually becomes generalized), chorea, athetosis, and Parkinsonism are also part of the neurologic picture.[182–186] Peripheral neuropathy is a rare complication.[187] Death occurs in the second decade due to progressive dysphagia and inanition.

DIAGNOSIS In the setting of characteristic symptoms, biochemical testing is most useful. Cultured fibroblasts are tested for abnormal esterification of exogenous cholesterol and accumulation in lysosomes (seen with filipin staining). MRI of the brain in Niemann–Pick type C ranges from normal to mild posterior periventricular white matter hyperintensity. Bone marrow testing, which shows foamy cells or sea-blue histiocytes, is rarely needed. Sphingomyelinase activity is normal in cultured skin fibroblasts and peripheral leukocytes. Gene testing is recommended.[179]

TREATMENT There is no specific treatment for this disorder. Miglustat, an iminosugar that inhibits glucosylceramide synthase, improved or stabilized several clinical markers.[188]

GAUCHER DISEASE

GD is the most common of the lysosomal storage disorders. The disorder is an autosomal recessive trait resulting from defects of acid β-glucosidase (chromosome 1q21; more than 200 mutations) with the subsequent accumulation of its substrate glucocerebroside. GD is divided into three conventional types, with visceral involvement in all and neuronopathic symptoms in two of the three forms.[189,190] Diagnosis is usually based on the presence of Gaucher cells in the bone marrow aspirate and confirmation by enzymatic assay and molecular analysis. Gaucher-like cells can also be found in hematologic disorders such as leukemia, Hodgkin's lymphoma, and multiple myeloma. *Type 1 (nonneuronopathic)* is the most common form. Clinically, it is a chronic nonneurologic disorder with hepatosplenomegaly and hematologic (anemia, thrombocytopenia, leukopenia) problems. Extensive skeletal disease is typical. *Type 2 (acute neuronopathic),* the rarest and most severe form, is found in infants and is characterized by hepatosplenomegaly, progressive severe CNS deterioration, and death by age 5 years.[191] Neurologic signs include myoclonus, myoclonic epilepsy, supranuclear ocular paresis, rigidity, cervico-facial dystonia, mild spastic paraparesis, slow mental deterioration, Parkinson-like symptoms, and generalized epilepsy.[192,193] Numerous genotypes and clinical phenotypes are associated with type 2 GD. Necroptosis has been proposed as a possible pathophysiological mechanism, e.g., continued accumulation of glucocerebroside reaches a threshold and triggers a rapid cascade leading to neuroinflammation and neurodegeneration.[194] *Type 3 (chronic neuronopathic)* is more heterogeneous, occurring in children or adults, with affected individuals having organomegaly, Gaucher cells in the bone marrow, and some form of neurologic involvement. Several treatments are available for Type 1 GD including enzyme replacement and substrate reduction therapies.[189] Enzyme replacement therapy reverses most of the systemic manifestations, but rarely the neurologic deficits because it does not cross the blood–brain barrier.[195] Intraventricular delivery has been tried without success[196] and substrate reduction therapy with Miglustat did not benefit neurological manifestations.[197]

NEURONAL CEROID LIPOFUSCINOSES

Neuronal ceroid lipofuscinoses (NCLs), also known as Batten disease, are a group of neurodegenerative diseases usually beginning in childhood. The NCLs are autosomal recessive, lysosomal storage disorders that are characterized by the accumulation of autofluorescent ceroid lipopigment in brain tissue and various organs, including sweat glands and muscle. Historically, three classic forms were described in children based on the age of onset, clinical symptoms, and electron microscopic evaluation of the storage material[198] and included: infantile NCL (Haltia–Santavuori disease) with granular osmiophilic deposits; late-infantile NCL (Jansky–Bielschowsky disease) with accumulations having curvilinear profiles; and juvenile NCL (Batten or Spielmeyer–Vogt–Sjögren disease) with fingerprint profiles observed in biopsy material and in lymphocytes. More recently, a genetic classification, based on the gene defect for each disorder, has been implemented.

NCL disorders result from mutations in different *CLN* genes (*CLN1–CLN14*) (Table 17.3).[198–200] Several of the genes have been shown to encode soluble and transmembrane proteins located in endosomes/lysosomes or the endoplasmic reticulum.[201] Unfortunately, mutations do not strictly coincide with clinical classifications based on age of presentation, symptoms, or type of inclusion. For example, mutations in the *CLN1* gene can be associated with infantile, late-infantile, juvenile, or adult variants of the disease and different mutations can cause the same variant (e.g., CLN 1, 2, 5, 6, 7, and 8 cause the late-infantile variant). Most experts recommend primary classification by gene or protein abnormality, however, a new more extensive taxonomy has been proposed.[202]

i. *CLN1 disease*: Mutations in *CLN1* cause the classic infantile onset form. The *CLN1* gene encodes the enzyme palmitoyl protein thioesterase 1 (PPT1), which removes fatty acids from a variety of fatty acylated proteins. PPT1 deficiency leads to caspase 9 activation[203] and impairs synaptic vesicle recycling of nerve terminals.[204] In infantile NCL, onset is between 6 and 24 months. Typically, following an initial period of normal development, there is a rapid regression of developmental milestones, deceleration of head growth, hypotonia, motor clumsiness, ataxia, irritability, seizures, and visual failure. By age 2–3 years, affected children have lost all motor and social skills and are blind. Death occurs before the early teenage years. A late-infantile variant of CLN1 disease begins between 2 and 4 years of age and is characterized by visual and cognitive decline followed by the development of ataxia and myoclonus.[198] The juvenile variant usually starts between 5 and 10 years of age, with cognitive decline followed by seizures, motor decline, and visual failure due to pigmentary retinal degeneration. A rarer adult-onset form of CLN1 has been described with onset after age 18 years, cognitive decline and depression, followed by ataxia, Parkinsonism, and loss of vision.[205] In all forms of CLN1, storage granules have osmophillic deposits and correlate with PPT1 deficiency.

ii. *CLN2 disease*: CLN2 disease is the classic late-infantile form. The *CLN2* gene codes for tripeptidyl peptidase 1, a soluble lysosomal protein. Classic CLN2 disease usually presents between ages 1 and 4 years with developmental standstill or psychomotor regression, followed by refractory epilepsy of various types, ataxia, myoclonus, spastic quadriparesis, and visual loss (macular degeneration). Children with CLN2 disease onset after 4 years of age tend to have a milder course with more prominent ataxia and less prominent epilepsy.

TABLE 17.3   Classification of NCLs

Gene	Age of onset	Chromosome	Protein	Ultrastructure
CLN1	Infantile, but also late-infantile, juvenile, and adult	1p32	PPT 1	GRODS
CLN2	Late-infantile, but also juvenile	11p15	TPP 1	Curvilinear profiles
CLN3	Juvenile	16p12	Lysosomal transmembrane protein	Fingerprint profiles
CLN4 (DNAJC5)	Adult (Parry)	20q13.33	Cysteine string protein	Rectilinear profiles
CLN5	Late-infantile (Finnish variant)	13q22	Soluble lysosomal protein	Rectilinear profiles, curvilinear profiles, fingerprint profiles
CLN6	Late-infantile adult (Kufs Type A)	15q21	Transmembrane protein of ER	Rectilinear profiles, curvilinear profiles, fingerprint profiles
CLN7	Late-infantile, Turkish variant	4q28	MFSD8, lysosomal membrane protein	Fingerprint profiles
CLN8	Late-infantile, Northern epilepsy	8q23	Transmembrane protein of ER	Curvilinear profiles
CLN10	Congenital	11p15	Cathepsin D	GRODS?
CLN11	Adult	17q21.31	Progranulin	–
CLN12	Juvenile	1p36.13	ATP13A2 protein	–
CLN13	Adult	11q13	Cathepsin F	–
CLN14	Late-infantile	7q11.21	Potassium channel tetramerization domain containing protein 7	–

Modified from Mink et al.[198] and Schulz et al.[200]
ER, endoplasmic reticulum; GRODS, granular osmiophilic deposits; NCLs, neuronal ceroid lipofuseinoses.

iii. *CLN3 Disease*: CLN3 disease is the classic juvenile-onset form of NCL. The CLN3 protein is a lysosomal transmembrane protein of unknown function. Onset in CLN3 disease is between 4 and 7 years, with insidious, but rapidly progressive, vision loss, followed by cognitive decline, behavioral problems, and seizures (usually generalized tonic-clonic). The movement disorder in CLN3 is Parkinsonism, sometimes responsive to L-dopa. Dysarthria is prominent after age 10 years.

iv. *CLN4 disease*: An autosomal-dominant form, now classified as "Parry disease," named after the family in which it was first described. CLN4 is due to a mutation in the *DNAJC5* gene that codes for a cysteine string protein. Onset of symptoms is after age 30 years with clinical features including ataxia, progressive dementia, seizures, and myoclonus with no visual loss.

v. *CLN5 disease*: A late-infantile NCL referred to as the "Finnish variant" but occurs worldwide. The CLN5 protein is a soluble lysosomal glycoprotein of unknown function. The mean age of onset is 5.6 years (range 4–17 years). Clinical features include psychomotor regression, ataxia, myoclonic epilepsy, and visual failure, often the presenting sign.

vi. *CLN6 disease*: This disorder has a variable onset, ranging from 18 months to 8 years. The CLN6 protein is a transmembrane protein of unknown function. Clinical features include vision loss, motor developmental delay, dysarthria, ataxia, and seizures. There is rapid deterioration and death usually occurs between 5 and 12 years of age. *CLN6* mutations have been shown to cause autosomal recessive Kufs A disease (formerly CLN4). Kufs disease has been subclassified as types A and B.[206] Type A begins with a progressive myoclonic epilepsy, with later development of dementia and ataxia.

vii. *CLN7 disease*: Called the Turkish variant, but occurs worldwide. The CLN7 protein, encoded by the *MFSD8* gene, is a lysosomal membrane protein that belongs to the "major facilitator" superfamily of transporter proteins. Onset for CLN7 disease is typically between 2 and 7 years. Initial symptoms are typically seizures, followed by motor decline, myoclonus, and dementia. Vision loss is usually preserved.

viii. *CLN8 disease*: Mutations in *CLN8* cause a variant of late-infantile NCL and a form of progressive myoclonic epilepsy ("Northern epilepsy"). The disorder is due to mutations in a transmembrane protein of the endoplasmic reticulum with an unknown function. In the late-infantile form, onset is usually between 5 and 10 years of age, with a presentation of myoclonic seizures, progressive motor and cognitive decline, and vision loss. "Northern epilepsy," in addition to seizures, has cognitive and motor decline, but no visual loss.

ix. *CLN10 disease*: CLN10 disease is the only form in which patients are severely affected at birth. It is caused by mutations in the lysosomal aspartic protease cathepsin D gene (*CTSD*). Infants are microcephalic, have intrauterine or early postnatal seizures, absence of neonatal reflexes, and respiratory insufficiency. Death is in early infancy.

x. *CLN11 disease*: This variant has an adult onset[207] and is due to homozygous mutations in the progranulin gene that encodes a glycoprotein of unknown function. Progranulin has roles in inflammation, early embryogenesis, cell motility, and tumorigenesis.[208]

xi. *CLN12 disease*: CLN12 has a juvenile onset, presents with learning difficulties[209] and is due to mutations in the *ATP13A2* gene which encodes a lysosomal type 5 P-type ATPase. Also associated with Parkinsonism, this finding emphasizes an overlap between Parkinson's disease and NCLs.[210,211]

xii. *CLN13 disease*: Adult onset (Kufs B). Type B is characterized by dementia with cerebellar and/or extrapyramidal motor symptoms without visual loss.[206] Age of onset is around 30 years. The disease is associated with mutations in the *cathepsin F (CTSF or CLN13)* gene; the physiological function of CTSF is unclear.[212]

xiii. *CLIN14 disease*: Infantile onset. Two infant siblings presented with myoclonus, developmental regression, and visual failure.[213] A mutation in the *KCTD7* gene was identified; encodes the potassium channel tetramerization domain containing protein 7 with a suggested function being modulation of transporter subunits.[201]

V. SELECTED SECONDARY MOVEMENT DISORDERS

DIAGNOSIS The diagnosis of NCLs is based on clinical presentation, ophthalmologic findings, electroretinography, MRI, evidence of storage (electron microscopy of leukocytes, skin, or conjunctival biopsy), measurement of *PPT1* and TPP1 activities, and additional molecular genetic studies. Prenatal testing using a combination of enzyme assay and mutation testing is reliable in families where the biochemical and genetic diagnosis is established. A diagnostic algorithm for the evaluation of NCL has been published.[200] There is no effective treatment for the NCL disorders.

White Matter Disorders

Disorders primarily affecting white matter typically manifest with symptoms and signs of progressive motor difficulties, spasticity, peripheral neuropathy, and optic atrophy whereas extrapyramidal symptoms are generally uncommon. For example, metachromatic leukodystrophy (MLD), with deficient arylsulfatase A, has the accumulation of sulfatides in central and peripheral myelin and a combination of upper and lower motor neuron findings. Nevertheless, a dystonic phenotype has been reported in an individual with juvenile MLD.[214] Two disorders, Pelizaeus–Merzbacher disease and Canavan disease, both with leukoencephalopathies and potential extrapyramidal findings are included in this review.

PELIZAEUS–MERZBACHER DISEASE

Pelizaeus–Merzbacher disease is an X-linked recessive disorder of CNS myelin caused by a mutation in the proteolipid protein (PLP1) gene on Xq22.2.[215] The gene has two major transcripts, PLP1 and DM20, which are developmentally regulated in the CNS and peripheral nervous system.[216] Gene duplication is the most common mutation with missense mutations, insertions, and deletions being less common. PLP is a major CNS myelin protein and its excessive production or conformational change can have a critical role in the maturation and maintenance of central myelin. Pelizaeus–Merzbacher disease has two clinical forms: *type 1* begins in infancy with abnormal eye movements (irregular oscillations, horizontal, or vertical nystagmus) and laryngeal stridor. Later, generally within the first 6 months, psychomotor development slows, with a greater involvement of motor function, especially in the lower extremities due to progressive spasticity.[217] Choreiform movements of the limbs may be present, and seizures have been reported.[218,219] MRI scans typically show a lack of myelin with low intensity on T1-weighted and high intensity on T2-weighted images. The proton MRS profile differs from other commonly observed demyelinating disorders and can aid in diagnosis.[220] Females heterozygous for the mutation have been reported with progressive pendular nystagmus, athetosis, spastic gait, and dysarthria.[221] *Type 2* is an X-linked spastic paraplegia. Treatment is symptomatic and new clinical treatments are under review.[215]

CANAVAN DISEASE (VAN BOGAERT, BERTRAND DISEASE)

Canavan disease, also called spongy degeneration of the CNS, is a progressive autosomal recessive leukodystrophy caused by a deficiency in aspartoacylase, localized in oligodendrocytes, which catalyzes the deacetylation of *N*-acetyl-L-aspartate to form aspartate and acetate.[222,223] Various mutations in the asparto-acylase gene, localized on chromosome 17pter-p13, have been identified. The *classic form* manifests in infancy, at about 3–6 months, with lethargy, irritability, hypotonia, head lag, and decreased motor activity.[224] Macrocephaly becomes apparent in the first year. Over time, the child develops dystonia and spasticity. Increased irritability, nystagmus, optic atrophy, seizures, and cognitive symptoms are common. Death usually occurs in the first decade. Congenital, juvenile, and mild variants have been reported.[225-227] Diagnosis is based on detection of elevated levels of *N*-acetyl aspartic acid (NAA) in urine, CSF, and brain (elevated NAA to creatine ratio on magnetic resonance spectroscopy), and enzyme activity measurement in fibroblasts. MRI shows decreased signal on T1-weighted and increased signal on T2-weighted images in white matter, primarily in cerebral hemispheres, globus pallidus, and thalamus. Histology demonstrates spongiform degeneration of the cortex and subcortical white matter. The mechanism by which elevated NAA or its related dipeptide *N*-acetyl-aspartyl-glutamate (NAAG) leads to underlying pathophysiological changes remains unclear.[222] Management is strictly supportive. Lithium, which reduces NAA levels in the brain, has been reported to improve alertness and social interactions.[228] Gene therapy with an AAV vector carrying the ASPA gene was beneficial in slowing the course of the disorder.[229]

Amino Acid Disorders

Homocysteinuria

In the most common form of homocysteinuria, the metabolic defect involves the enzyme cystathionine β-synthase encoded on chromosome 21, which catalyzes the formation of cystathionine from homocysteine and serine (Figure 17.8). Clinically, two phenotypes have

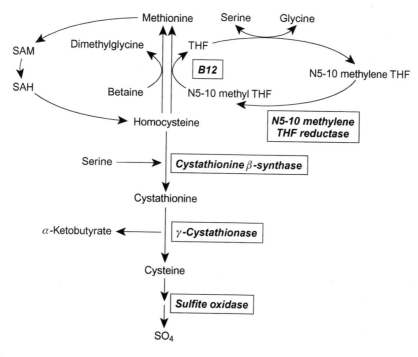

FIGURE 17.8 Metabolism of homocysteine.

been described; a milder pyridoxyl phosphate (Vit B$_6$) responsive form and a more severe pyridoxyl phosphate nonresponsive variant. The primary pathologic alterations are intimal thickening and fibrosis in vessels of all calibers, which lead to arterial and venous thromboses occurring in multiple organs, including skeletal, ophthalmologic, and nervous systems. CNS dysfunction includes intellectual retardation, motor delays, and stroke syndromes. Extrapyramidal abnormalities, primarily dystonia, oromandibular dyskinesia, spasmodic dysphonia, tremor, bradykinesia, have occurred in both children and adolescents with homocysteinuria.[230-232] Seizures and psychiatric disturbances can also be present. MRI studies have shown cerebral infarction, atrophy, venous occlusions, and bilateral low-intensity lesions in the basal ganglia on T2-weighted imaging. Leukoencephalopathy is an uncommon finding.[233] Several hypotheses have been proposed for the pathophysiology in classic homocysteinuria including dysfunctions of *S*-adenosylmethionine, serine, and glutathione metabolism. The treatment of homocysteinuria-related dystonia can be difficult and DBS has been tried.[234]

Homocysteinuria can also be due to remethylation defects, such as cobalamin C disease,[235] methionine synthase deficiency (CblG), or methylene tetrahydrofolate reductase deficiency. In these disorders, in contrast to deficiencies of cystathionine β-synthase, plasma methionine concentrations are low, and there is neither skeletal involvement nor ectopia lentis. In these variants, patients have a wide range of neurologic problems including psychomotor delay, cognitive impairment, seizures, and microcephaly. A deficiency of choline-containing compounds has been identified in the brain, possibly due to depletion of labile methyl groups produced by the transmethylation pathway.[236]

Hartnup Disease

Hartnup disease is an inherited autosomal recessive defect in amino acid transport due to mutations in the *SLC6A19* gene.[237] This gene encodes a neutral amino acid transporter (B(0)AT1) that mediates neutral amino acid transport from the luminal compartment into the cells. Affected individuals have a selective monoamino-monocarboxylic (neutral) aminoaciduria (alanine, asparagine, citrulline, glutamine, histidine, isoleucine, leucine, phenylalanine, serine, threonine, tyrosine, tryptophan, and valine), but with normal or low levels in plasma. Skin changes, resembling findings in pellagra (light-sensitive dermatitis due to nicotinamide deficiency), are usually the first clinical signs, occurring in the late-infantile or juvenile period. Neurologic and psychiatric issues begin about 2–10 years after the appearance of dermatologic changes. Intermittent recurrent ataxia lasting for days to weeks is the most common neurologic symptom with exacerbations of variable intensity. Other, less common symptoms include spasticity, intention tremor, dysarthria, headaches, and psychiatric symptoms ranging from emotional lability to acute psychosis. One case with intermittent dystonia and two cases with dystonic features have been reported.[238,239] Nicotinamide therapy improves the dermatitis and neurologic problems, but spontaneous improvement also occurs with maturation.

Maple Syrup Urine Disease

This disease is an autosomal recessive disorder caused by defective activity of the branched-chain α-ketoacid dehydrogenase enzyme complex. This α-ketoacid dehydrogenase complex consists of three catalytic components (a thiamine pyrophosphate-dependent carboxylase (E1), a transacylase (E2), and a dehydrogenase (E3)) and two regulatory enzymes (a kinase and a phosphatase). This mitochondrial complex catalyzes the oxidative decarboxylation of branched-chain ketoacids derived from the transamination of the branched-chain amino acids, leucine, isoleucine, and valine[240] (Figure 17.9). The defect results in the marked increase of these three essential amino acids, their corresponding α-ketoacids and hydroxy acid derivatives in serum, urine, and CSF. Proposed mechanisms for brain dysfunction include branch-chain amino acid accumulation causing neurotransmitter deficiencies and growth restriction and branched-chain ketoacid accumulation causing energy deprivation through disruption of the Krebs cycle.[241] Clinically, there are four presentations with some overlap: (1) Classic maple syrup urine disease (MSUD) manifests in the newborn period with feeding difficulties, decreased responsiveness, metabolic acidosis, seizures, an abnormal odor of the urine, progressive coma, and cerebral edema. Fluctuating ophthalmoplegia has also been observed.[242] Movement disorders, especially paroxysmal ataxia or dystonia, have been reported during periods of decompensation and improve after appropriate dietary therapy.[240,243] Early recognition and treatment can result in improved neurologic outcome. In adults with treated MSUD, 12/17 had a movement

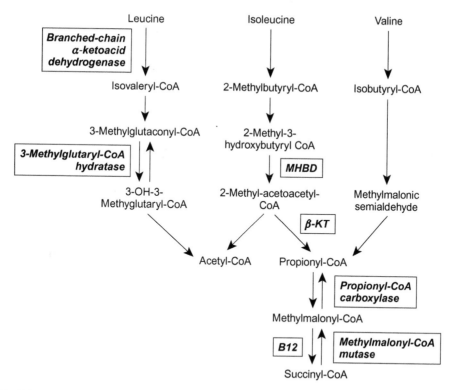

FIGURE 17.9 Catabolism of branched-chain amino acids. Abbreviations: MHBD, 2-methyl-3-hydroxylbutyl-CoA-dehydrogenase; β-KT, β-ketothiolase.

disorder, primarily tremor or dystonia, and some had pyramidal signs and a spastic dystonic gait.[244] (2) Intermittent MSUD with recurrent episodes precipitated by intercurrent illness. (3) Intermediate MSUD with symptoms beginning in infancy or childhood and progressing to include failure to thrive, motor delays, dystonia, autistic features, and seizures.[245] (4) Thiamine-responsive MSUD[246]—MRI shows cerebral edema, delayed myelin maturation, and symmetrical signal abnormalities in the globus pallidus, and brainstem.[247] Diagnosis is confirmed by detection of increased concentrations of leucine, isoleucine and valine, and/or the increased urinary excretion of α-ketoacids and hydroxy acids. Long-term treatment is based on dietary restriction of branched-chain amino acids.

Phenylketonuria

PKU is an autosomal recessive disorder caused by a deficiency of hepatic PAH, the enzyme required to metabolize phenylalanine to tyrosine (Figure 17.10). Most cases are associated with mutations in the *PAH* gene located on chromosome 12q24.1. PKU is classified into the classic and mild forms. Untreated infants have growth failure, seizures, developmental delay, and microcephaly as the result of the accumulation of toxic by-products of phenylalanine, a deficiency of tyrosine and its products including melanin, L-thyroxine, and catecholamines,[248] and possibly stimulation of peroxisome proliferator-activated receptor-gamma receptors.[249] In older patients, pyramidal signs (increased tone, hyperreflexia, and extensor plantar responses) and an irregular, rapid, small-amplitude tremors of the hands are common. Bizarre twisting movements, repetitious movements of the fingers, stereotypies, and overt Parkinsonian features may also be present.[250,251] A meta-analysis of neuropsychological symptoms in treated adolescents and adults showed significant reductions in full-scale IQ, processing speed, reduced attention, and control and inhibitory activities.[252] Psychological and psychiatric problems commonly affect social competence, autonomy, self-esteem, mood, and anxiety.[253] White matter abnormalities have been identified in the brains of adults with PKU.[254] Reduced cerebral fluorodopa uptake has been identified in adult patients.[255] In general, the level of disability remains stable after early childhood, but there are cases of neurologic deterioration in adulthood.[256] It has been suggested that women with PKU start a phenylalanine-restricted diet before conception.[257]

As reviewed in the section on pediatric neurotransmitter disorders, hyperphenylalaninemia can have other etiologies. Treatment is based on early detection with routine newborn screening and prevention of neurologic consequences by early initiation of a phenylalanine-free diet, the administration of large neutral amino acids to prevent phenylalanine entry into the brain, and tetrahydropterin, a cofactor capable of increasing residual PAH activity.[258,259]

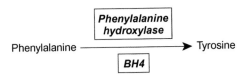

FIGURE 17.10   Phenylalanine metabolism. Abbreviation: BH4, tetrahydrobiopterin.

Organic Acid Disorders

Organic acids are produced from the catabolism of amino acids and are intermediates in metabolic pathways. They contain one or more carboxylic acid or acid phenolic groups without basic amino groups. Organic acidurias are generally considered inborn errors of protein metabolism, a defect in metabolism resulting in an elevation of the organic acid, and an intoxication-like clinical presentation. Neurologic manifestations are extremely common in organic acid disorders and in some can represent the presenting or primary feature. Organic acidurias can be roughly divided into classical and cerebral groups, recognizing the limitation that many forms also have later onset variants. Those with classical organic acidurias usually present with an acute metabolic deterioration after a short symptom-free period at birth. In contrast, cerebral organic acidurias present with neurological symptoms in the absence of severe metabolic disturbances.

Classical Organic Acidurias

METHYLMALONIC ACIDEMIA (AUTOSOMAL RECESSIVE)

In genetic forms of methylmalonic acidemia (MMA), the conversion of methylmalonyl-CoA to succinyl-CoA is impaired secondary to a genetic abnormality in the mitochondrial apoenzyme, methylmalonyl-CoA mutase, or reduction of its adenosylcobalamin cofactor (due to abnormal biosynthesis, deficient cobalamin transport, or acquired deficiency) (Figure 17.9). Infants with absence of the apoenzyme (classic form) become symptomatic in the first week of life with hypotonia, lethargy, respiratory distress, vomiting, metabolic acidosis, and ketosis. Laboratory tests show metabolic acidosis and ketosis with many having hyperammonemia and hypoglycemia. Diagnosis is made by analysis of urine organic acids, which show elevated methylmalonic acid; propionic acid may also be increased because of a secondary inhibition of propionyl-CoA carboxylase. Enzyme assays can be performed on leukocytes and all cases should be tested for responsiveness to vitamin B_{12} (cobalamin). Survivors typically have severe residual neurologic impairments, including dystonia.[260] MRI studies show alterations in myelination and changes in the basal ganglia.[261] Pathologically, there is necrosis of the putamen or globus pallidus. Less frequently, especially in those with cobalamin cofactor deficiencies, onset is delayed to the late-infantile or juvenile period. In general, the vitamin B_{12}-responsive group has a milder course and better outcome. The latter may be characterized by recurrent episodes of ketoacidosis, hyperammonemia, leukopenia, thrombocytopenia, and anemia, which can result in multiple organ failure and even death.[262] The enzymatic defect is treated with protein restriction, cobalamin supplementation, and metronidazole to suppress microbial propionate production. Therapy directed toward extrapyramidal findings generally has a limited response.

PROPIONIC ACIDEMIA (AUTOSOMAL RECESSIVE)

Propionic acidemia is caused by a deficiency of propionyl-CoA carboxylase, a mitochondrial biotin-dependent enzyme, resulting in elevation of serum and urine propionic acid (see Figure 17.9). There are several presentations including severe neonatal, chronic intermittent, and gradually progressive.[263] The presentation of this disorder in early infancy mimics that of methylmalonic aciduria—i.e., recurrent episodes of ketoacidosis, hyperammonemia, hyperglycinemia, hypoglycemia, and seizures. Symptoms of chronic disease are failure to thrive, microcephaly, intellectual disability, spastic quadriplegia, athetosis, dysto-nia, chorea, myoclonus, seizures, optic neuropathy, and myopathy.[263,264] Two children with treated neonatal onset proprionic aciduria developed acute psychotic episodes as teenag-ers.[265] A variant of this disorder has been reported with hypotonia, spastic quadriparesis, and choreoathetosis, but lacking the typical metabolic crises.[266] Metabolites and physiologi-cal stressors are thought to account for many of the disease manifestations. Most autopsies revealed no gross CNS abnormalities. Neuroimaging has been variable and may correlate with the degree of compliance to therapy.[263]

High levels of propionic acid and its derivatives (3-hydroxypropionate, propionylglycine, and tiglic acid) are excreted in the urine. Since propionate accumulates in propionic aciduria as well as MMA, the diagnosis should be confirmed by documentation of reduced activity of propionyl-CoA carboxylase in fibroblasts or leukocytes. Long-term treatment includes a low-protein diet, supplementation with biotin and L-carnitine, and the use of metronidazole to reduce the amount of propionate in tissues. Orthotopic liver transplantation has been used in patients with propionic academia who fail maximum medical therapy.[267]

3-METHYLGLUTACONIC ACIDURIAS

3-Methylglutaconic acidemia is actually a group of four metabolic disorders character-ized by the increased urinary excretion of 3-methylglutaconic acid and 3-methylglutaric acid.[246,268] In 3-methylglutaconic acidemia type 1 (primary), the conversion of 3-methylglu-taryl-CoA to 3-OH-methylglutaryl-CoA is impaired due to a defect of 3-methylglutaryl-CoA hydratase (see Figure 17.9). Defective enzyme activity results in a wide spectrum of clinical abnormalities ranging from mild speech delay to severe encephalopathy with basal ganglia involvement. Several other secondary 3-methylglutaconic acidurias have been described, including type II (Barth syndrome), an X-linked neuromuscular disease with cardiomyopa-thy; type III (*Costeff syndrome*) with symptoms of bilateral optic atrophy, chorea, ataxia, spas-ticity, and cognitive effects[269,270]; and type IV, a mild nonsyndromic form associated with psychomotor retardation, spasticity, hypotonia, optic atrophy, and seizures.

METHYLHYDROXYBUTYRYL-COA DEHYDROGENASE DEFICIENCY

This is one of several inborn errors in the pathway of isoleucine degradation (see Figure 17.9).[246,271] Deficiency of 2-methyl-3-hydroxybutyryl-CoA dehydrogenase (MHBD) has a predominantly neurologic presentation ranging from a static encephalopathy to a progres-sive global neurodegenerative disorder. Normal development in the early months may be followed by regression and loss of previously acquired skills. Neurologic features have included ataxia, dystonia, choreoathetosis, spasticity, optic atrophy, and a retinopathy. MRIs have been variable, ranging from normal to cortical atrophy with signal changes in the basal ganglia.[272]

METHYLACETOACETYL-COA OR ACETOACETYL-COA THIOLASE (β-KETOTHIOLASE) DEFICIENCY

β-Ketothiolase (B-KT) deficiency is a rare autosomal recessive disorder that affects the metabolism of isoleucine and ketone bodies, and typically manifests with an episode of ketoacidosis (see Figure 17.9).[271] 2-Methyl-3-hydroxybutyric acid is the characteristic metab-olite in the urine, but additional metabolic complications may include hyperammonemia and hyperglycinemia. The gene for the hepatic mitochondrial acetoacetyl-CoA thiolase has been mapped to 11q22.3-q23.1. The disorder usually manifests in childhood, between 6 and 24 months, with recurrent episodes of ketoacidosis, vomiting, and dehydration. Episodes usually resolve after symptomatic treatment with glucose and bicarbonate and most patients recover fully. Some patients, especially those with prolonged crises, have had long-term neurologic sequelae. Four patients were reported with developmental delay and radiographic abnormalities involving the putamen preceding the first episode of ketoacidosis.[273] A single case had generalized and intractable dystonia associated with a linear area of increased signal intensity on T2-weighted images in the globus pallidus bilaterally[274] and a second presented with nonprogressive chorea since infancy and stable MRI basal ganglia abnormalities.[275]

Cerebral Organic Acidurias

GLUTARIC ACIDURIA TYPE 1 (AUTOSOMAL RECESSIVE)

Glutaric aciduria type 1 (GA-1) is caused by a defect in the gene localized on chromosome 19p13.2 that codes for glutaryl-CoA dehydrogenase (GCDH), which catalyzes the formation of crotonyl-CoA from glutaryl-CoA (Figure 17.11).[276,277] Biochemically, deficiency of GCDH activity results in the accumulation and excretion of glutaric acid and 3-hydroxyglutaric acid, detectable in the urine, blood, and CSF. Due to the limited permeability of the blood–brain barrier to dicarboxylic acids (glutaric acid) they heavily accumulate in the brain.[246] The diagnosis is confirmed by documentation of deficient GCDH activity in cultured skin fibroblasts. Glutarylcarnitine can be identified on newborn screen by tandem mass spectrometry, if carnitine is not significantly reduced. The disorder has a predilection for the basal ganglia.

Clinically, there are several types of presentation, and phenotypic heterogeneity occurs within families.[278,279] In the majority, macrocephalus is present at or shortly after birth, with rapid changes in head circumference reaching a peak in the first 6 months. Most infants are hypotonic, irritable, jittery, and have feeding difficulties, although cognitive development may be appropriate. Others have global developmental delay and progressive hyperkinetic

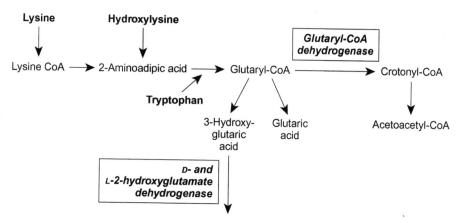

FIGURE 17.11   Catabolism of lysine, hydroxylysine, and tryptophan.

movement problems. Typically, around 6–18 months of age, there is an acute deterioration of motor function in association with an infection, a minor head injury, or following an immunization. Although the child appears to be alert, hypotonia, dystonia, choreoathetosis, and generalized seizures may be present. Extrapyramidal movements are often residual symptoms. Severe episodes of dystonia ("dystonic storm" or "status dystonicus") can be accompanied by hyperthermia and rhabdomyolysis. Other variants of this disorder include normal development until about 2 years of age, a form that mimics the presentation of extrapyramidal cerebral palsy, and even single cases over age 6 years without neurologic symptoms.[280] Infants are also prone to suffer acute subdural hemorrhages after mild head injury.[281] GA-1 has manifested in adulthood with leukoencephalopathy.[282]

Neuroimaging studies show widening of the Sylvian fissure ("bat-winged" dilation), ventriculomegaly, enlarged subdural fluid spaces, and delayed myelination.[283] Additional findings may include "bilateral symmetric" hypodensities in the lenticular nuclei, caudate degeneration, bilateral temporal arachnoid cysts, and mild leukodystrophy that spares U-fibers.

More than 200 mutations in the *GCDH* gene have been identified and no molecular basis differentiates the groups. Clinical variability does not appear to correlate with the extent of residual enzyme activity. The pathological mechanism in glutaric aciduria is unclear with hypotheses including 3-hydroxyglutaric acid stimulation of glutamatergic NMDA receptors causing excitatory neurotoxicity and an inhibitory effect of glutaric acid, glutaconic acid, and 3-hydroxyglutaric acid on the inhibitory neurotransmitter GABA.

In patients diagnosed during the neonatal period, striatal injury can be prevented by metabolic therapy including a low-protein diet (restriction of the glutarigenic amino acids (lysine, tryptophan, and hydroxylysine), carnitine supplementation, and aggressive treatment during acute episodes of intercurrent illnesses. GA-1 affects fine motor skills and speech regardless of early treatment, but not IQ scores.[284] Dystonia is treated empirically and pallidotomy has been tried in cases with severe striatal injury, with limited benefit.

HYDROXYGLUTARIC ACIDURIAS

Two different clinical entities, identified respectively by an increase in either the L- or D-isoform of hydroxyglutaric acidemia, have been identified. The D-form produces a severe neonatal neurologic syndrome, whereas the L-form has a later onset and more variable presentation. A combined L- and D-form with neonatal onset represents an additional variant.[285]

L-2-HYDROXYGLUTARIC ACIDURIA

L-2-hydroxyglutaric aciduria (L2HGA) is a rare autosomal recessive neurometabolic disorder of childhood (see Figure 17.11). The disease is caused by a deficiency of the mitochondrial enzyme L-2-hydroxyglutarate dehydrogenase which converts L-2-hydroxyglutarate to oxoglutarate. Mutations have been identified in a gene called *duranin/C14orf160*, localized on chromosome 14q22.1.[286] Most patients appear normal until early childhood, when symptoms of cognitive deterioration, speech difficulties, progressive truncal or gait ataxia, intention tremor, dystonia, myoclonus, and pyramidal signs become apparent. Seizures are often a presenting sign and macrocephaly is present in most cases.[287–291] A child with migraine and no other manifestations except seizures has been described.[292] Neuroimaging shows symmetrical subcortical white matter abnormalities with sparing of the internal capsule, corpus callosum, cerebellar white matter and brainstem, bilateral increased densities in the basal ganglia (globus pallidus more than caudate or putamen) and dentate nucleus, and progressive cerebellar atrophy.[293] The severity of symptoms may vary within families and diagnosis may be delayed until adulthood because of mild clinical symptoms.

Diagnosis is established by the identification of elevated levels of L-2-hydroxyglutaric acid in urine, CSF, or plasma. It has been postulated that excess L-2-hydroxyglutaric acid is toxic to neurons.[289] Individuals with L2HGA are at increased risk for developing glioblastoma multiforme and primitive neuroectodermal tumors.[294] Treatment has included protein restriction, riboflavin, flavin adenine dinucleotide, and levocarnitine chloride.

D-2-HYDROXYGLUTARIC ACIDURIA

D-2-hydroxyglutaric aciduria (D2HGA) is a rare autosomal recessive disorder divided into two types, I and II. Type I is caused by a deficiency of the mitochondrial enzyme D-2-hydroxyglutarate dehydrogenase (converts G-2-hydroxyglutarate to 2-oxoglutarate) whereas type II is due to deficiency of mitochondrial isocitrate dehydrogenase.[246,286] D-2-Hydroxyglutaric acid inhibits cytochrome c oxidase and ATP synthase activity and is presumed to impair energy metabolism.[295] Patients with both types I and II exhibit variable phenotypes ranging from severely affected to having no or minimal symptoms. There is no genotypic:phenotypic correlation. Severe cases have a neonatal onset with intractable epilepsy, hypotonia, persistent involuntary movements including dystonia and choreoathetosis, cortical blindness, and profound developmental delay.[296,297] Milder cases have developmental motor and speech delay.[297,298] Neuroimaging has shown reduced myelination and gyration, ventriculomegaly, and caudate cysts. Diagnosis is confirmed by a large excretion of D-2-hydroxyglutaric acid in the urine and accumulation in plasma and CSF. Demonstration of elevated levels of D-2-hydroxyglutaric acid should be followed by differential quantitation of the two isomers L- and D-2-hydroxyglutaric acid. There is no specific therapy.

Glycolysis, Pyruvate Metabolism, and Krebs Cycle Disorders

The major energy source of most cells is glucose, which is metabolized by the glycolytic pathway. Glycolysis is a sequence of reactions that convert glucose into pyruvate. Pyruvate is a crucial metabolite in cells that are metabolized by four different enzymes: pyruvate carboxylase (PC), pyruvate dehydrogenase complex (PDH), lactate dehydrogenase (LDH), and alanine aminotransferase (ALT). The tricarboxylic acid cycle (TCA, Krebs cycle) occurs in the matrix of the mitochondrion and converts acetyl-CoA to carbon dioxide and energy (GTP and reduced cofactors of nicotinamide adenine dinucleotide (NADH) and flavin adenine dinucleotide (FADH2)). These cofactors, in turn, feed into the electron transport chain to generate ATP (Figure 17.12).

Triosephosphate Isomerase Deficiency

Triosephosphate isomerase (TPI) deficiency is an autosomal recessive disorder of glycolysis. TPI, encoded at chromosome 12p13, catalyzes the interconversion of glyceraldehyde-3-phosphate and dihydroxyacetone phosphate, and its deficiency results in the accumulation of dihydroxyacetone phosphate, especially in red blood cells

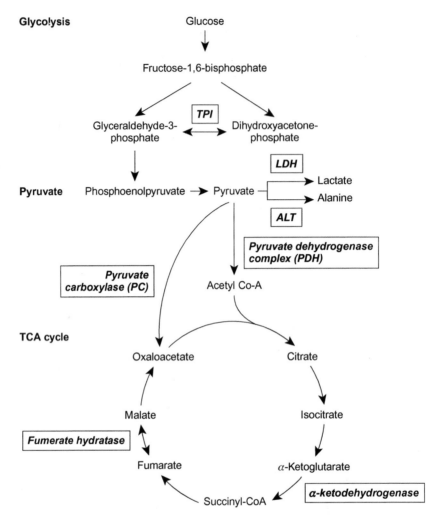

FIGURE 17.12   Glycolysis, pyruvate metabolism, and TCA cycle. Abbreviations: TPI, triosephosphate isomerase; LDH, lactate dehydrogenase; ALT, alanine aminotransferase.

(RBCs), and oxidative stress. A variety of gene mutations have been identified with little phenotypic:genotypic correlation.[299] This rare multisystem disease is characterized by a triad of symptoms including nonspherocytic hemolytic anemia, recurrent infections, and progressive neurologic dysfunction. Neurological symptoms become evident after age 2 and may include dystonia, tremor, dyskinesia, opisthotonos, pyramidal tract signs, myopathy, neuropathy, and evidence of spinal motor neuron involvement.[299–302] A patient with a TPI deficiency, resulting from a compound heterozygote mutation, had a biopsy-proven chronic axonal neuropathy.[303] Most patients die within the first 6 years.

Pyruvate Carboxylase (PC) Deficiency

PC is a biotin-containing mitochondrial enzyme that catalyzes the conversion of pyruvate and CO_2 to oxaloacetate, controls the first step in hepatic gluconeogenesis, and is involved in lipogenesis (Figure 17.12).[304,305] PC deficiency is an autosomal recessive disorder with three phenotypes based on clinical presentation. The *type A* (infantile or North American) group is common in North American Indians and characterized by onset at 2–5 months with mild to moderate lactic acidemia, hypoglycemia, severe developmental retardation, failure to thrive, hypotonia, ataxia, pyramidal tract signs, and convulsions. The prognosis is poor and most die in early childhood. *Type B* (neonatal or French form) was first described in France and is the severe neonatal variant. Patients present in the first 72 h of life with hypotonia, lactic acidosis, hypoglycemia, hyperammonemia, and hypercitrullinemia. Clinically, patients have hypothermia, lethargy, a combination of rigidity and hypokinesia (hypokinetic-rigid syndrome), abnormal eye movements, seizures, pyramidal tract dysfunction, and developmental delay. CSF and postmortem analyses have identified hypo-dopaminergic and altered GABAergic transmission.[306] Almost all die in the first 3 months. Type C (benign form) has been reported in a small number of individuals. Onset is in the first year with episodic metabolic acidosis associated with lactic acidosis. Neurological development is only mildly impaired with some having dystonia, episodic ataxia, dysarthria, transitory hemiparesis, and seizures.[304] Neuroradiographic findings in Type A and B include periventricular leukomalacia, subcortical leukodystrophy, cystic brain degeneration, and delayed myelination.[307] Treatment is primarily symptomatic, although triheptanoin, an odd-carbon triglyceride, has been beneficial.[308]

Pyruvate Dehydrogenase Complex (PDH) Deficiency

The PDH is a mitochondrial matrix multienzyme complex that provides the link between glycolysis and the TCA cycle by catalyzing the conversion of pyruvate into acetyl-CoA (Figure 17.12). The complex has three main components and most cases are secondary to mutations encoding the E1α-subunit on chromosome Xp22. PDH deficiency is a commonly identified cause of lactic acidosis in children with metabolic symptoms that vary from mild to severe. The clinical spectrum is broad, although neurodevelopmental delay and hypotonia are most common. Neurological manifestations include hypotonia, weakness, ataxia, spasticity, cerebellar degeneration, seizures, and mental retardation.[305,309–311] Ataxia can be intermittent with its median age at onset being about 18 months. Other motor symptoms can include recurrent acute dystonia,[312] complex extrapyramidal movements in adults,[313] and episodic peripheral weakness mimicking Guillain–Barré syndrome.[314,315] Structural brain abnormalities frequently include ventriculomegaly, microcephaly, agenesis of the corpus callosum, and bilaterally symmetrical lesions in the basal ganglia, thalamus, and brainstem. Laboratory studies show elevated lactate and pyruvate levels in plasma and urine, although cases with normal blood, and even CSF, values have been reported.[309,315,316] Definitive diagnosis requires documentation of diminished PDH activity in muscle, white blood cells, cultured fibroblasts, and other tissue. Treatments include addressing the acidosis, a ketogenic diet, thiamine supplementation, and use of dichloroacetate (an inhibitor of pyruvate dehydrogenase kinases and activator of PDH).

2-Ketoglutarate Dehydrogenase Deficiency

2-Ketodehydrogenase is a multienzyme complex consisting of three protein subunits that catalyze the oxidative decarboxylation of 2-ketoglutarate to succinyl-CoA. The onset of symptoms has varied from neonatal to 16 months. Clinical presentation involves severe neurologic impairment with failure to thrive, hypotonia, weakness, developmental delay, seizures, extrapyramidal symptoms, ataxia, and increased tone.[317,318] Patients have elevated serum lactate levels, a high lactate/pyruvate ratio, ketoglutaric aciduria, and ketoacidosis. A 14-month-old child with intermittently normal excretion of 2-ketoglutarate and mild clinical findings has been reported.[318] Secondary reductions in α-ketoglutarate dehydrogenase have been reported in a putative case of H protein-derived lipoic acid attachment due to *LIPT1* mutations.[319]

Fumarase (Fumarate Hydratase) Deficiency

Fumarase deficiency is an autosomal recessive inborn error of the Krebs cycle; fumarase catalyzes the reversible interconversion of fumarate and malate. There are two isoforms of fumarase (coded on the same region of chromosome 1q.42.1), mitochondrial and cytosolic, with similar structures except for the amino-terminal residue.[320] Variable clinical presentations have been reported.[321,322] Early-onset cases have a progressive encephalopathy with failure to thrive, microcephaly, hypotonia, seizures, and fumaric aciduria. Some patients have craniofacial dysmorphism including microcephaly, frontal bossing, hypertelorism, and a depressed nasal bridge.[323] Other manifestations have included muscular atrophy, pyramidal syndromes, dystonia, and paralysis of upgaze.[324] Cerebral malformations have encompassed agenesis of the corpus callosum and ventriculomegaly with polymicrogyria, hypomyelination, or periventricular cysts.[325] Outcome is frequently fatal in infancy or childhood. Laboratory studies show elevated plasma pyruvate and lactate and elevated amounts of fumaric acid in the urine. It has been suggested that fumarate excretion does not correlate with residual enzyme activity or clinical severity, prompting a need for measurement of fumarate hydratase enzyme activity or molecular genetic testing.[321] Heterozygote mutations of the fumarate hydratase gene are associated with renal cell cancer and hereditary leiomyomatosis.[326] There is no effective specific treatment.

Mitochondrial Disorders

Mitochondrial diseases[327–331] represent a variety of inherited disorders of energy metabolism with a wide range of symptoms and presentations. In a 20-year review,[332] patients fell into seven phenotypic categories: neonatal-onset lactic acidosis (fulminant acidosis), Leigh syndrome (LS), nonspecific encephalopathy, mitochondrial (encephalo)myopathy (MERRF, MELAS, MNGIE, Kearne-Sayne), intermittent neurologic (ataxia or weakness), visceral (liver, cardiac), and Leber hereditary optic neuropathy (LHON). Disorders involve mitochondrial abnormalities involving pyruvate metabolism (discussed previously) and respiratory chain defects.

Components of oxidative phosphorylation (OXPHOS) include five protein-lipid enzyme complexes, designated complex I, complex II, complex III, complex IV (cytochrome *c* oxidase), and complex V (ATP synthase), which are located in the mitochondrial inner membrane (Figure 17.13). These enzymes contain flavins, coenzyme Q_{10} (ubiquinone), iron-sulfur

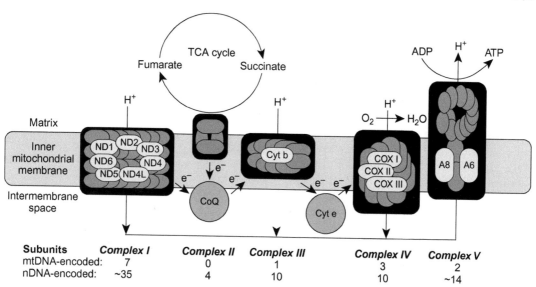

FIGURE 17.13   Respiratory chain. Abbreviations: ND1, NADH dehydrogenase 1; Cyt b, cytochrome b; COX 1, cytochrome C oxidase.

clusters, hemes, and protein-bound copper. Complexes I and II collect electrons from the catabolism of fats, proteins, and carbohydrates and transfer them sequentially to coenzyme Q_{10}, complex III, and complex IV. Complexes I, III, and IV utilize the energy in electron transfer to pump protons across the inner mitochondrial membrane, producing a proton gradient that is used by complex V to condense ADP and inorganic phosphate into ATP. Complexes I through V are unique enzymes in the body in that they are derived from genes from both the nuclear DNA and from the mtDNA.[333]

Elevations of lactate, pyruvate, lactate/pyruvate ratio (greater than 20), alanine, TCA intermediates, dicarboxylic acids, and/or a generalized amino aciduria can be important diagnostic clues to the presence of an OXPHOS disease. Other metabolites that may also be increased include tiglylglycine, ethylmalonic acid, 3-methylglutaconic acid, 2-ethylhydracrylic acid, 2-methylsuccinate, butyrylglycine, isovaleryl glycine, and ammonia. Analysis of lactate, pyruvate, and amino acids in venous blood can be complicated by technical factors, such as duration of tourniquet application, recent seizures, vigorous crying and struggling that occurs during venipuncture, and delays in sample processing. Further, isolated normal plasma lactate concentrations have been identified in subjects with chronic lactic acidemia. CSF analysis (cell count, protein, glucose, lactate, pyruvate, and amino acids) is less variable and very important in patients with evidence of CNS involvement.

Leigh Syndrome (LS)

LS (subacute necrotizing encephalomyelopathy) is a complex of progressive neurodegenerative disorders caused by several defects of energy metabolism, including the PDH (E1α subunit gene), PC, and deficiencies in respiratory complexes I (nDNA-encoded NADH-Ubiquinone oxidoreductase Fe-S protein (NDUFS) gene subunit), II (nDNA-encoded flavoprotein subunit), IV (assembly protein), and V (mtDNA-encoded A6 subunit) (see Figure 17.13).[334–336] The most common defect, affecting about one quarter of patients, involves cytochrome *c* oxidase or COX deficiency (complex IV). In some cases, the defect in COX-deficient Leigh disease has been mapped to chromosomal locus 9q34 with the putative candidate gene (SURF-1) shown to encode an assembly or maintenance factor.[337] All of the aforementioned defects impair brain metabolism, the brain and brainstem being especially vulnerable.

A recently proposed definition for LS includes the presence of (i) a neurodegenerative disease with variable symptoms due to (ii) mitochondrial dysfunction caused by a hereditary genetic defect accompanied by (iii) bilateral CNS lesions that are associated with abnormalities in diagnostic imaging.[338] LS usually manifests in infancy or early childhood (7 months to 2 years) with psychomotor delay and hypotonia. As this multisystem disorder progresses, feeding and swallowing defects, nystagmus, ophthalmoplegia, optic atrophy, ataxia, pyramidal signs, respiratory problems, and seizures become apparent.[339–341] Movement disorders, such as dystonia, choreoathetosis, and myoclonus, have been prominent in some cases and, at times, may be the initial sign.[342–344] A total of 19 of 34 cases with LS had multifocal or generalized dystonia at presentation.[343] Acute exacerbations are associated with infection, respiratory complications, stroke-like episodes, and poor hydration.[341] Nonneurologic features in LS can include short stature, dysmorphism, endocrine, gastrointestinal, and cardiac problems.[340] Pathologic findings contain symmetric necrotic lesions (spongy degeneration) with demyelination, vascular proliferation, and gliosis affecting the basal ganglia, diencephalon, cerebellum, and brainstem. The term "Leigh-like syndrome" should be reserved for situations where clinical criteria are only partially met, or when patients present with atypical symptoms, laboratory findings, or radiological features, but the overall clinical picture is indicative of LS.[338,340]

It is important to exclude disorders that mimic LS, especially those that can be treated such as *biotin-responsive basal ganglia disease* (see later discussion). The diagnosis of LS is based on clinical features, the presence of elevated arterial or CSF lactate levels, and T2-weighted MR images showing symmetric areas of increased signal in the putamen, or occasionally the caudate, globus pallidus, substantia nigra, thalamus, and brainstem.[340,345] Lactic acidosis is not always present in LS patients.[341] Additional helpful diagnostic testing includes a muscle biopsy for the presence of ragged red fibers and biochemical analysis, mitochondrial DNA analysis, magnetic resonance spectroscopy of the brain, and phosphorus magnetic resonance spectroscopy of muscle. There is no specific therapy for mitochondrial diseases. Various therapies, including vitamins, coenzyme Q, and dichloroacetate, improve metabolic indices, but have not been shown to significantly improve clinical outcome.[338,346]

OTHER MITOCHONDRIAL SYNDROMES

The classic syndrome of *mitochondrial encephalomyopathy, lactic acidosis, and stroke-like episodes* (MELAS) is generally associated with a mitochondrial gene *MTTL1* A3243G mutation. The load of mutant mtDNA is believed to be responsible for varied clinical expression.[347] Onset is between the ages of 2 and 10 years, although later onsets have been described.[331] The most common presenting symptoms in children younger than age 6 are developmental delay, deafness, and weakness whereas in older children muscle cramping or pain.[348,349] Stroke-like lesions occur in about 90% of MELAS patients and correlate with clinical focality. Additional symptoms in MELAS include ataxia, progressive external ophthalmoplegia, and seizures.[350] Over the course of years, the progressive episodic deterioration in neuropsychological and neurological signs and symptoms is due to stroke-like events. MRI often shows signal lesions in the cerebellum. The 3243 mutation is not specific for this disorder, since it has been reported with a wide range of clinical phenotypes, including sensorineural hearing loss, diabetes, myopathy, and cardiomyopathy.[351,352]

Myoclonic epilepsy with ragged red fibers (MERRF) is associated with an mtDNA mutation at 8344. Clinical features include cortical myoclonus with or without epilepsy, myopathy, and encephalopathy. Ataxia is commonly present and is sometimes associated with a photomyoclonic response. Multifocal dystonia was the presenting and salient feature in a patient with myopathy, ragged red fibers, progressive ophthalmoplegia, and a sensorineural hearing loss but with a 3243 mtDNA mutation.[353] Neuromuscular problems include weakness, exercise intolerance, ptosis, ophthalamoparesis, and elevated CPK.

Mitochondrial neurogastrointestinal encephalopathy (MNGIE) is a rare autosomal recessive disorder caused by mutations in the thymidine phosphorylase (*ECGF1*) gene. Patients usually have gastrointestinal problems (diarrhea, vomiting, and pseudo-obstruction), cachexia, ptosis, ophthalmoparesis, myopathy, and sensorimotor neuropathy. MRI shows a leukoencephalopathy.[354–356]

Neurogenic weakness, ataxia, and retinitis pigmentosa (NARP): NARP is a maternally inherited syndrome in which the cardinal manifestations are ataxia (more of a sensory ataxia), retinitis pigmentosa, and a sensory neuropathy.[331,357] The disorder is associated with mutations in MT-ATP6, which encodes subunit 6 of ATPase. The phenotype is variable and may also include sensorineural hearing loss, seizures, cognitive loss, progressive external ophthalmoplegia, and cardiac conduction defects. MRI shows diffuse atrophy and in severely affected patients symmetric lesions of the basal ganglia. Analysis of mtDNA can be performed in peripheral blood, but may be absent if the mutation is undetectable in leukocytes.

Other: The high energy requirement of the brain makes it vulnerable to various other mitochondrial mutations. Hence, numerous other mitochondrial DNA defects have been described that affect the nervous system.[331] For example, a patient with dementia, ataxia, and chorea had a mutation in tRNA at position 5549.[358]

Leber Hereditary Optic Neuropathy (LHON) Plus Dystonia

LHON plus dystonia is a mitochondrial disorder associated with vision loss and progressive dystonia. It is caused by mutations in the mitochondrial genes that encode subunits of the NADH dehydrogenase (ND) gene. The disorder is characterized by a variable combination of progressive dystonia and visual loss, occasionally accompanied by pyramidal tract signs and intellectual impairment.[359] Several pediatric cases, including members of a single family, began with progressive spastic dystonia in childhood with the later development of visual problems.[359,360] MRI lesions are similar to those seen in LS.[361,362] A G14459A mitochondrial mutation in the ND6 gene has been identified in individuals with LHON alone and with dystonia, as well as in a family with bilateral striatal necrosis and pediatric onset dystonia.[363]

Mohr–Tranebjaerg Syndrome

Mohr–Tranebjaerg syndrome (MTS), or deafness-dystonia-optic neuropathy syndrome, is a mitochondrial disorder, but not one that is associated with a defect of energy generation. Gene mutations are linked to the nuclear-encoded deafness dystonia peptide1 (DDP1)/translocase of mitochondrial inner membrane 8A (TIMM8A) gene on Xq21.3-22.[364,365] TIMM8a, a protein product of the DDP1 gene, is part of a multiprotein complex located in the intermembrane space of the mitochondrial inner membrane. Truncated peptides lead to impairment of the import of nuclear-encoded proteins into the inner membrane of carrier protein and insertion into the mitochondrial inner membrane.[366]

Clinically, MTS is a rare neurodegenerative disorder. Symptoms are characterized by the childhood onset of sensorineural deafness and appearance of progressive dystonia beginning in adolescence.[367–369] The dystonia tends to be focal, segmental, or multifocal at onset (primarily in the upper body, variably involving the head, neck, and upper limbs) with progressive generalization.[370] The median time from onset to the development of moderately severe dystonia was 11 years. Other symptoms consist of visual loss, varying degrees of cognitive impairment, behavioral problems, and spasticity. PET and MRI studies show hypometabolic areas in the striatum and cortex and atrophy of the occipital lobes.[368] Dystonia has been reported in female carriers of MTS.[371]

Disorders of Purine Metabolism

Lesch–Nyhan Disease

LND is an X-linked recessive disorder associated with heterogeneous mutations (substitutions, deletions, early stops, insertions) in the gene for the enzyme hypoxanthine-guanine phosphoribosyltransferase (HPRT) located on Xq26-27.[372] A given mutation of the HRPT gene may lead to different phenotypes.[373] The biochemical defect is a deficiency of HPRT, which converts the free purine bases hypoxanthine and guanine into their respective nucleotides (Figure 17.14). In addition to this recycling defect, there is also a secondary increased activity in the *de novo* purine synthesis pathway. Purines are important intermediaries in energy-dependent reactions, cofactor-requiring reactions, and intercellular-intracellular signaling. In the absence of HPRT, hypoxanthine and guanine cannot be recycled and are degraded and excreted as uric acid. HPRT activity in classic cases is less than 1% of normal, but patients with partial syndromes and higher levels of residual enzyme have been described (Table 17.4).[372,374]

Clinically, the three major features of LND are hyperuricemia, self-injurious behaviors (SIBs), and neurological problems. Although the full syndrome is most typical, individual components may occur in isolation. Overproduction of uric acid leads to hyperuricemia, and if not treated, to renal stones and gouty arthritis. SIBs (e.g., self-biting, head banging, eye poking, arm flinging) are a hallmark, but nondiagnostic, feature of this disorder. SIBs typically appear at about age 2–3 years, although in some may not emerge until the late-teenage years. Neurologic abnormalities have been variably described in the literature. In three older series, the cardinal features were described as mental retardation, choreoathetosis, and spasticity or dystonia with hypotonia.[375–377] In a study of 17 patients (age range 8–38 years) with LND, performed with particular attention to motor features, dysfunction was

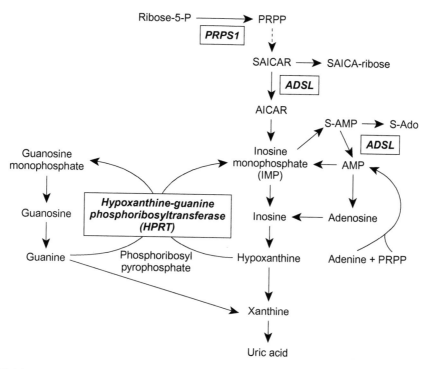

FIGURE 17.14   Disorders of purine metabolism. Abbreviations: PRPP, phosphoribosylpyrophosphate; PRPS1, phosphoribosylpyrophosphate synthetase 1; SAICAR, succinylaminoimidazolecarboxamide ribotide; AICAR, aminoimidazolecarboxamide ribotide; S-AMP, adenylosuccinate; S-Ado, succinyladenosine; AMP, adenosine monophosphate; ADSL, adenylosuccinate lyase.

best described as severe dystonia superimposed on hypotonia.[378] Dystonia, present in all subjects, was typically absent at rest and increased with excitement or attempted purposeful movements. Choreiform movements were present in about half the subjects and ballismus of the upper extremity in about one quarter. Pyramidal signs were observed in a minority of cases. In patients with severe enzyme deficiency, ocular motility is grossly abnormal; fixation interrupted by unwanted saccades and voluntary saccades preceded by head movement or eye blink.[379]

In addition to the classical LND, two groups of attenuated variants with incomplete or milder phenotypes have been described, both having overproduction of uric acid.[374,380,381] Individuals with *HRPT-related hyperuricemia* have no motor or cognitive abnormalities whereas those with *HRPT-related neurological dysfunction* have milder neurological and behavioral problems, but self-injury is absent.[372,382] Patients with intermediate phenotypes often have difficulty with muscle control ranging from incapacitating to minor clumsiness/stiffness.

The pathogenesis of the neurological and neurobehavioral manifestation in LND is not well understood. Autopsy studies have identified no overt morphological defects or

TABLE 17.4   Disorders of Purine Metabolism

Disorder	Enzyme	Neurological features	Other clinical features
Lesch–Nyhan disease (LND)	HPRT	Motor disability: dystonia, choreoathetosis, pyramidal signs	Hyperuricemia, gout, nephrolithiasis
		Self-injurious behavior (SIB) intellectual disability	
Adenylosuccinate synthase deficiency	ADSL	Seizures, autism, intellectual disability	Growth retardation
Phosphoribosylpyrophosphate synthase superactivity	PRPP synthase	Neurodevelopmental impairment, sensorineural deafness, and ataxia	Hyperuricemia, gout
Phosphoribosylpyrophosphate synthase deficiency	PRPP synthase	i. Hypotonia, ataxia, delayed motor development, and optic atrophy, recurrent infection ii. Optic atrophy, hearing loss, polyneuropathy	Hypouricemia
AICR-transformylase/ IMP-cyclohydrolase	ATIC	Intellectual disability, blindness, epilepsy	Facial dysmorphism
5′-Nucleotidase pervasive developmental disorder	5′-Nucleotidase	Language delay, behavioral problems, epilepsy, ataxia, poor manual dexterity	Recurrent infections
Myoadenylate deaminase deficiency	mAMPD	Muscle cramps/myalgias after exercise	

evidence of neurodegeneration.[383] Involvement of dopaminergic pathways has been postulated based on: reduced CSF levels of dopamine and HVA,[384] reduction of dopamine in postmortem brain limbic and striatal regions,[385] increased dopamine D2-receptor immunoreactivity in the putamen,[386] and PET scans showing reduced fluorodopa uptake and [^{11}C] WIN 35,428 binding to dopamine transporters. Despite the identified reductions of dopaminergic activity, patients with LND are hyperkinetic rather than Parkinsonian.

Diagnosis is made based on clinical presentation plus elevated uric acid in urine. Since hyperuricemia may not be present in all patients, measures of 24-h urinary uric acid excretion, demonstration of reduced HGRT enzyme activity in blood cells or fibroblasts, and documentation of a pathogenic mutation in the HPRT gene may be required for confirmation.[372] Therapy is directed to reducing hyperuricemia (generous hydration and allopurinol) and to preventing self-injury (protective measures), behavior modification therapy, and possibly pharmacotherapy (benzodiazepines, neuroleptics, gabapentin, or carbamazepine). Although no adequate controlled trials have been performed, available reports suggest that extrapyramidal signs do not uniformly improve with levodopa, neuroleptics, or tetrabenazine. In investigations of levodopa therapy, some patients failed, others had unacceptable side effects, and a child with LND and low CSF HVA improved.[387]

Adenylosuccinate Lyase Deficiency

Adenylosuccinate lyase (ADSL) catalyzes two steps in the synthesis of purine nucleotides: the conversion of succinyl aminoimidazole carboxamide ribotide (SAICAR) into aminoimidazole carboxamide ribotide (AICAR) along the *de novo* pathway of purine synthesis and the conversion of adenylosuccinate (s-AMP) into AMP (see Figure 17.14). The ADSL gene has been mapped to chromosome region 22q13.1-q13.2.[388] Clinical disorders of ADSL deficiency (autosomal recessive) have a variable spectrum ranging from an acute presentation within the first several weeks of life and rapid demise to minimally delayed cognitive and motor development.[389–392] Common features include psychomotor retardation, autistic features, hypotonia, epilepsy, feeding problems, and growth retardation. Microcephaly is often present, but only very rarely are there other dysmorphic features. Variability in enzyme loss and a nonparallel loss of both activities of ADSL likely explain differences in phenotype. The pathogenesis of ADSL deficiency is unclear with hypotheses ranging from an impaired synthesis of purine nucleotides to toxic effects of accumulating succinyl purines.[372]

Diagnosis is based on the presence in urine and CSF of succinyl purines adenosine (s-Ado) and SAICAR; both normally absent. Several methodologies are used for detection including high-performance liquid chromatography with ultraviolet detection and spectral analysis[393] and the modified Bratton–Marshall test.[394] Patients with higher s-Ado/SAICAR ratios tend to do better and have survival into adulthood. Treatment with adenine, with the goal of replacing deficient adenine nucleotides, and allopurinol, to avoid conversion into poorly soluble 2,8-dihydroxyadenine, has not been successful.[389] Oral administration of D-ribose does not appear to be effective.[395]

Phosphoribosylpyrophosphate Synthase Superactivity

Phosphoribosylpyrophosphate synthetase (PRPS1) superactivity syndrome is characterized by hyperuricemia and hyperuricosuria and divided into a severe form with infantile or early-childhood onset and a milder phenotype with later onset. PRPS1 catalyzes the phosphoribosylation of ribose 5-phosphate to 5-phosphoribosyl-1-pyrophosphate (PRPP)—a necessary step for the *de novo* and salvage pathways of purine and pyrimidine biosynthesis (Figure 17.14). Superactivity of PRPS1, located on the X chromosome (Xq22-q24), is due to a gene mutation causing an increase in PRPS1 reaction velocity.[396,397] In the more severe form, affected males present with neurodevelopmental impairment, hyperuricemia, gout, sensorineural deafness, and ataxia.[396,398,399] The late-onset form has only gout and urolithiasis. Therapies designed to reduce uric acid production and increase its excretion have no beneficial effect on neurodevelopmental problems, ataxia, or deafness.

Phosphoribosylpyrophosphate Synthase Deficiency

Two disorders identified with PRPS1 deficiency are: (1) *Arts syndrome* with mental retardation, early-onset hypotonia, ataxia, delayed motor development, and optic atrophy. A predisposure for infections can lead to early death.[400,401] (2) *Charcot–Marie–Tooth disease-5* with a triad of optic atrophy, sensorineural hearing loss, and peripheral sensorimotor polyneuropathy.[402,403]

Disorders of Creatine Metabolism

Creatine metabolism is involved in the storage and transmission of phosphate-bound energy and has an essential role in sites of high energy utilization such as the brain and muscles. Creatine is synthesized in the liver and pancreas, stored in the muscle and brain, and nonenzymatically converted to creatinine. There are three creatine deficiency disorders: two autosomal recessive disorders that affect the biosynthesis of creatine (guanidinoacetate methyltransferase (GAMT) and arginine:glycine amidinotransferase (AGAT) deficiency) and an X-linked creatine transporter (CrT) defect. Developmental delay, speech disturbances, mental retardation, and autistic behavior are common symptoms in all creatine deficiency syndromes (CDSs).[404,405]

Guanidinoacetate Methyltransferase (GAMT) Deficiency

GAMT converts guanidinoacetate to creatine and deficiency of this enzyme results in creatine depletion and accumulation of guanidinoacetate (Figure 17.15). The disorder, transmitted in an autosomal recessive fashion, is localized to mutations on chromosome 19p13.3. GAMT deficiency manifests in infancy after an unremarkable postnatal period. Symptoms are characterized by developmental arrest, medication-resistant epilepsy (myoclonic, generalized tonic-clonic, partial complex, atonic), severe speech impairment, progressive dystonia, dyskinesias, hypotonia, ataxia, and autistic-like behavior, although each can occur to a varying degree.[406-410] MRI imaging has ranged from showing delayed myelination and/or bilateral hyperintensities in the globus pallidus on T2-weighted imaging to being normal. Brain magnetic resonance spectroscopy is diagnostic with diminished creatine and phosphocreatine peaks. Neurologic manifestations are believed to reflect a combination of cerebral energy deficiency, due to a depletion of brain creatine/phosphocreatine, and the neurotoxic effect of excess brain guanidinoacetate. Since the other two CDSs lack extrapyramidal problems, it has been suggested that basal ganglia involvement may arise specifically from the neurotoxic effect of guanidinoacetate.

Diagnosis of GAMT deficiency is established by detection of a creatine deficiency (absence of creatine peak) in the brain by MR spectroscopy, the measurement of guanidino compounds (decreased creatine and increased guanidinoacetate) in CSF and urine, low plasma and urine creatinine, and defective GAMT activity in fibroblasts or liver tissue.

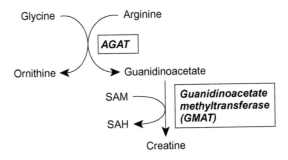

FIGURE 17.15   GMAT-mediated reactions. Abbreviations: AGAT, L-arginine:glycine amidinotransferase; SAM, S-adenosylmethionine; SAH, S-adenosylhomocysteine; THF, tetrahydrofolate.

Biochemical and neuroradiological abnormalities respond to treatment with oral creatine supplementation and the use of guanidine-lowering strategies, but clinical improvement may be incomplete.[411] Dietary treatment with arginine restriction and ornithine supplementation has reduced EEG epileptogenic activity.[404,412]

Arginine: Glycine Amidinotransferase (AGAT) Deficiency

AGAT catalyzes the first and rate limiting step in creatine synthesis; the reversible transfer of the guanidine group from L-arginine to glycine forming guanidinoacetate and ornithine. AGAT is an autosomal recessive disorder and the gene is located at 15q15.3.[405] Based on only a limited number of patients, symptoms appeared in the first year of life and included developmental delay, poor speech acquisition, and mild to moderate mental retardation.[413,414] Other than febrile seizures, epilepsy has not been observed and no abnormalities have been reported on MRI.[404] In AGAT, urine guanidinoacetate concentration and the creatine/creatinine ratio is decreased. MR spectroscopy, as in the other CDS, shows virtual complete absence of creatine and phosphocreatine. Creatine supplementation in AGAT deficiency has been beneficial.[415]

Creatine Transporter Deficiency

The sodium- and chloride-dependent creatinetransporter (CrT) a member of the solute carrier 6 (SLC6) neurotransporter family of transporters, is required to move creatine into the brain and muscle against a high gradient. The CrT1 gene (SLC6A8) is located at Xq28 and is highly expressed in skeletal muscle and kidneys.[405] Most males had the exact features of CDS, delayed development, language impairment, and cognitive delays with some having seizures, behavioral problems, macrocephaly or microcephaly, and facial dysmorphism.[414,416–419] Brain MRI may be normal or show myelination delay and signal changes in the pallidum and paratrigonal white matter. In the CrT defect, urine guanidinoacetate is normal and the creatine/creatinine ratio is increased. Brain spectroscopy is abnormal. Treatment for the CrT defect remains to be identified.

Congenital Disorders of Glycosylation

Congenital disorders of glycosylation (CDG; formerly named Carbohydrate-Deficient Glycoprotein Syndrome) represent an expanding group of inherited (autosomal recessive) disorders that are characterized by defects in the synthesis of the glycan (sugar chain) moiety of glycoproteins or glycolipids and in the attachment of these glycans to proteins and lipids.[420,421] The two main types of protein glycosylation are N- and O-glycosylation of proteins and subsequent aberrant formation of glycoproteins. In brief, proteins synthesized in the rough endoplasmic reticulum (RER) that are to be secreted or destined to become membrane proteins must be glycosylated. In order to become glycosylated, during the process of protein translation, the N-terminal portion of the protein is translocated from the outer to the inner side of the RER membrane, and, in turn, a preassembled oligosaccharide is attached. The oligosaccharide itself is a branched structure consisting of two N-acetylglucosamines, nine mannoses, and three glucose residues (Figure 17.16). In CDG I disorders, the defect resides in the assembly of the oligosaccharide precursor, which results in partial or complete underglycosylation of proteins.[422,423]

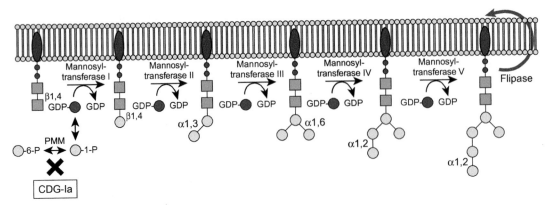

FIGURE 17.16   Construction of the transferred oligosaccharide. Squares are N-acetylglucosamine residues. Circles are mannose. CDG-1a, congenital disorders of glycosylation-1a; GDP guanosine diphosphate. *From Marquardt and Denecke.*[423]

The CDGs are a rapidly expanding group of disorders. In the past, all CDG types were grouped into types I and II; however, newer classifications include divisions into defects of N-linked glycosylation, O-linked glycosylation, glycosphingolipid and glycosylphosphatidylinositol anchor glycosylation, combined N- and O-glycosylation; dolichol biosynthesis or recycling, and other.[420,424] The total number of disorders within these categories exceeds 60 and new defects continue to be reported.[424,425] One of the more common N-glycosylation disorders is a deficiency in the enzyme phosphomannomutase 2 (PMM2) caused by a mutation in the *PMM2* gene located on chromosome 16.[426]

The presentations of patients with CDG range from multisystem disorders to those affecting specific organs.[422,423,427] Common neurologic features include delayed development, hypotonia, strabismus/other oculomotor abnormalities, ataxia, areflexia-polyneuropathy, and seizures. Some patients have feeding problems, failure to thrive, dysmorphic features facies, bilaterally inverted nipples, and mild clinodactyly, and areas of lipohypertrophy and lipoatrophy on the buttocks and arms. Retinitis pigmentosa, cardiomyopathy, hepatic dysfunction, stroke-like episodes, and a coagulopathy characterized by low levels of protein C, protein S, antithrombin III, and factor XI may be present. MRI studies typically show hypoplasia of the vermis and cerebellar hemispheres, thin or absent corpus callosum, and leukoencephalopathy. Other, less frequently appearing radiographic abnormalities include moderate global atrophy, olivopontocerebellar hypoplasia, and brainstem hypoplasia. Diagnosis is based on electrophoretic mobility of the serum protein transferrin and the detection of unusual isoforms. GC/mass spectroscopy is used to identify defective N-glycans or glycoforms of transferrin.[428–430] Effective treatments are not available except for a case of phosphomannose isomerase deficiency successfully treated with mannose and in another liver transplantation.[431]

Disorders Involving Cofactors, Minerals, Vitamins

Molybdenum Cofactor (Sulfite Oxidase) Deficiency

A molybdenum-containing pterin molecule is a cofactor for three mammalian enzymes; sulfite oxidase (essential for detoxifying sulfites), xanthine dehydrogenase (role in purine metabolism and formation of uric acid from xanthine and hypoxanthine), and aldehyde dehydrogenase (catalyzes conversion of aldehydes to acids). Molybdenum cofactor deficiency is a rare neurodegenerative condition that primarily affects the CNS by altering sulfite oxidase activity. Sulfite oxidase is a mitochondrial enzyme responsible for catalyzing the oxidation of sulfites; the latter are produced from metabolites of sulfur containing amino acids and sulfates. Deficit enzyme activity can be secondary to a defect in the enzyme (autosomal recessive) or secondary to defects in the production of its cofactor. Clinical manifestations induced by cofactor deficiency are indistinguishable from those caused by an isolated sulfite oxidase enzyme deficiency. In both, the disorder starts in the neonatal period with feeding difficulties, encephalopathy, and intractable seizures. Other manifestations include axial hypotonia, hypomotility, limb rigidity, dislocated lenses, and profound developmental delay.[432] Dystonia and bilateral basal ganglia changes have been reported early in the presentation,[433] and survivors have a variety of extrapyramidal movements. Brain imaging may show multiple cystic white matter cavities in basal ganglia, brainstem, and cerebellum, loss of brain volume, and cessation of myelination. Isolated sulfite oxidase deficiency has also manifested with a progressive leukoencephalopathy and lactic academia.[434]

Diagnosis is suspected by excess urinary excretion of sulfite (detectable by dipstick), thiosulfate, and S-sulfocysteine (detectable by anion exchange chromatography). Plasma cystine and homocysteine levels are reduced due to sulfite conjugation with cystine, forming sulfocysteine, and to homocysteine.[434] False-negative urinary screens for sulfite can occur if the urine is not fresh (sulfites convert to sulfates) and false-positive results can be due to treatment with sulfur-containing medications. Enzymatic diagnosis can be confirmed in fibroblasts and liver. A short-term response to dietary methionine restriction with cysteine supplementation has been reported.[435]

Cerebral Folate Deficiency Syndromes

Cerebral folate deficiency (CFD) is characterized by low levels of 5-methyltetrahydrofolate (5MTF) in the CSF with normal folate levels in the plasma and RBCs.[436–438] CFD has been associated with antibodies against a folate receptor, deficiencies of 5, 10-methylene-tetrahydrofolate reductase, 3-phosphoglycerate dehydrogenase, dihydrofolate reductase, and DHPR mutations in the folate receptor *FOLR1* gene,[439] hereditary folate malabsorption, and mitochondrial disorders. Hence, the question whether CFD represents a clear-cut clinical syndrome has been questioned.[440] In contrast, others have reported clinical CFD phenotypes associated with the presence of serum antibodies directed against folate receptor-α (FRα).[436]

Pathophysiologically, it is proposed that anti-FRα antibodies inhibit N^5-methyltetrahydrofolate (MTHF) transport across the choroid plexus. Resultant clinical phenotypes of CFD deficiency due to folate receptor antibodies have been variable[436]: an *infantile-onset* type begins at 4–6 months, and requirements include meeting more than three out of seven major criteria: irritability/insomnia, deceleration of head growth, developmental delay/regression, hypotonia/ataxia, pyramidal signs, dyskinesias (choreoathetosis and hemiballismus), and epilepsy. The full-blown clinical pattern does not manifest until 2.5 years. MRI may be normal or show moderate frontotemporal atrophy, delayed myelination, or periventricular and subcortical demyelination. Other phenotypes include a *Spastic-ataxic syndrome* that begins after age 1 year; *Autism* with or without other neurological deficits seen in the infantile-onset group; and a *Dystonia/pyramidal syndrome*. After identification of FRα antibodies, the treatment of choice is high doses of folinic acid.

Biotin-Responsive Basal Ganglia Disease

Biotin-responsive basal ganglia disease is caused by mutations in the SLC19A3 gene that encodes a thiamine transporter.[441,442] The age of onset is variable, but commonly occurs between 3 and 4 years. Presentation is that of a fever-triggered, subacute encephalopathy (confusion, drowsiness, altered consciousness), with seizures, and ataxia. Dystonia and dysarthria are common, as are pyramidal signs. MRI findings include abnormal signal intensity in the caudate and putamen and diffuse involvement of cortical and subcortical white matter. Neurological outcome is dependent on the time of diagnosis and initiation of thiamine and biotin treatment.[441,443]

Other

Glucose Transport Defect (GLUT1 Deficiency)

The glucose transport defect (GLUT1) is an autosomal-dominant disorder of glucose transport across the blood–brain barrier.[444–446] The affected gene, located at 1p35-p31.3, solute carrier member 2, family 1 (SLC2A1), encodes a facilitator glucose transporter in the blood–brain barrier. Several clinical phenotypes have been described. The classical form presents with infantile seizures, typically unresponsive to antiepileptic drugs, a developmental encephalopathy with mild to severe mental retardation, acquired microcephaly, hypotonia, spasticity, and a movement disorder consisting of ataxia and dystonia.[447] Several atypical presentations have occurred without seizures, but with prominent movement disorders. These include three phenotypes characterized by: (1) mental retardation, dysarthric speech, and intermittent ataxia; (2) choreoathetosis and dystonia; and (3) paroxysmal exercise induced dyskinesias, with or without seizures.[416,447–453] Based on a review of 57 patients with Glut1 deficiency the frequency of movement disorders included gait disturbance (89%), dystonia (86%), chorea (75%), cerebellar action tremor (70%), myoclonus (16%), and dyspraxia (21%).[450]

The pathogenesis of GLUT1 deficiency is believed to be due to decreased glucose in the brain, with glucose acting as both a source of energy and a signaling molecule.[454] Diagnosis is confirmed by measurement of CSF glucose and lactate levels and whole-exome sequencing. GLUT1 deficiency syndrome is defined by hypoglycorrhachia in combination with a decreased CSF to blood glucose ratio. In reported cases, CSF glucose levels ranged from 16.2 to 50.5 mg/dL and CSF to blood glucose ratios from 0.19 to 0.59.[455] Reliance solely on whole exome sequencing is not recommended, since in about 10% of cases a SLC2A1 mutation was not identified.[456,457] The ketogenic diet has been successfully used to treat seizures and paroxysmal movements.[446,455,458] Food grade triheptanoin, a naturally occurring medium-chain triglyceride, is currently under investigation.[459]

Neuroacanthocytosis Syndromes

Acanthocytes (Greek for "thorn," deformed erythrocytes with spicules of varying sizes) are seen in the peripheral smear in patients with several hereditary neurological disorders labeled as neuroacanthocytoses. The "core" neuroacanthocyte syndromes (chorea-acanthocytosis and McLeod syndrome) are characterized by involvement of the basal ganglia, movement disorders, and psychiatric features whereas others disorders (abetalipoproteinemia and hypobetalipoproteinemia) involve lipoprotein metabolism and lead to vitamin E

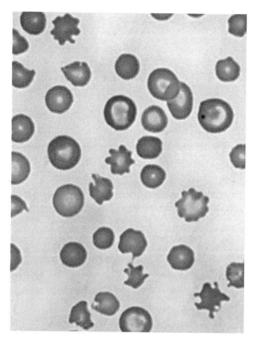

FIGURE 17.17 Acanthocytes (Greek for "thorn," deformed erythrocytes with spicules of varying sizes) are seen in the peripheral smear in patients with at least three hereditary neurologic disorders labeled as neuroacanthocytoses.

malabsorption and clinical symptoms of peripheral neuropathy and sensory ataxia.[460] Acanthocytes are also found in PKAN and HARP syndromes (Figure 17.17).

CHOREA-ACANTHOCYTOSIS

Chorea-acanthocytosis (ChAc) is an autosomal recessive disorder characterized by the presence of progressive hyperkinetic movements (orofacial dyskinesias, limb chorea, dystonia, motor and phonic tics), acanthocytosis, and the absence of any lipid abnormality.[460,461] The disorder is caused by mutations in the *VPS13A* gene on chromosome 9 leading to altered production of chorein located in human brain and erythrocytes.[462,463] The mean age of onset is in the twenties, but the disorder has been reported in children less than 10 years old. Many patients have psychiatric issues, including obsessive-compulsive disorder, several years prior to onset of neurological problems.[464] Chorea is the most characteristic movement abnormality, primarily affecting the lower extremities. Patients have an unusual feeding dystonia (tongue protrusions push food out of the mouth), orofacial dyskinesias, vocalizations, dysarthria, and tongue and lip biting. They may also have truncal instability with near falls and sudden truncal spasms, termed the "rubber man appearance."[461] Dystonia of the limbs is common and may be a presenting symptom in some cases.[465] The aforementioned hyperkinetic states occasionally progress to Parkinsonism or akinetic mutism. Chorea-acanthocytosis is associated with seizures (about 50%), dementia,

SIBs, impaired executive function skills, cognitive decline, and psychiatric features. Muscle creatine kinase and/or liver transaminase levels are increased, muscle wasting or weakness is common, and tendon reflexes are reduced due to a sensorimotor polyneuropathy. Muscle biopsies have shown signs of denervation and peripheral nerve biopsies demonstrate depletion of large myelinated fibers.[465,466] Pathologically, the caudate and putamen are atrophic with depletion of small and medium-sized spiny neurons.[467] MRI has shown symmetric abnormalities in the basal ganglia, with increased signal on T2-weighted scans of the striatum with predilection to the head of the caudate.[465,468–470] PET studies show a reduction in blood flow and glucose utilization in frontal-subcortical regions and dysfunction of dopaminergic neurons projecting from the substantia nigra to the striatum.[468,471,472] Diagnostically, the presence of acanthocytes is not a reliable marker and testing should include Western blot measurement of chorein in RBC membranes (should be absent) and genetic testing for mutations of *VPS13A*.[461,462,473]

McLEOD SYNDROME

McLeod syndrome is an X-linked multisystem disorder caused by mutations of the *XK* gene located on Xp21.1 encoding the XK protein, the exact function of which is unknown.[474,475] Hematologic findings include acanthocytes, compensated hemolysis, the absence of RBC Kx antigen, and weak expression of Kell antigens on RBC. Onset of neurologic signs ranges from 25 to 60 years and duration may be more than 30 years. The CNS phenotype is similar to Huntington's disease with choreic movements, neurobehavioral problems, psychiatric difficulties, and seizures.[460,461] Initial abnormal movements may be subtle and include increased restlessness, postural adjustments, or facial tic–like movements.[476] Facial dyskinesia, dysarthria, and involuntary vocalizations may also be present. A case progressing from chorea to Parkinsonism has been reported.[477] Affected individuals also have neuromuscular manifestations with myopathy, sensorimotor axonal neuropathy, and cardiomyopathy. Cognitive impairment is not a typical feature. MRI shows atrophy of the caudate nucleus and putamen.[478] PET of ^{18}F-fluorodeoxyglucose shows impaired glucose metabolism in the striatum.[479] Diagnosis is based on the absence of Kx antigen and reduced Kell antigens and analysis of the XK gene.

BASSEN–KORNZWEIG SYNDROME (ABETALIPOPROTEINEMIA)

Abetalipoproteinemia is an autosomal recessive disorder characterized by acanthocytes, fat malabsorption, hypocholesterolemia, ataxia, neuropathy, and pigmentary retinal degeneration.[480–482] It is caused by mutations in the gene encoding microsomal triglyceride transfer protein located on chromosome 4q22-24. The protein functions in the assembly of apolipoprotein B containing low-density lipoproteins and chylomicrons.[483,484] Absent serum apolipoprotein B containing lipoproteins, low-density, and very-low-density lipoproteins cause impaired fat absorption and intestinal transport that, in turn, results in very low serum levels of cholesterol and triglycerides. The disorder may manifest in early childhood with malabsorption whereas neurological problems begin before age 20 with progressive ataxia, visual problems, and neuropathy. Neurological symptoms are due to deficient absorption of fat-soluble vitamin E, involve the posterior columns and spinocerebellar tracts, and can be prevented or treated with vitamin A and E administration.[485] Retinal degeneration is due to a combined deficiency of vitamins A and E.

Aicardi–Goutières Syndrome (AGS)

AGS is an autosomal recessive encephalopathy associated with mutations in several genes including those that encode the exonuclease TREX1, subunits of the human ribonuclease H2 complex (RNASEH2-A, B, or C), or SAMHD1.[486–488] It is believed that these mutated genes cause an accumulation of immune stimulatory nucleic acids and activation of innate cellular immunity. The Aicardi–Goutières syndrome can be broadly divided into two types: (1) a neonatal form with poor feeding, jitteriness, seizures, and often hepatosplenomegaly and thrombocytopenia—the latter reminiscent of a congenital infection; and (2) a late-onset form, ranging from later in infancy to after age 1, presenting with a more subacute onset and greater clinical heterogeneity.[489–491] Severely affected individuals have profound psychomotor developmental delay, spasticity, progressive microcephaly, dystonic posturing, and death in early childhood. Chilblains, small itchy, painful lumps that develop on the skin in response to cold, are seen in about 40% of patients. CSF studies show a variable lymphocytosis, an elevated interferon-α (early in the clinical course), and high levels of neopterin.[492] Radiographic imaging shows intracranial calcifications (especially basal ganglia), abnormal cerebral white matter (diffuse or with an anteroposterior gradient), possible frontotemporal cysts, and cerebral atrophy involving both hemispheres and brainstem.[487] Evidence for the use of steroids or immunosuppressents is equivocal.[490,493]

References

1. Pearl PL. Monoamine neurotransmitter deficiencies. *Handb Clin Neurol.* 2013;113:1819–1825.
2. Ng J, Heales SJ, Kurian MA. Clinical features and pharmacotherapy of childhood monoamine neurotransmitter disorders. *Paediatr Drugs.* 2014;16(4):275–291.
3. Marecos C, Ng J, Kurian MA. What is new for monoamine neurotransmitter disorders? *J Inherit Metab Dis.* 2014;37(4):619–626.
4. Hyland K. Inherited disorders affecting dopamine and serotonin: critical neurotransmitters derived from aromatic amino acids. *J Nutr.* 2007;137(6 suppl 1) [1568S-1572S; discussion 1573S-1575S].
5. Hyland K. Presentation, diagnosis, and treatment of the disorders of monoamine neurotransmitter metabolism. *Semin Perinatol.* 1999;23(2):194–203.
6. Blau N, Thony B, Cotton RG, Hyland K. Disorders of tetrahydrobiopterin and related biogenic aminesScriver C.Beaudet AL, Sly WS, Valle D, editors. *The metabolic and molecular bases of inherited disease,* Vol 8. New York: McGraw-Hill; 2001:1725–1776.
7. Hyland K. Abnormalities of biogenic amine metabolism. *J Inherit Metab Dis.* 1993;16(4):676–690.
8. Swoboda KJ, Hyland K. Diagnosis and treatment of neurotransmitter-related disorders. *Neurol Clin.* 2002;20(4):1143–1161.
9. Kaufman S, Holtzman NA, Milstien S, Butler LJ, Krumholz A. Phenylketonuria due to a deficiency of dihydropteridine reductase. *N Engl J Med.* 1975;293(16):785–790.
10. Smith KJ, Hall SM, Schauf CL. Vesicular demyelination induced by raised intracellular calcium. *J Neurol Sci.* 1985;71(1):19–37.
11. Dudesek A, Roschinger W, Muntau AC, et al. Molecular analysis and long-term follow-up of patients with different forms of 6-pyruvoyl-tetrahydropterin synthase deficiency. *Eur J Pediatr.* 2001;160(5):267–276.
12. Pearl PL, Taylor JL, Trzcinski S, Sokohl A. The pediatric neurotransmitter disorders. *J Child Neurol.* 2007;22(5):606–616.
13. Niederwieser A, Shintaku H, Leimbacher W, et al. "Peripheral" tetrahydrobiopterin deficiency with hyperphenylalaninaemia due to incomplete 6-pyruvoyl tetrahydropterin synthase deficiency or heterozygosity. *Eur J Pediatr.* 1987;146(3):228–232.
14. Larnaout A, Belal S, Miladi N, et al. Juvenile form of dihydropteridine reductase deficiency in 2 Tunisian patients. *Neuropediatrics.* 1998;29(6):322–323.

15. Opladen T, Hoffmann G, Horster F, et al. Clinical and biochemical characterization of patients with early infantile onset of autosomal recessive GTP cyclohydrolase I deficiency without hyperphenylalaninemia. *Mov Disord.* 2011;26(1):157–161.

16. Blau N, Bonafe L, Thony B. Tetrahydrobiopterin deficiencies without hyperphenylalaninemia: diagnosis and genetics of dopa-responsive dystonia and sepiapterin reductase deficiency. *Mol Genet Metab.* 2001;74(1-2):172–185.

17. Ichinose H, Inagaki H, Suzuki T, Ohye T, Nagatsu T. Molecular mechanisms of hereditary progressive dystonia with marked diurnal fluctuation, Segawa's disease. *Brain Dev.* 2000;22(Suppl 1):S107–110.

18. Ichinose H, Nagatsu T. Molecular genetics of DOPA-responsive dystonia. *Adv Neurol.* 1999;80:195–198.

19. Steinberger D, Weber Y, Korinthenberg R, et al. High penetrance and pronounced variation in expressivity of GCH1 mutations in five families with dopa-responsive dystonia. *Ann Neurol.* 1998;43(5):634–639.

20. Segawa M. Hereditary progressive dystonia with marked diurnal fluctuation. *Brain Dev.* 2011;33(3):195–201.

21. Bandmann O, Wood NW. Dopa-responsive dystonia -- the story so far. *Neuropediatrics.* 2002;33(1):1–5.

22. Leuzzi V, Carducci C, Cardona F, Artiola C, Antonozzi I. Autosomal dominant GTP-CH deficiency presenting as a dopa-responsive myoclonus-dystonia syndrome. *Neurology.* 2002;59(8):1241–1243.

23. Van Hove JL, Steyaert J, Matthijs G, et al. Expanded motor and psychiatric phenotype in autosomal dominant Segawa syndrome due to GTP cyclohydrolase deficiency. *J Neurol Neurosurg Psychiatry.* 2006;77(1):18–23.

24. Jarman PR, Bandmann O, Marsden CD, Wood NW. GTP cyclohydrolase I mutations in patients with dystonia responsive to anticholinergic drugs. *J Neurol Neurosurg Psychiatry.* 1997;63(3):304–308.

25. Hyland K, Arnold LA, Trugman JM. Defects of biopterin metabolism and biogenic amine biosynthesis: clinical diagnostic, and therapeutic aspects. *Adv Neurol.* 1998;78:301–308.

26. Hyland K, Fryburg JS, Wilson WG, et al. Oral phenylalanine loading in dopa-responsive dystonia: a possible diagnostic test. *Neurology.* 1997;48(5):1290–1297.

27. Saunders-Pullman R, Blau N, Hyland K, et al. Phenylalanine loading as a diagnostic test for DRD: interpreting the utility of the test. *Mol Genet Metab.* 2004;83(3):207–212.

28. Trender-Gerhard I, Sweeney MG, Schwingenschuh P, et al. Autosomal-dominant GTPCH1-deficient DRD: clinical characteristics and long-term outcome of 34 patients. *J Neurol Neurosurg Psychiatry.* 2009;80(8):839–845.

29. Tassin J, Durr A, Bonnet AM, et al. Levodopa-responsive dystonia. GTP cyclohydrolase I or parkin mutations? *Brain.* 2000;123(Pt 6):1112–1121.

30. Naumann M, Pirker W, Reiners K, Lange K, Becker G, Brucke T. [123I]beta-CIT single-photon emission tomography in DOPA-responsive dystonia. *Mov Disord.* 1997;12(3):448–451.

31. Kishore A, Nygaard TG, de la Fuente-Fernandez R, et al. Striatal D2 receptors in symptomatic and asymptomatic carriers of dopa- responsive dystonia measured with [11C]-raclopride and positron- emission tomography. *Neurology.* 1998;50(4):1028–1032.

32. Blau N, Thony B, Renneberg A, Arnold LA, Hyland K. Dihydropteridine reductase deficiency localized to the central nervous system. *J Inherit Metab Dis.* 1998;21(4):433–434.

33. Friedman J, Hyland K, Blau N, MacCollin M. Dopa-responsive hypersomnia and mixed movement disorder due to sepiapterin reductase deficiency. *Neurology.* 2006;67(11):2032–2035.

34. Friedman J, Roze E, Abdenur JE, et al. Sepiapterin reductase deficiency: a treatable mimic of cerebral palsy. *Ann Neurol.* 2012;71(4):520–530.

35. Leuzzi V, Carducci C, Tolve M, Giannini MT, Angeloni A, Carducci C. Very early pattern of movement disorders in sepiapterin reductase deficiency. *Neurology.* 2013;81(24):2141–2142.

36. Zorzi G, Redweik U, Trippe H, Penzien JM, Thony B, Blau N. Detection of sepiapterin in CSF of patients with sepiapterin reductase deficiency. *Mol Genet Metab.* 2002;75(2):174–177.

37. Grima B, Lamouroux A, Boni C, Julien JF, Javoy-Agid F, Mallet J. A single human gene encoding multiple tyrosine hydroxylases with different predicted functional characteristics. *Nature.* 1987;326(6114):707–711.

38. Yeung WL, Wong VC, Chan KY, et al. Expanding phenotype and clinical analysis of tyrosine hydroxylase deficiency. *J Child Neurol.* 2011;26(2):179–187.

39. Pons R, Syrengelas D, Youroukos S, et al. Levodopa-induced dyskinesias in tyrosine hydroxylase deficiency. *Mov Disord.* 2013;28(8):1058–1063.

40. Willemsen MA, Verbeek MM, Kamsteeg EJ, et al. Tyrosine hydroxylase deficiency: a treatable disorder of brain catecholamine biosynthesis. *Brain.* 2010;133(Pt 6):1810–1822.

41. Giovanniello T, Leuzzi V, Carducci C, et al. Tyrosine hydroxylase deficiency presenting with a biphasic clinical course. *Neuropediatrics.* 2007;38(4):213–215.

42. Ludecke B, Knappskog PM, Clayton PT, et al. Recessively inherited L-DOPA-responsive parkinsonism in infancy caused by a point mutation (L205P) in the tyrosine hydroxylase gene. *Hum Mol Genet*. 1996;5(7):1023–1028.

43. van den Heuvel LP, Luiten B, Smeitink JA, et al. A common point mutation in the tyrosine hydroxylase gene in autosomal recessive L-DOPA-responsive dystonia in the Dutch population. *Hum Genet*. 1998;102(6):644–646.

44. Furukawa Y, Graf WD, Wong H, Shimadzu M, Kish SJ. Dopa-responsive dystonia simulating spastic paraplegia due to tyrosine hydroxylase (TH) gene mutations. *Neurology*. 2001;56(2):260–263.

45. Chi CS, Lee HF, Tsai CR. Tyrosine hydroxylase deficiency in Taiwanese infants. *Pediatr Neurol*. 2012;46(2):77–82.

46. Tormenti MJ, Tomycz ND, Coffman KA, Kondziolka D, Crammond DJ, Tyler-Kabara EC. Bilateral subthalamic nucleus deep brain stimulation for dopa-responsive dystonia in a 6-year-old child. *J Neurosurg Pediatr*. 2011;7(6):650–653.

47. Lee HF, Tsai CR, Chi CS, Chang TM, Lee HJ. Aromatic L-amino acid decarboxylase deficiency in Taiwan. *Eur J Paediatr Neurol*. 2009;13(2):135–140.

48. Brun L, Ngu LH, Keng WT, et al. Clinical and biochemical features of aromatic L-amino acid decarboxylase deficiency. *Neurology*. 2010;75(1):64–71.

49. Tay SK, Poh KS, Hyland K, et al. Unusually mild phenotype of AADC deficiency in 2 siblings. *Mol Genet Metab*. 2007;91(4):374–378.

50. Abeling NG, van Gennip AH, Barth PG, van Cruchten A, Westra M, Wijburg FA. Aromatic L-amino acid decarboxylase deficiency: a new case with a mild clinical presentation and unexpected laboratory findings. *J Inherit Metab Dis*. 1998;21(3):240–242.

51. Hyland K, Surtees RA, Rodeck C, Clayton PT. Aromatic L-amino acid decarboxylase deficiency: clinical features, diagnosis, and treatment of a new inborn error of neurotransmitter amine synthesis. *Neurology*. 1992;42(10):1980–1988.

52. Mills PB, Surtees RA, Champion MP, et al. Neonatal epileptic encephalopathy caused by mutations in the PNPO gene encoding pyridox(am)ine 5′-phosphate oxidase. *Hum Mol Genet*. 2005;14(8):1077–1086.

53. Allen GF, Land JM, Heales SJ. A new perspective on the treatment of aromatic L-amino acid decarboxylase deficiency. *Mol Genet Metab*. 2009;97(1):6–14.

54. Chang YT, Sharma R, Marsh JL, et al. Levodopa-responsive aromatic L-amino acid decarboxylase deficiency. *Ann Neurol*. 2004;55(3):435–438.

55. Brunner HG, Nelen M, Breakefield XO, Ropers HH, van Oost BA. Abnormal behavior associated with a point mutation in the structural gene for monoamine oxidase A. *Science*. 1993;262(5133):578–580.

56. Rilstone JJ, Alkhater RA, Minassian BA. Brain dopamine-serotonin vesicular transport disease and its treatment. *N Engl J Med*. 2013;368(6):543–550.

57. Kurian MA, Li Y, Zhen J, et al. Clinical and molecular characterisation of hereditary dopamine transporter deficiency syndrome: an observational cohort and experimental study. *Lancet Neurol*. 2011;10(1):54–62.

58. Ng J, Zhen J, Meyer E, et al. Dopamine transporter deficiency syndrome: phenotypic spectrum from infancy to adulthood. *Brain*. 2014;137(Pt 4):1107–1119.

59. Kurian MA, Zhen J, Cheng SY, et al. Homozygous loss-of-function mutations in the gene encoding the dopamine transporter are associated with infantile parkinsonism-dystonia. *J Clin Invest*. 2009;119(6):1595–1603.

60. Knerr I, Gibson KM, Jakobs C, Pearl PL. Neuropsychiatric morbidity in adolescent and adult succinic semialdehyde dehydrogenase deficiency patients. *CNS Spectr*. 2008;13(7):598–605.

61. Pearl PL, Gibson KM, Acosta MT, et al. Clinical spectrum of succinic semialdehyde dehydrogenase deficiency. *Neurology*. 2003;60(9):1413–1417.

62. Pearl PL, Shukla L, Theodore WH, Jakobs C, Michael Gibson K. Epilepsy in succinic semialdehyde dehydrogenase deficiency, a disorder of GABA metabolism. *Brain Dev*. 2011;33(9):796–805.

63. Yamakawa Y, Nakazawa T, Ishida A, et al. A boy with a severe phenotype of succinic semialdehyde dehydrogenase deficiency. *Brain Dev*. 2012;34(2):107–112.

64. Pearl PL, Acosta MT, Wallis DD, et al. Dyskinetic features of succinate semialdehyde dehydrogenase deficiency, a GABA degradative defect. In: Fernandez-Alvarez E, Arzimanoglou A, Tolosa E, eds. *Pediatric Movement Disorders: Progress in Understanding*. : John Libbey Eurotext; 2005.

65. Knerr I, Gibson KM, Murdoch G, et al. Neuropathology in succinic semialdehyde dehydrogenase deficiency. *Pediatr Neurol*. 2010;42(4):255–258.

66. Pearl PL, Capp PK, Novotny EJ, Gibson KM. Inherited disorders of neurotransmitters in children and adults. *Clin Biochem*. 2005;38(12):1051–1058.

67. Gibson KM, Lee CF, Chambliss KL, et al. 4-Hydroxybutyric aciduria: application of a fluorometric assay to the determination of succinic semialdehyde dehydrogenase activity in extracts of cultured human lymphoblasts. *Clin Chim Acta*. 1991;196(2-3):219–221.

68. Akaboshi S, Hogema BM, Novelletto A, et al. Mutational spectrum of the succinate semialdehyde dehydrogenase (ALDH5A1) gene and functional analysis of 27 novel disease-causing mutations in patients with SSADH deficiency. *Hum Mutat*. 2003;22(6):442–450.

69. Hogema BM, Akaboshi S, Taylor M, et al. Prenatal diagnosis of succinic semialdehyde dehydrogenase deficiency: increased accuracy employing DNA, enzyme, and metabolite analyses. *Mol Genet Metab*. 2001;72(3):218–222.

70. Leuzzi V, Di Sabato ML, Deodato F, et al. Vigabatrin improves paroxysmal dystonia in succinic semialdehyde dehydrogenase deficiency. *Neurology*. 2007;68(16):1320–1321.

71. Sarkar B. Copper transport and its defect in Wilson disease: characterization of the copper-binding domain of Wilson disease ATPase. *J Inorg Biochem*. 2000;79(1-4):187–191.

72. Bandmann O, Weiss KH, Kaler SG. Wilson's disease and other neurological copper disorders. *Lancet Neurol*. 2015;14(1):103–113.

73. Dusek P, Roos PM, Litwin T, Schneider SA, Flaten TP, Aaseth J. The neurotoxicity of iron, copper and manganese in Parkinson's and Wilson's diseases. *Journal of trace elements in medicine and biology : organ of the Society for Minerals and Trace Elements (GMS)*. 2014

74. Kodama H, Fujisawa C, Bhadhprasit W. Pathology, clinical features and treatments of congenital copper metabolic disorders--focus on neurologic aspects. *Brain Dev*. 2011;33(3):243–251.

75. Brewer GJ. Recognition, diagnosis, and management of Wilson's disease. *Proc Soc Exp Biol Med*. 2000;223(1):39–46.

76. Kim JW, Kim JH, Seo JK, et al. Genetically confirmed Wilson disease in a 9-month old boy with elevations of aminotransferases. *World J Hepatol*. 2013;5(3):156–159.

77. Ala A, Borjigin J, Rochwarger A, Schilsky M. Wilson disease in septuagenarian siblings: Raising the bar for diagnosis. *Hepatology*. 2005;41(3):668–670.

78. Strickland GT, Leu ML. Wilson's disease. Clinical and laboratory maniestations in 40 patients. *Medicine (Baltimore)*. 1975;54(2):113–137.

79. Walshe JM. The eye in Wilson disease. *Birth Defects Orig Artic Ser*. 1976;12(3):187–194.

80. Merle U, Schaefer M, Ferenci P, Stremmel W. Clinical presentation, diagnosis and long-term outcome of Wilson's disease: a cohort study. *Gut*. 2007;56(1):115–120.

81. Wilson SAK. Progressive lenticular degeneration: A familial nervous disease associated with cirrhosis of the liver. *Brain*. 1912;34:295–309.

82. Stremmel W, Meyerrose KW, Niederau C, Hefter H, Kreuzpaintner G, Strohmeyer G. Wilson disease: clinical presentation, treatment, and survival. *Ann Intern Med*. 1991;115(9):720–726.

83. Walshe JM, Yealland M. Wilson's disease: the problem of delayed diagnosis. *J Neurol Neurosurg Psychiatry*. 1992;55(8):692–696.

84. Rosen JM, Kuntz N, Melin-Aldana H, Bass LM. Spasmodic muscle cramps and weakness as presenting symptoms in Wilson disease. *Pediatrics*. 2013;132(4):e1039–1042.

85. Taly AB, Meenakshi-Sundaram S, Sinha S, Swamy HS, Arunodaya GR. Wilson disease: description of 282 patients evaluated over 3 decades. *Medicine (Baltimore)*. 2007;86(2):112–121.

86. Svetel M, Potrebic A, Pekmezovic T, et al. Neuropsychiatric aspects of treated Wilson's disease. *Parkinsonism Relat Disord*. 2009;15(10):772–775.

87. Zimbrean PC, Schilsky ML. Psychiatric aspects of Wilson disease: a review. *Gen Hosp Psychiatry*. 2014;36(1):53–62.

88. Walshe JM, Dixon AK. Dangers of non-compliance in Wilson's disease. *Lancet*. 1986;1(8485):845–847.

89. Ingster-Moati I, Bui Quoc E, Pless M, et al. Ocular motility and Wilson's disease: a study on 34 patients. *J Neurol Neurosurg Psychiatry*. 2007;78(11):1199–1201.

90. Portala K, Waldenstrom E, von Knorring L, Westermark K. Psychopathology and personality traits in patients with treated Wilson disease grouped according to gene mutations. *Ups J Med Sci*. 2008;113(1):79–94.

91. Patel AD, Bozdech M. Wilson disease. *Arch Ophthalmol*. 2001;119(10):1556–1557.

92. Prashanth LK, Sinha S, Taly AB, Vasudev MK. Do MRI features distinguish Wilson's disease from other early onset extrapyramidal disorders? An analysis of 100 cases. *Mov Disord*. 2010;25(6):672–678.

93. Stefano Zagami A, Boers PM. Disappearing "face of the giant panda". *Neurology*. 2001;56(5):665.

94. Horoupian DS, Sternlieb I, Scheinberg IH. Neuropathological findings in penicillamine-treated patients with Wilson's disease. *Clin Neuropathol.* 1988;7(2):62–67.

95. Mak CM, Lam CW. Diagnosis of Wilson's disease: a comprehensive review. *Crit Rev Clin Lab Sci.* 2008;45(3):263–290.

96. Harada M. Pathogenesis and management of Wilson disease. *Hepatol Res.* 2014.

97. Walshe JM. Penicillamine: the treatment of first choice for patients with Wilson's disease. *Mov Disord.* 1999;14(4):545–550.

98. Brewer GJ. Zinc acetate for the treatment of Wilson's disease. *Expert Opin Pharmacother.* 2001;2(9):1473–1477.

99. Brewer GJ, Askari F, Dick RB, et al. Treatment of Wilson's disease with tetrathiomolybdate: V. Control of free copper by tetrathiomolybdate and a comparison with trientine. *Translational research : the journal of laboratory and clinical medicine.* 2009;154(2):70–77.

100. Schilsky ML. Liver transplantation for Wilson's disease. *Ann N Y Acad Sci.* 2014;1315:45–49.

101. Hedera P. Treatment of Wilson's disease motor complications with deep brain stimulation. *Ann N Y Acad Sci.* 2014;1315:16–23.

102. Zhang S, Chen S, Li W, et al. Rescue of ATP7B function in hepatocyte-like cells from Wilson's disease induced pluripotent stem cells using gene therapy or the chaperone drug curcumin. *Hum Mol Genet.* 2011;20(16):3176–3187.

103. Roybal JL, Endo M, Radu A, et al. Early gestational gene transfer with targeted ATP7B expression in the liver improves phenotype in a murine model of Wilson's disease. *Gene therapy.* 2012;19(11):1085–1094.

104. Huppke P, Brendel C, Kalscheuer V, et al. Mutations in SLC33A1 cause a lethal autosomal-recessive disorder with congenital cataracts, hearing loss, and low serum copper and ceruloplasmin. *Am J Hum Genet.* 2012;90(1):61–68.

105. Stamelou M, Tuschl K, Chong WK, et al. Dystonia with brain manganese accumulation resulting from SLC30A10 mutations: a new treatable disorder. *Mov Disord.* 2012;27(10):1317–1322.

106. Tuschl K, Clayton PT, Gospe Jr. SM, et al. Syndrome of hepatic cirrhosis, dystonia, polycythemia, and hypermanganesemia caused by mutations in SLC30A10, a manganese transporter in man. *Am J Hum Genet.* 2012;90(3):457–466.

107. Di Toro Mammarella L, Mignarri A, Battisti C, et al. Two-year follow-up after chelating therapy in a patient with adult-onset parkinsonism and hypermanganesaemia due to SLC30A10 mutations. *J Neurol.* 2014;261(1):227–228.

108. Kurian MA, Hayflick SJ. Pantothenate kinase-associated neurodegeneration (PKAN) and PLA2G6-associated neurodegeneration (PLAN): review of two major neurodegeneration with brain iron accumulation (NBIA) phenotypes. *Int Rev Neurobiol.* 2013;110:49–71.

109. Hartig M, Prokisch H, Meitinger T, Klopstock T. Mitochondrial membrane protein-associated neurodegeneration (MPAN). *Int Rev Neurobiol.* 2013;110:73–84.

110. Levi S, Finazzi D. Neurodegeneration with brain iron accumulation: update on pathogenic mechanisms. *Frontiers in pharmacology.* 2014;5:99.

111. Brunetti D, Dusi S, Morbin M, et al. Pantothenate kinase-associated neurodegeneration: altered mitochondria membrane potential and defective respiration in Pank2 knock-out mouse model. *Hum Mol Genet.* 2012;21(24):5294–5305.

112. Kazek B, Jamroz E, Gencik M, Jezela Stanek A, Marszal E, Wojaczynska-Stanek K. A novel PANK2 gene mutation: clinical and molecular characteristics of patients short communication. *J Child Neurol.* 2007;22(11):1256–1259.

113. Gregory A, Hayflick SJ. Neurogeneration with brain iron accumulation. *Folia Neuropathol.* 2005;43(4):286–296.

114. Hayflick SJ, Westaway SK, Levinson B, et al. Genetic, clinical, and radiographic delineation of Hallervorden-Spatz syndrome. *N Engl J Med.* 2003;348(1):33–40.

115. Szanto J, Gallyas F. A study of iron metabolism in neuropsychiatric patients. Hallervorden- Spatz disease. *Arch Neurol.* 1966;14(4):438–442.

116. Morphy MA, Feldman JA, Kilburn G. Hallervorden-Spatz disease in a psychiatric setting. *J Clin Psychiatry.* 1989;50(2):66–68.

117. Guimaraes J, Santos JV. Generalized freezing in Hallervorden-Spatz syndrome: case report. *Eur J Neurol.* 1999;6(4):509–513.

118. Hayflick SJ, Penzien JM, Michl W, Sharif UM, Rosman NP, Wheeler PG. Cranial MRI changes may precede symptoms in Hallervorden-Spatz syndrome. *Pediatr Neurol.* 2001;25(2):166–169.

119. Gallucci M, Splendiani A, Bozzao A, et al. MR imaging of degenerative disorders of brainstem and cerebellum. *Magn Reson Imaging.* 1990;8(2):117–122.

120. Delgado RF, Sanchez PR, Speckter H, et al. Missense PANK2 mutation without "eye of the tiger" sign: MR findings in a large group of patients with pantothenate kinase-associated neurodegeneration (PKAN). *J Magn Reson Imaging.* 2012;35(4):788–794.

121. Zupanc ML, Chun RW, Gilbert-Barness EF. Osmiophilic deposits in cytosomes in Hallervorden-Spatz syndrome. *Pediatr Neurol.* 1990;6(5):349–352.

122. Abbruzzese G, Cossu G, Balocco M, et al. A pilot trial of deferiprone for neurodegeneration with brain iron accumulation. *Haematologica.* 2011;96(11):1708–1711.

123. Zorzi G, Zibordi F, Chiapparini L, et al. Iron-related MRI images in patients with pantothenate kinase-associated neurodegeneration (PKAN) treated with deferiprone: results of a phase II pilot trial. *Mov Disord.* 2011;26(9):1756–1759.

124. Albright AL. Intrathecal baclofen in cerebral palsy movement disorders. *J Child Neurol.* 1996;11(suppl 1):S29–35.

125. Timmermann L, Pauls KA, Wieland K, et al. Dystonia in neurodegeneration with brain iron accumulation: outcome of bilateral pallidal stimulation. *Brain.* 2010;133(Pt 3):701–712.

126. Tsukamoto H, Inui K, Taniike M, et al. A case of Hallervorden-Spatz disease: progressive and intractable dystonia controlled by bilateral thalamotomy. *Brain Dev.* 1992;14(4):269–272.

127. Justesen CR, Penn RD, Kroin JS, Egel RT. Stereotactic pallidotomy in a child with Hallervorden-Spatz disease. Case report. *J Neurosurg.* 1999;90(3):551–554.

128. Mikati MA, Yehya A, Darwish H, Karam P, Comair Y. Deep brain stimulation as a mode of treatment of early onset pantothenate kinase-associated neurodegeneration. *Eur J Paediatr Neurol.* 2008.

129. Balsinde J, Balboa MA. Cellular regulation and proposed biological functions of group VIA calcium-independent phospholipase A2 in activated cells. *Cellular signalling.* 2005;17(9):1052–1062.

130. Kurian MA, Morgan NV, MacPherson L, et al. Phenotypic spectrum of neurodegeneration associated with mutations in the PLA2G6 gene (PLAN). *Neurology.* 2008;70(18):1623–1629.

131. Maawali AL, Yoon G, Halliday W, et al. *Hypertrophy of the clava, a new MRI sign in patients with PLA2G6 mutations.* Paper presented at: American Society of Human Genetics. Montreal, Canada; 2011.

132. Gregory A, Westaway SK, Holm IE, et al. Neurodegeneration associated with genetic defects in phospholipase A(2). *Neurology.* 2008;71(18):1402–1409.

133. Gregory A, Polster BJ, Hayflick SJ. Clinical and genetic delineation of neurodegeneration with brain iron accumulation. *J Med Genet.* 2009;46(2):73–80.

134. Mubaidin A, Roberts E, Hampshire D, et al. Karak syndrome: a novel degenerative disorder of the basal ganglia and cerebellum. *J Med Genet.* 2003;40(7):543–546.

135. Gregory A, Hayflick S. Neurodegeneration with Brain Iron Accumulation Disorders Overview All rights reserved. In: Pagon RA, Adam MP, Ardinger HH, eds. *GeneReviews(R).* Seattle: Seattle University of Washington; 2014.

136. Hayflick SJ, Kruer MC, Gregory A, et al. beta-Propeller protein-associated neurodegeneration: a new X-linked dominant disorder with brain iron accumulation. *Brain.* 2013;136(Pt 6):1708–1717.

137. Haack TB, Hogarth P, Gregory A, Prokisch H, Hayflick SJ. BPAN: the only X-linked dominant NBIA disorder. *Int Rev Neurobiol.* 2013;110:85–90.

138. Curtis AR, Fey C, Morris CM, et al. Mutation in the gene encoding ferritin light polypeptide causes dominant adult-onset basal ganglia disease. *Nat Genet.* 2001;28(4):350–354.

139. Chinnery PF, Curtis AR, Fey C, et al. Neuroferritinopathy in a French family with late onset dominant dystonia. *J Med Genet.* 2003;40(5):e69.

140. Keogh MJ, Singh B, Chinnery PF. Early neuropsychiatry features in neuroferritinopathy. *Mov Disord.* 2013;28(9):1310–1313.

141. Maciel P, Cruz VT, Constante M, et al. Neuroferritinopathy: missense mutation in FTL causing early-onset bilateral pallidal involvement. *Neurology.* 2005;65(4):603–605.

142. Kerkhof M, Honkoop P. Never forget aceruloplasminemia in case of highly suggestive Wilson's disease score. *Hepatology.* 2014;59(4):1645–1647.

143. Kono S. Aceruloplasminemia: an update. *Int Rev Neurobiol.* 2013;110:125–151.

144. Nittis T, Gitlin JD. The copper-iron connection: hereditary aceruloplasminemia. *Semin Hematol.* 2002;39(4):282–289.

145. Kono S, Miyajima H. Molecular and pathological basis of aceruloplasminemia. *Biol Res.* 2006;39(1):15–23.

146. McNeill A. PLA2G6 mutations and other rare causes of neurodegeneration with brain iron accumulation. *Current drug targets.* 2012;13(9):1204–1206.

147. Radi E, Formichi P, Di Maio G, Battisti C, Federico A. Altered apoptosis regulation in Kufor-Rakeb syndrome patients with mutations in the ATP13A2 gene. *J Cell Mol Med.* 2012;16(8):1916–1923.

148. Zaki MS, Selim L, Mansour L, et al. Mutations in FA2H in three Arab families with a clinical spectrum of neurodegeneration and hereditary spastic paraparesis. *Clin Genet.* 2014.

149. Schneider SA, Hardy J, Bhatia KP. Syndromes of neurodegeneration with brain iron accumulation (NBIA): an update on clinical presentations, histological and genetic underpinnings, and treatment considerations. *Mov Disord.* 2012;27(1):42–53.

150. Ben-Omran T, Ali R, Almureikhi M, et al. Phenotypic heterogeneity in Woodhouse-Sakati syndrome: two new families with a mutation in the C2orf37 gene. *Am J Med Genet A.* 2011;155a(11):2647–2653.

151. Steindl K, Alazami AM, Bhatia KP, et al. A novel C2orf37 mutation causes the first Italian cases of Woodhouse Sakati syndrome. *Clin Genet.* 2010;78(6):594–597.

152. Higgins JJ, Patterson MC, Papadopoulos NM, Brady RO, Pentchev PG, Barton NW. Hypoprebetalipoproteinemia, acanthocytosis, retinitis pigmentosa, and pallidal degeneration (HARP syndrome). *Neurology.* 1992;42(1):194–198.

153. Malandrini A, Cesaretti S, Mulinari M, et al. Acanthocytosis, retinitis pigmentosa, pallidal degeneration. Report of two cases without serum lipid abnormalities. *J Neurol Sci.* 1996;140(1-2):129–131.

154. Boustany RM. Lysosomal storage diseases--the horizon expands. *Nature reviews. Neurology.* 2013;9(10):583–598.

155. Singer HS, Nankervis GA, Schafer IA. Leukocyte beta-galactosidase activity in the diagnosis of generalized GM 1 gangliosidosis. *Pediatrics.* 1972;49(3):352–361.

156. Patterson MC. Gangliosidoses. *Handb Clin Neurol.* 2013;113:1707–1708.

157. Brunetti-Pierri N, Scaglia F. GM1 gangliosidosis: review of clinical, molecular, and therapeutic aspects. *Mol Genet Metab.* 2008;94(4):391–396.

158. Chen CC, Chiu PC, Shieh KS. Type 1 GM1 gangliosidosis with basal ganglia calcification: a case report. *Zhonghua Yi Xue Za Zhi (Taipei).* 1999;62(1):40–45.

159. Uyama E, Terasaki T, Watanabe S, et al. Type 3 GM1 gangliosidosis: characteristic MRI findings correlated with dystonia. *Acta Neurol Scand.* 1992;86(6):609–615.

160. Yoshida K, Oshima A, Sakuraba H, et al. GM1 gangliosidosis in adults: clinical and molecular analysis of 16 Japanese patients. *Ann Neurol.* 1992;31(3):328–332.

161. Tanaka R, Momoi T, Yoshida A, et al. Type 3 GM1 gangliosidosis: clinical and neuroradiological findings in an 11-year-old girl. *J Neurol.* 1995;242(5):299–303.

162. Campdelacreu J, Munoz E, Gomez B, Pujol T, Chabas A, Tolosa E. Generalised dystonia with an abnormal magnetic resonance imaging signal in the basal ganglia: a case of adult-onset GM1 gangliosidosis. *Mov Disord.* 2002;17(5):1095–1097.

163. Yoshida K, Ikeda S, Kawaguchi K, Yanagisawa N. Adult GM1 gangliosidosis: immunohistochemical and ultrastructural findings in an autopsy case. *Neurology.* 1994;44(12):2376–2382.

164. Platt FM. Sphingolipid lysosomal storage disorders. *Nature.* 2014;510(7503):68–75.

165. Bisel B, Pavone FS, Calamai M. GM1 and GM2 gangliosides: recent developments. *Biomolecular concepts.* 2014;5(1):87–93.

166. Hall P, Minnich S, Teigen C, Raymond K. Diagnosing Lysosomal Storage Disorders: The GM2 Gangliosidoses. *Current protocols in human genetics/editorial board, Jonathan L. Haines ... [et al.].* 2014;83 17.16.11-18.

167. Mugikura S, Takahashi S, Higano S, Kurihara N, Kon K, Sakamoto K. MR findings in Tay-Sachs disease. *J Comput Assist Tomogr.* 1996;20(4):551–555.

168. Nardocci N, Bertagnolio B, Rumi V, Angelini L. Progressive dystonia symptomatic of juvenile GM2 gangliosidosis. *Mov Disord.* 1992;7(1):64–67.

169. Navon R, Khosravi R, Melki J, et al. Juvenile-onset spinal muscular atrophy caused by compound heterozygosity for mutations in the HEXA gene. *Ann Neurol.* 1997;41(5):631–638.

170. Rondot P, Navon R, Eymard B, et al. [Juvenile GM2 gangliosidosis with progressive spinal muscular atrophy onset]. *Rev Neurol (Paris).* 1997;153(2):120–123.

171. Karni A, Navon R, Sadeh M. Hexosaminidase A deficiency manifesting as spinal muscular atrophy of late onset. *Ann Neurol.* 1988;24(3):451–453.

172. Salman MS, Clarke JT, Midroni G, Waxman MB. Peripheral and autonomic nervous system involvement in chronic GM2-gangliosidosis. *J Inherit Metab Dis*. 2001;24(1):65–71.

173. MacQueen GM, Rosebush PI, Mazurek MF. Neuropsychiatric aspects of the adult variant of Tay-Sachs disease. *J Neuropsychiatry Clin Neurosci*. 1998;10(1):10–19.

174. Higaki K, Li L, Bahrudin U, et al. Chemical chaperone therapy: chaperone effect on mutant enzyme and cellular pathophysiology in beta-galactosidase deficiency. *Hum Mutat*. 2011;32(7):843–852.

175. Matsuoka K, Tamura T, Tsuji D, et al. Therapeutic potential of intracerebroventricular replacement of modified human beta-hexosaminidase B for GM2 gangliosidosis. *Molecular therapy : the journal of the American Society of Gene Therapy*. 2011;19(6):1017–1024.

176. Masciullo M, Santoro M, Modoni A, et al. Substrate reduction therapy with miglustat in chronic GM2 gangliosidosis type Sandhoff: results of a 3-year follow-up. *J Inherit Metab Dis*. 2010;33(suppl 3):S355–361.

177. Vanier MT. Complex lipid trafficking in Niemann-Pick disease type C. *J Inherit Metab Dis*. 2014.

178. Klein AD, Alvarez A, Zanlungo S. The unique case of the Niemann-Pick type C cholesterol storage disorder. *Pediatric endocrinology reviews: PER*. 2014;12(suppl 1):166–175.

179. Vanier MT. Niemann-Pick diseases. *Handb Clin Neurol*. 2013;113:1717–1721.

180. Ory DS. Niemann-Pick type C: a disorder of cellular cholesterol trafficking. *Biochim Biophys Acta*. 2000;1529(1-3):331–339.

181. Tang Y, Li H, Liu JP. Niemann-Pick Disease Type C: from molecule to clinic. *Clinical and experimental pharmacology & physiology*. 2010;37(1):132–140.

182. Longstreth Jr. WT, Daven JR, Farrell DF, Bolen JW, Bird TD. Adult dystonic lipidosis: clinical, histologic, and biochemical findings of a neurovisceral storage disease. *Neurology*. 1982;32(11):1295–1299.

183. Fink JK, Filling-Katz MR, Sokol J, et al. Clinical spectrum of Niemann-Pick disease type C. *Neurology*. 1989;39(8):1040–1049.

184. Natowicz MR, Stoler JM, Prence EM, Liscum L. Marked heterogeneity in Niemann-Pick disease, type C. Clinical and ultrastructural findings. *Clin Pediatr (Phila)*. 1995;34(4):190–197.

185. Schiffmann R. Niemann-Pick disease type C. From bench to bedside. *Jama*. 1996;276(7):561–564.

186. Uc EY, Wenger DA, Jankovic J. Niemann-Pick disease type C: two cases and an update. *Mov Disord*. 2000;15(6):1199–1203.

187. Zafeiriou DI, Triantafyllou P, Gombakis NP, Vargiami E, Tsantali C, Michelakaki E. Niemann-Pick type C disease associated with peripheral neuropathy. *Pediatr Neurol*. 2003;29(3):242–244.

188. Patterson MC, Hendriksz CJ, Walterfang M, Sedel F, Vanier MT, Wijburg F. Recommendations for the diagnosis and management of Niemann-Pick disease type C: an update. *Mol Genet Metab*. 2012;106(3):330–344.

189. Bennett LL, Mohan D. Gaucher disease and its treatment options. *Ann Pharmacother*. 2013;47(9):1182–1193.

190. Chen M, Wang J. Gaucher disease: review of the literature. *Arch Pathol Lab Med*. 2008;132(5):851–853.

191. Weiss K, Gonzalez AN, Lopez G, Pedoeim L, Groden C, Sidransky E. The clinical management of type 2 Gaucher disease. *Mol Genet Metab*. 2014.

192. Cox TM, Schofield JP. Gaucher disease: clinical features and natural history. *Baillieres Clin Hematol*. 1997;10:657–689.

193. Park JK, Orvisky E, Tayebi N, et al. Myoclonic epilepsy in Gaucher disease: genotype-phenotype insights from a rare patient subgroup. *Pediatr Res*. 2003;53(3):387–395.

194. Farfel-Becker T, Vitner EB, Kelly SL, et al. Neuronal accumulation of glucosylceramide in a mouse model of neuronopathic Gaucher disease leads to neurodegeneration. *Hum Mol Genet*. 2014;23(4):843–854.

195. Vellodi A, Tylki-Szymanska A, Davies EH, et al. Management of neuronopathic Gaucher disease: revised recommendations. *J Inherit Metab Dis*. 2009;32(5):660–664.

196. Bembi B, Ciana G, Bottega M, Pelos G, Gornati R, Berra B. Cerebrospinal fluid infusion of alglucerase in the treatment of acute neuronopathic Gaucher's disease. *Pediatr Res*. 1995;38:425.

197. Schiffmann R, Fitzgibbon EJ, Harris C, et al. Randomized, controlled trial of miglustat in Gaucher's disease type 3. *Ann Neurol*. 2008;64(5):514–522.

198. Mink JW, Augustine EF, Adams HR, Marshall FJ, Kwon JM. Classification and natural history of the neuronal ceroid lipofuscinoses. *J Child Neurol*. 2013;28(9):1101–1105.

199. Dolisca SB, Mehta M, Pearce DA, Mink JW, Maria BL. Batten disease: clinical aspects, molecular mechanisms, translational science, and future directions. *J Child Neurol*. 2013;28(9):1074–1100.

200. Schulz A, Kohlschutter A, Mink J, Simonati A, Williams R. NCL diseases - clinical perspectives. *Biochim Biophys Acta*. 2013;1832(11):1801–1806.

201. Kollmann K, Uusi-Rauva K, Scifo E, Tyynela J, Jalanko A, Braulke T. Cell biology and function of neuronal ceroid lipofuscinosis-related proteins. *Biochim Biophys Acta*. 2013;1832(11):1866–1881.

202. Williams RE, Mole SE. New nomenclature and classification scheme for the neuronal ceroid lipofuscinoses. *Neurology*. 2012;79(2):183–191.

203. Kim SJ, Zhang Z, Lee YC, Mukherjee AB. Palmitoyl-protein thioesterase-1 deficiency leads to the activation of caspase-9 and contributes to rapid neurodegeneration in INCL. *Hum Mol Genet*. 2006;15(10):1580–1586.

204. Kim SJ, Zhang Z, Sarkar C, et al. Palmitoyl protein thioesterase-1 deficiency impairs synaptic vesicle recycling at nerve terminals, contributing to neuropathology in humans and mice. *J Clin Invest*. 2008;118(9):3075–3086.

205. Ramadan H, Al-Din AS, Ismail A, et al. Adult neuronal ceroid lipofuscinosis caused by deficiency in palmitoyl protein thioesterase 1. *Neurology*. 2007;68(5):387–388.

206. Berkovic SF, Andermann F, Andermann E, Carpenter S, Wolfe L. Kufs disease: clinical features and forms. *Am J Med Genet Suppl*. 1988;5:105–109.

207. Smith KR, Damiano J, Franceschetti S, et al. Strikingly different clinicopathological phenotypes determined by progranulin-mutation dosage. *Am J Hum Genet*. 2012;90(6):1102–1107.

208. Toh H, Chitramuthu BP, Bennett HP, Bateman A. Structure, function, and mechanism of progranulin; the brain and beyond. *J Mol Neurosci*. 2011;45(3):538–548.

209. Bras J, Verloes A, Schneider SA, Mole SE, Guerreiro RJ. Mutation of the parkinsonism gene ATP13A2 causes neuronal ceroid-lipofuscinosis. *Hum Mol Genet*. 2012;21(12):2646–2650.

210. Di Fonzo A, Chien HF, Socal M, et al. ATP13A2 missense mutations in juvenile parkinsonism and young onset Parkinson disease. *Neurology*. 2007;68(19):1557–1562.

211. Djarmati A, Hagenah J, Reetz K, et al. ATP13A2 variants in early-onset Parkinson's disease patients and controls. *Mov Disord*. 2009;24(14):2104–2111.

212. Smith KR, Dahl HH, Canafoglia L, et al. Cathepsin F mutations cause Type B Kufs disease, an adult-onset neuronal ceroid lipofuscinosis. *Hum Mol Genet*. 2013;22(7):1417–1423.

213. Staropoli JF, Karaa A, Lim ET, et al. A homozygous mutation in KCTD7 links neuronal ceroid lipofuscinosis to the ubiquitin-proteasome system. *Am J Hum Genet*. 2012;91(1):202–208.

214. Lang AE, Clarke JTR, Rosch L. Progressive longstanding "pure" dystonia: A new phenotype of juvenile metachromatic leukodystrophy. *Neurology*. 1985;35(suppl 1):194.

215. Torii T, Miyamoto Y, Yamauchi J, Tanoue A. Pelizaeus-Merzbacher disease: cellular pathogenesis and pharmacologic therapy. *Pediatr Int*. 2014;56(5):659–666.

216. Lassuthova P, Zaliova M, Inoue K, et al. Three New PLP1 Splicing Mutations Demonstrate Pathogenic and Phenotypic Diversity of Pelizaeus-Merzbacher Disease. *J Child Neurol*. 2013;29(7):924–931.

217. Golomb MR, Walsh LE, Carvalho KS, Christensen CK, DeMyer WE. Clinical findings in Pelizaeus-Merzbacher disease. *J Child Neurol*. 2004;19(5):328–331.

218. Berger J, Moser HW, Forss-Petter S. Leukodystrophies: recent developments in genetics, molecular biology, pathogenesis and treatment. *Curr Opin Neurol*. 2001;14(3):305–312.

219. Koeppen AH, Robitaille Y. Pelizaeus-Merzbacher disease. *J Neuropathol Exp Neurol*. 2002;61(9):747–759.

220. Hanefeld FA, Brockmann K, Pouwels PJ, Wilken B, Frahm J, Dechent P. Quantitative proton MRS of Pelizaeus-Merzbacher disease: evidence of dys- and hypomyelination. *Neurology*. 2005;65(5):701–706.

221. Nezu A, Kimura S, Uehara S, et al. Pelizaeus-Merzbacher-like disease: female case report. *Brain Dev*. 1996;18(2):114–118.

222. Hoshino H, Kubota M. Canavan disease: clinical features and recent advances in research. *Pediatr Int*. 2014;56(4):477–483.

223. Rodriguez D. Leukodystrophies with astrocytic dysfunction. *Handb Clin Neurol*. 2013;113:1619–1628.

224. Surendran S, Michals-Matalon K, Quast MJ, et al. Canavan disease: a monogenic trait with complex genomic interaction. *Mol Genet Metab*. 2003;80(1-2):74–80.

225. Matalon R, Kaul R, Michals K. Canavan disease: biochemical and molecular studies. *J Inherit Metab Dis*. 1993;16(4):744–752.

226. Toft PB, Geiss-Holtorff R, Rolland MO, et al. Magnetic resonance imaging in juvenile Canavan disease. *Eur J Pediatr*. 1993;152(9):750–753.

227. Nguyen HV, Havalad V, Aponte-Patel L, et al. Temporary biventricular pacing decreases the vasoactive-inotropic score after cardiac surgery: a substudy of a randomized clinical trial. *J Thorac Cardiovasc Surg*. 2013;146(2):296–301.

228. Assadi M, Janson C, Wang DJ, et al. Lithium citrate reduces excessive intra-cerebral N-acetyl aspartate in Canavan disease. *Eur J Paediatr Neurol*. 2010;14(4):354–359.

229. Ahmed SS, Li H, Cao C, et al. A single intravenous rAAV injection as late as P20 achieves efficacious and sustained CNS Gene therapy in Canavan mice. *Molecular therapy : the journal of the American Society of Gene Therapy*. 2013;21(12):2136–2147.

230. Ekinci B, Apaydin H, Vural M, Ozekmekci S. Two siblings with homocystinuria presenting with dystonia and parkinsonism. *Mov Disord*. 2004;19(8):962–964.

231. Sinclair AJ, Barling L, Nightingale S. Recurrent dystonia in homocystinuria: a metabolic pathogenesis. *Mov Disord*. 2006;21(10):1780–1782.

232. Varlibas F, Cobanoglu O, Ergin B, Tireli H. Different phenotypy in three siblings with homocystinuria. *The neurologist*. 2009;15(3):144–146.

233. Vatanavicharn N, Pressman BD, Wilcox WR. Reversible leukoencephalopathy with acute neurological deterioration and permanent residua in classical homocystinuria: A case report. *J Inherit Metab Dis*. 2008.

234. Aydin S, Abuzayed B, Varlibas F, et al. Treatment of homocystinuria-related dystonia with deep brain stimulation: a case report. *Stereotact Funct Neurosurg*. 2011;89(4):210–213.

235. Thauvin-Robinet C, Roze E, Couvreur G, et al. The adolescent and adult form of cobalamin C disease: clinical and molecular spectrum. *J Neurol Neurosurg Psychiatry*. 2008;79(6):725–728.

236. Debray FG, Boulanger Y, Khiat A, et al. Reduced brain choline in homocystinuria due to remethylation defects. *Neurology*. 2008;71(1):44–49.

237. Seow HF, Broer S, Broer A, et al. Hartnup disorder is caused by mutations in the gene encoding the neutral amino acid transporter SLC6A19. *Nat Genet*. 2004;36(9):1003–1007.

238. Tahmoush AJ, Alpers DH, Feigin RD, Armbrustmacher V, Prensky AL. Hartnup disease. Clinical, pathological, and biochemical observations. *Arch Neurol*. 1976;33(12):797–807.

239. Darras BT, Ampola MG, Dietz WH, Gilmore HE. Intermittent dystonia in Hartnup disease. *Pediatr Neurol*. 1989;5(2):118–120.

240. Chuang DT, Shih VE. Maple syrup urine disease (branched-chain ketoaciduria). In: Scriver CR, Beaudet AL, Sly WS, Valle D, eds. *The metabolic and molecular bases of inherited disease*. New York: McGraw-Hill; 2001:1971–2005.

241. Zinnanti WJ, Lazovic J, Griffin K, et al. Dual mechanism of brain injury and novel treatment strategy in maple syrup urine disease. *Brain*. 2009;132(Pt 4):903–918.

242. Zee DS, Freeman JM, Holtzman NA. Ophthalmoplegia in maple syrup urine disease. *J Pediatr*. 1974;84(1):113–115.

243. Temudo T, Martins E, Pocas F, Cruz R, Vilarinho L. Maple syrup disease presenting as paroxysmal dystonia. *Ann Neurol*. 2004;56(5):749–750.

244. Carecchio M, Schneider SA, Chan H, et al. Movement disorders in adult surviving patients with maple syrup urine disease. *Mov Disord*. 2011;26(7):1324–1328.

245. Nellis MM, Kasinski A, Carlson M, et al. Relationship of causative genetic mutations in maple syrup urine disease with their clinical expression. *Mol Genet Metab*. 2003;80(1-2):189–195.

246. Hoffmann GF, Kolker S. Defects in amino acid catabolism and the urea cycle. *Handb Clin Neurol*. 2013;113:1755–1773.

247. Bindu PS, Shehanaz KE, Christopher R, Pal PK, Ravishankar S. Intermediate maple syrup urine disease: neuroimaging observations in 3 patients from South India. *J Child Neurol*. 2007;22(7):911–913.

248. Williams RA, Mamotte CD, Burnett JR. Phenylketonuria: an inborn error of phenylalanine metabolism. *Clin Biochem Rev*. 2008;29(1):31–41.

249. Schumacher U, Lukacs Z, Kaltschmidt C, et al. High concentrations of phenylalanine stimulate peroxisome proliferator-activated receptor gamma: Implications for the pathophysiology of phenylketonuria. *Neurobiol Dis*. 2008.

250. Paine R. The Variability in Manifestation of untreated patients with phenylketonuria (phenylpyruvic aciduria). *Pediatrics*. 1957;26:290.

251. French JH, Clark D, Butler HG, et al. Phenylketonuria: some obersvations on reflex activity. *J Pediatr*. 1961;58:16.

252. Moyle JJ, Fox AM, Arthur M, Bynevelt M, Burnett JR. Meta-Analysis of Neuropsychological Symptoms of Adolescents and Adults with PKU. *Neuropsychol Rev*. 2007;17(2):91–101.

253. Bone A, Kuehl AK, Angelino AF. A neuropsychiatric perspective of phenylketonuria I: overview of phenylketonuria and its neuropsychiatric sequelae. *Psychosomatics*. 2012;53(6):517–523.

254. Vermathen P, Robert-Tissot L, Pietz J, Lutz T, Boesch C, Kreis R. Characterization of white matter alterations in phenylketonuria by magnetic resonance relaxometry and diffusion tensor imaging. *Magn Reson Med*. 2007;58(6):1145–1156.

255. Landvogt C, Mengel E, Bartenstein P, et al. Reduced cerebral fluoro-L-dopamine uptake in adult patients suffering from phenylketonuria. *J Cereb Blood Flow Metab*. 2008;28(4):824–831.

256. Pitt DB, Danks DM. The natural history of untreated phenylketonuria over 20 years. *J Paediatr Child Health*. 1991;27(3):189–190.

257. Maillot F, Lilburn M, Baudin J, Morley DW, Lee PJ. Factors influencing outcomes in the offspring of mothers with phenylketonuria during pregnancy: the importance of variation in maternal blood phenylalanine. *Am J Clin Nutr*. 2008;88(3):700–705.

258. Strisciuglio P, Concolino D. New Strategies for the Treatment of Phenylketonuria (PKU). *Metabolites*. 2014;4(4):1007–1017.

259. Camp KM, Parisi MA, Acosta PB, et al. Phenylketonuria Scientific Review Conference: state of the science and future research needs. *Mol Genet Metab*. 2014;112(2):87–122.

260. van der Meer SB, Poggi F, Spada M, et al. Clinical outcome of long-term management of patients with vitamin B12-unresponsive methylmalonic acidemia. *J Pediatr*. 1994;125(6 Pt 1):903–908.

261. Brismar J, Ozand PT. CT and MR of the brain in disorders of the propionate and methylmalonate metabolism. *AJNR Am J Neuroradiol*. 1994;15(8):1459–1473.

262. Morath MA, Okun JG, Muller IB, et al. Neurodegeneration and chronic renal failure in methylmalonic aciduria--a pathophysiological approach. *J Inherit Metab Dis*. 2008;31(1):35–43.

263. Schreiber J, Chapman KA, Summar ML, et al. Neurologic considerations in propionic acidemia. *Mol Genet Metab*. 2012;105(1):10–15.

264. Pena L, Franks J, Chapman KA, et al. Natural history of propionic acidemia. *Mol Genet Metab*. 2012;105(1):5–9.

265. Dejean de la Batie C, Barbier V, Valayannopoulos V, et al. Acute psychosis in propionic acidemia: 2 case reports. *J Child Neurol*. 2014;29(2):274–279.

266. Nyhan WL, Bay C, Beyer EW, Mazi M. Neurologic nonmetabolic presentation of propionic acidemia. *Arch Neurol*. 1999;56(9):1143–1147.

267. Barshes NR, Vanatta JM, Patel AJ, et al. Evaluation and management of patients with propionic acidemia undergoing liver transplantation: a comprehensive review. *Pediatr Transplant*. 2006;10(7):773–781.

268. Wortmann SB, Kluijtmans LA, Rodenburg RJ, et al. 3-Methylglutaconic aciduria--lessons from 50 genes and 977 patients. *J Inherit Metab Dis*. 2013;36(6):913–921.

269. Elpeleg ON, Costeff H, Joseph A, Shental Y, Weitz R, Gibson KM. 3-Methylglutaconic aciduria in the Iraqi-Jewish 'optic atrophy plus' (Costeff) syndrome. *Dev Med Child Neurol*. 1994;36(2):167–172.

270. Kleta R, Skovby F, Christensen E, Rosenberg T, Gahl WA, Anikster Y. 3-Methylglutaconic aciduria type III in a non-Iraqi-Jewish kindred: clinical and molecular findings. *Mol Genet Metab*. 2002;76(3):201–206.

271. Korman SH. Inborn errors of isoleucine degradation: a review. *Mol Genet Metab*. 2006;89(4):289–299.

272. Sass JO, Forstner R, Sperl W. 2-Methyl-3-hydroxybutyryl-CoA dehydrogenase deficiency: impaired catabolism of isoleucine presenting as neurodegenerative disease. *Brain Dev*. 2004;26(1):12–14.

273. Ozand PT, Nyhan WL, al Aqeel A, Christodoulou J. Malonic aciduria. *Brain Dev*. 1994;suppl:7–11:16.

274. Yalcinkaya C, Apaydin H, Ozekmekci S, Gibson KM. Delayed-onset dystonia associated with 3-oxothiolase deficiency. *Mov Disord*. 2001;16(2):372–375.

275. Buhas D, Bernard G, Fukao T, Decarie JC, Chouinard S, Mitchell GA. A treatable new cause of chorea: beta-ketothiolase deficiency. *Mov Disord*. 2013;28(8):1054–1056.

276. Hoffmann GF, Zschocke J. Glutaric aciduria type I: from clinical, biochemical and molecular diversity to successful therapy. *J Inherit Metab Dis*. 1999;22(4):381–391.

277. Gitiaux C, Roze E, Kinugawa K, et al. Spectrum of movement disorders associated with glutaric aciduria type 1: a study of 16 patients. *Mov Disord*. 2008;23(16):2392–2397.

278. Hauser SE, Peters H. Glutaric aciduria type 1: an underdiagnosed cause of encephalopathy and dystonia-dyskinesia syndrome in children. *J Paediatr Child Health*. 1998;34(3):302–304.

279. Zafeiriou DI, Zschocke J, Augoustidou-Savvopoulou P, et al. Atypical and variable clinical presentation of glutaric aciduria type I. *Neuropediatrics*. 2000;31(6):303–306.

V. SELECTED SECONDARY MOVEMENT DISORDERS

280. Haworth JC, Booth FA, Chudley AE, et al. Phenotypic variability in glutaric aciduria type I: Report of fourteen cases in five Canadian Indian kindreds. *J Pediatr*. 1991;118(1):52–58.

281. Zielonka M, Braun K, Bengel A, Seitz A, Kolker S, Boy N. Severe Acute Subdural Hemorrhage in a Patient With Glutaric Aciduria Type I After Minor Head Trauma: A Case Report. *J Child Neurol*. 2014.

282. Bahr O, Mader I, Zschocke J, Dichgans J, Schulz JB. Adult onset glutaric aciduria type I presenting with a leukoencephalopathy. *Neurology*. 2002;59(11):1802–1804.

283. Harting I, Neumaier-Probst E, Seitz A, et al. Dynamic changes of striatal and extrastriatal abnormalities in glutaric aciduria type I. *Brain*. 2009;132(Pt 7):1764–1782.

284. Brown A, Crowe L, Beauchamp MH, Anderson V, Boneh A. Neurodevelopmental Profiles of Children with Glutaric Aciduria Type I Diagnosed by Newborn Screening: A Follow-Up Case Series. *JIMD Rep*. 2014.

285. Muntau AC, Roschinger W, Merkenschlager A, et al. Combined D-2- and L-2-hydroxyglutaric aciduria with neonatal onset encephalopathy: a third biochemical variant of 2-hydroxyglutaric aciduria? *Neuropediatrics*. 2000;31(3):137–140.

286. Kranendijk M, Struys EA, Salomons GS, Van der Knaap MS, Jakobs C. Progress in understanding 2-hydroxyglutaric acidurias. *J Inherit Metab Dis*. 2012;35(4):571–587.

287. Barth PG, Hoffmann GF, Jaeken J, et al. L-2-hydroxyglutaric acidemia: a novel inherited neurometabolic disease. *Ann Neurol*. 1992;32(1):66–71.

288. Barbot C, Fineza I, Diogo L, et al. L-2-Hydroxyglutaric aciduria: clinical, biochemical and magnetic resonance imaging in six Portuguese pediatric patients. *Brain Dev*. 1997;19(4):268–273.

289. Moroni I, D'Incerti L, Farina L, Rimoldi M, Uziel G. Clinical, biochemical and neuroradiological findings in L-2-hydroxyglutaric aciduria. *Neurol Sci*. 2000;21(2):103–108.

290. Sztriha L, Gururaj A, Vreken P, Nork M, Lestringant G. L-2-hydroxyglutaric aciduria in two siblings. *Pediatr Neurol*. 2002;27(2):141–144.

291. Cachia D, Stine C. Child Neurology: cognitive delay in a 7-year-old girl. *Neurology*. 2013;81(20):e148–150.

292. Kossoff EH, Keswani SC, Raymond GV. L-2-hydroxyglutaric aciduria presenting as migraine. *Neurology*. 2001;57(9):1731–1732.

293. Yang E, Prabhu SP. Imaging manifestations of the leukodystrophies, inherited disorders of white matter. *Radiologic clinics of North America*. 2014;52(2):279–319.

294. Moroni I, Bugiani M, D'Incerti L, et al. L-2-hydroxyglutaric aciduria and brain malignant tumors: a predisposing condition? *Neurology*. 2004;62(10):1882–1884.

295. Latini A, da Silva CG, Ferreira GC, et al. Mitochondrial energy metabolism is markedly impaired by D-2-hydroxyglutaric acid in rat tissues. *Mol Genet Metab*. 2005;86(1-2):188–199.

296. Craigen WJ, Jakobs C, Sekul EA, et al. D-2-hydroxyglutaric aciduria in neonate with seizures and CNS dysfunction. *Pediatr Neurol*. 1994;10(1):49–53.

297. van der Knaap MS, Jakobs C, Hoffmann GF, et al. D-2-hydroxyglutaric aciduria: further clinical delineation. *J Inherit Metab Dis*. 1999;22(4):404–413.

298. Nyhan WL, Shelton GD, Jakobs C, et al. D-2-hydroxyglutaric aciduria. *J Child Neurol*. 1995;10(2):137–142.

299. Serdaroglu G, Aydinok Y, Yilmaz S, Manco L, Ozer E. Triosephosphate isomerase deficiency: a patient with Val231Met mutation. *Pediatr Neurol*. 2011;44(2):139–142.

300. Poll-The BT, Aicardi J, Girot R, Rosa R. Neurological findings in triosephosphate isomerase deficiency. *Ann Neurol*. 1985;17(5):439–443.

301. Linarello RE, Shetty AK, Thomas T, Warrier RP. Triosephosphate isomerase deficiency in a child with congenital hemolytic anemia and severe hypotonia. *Pediatr Hematol Oncol*. 1998;15(6):553–556.

302. Bardosi A, Eber SW, Hendrys M, Pekrun A. Myopathy with altered mitochondria due to a triosephosphate isomerase (TPI) deficiency. *Acta Neuropathol*. 1990;79(4):387–394.

303. Wilmshurst JM, Wise GA, Pollard JD, Ouvrier RA. Chronic axonal neuropathy with triosephosphate isomerase deficiency. *Pediatr Neurol*. 2004;30(2):146–148.

304. Marin-Valencia I, Roe CR, Pascual JM. Pyruvate carboxylase deficiency: mechanisms, mimics and anaplerosis. *Mol Genet Metab*. 2010;101(1):9–17.

305. De Meirleir L. Disorders of pyruvate metabolism. *Handb Clin Neurol*. 2013;113:1667–1673.

306. Ortez C, Jou C, Cortes-Saladelafont E, et al. Infantile parkinsonism and GABAergic hypotransmission in a patient with pyruvate carboxylase deficiency. *Gene*. 2013;532(2):302–306.

307. Saudubray JM, Marsac C, Cathelineau CL, Besson Leaud M, Leroux JP. Neonatal congenital lactic acidosis with pyruvate carboxylase deficiency in two siblings. *Acta Paediatr Scand*. 1976;65(6):717–724.

308. Mochel F, DeLonlay P, Touati G, et al. Pyruvate carboxylase deficiency: clinical and biochemical response to anaplerotic diet therapy. *Mol Genet Metab.* 2005;84(4):305–312.

309. Patel KP, O'Brien TW, Subramony SH, Shuster J, Stacpoole PW. The spectrum of pyruvate dehydrogenase complex deficiency: clinical, biochemical and genetic features in 371 patients. *Mol Genet Metab.* 2012;105(1):34–43.

310. Prasad C, Rupar T, Prasad AN. Pyruvate dehydrogenase deficiency and epilepsy. *Brain Dev.* 2011;33(10):856–865.

311. DeBrosse SD, Okajima K, Zhang S, et al. Spectrum of neurological and survival outcomes in pyruvate dehydrogenase complex (PDC) deficiency: lack of correlation with genotype. *Mol Genet Metab.* 2012;107(3):394–402.

312. Head RA, de Goede CG, Newton RW, et al. Pyruvate dehydrogenase deficiency presenting as dystonia in childhood. *Dev Med Child Neurol.* 2004;46(10):710–712.

313. Mellick G, Price L, Boyle R. Late-onset presentation of pyruvate dehydrogenase deficiency. *Mov Disord.* 2004;19(6):727–729.

314. Strassburg HM, Koch J, Mayr J, Sperl W, Boltshauser E. Acute flaccid paralysis as initial symptom in 4 patients with novel E1alpha mutations of the pyruvate dehydrogenase complex. *Neuropediatrics.* 2006;37(3):137–141.

315. Debray FG, Lambert M, Gagne R, et al. Pyruvate dehydrogenase deficiency presenting as intermittent isolated acute ataxia. *Neuropediatrics.* 2008;39(1):20–23.

316. Brown GK, Haan EA, Kirby DM, et al. "Cerebral" lactic acidosis: defects in pyruvate metabolism with profound brain damage and minimal systemic acidosis. *Eur J Pediatr.* 1988;147(1):10–14.

317. Bonnefont JP, Chretien D, Rustin P, et al. Alpha-ketoglutarate dehydrogenase deficiency presenting as congenital lactic acidosis. *J Pediatr.* 1992;121(2):255–258.

318. Dunckelmann RJ, Ebinger F, Schulze A, Wanders RJ, Rating D, Mayatepek E. 2-ketoglutarate dehydrogenase deficiency with intermittent 2-ketoglutaric aciduria. *Neuropediatrics.* 2000;31(1):35–38.

319. Soreze Y, Boutron A, Habarou F, et al. Mutations in human lipoyltransferase gene LIPT1 cause a Leigh disease with secondary deficiency for pyruvate and alpha-ketoglutarate dehydrogenase. *Orphanet J Rare Dis.* 2013;8:192.

320. Ottolenghi C, Hubert L, Allanore Y, et al. Clinical and biochemical heterogeneity associated with fumarase deficiency. *Hum Mutat.* 2011;32(9):1046–1052.

321. Saini AG, Singhi P. Infantile metabolic encephalopathy due to fumarase deficiency. *J Child Neurol.* 2013;28(4):535–537.

322. Allegri G, Fernandes MJ, Scalco FB, et al. Fumaric aciduria: an overview and the first Brazilian case report. *J Inherit Metab Dis.* 2010;33(4):411–419.

323. Gellera C, Uziel G, Rimoldi M, et al. Fumarase deficiency is an autosomal recessive encephalopathy affecting both the mitochondrial and the cytosolic enzymes. *Neurology.* 1990;40(3 Pt 1):495–499.

324. Lyon G, Adams RD, Kolodny EH. *Neurology of Hereditary Metabolic Diseases of Children.* 2nd ed. New York: McGraw-Hill; 1996.

325. Loeffen J, Smeets R, Voit T, Hoffmann G, Smeitink J. Fumarase deficiency presenting with periventricular cysts. *J Inherit Metab Dis.* 2005;28(5):799–800.

326. Toro JR, Nickerson ML, Wei MH, et al. Mutations in the fumarate hydratase gene cause hereditary leiomyomatosis and renal cell cancer in families in North America. *Am J Hum Genet.* 2003;73(1):95–106.

327. Chaussenot A, Paquis-Flucklinger V. An overview of neurological and neuromuscular signs in mitochondrial diseases. *Rev Neurol (Paris).* 2014;170(5):323–338.

328. Milone M, Benarroch EE. Mitochondrial dynamics: general concepts and clinical implications. *Neurology.* 2012;78(20):1612–1619.

329. Delonlay P, Rotig A, Sarnat HB. Respiratory chain deficiencies. *Handb Clin Neurol.* 2013;113:1651–1666.

330. Zeviani M, Simonati A, Bindoff LA. Ataxia in mitochondrial disorders. *Handb Clin Neurol.* 2012;103:359–372.

331. Haas RH, Zolkipli Z. Mitochondrial disorders affecting the nervous system. *Semin Neurol.* 2014;34(3):321–340.

332. Debray FG, Lambert M, Chevalier I, et al. Long-term outcome and clinical spectrum of 73 pediatric patients with mitochondrial diseases. *Pediatrics.* 2007;119(4):722–733.

333. Wallace DC, Murdock DG. Mitochondria and dystonia: the movement disorder connection? *Proc Natl Acad Sci U S A.* 1999;96(5):1817–1819.

334. DiMauro S, De Vivo DC. Genetic heterogeneity in Leigh syndrome. *Ann Neurol.* 1996;40(1):5–7.

335. De Vivo DC. Leigh syndrome: historical perspective and clinical variations. *Biofactors.* 1998;7(3):269–271.

336. Vu TH, Hirano M, DiMauro S. Mitochondrial diseases. *Neurol Clin.* 2002.

337. Zhu Z, Yao J, Johns T, et al. SURF1, encoding a factor involved in the biogenesis of cytochrome c oxidase, is mutated in Leigh syndrome. *Nat Genet*. 1998;20(4):337–343.

338. Baertling F, Rodenburg RJ, Schaper J, et al. A guide to diagnosis and treatment of Leigh syndrome. *J Neurol Neurosurg Psychiatry*. 2014;85(3):257–265.

339. Zeviani M, Bertagnolio B, Uziel G. Neurological presentations of mitochondrial diseases. *J Inherit Metab Dis*. 1996;19(4):504–520.

340. Finsterer J. Leigh and leigh-like syndrome in children and adults. *Pediatr Neurol*. 2008;39(4):223–235.

341. Sofou K, De Coo IF, Isohanni P, et al. A multicenter study on Leigh syndrome: disease course and predictors of survival. *Orphanet J Rare Dis*. 2014;9:52.

342. Campistol J, Cusi V, Vernet A, Fernandez-Alvarez E. Dystonia as a presenting sign of subacute necrotising encephalomyelopathy in infancy. *Eur J Pediatr*. 1986;144(6):589–591.

343. Macaya A, Munell F, Burke RE, De Vivo DC. Disorders of movement in Leigh syndrome. *Neuropediatrics*. 1993;24(2):60–67.

344. Cacic M, Wilichowski E, Mejaski-Bosnjak V, et al. Cytochrome c oxidase partial deficiency-associated Leigh disease presenting as an extrapyramidal syndrome. *J Child Neurol*. 2001;16(8):616–619.

345. Barkovich AJ, Good WV, Koch TK, Berg BO. Mitochondrial disorders: analysis of their clinical and imaging characteristics. *AJNR Am J Neuroradiol*. 1993;14(5):1119–1137.

346. Scarpelli M, Todeschini A, Rinaldi F, Rota S, Padovani A, Filosto M. Strategies for treating mitochondrial disorders: An update. *Mol Genet Metab*. 2014;113(4):253–260.

347. Mehrazin M, Shanske S, Kaufmann P, et al. Longitudinal changes of mtDNA A3243G mutation load and level of functioning in MELAS. *Am J Med Genet A*. 2009;149a(4):584–587.

348. Kaufmann P, Engelstad K, Wei Y, et al. Natural history of MELAS associated with mitochondrial DNA m.3243A> G genotype. *Neurology*. 2011;77(22):1965–1971.

349. Hirano M, Pavlakis SG. Mitochondrial myopathy, encephalopathy, lactic acidosis, and strokelike episodes (MELAS): current concepts. *J Child Neurol*. 1994;9(1):4–13.

350. Thambisetty M, Newman NJ, Glass JD, Frankel MR. A Practical Approach to the Diagnosis and Management of MELAS: Case Report and Review. *Neurolog*. 2002;8(5):302–312.

351. Moraes CT, Ciacci F, Silvestri G, et al. Atypical clinical presentations associated with the MELAS mutation at position 3243 of human mitochondrial DNA. *Neuromuscul Disord*. 1993;3(1):43–50.

352. Tan TM, Caputo C, Medici F, et al. MELAS syndrome, diabetes and thyroid disease: the role of mitochondrial oxidative stress. *Clin Endocrinol (Oxf)*. 2009;70(2):340–341.

353. Sudarsky L, Plotkin GM, Logigian EL, Johns DR. Dystonia as a presenting feature of the 3243 mitochondrial DNA mutation. *Mov Disord*. 1999;14(3):488–491.

354. Nishino I, Spinazzola A, Papadimitriou A, et al. Mitochondrial neurogastrointestinal encephalomyopathy: an autosomal recessive disorder due to thymidine phosphorylase mutations. *Ann Neurol*. 2000;47(6):792–800.

355. Schupbach WM, Vadday KM, Schaller A, et al. Mitochondrial neurogastrointestinal encephalomyopathy in three siblings: clinical, genetic and neuroradiological features. *J Neurol*. 2007;254(2):146–153.

356. Monroy N, Macias Kauffer LR, Mutchinick OM. Mitochondrial neurogastrointestinal encephalomyopathy (MNGIE) in two Mexican brothers harboring a novel mutation in the ECGF1 gene. *Eur J Med Genet*. 2008;51(3):245–250.

357. Cohen BH. Neuromuscular and systemic presentations in adults: diagnoses beyond MERRF and MELAS. *Neurotherapeutics*. 2013;10(2):227–242.

358. Nelson KB, Willoughby RE. Infection, inflammation and the risk of cerebral palsy. *Curr Opin Neurol*. 2000;13(2):133–139.

359. Saracchi E, Difrancesco JC, Brighina L, et al. A case of Leber hereditary optic neuropathy plus dystonia caused by G14459A mitochondrial mutation. *Neurol Sci*. 2013;34(3):407–408.

360. Wang K, Takahashi Y, Gao ZL, et al. Mitochondrial ND3 as the novel causative gene for Leber hereditary optic neuropathy and dystonia. *Neurogenetics*. 2009;10(4):337–345.

361. Novotny Jr. EJ, Singh G, Wallace DC, et al. Leber's disease and dystonia: a mitochondrial disease. *Neurology*. 1986;36(8):1053–1060.

362. Johns DR, Heher KL, Miller NR, Smith KH. Leber's hereditary optic neuropathy. Clinical manifestations of the 14484 mutation. *Arch Ophthalmol*. 1993;111(4):495–498.

363. Kim IS, Ki CS, Park KJ. Pediatric-onset dystonia associated with bilateral striatal necrosis and G14459A mutation in a Korean family: a case report. *J Korean Med Sci*. 2010;25(1):180–184.

364. Jin H, May M, Tranebjaerg L, et al. A novel X-linked gene, DDP, shows mutations in families with deafness (DFN-1), dystonia, mental deficiency and blindness. *Nat Genet*. 1996;14(2):177–180.

365. Blesa JR, Solano A, Briones P, Prieto-Ruiz JA, Hernandez-Yago J, Coria F. Molecular genetics of a patient with Mohr-Tranebjaerg Syndrome due to a new mutation in the DDP1 gene. *Neuromolecular Med*. 2007;9(4): 285–291.

366. Rothbauer U, Hofmann S, Muhlenbein N, et al. Role of the deafness dystonia peptide 1 (DDP1) in import of human Tim23 into the inner membrane of mitochondria. *J Biol Chem*. 2001;276(40):37327–37334.

367. Tranebjaerg L, Schwartz C, Eriksen H, et al. A new X linked recessive deafness syndrome with blindness, dystonia, fractures, and mental deficiency is linked to Xq22. *J Med Genet*. 1995;32(4):257–263.

368. Binder J, Hofmann S, Kreisel S, et al. Clinical and molecular findings in a patient with a novel mutation in the deafness-dystonia peptide (DDP1) gene. *Brain*. 2003;126(Pt 8):1814–1820.

369. Kim HT, Edwards MJ, Tyson J, Quinn NP, Bitner-Glindzicz M, Bhatia KP. Blepharospasm and limb dystonia caused by Mohr-Tranebjaerg syndrome with a novel splice-site mutation in the deafness/dystonia peptide gene. *Mov Disord*. 2007;22(9):1328–1331.

370. Lerner A, Bagic A, Simmons JM, et al. Widespread abnormality of the gamma-aminobutyric acid-ergic system in Tourette syndrome. *Brain*. 2012;135(Pt 6):1926–1936.

371. Swerdlow RH, Wooten GF. A novel deafness/dystonia peptide gene mutation that causes dystonia in female carriers of Mohr-Tranebjaerg syndrome. *Ann Neurol*. 2001;50(4):537–540.

372. Jinnah HA, Sabina RL, Van Den Berghe G. Metabolic disorders of purine metabolism affecting the nervous system. *Handb Clin Neurol*. 2013;113:1827–1836.

373. Hladnik U, Nyhan WL, Bertelli M. Variable expression of HPRT deficiency in 5 members of a family with the same mutation. *Arch Neurol*. 2008;65(9):1240–1243.

374. Greene ML. Clinical features of patients with the "partial" deficiency of the X-linked uricaciduria enzyme. *Arch Intern Med*. 1972;130(2):193–198.

375. Christie R, Bay C, Kaufman IA, Bakay B, Borden M, Nyhan WL. Lesch-Nyhan disease: clinical experience with nineteen patients. *Dev Med Child Neurol*. 1982;24(3):293–306.

376. Watts RW, Spellacy E, Gibbs DA, Allsop J, McKeran RO, Slavin GE. Clinical, post-mortem, biochemical and therapeutic observations on the Lesch-Nyhan syndrome with particular reference to the Neurological manifestations. *Q J Med*. 1982;51(201):43–78.

377. Mizuno T. Long-term follow-up of ten patients with Lesch-Nyhan syndrome. *Neuropediatrics*. 1986;17(3):158–161.

378. Jinnah HA, Harris JC, Reich SG, Visser JE, Garabas G, Eddey GE. The motor disorder of Lesch-Nyhan disease. *Mov Disord*. 1998;13(suppl 2):98.

379. Jinnah HA, Lewis RF, Visser JE, Eddey GE, Barabas G, Harris JC. Ocular motor dysfunction in Lesch-Nyhan disease. *Pediatr Neurol*. 2001;24(3):200–204.

380. Jinnah HA, Ceballos-Picot I, Torres RJ, et al. Attenuated variants of Lesch-Nyhan disease. *Brain*. 2010;133(Pt 3):671–689.

381. Puig JG, Torres RJ, Mateos FA, et al. The spectrum of hypoxanthine-guanine phosphoribosyltransferase (HPRT) deficiency. Clinical experience based on 22 patients from 18 Spanish families. *Medicine (Baltimore)*. 2001;80(2):102–112.

382. Torres RJ, Puig JG, Jinnah HA. Update on the phenotypic spectrum of Lesch-Nyhan disease and its attenuated variants. *Current rheumatology reports*. 2012;14(2):189–194.

383. Del Bigio MR, Halliday WC. Multifocal atrophy of cerebellar internal granular neurons in lesch-nyhan disease: case reports and review. *J Neuropathol Exp Neurol*. 2007;66(5):346–353.

384. Jankovic J, Caskey TC, Stout JT, Butler IJ. Lesch-Nyhan syndrome: a study of motor behavior and cerebrospinal fluid neurotransmitters. *Ann Neurol*. 1988;23(5):466–469.

385. Lloyd KG, Hornykiewicz O, Davidson L, et al. Biochemical evidence of dysfunction of brain neurotransmitters in the Lesch-Nyhan syndrome. *N Engl J Med*. 1981;305(19):1106–1111.

386. Saito Y, Ito M, Hanaoka S, Ohama E, Akaboshi S, Takashima S. Dopamine receptor upregulation in Lesch-Nyhan syndrome: a postmortem study. *Neuropediatrics*. 1999;30(2):66–71.

387. Serrano M, Perez-Duenas B, Ormazabal A, et al. Levodopa therapy in a Lesch-Nyhan disease patient: pathological, biochemical, neuroimaging, and therapeutic remarks. *Mov Disord*. 2008;23(9):1297–1300.

388. Stone RL, Aimi J, Barshop BA, et al. A mutation in adenylosuccinate lyase associated with mental retardation and autistic features. *Nat Genet*. 1992;1(1):59–63.

389. Jaeken J, Wadman SK, Duran M, et al. Adenylosuccinase deficiency: an inborn error of purine nucleotide synthesis. *Eur J Pediatr.* 1988;148(2):126–131.
390. Spiegel EK, Colman RF, Patterson D. Adenylosuccinate lyase deficiency. *Mol Genet Metab.* 2006;89(1-2):19–31.
391. Mouchegh K, Zikanova M, Hoffmann GF, et al. Lethal fetal and early neonatal presentation of adenylosuccinate lyase deficiency: observation of 6 patients in 4 families. *J Pediatr.* 2007.
392. Jurecka A, Zikanova M, Tylki-Szymanska A, et al. Clinical, biochemical and molecular findings in seven Polish patients with adenylosuccinate lyase deficiency. *Mol Genet Metab.* 2008;94(4):435–442.
393. Van den Berghe G, Jaeken J. In: Scriver C, Beaudet AL, Sly WS, Valle D, eds. *The Metabolic and Molecular Bases of Inherited Disease.* : McGraw-Hill; 2001:2653–2662.
394. Laikind PK, Seegmiller JE, Gruber HE. Detection of 5′-phosphoribosyl-4-(N-succinylcarboxamide)-5-aminoimidazole in urine by use of the Bratton-Marshall reaction: identification of patients deficient in adenylosuccinate lyase activity. *Anal Biochem.* 1986;156(1):81–90.
395. Jurecka A, Tylki-Szymanska A, Zikanova M, Krijt J, Kmoch S. D: -Ribose therapy in four Polish patients with adenylosuccinate lyase deficiency: Absence of positive effect. *J Inherit Metab Dis.* 2008.
396. Becker MA, Taylor W, Smith PR, Ahmed M. Overexpression of the normal phosphoribosylpyrophosphate synthetase 1 isoform underlies catalytic superactivity of human phosphoribosylpyrophosphate synthetase. *J Biol Chem.* 1996;271(33):19894–19899.
397. Becker MA, Losman MJ, Rosenberg AL, Mehlman I, Levinson DJ, Holmes EW. Phosphoribosylpyrophosphate synthetase superactivity. A study of five patients with catalytic defects in the enzyme. *Arthritis Rheum.* 1986;29(7):880–888.
398. Nyhan WL. Disorders of purine and pyrimidine metabolism. *Mol Genet Metab.* 2005;86(1-2):25–33.
399. Moran R, Kuilenburg AB, Duley J, et al. Phosphoribosylpyrophosphate synthetase superactivity and recurrent infections is caused by a p.Val142Leu mutation in PRS-I. *Am J Med Genet A.* 2012;158a(2):455–460.
400. Arts WF, Loonen MC, Sengers RC, Slooff JL. X-linked ataxia, weakness, deafness, and loss of vision in early childhood with a fatal course. *Ann Neurol.* 1993;33(5):535–539.
401. de Brouwer AP, Williams KL, Duley JA, et al. Arts syndrome is caused by loss-of-function mutations in PRPS1. *Am J Hum Genet.* 2007;81(3):507–518.
402. Rosenberg RN, Chutorian A. Familial opticoacoustic nerve degeneration and polyneuropathy. *Neurology.* 1967;17(9):827–832.
403. Kim HJ, Sohn KM, Shy ME, et al. Mutations in PRPS1, which encodes the phosphoribosyl pyrophosphate synthetase enzyme critical for nucleotide biosynthesis, cause hereditary peripheral neuropathy with hearing loss and optic neuropathy (cmtx5). *Am J Hum Genet.* 2007;81(3):552–558.
404. Schulze A. Creatine deficiency syndromes. *Handb Clin Neurol.* 2013;113:1837–1843.
405. Comeaux MS, Wang J, Wang G, et al. Biochemical, molecular, and clinical diagnoses of patients with cerebral creatine deficiency syndromes. *Mol Genet Metab.* 2013;109(3):260–268.
406. Ganesan V, Johnson A, Connelly A, Eckhardt S, Surtees RA. Guanidinoacetate methyltransferase deficiency: new clinical features. *Pediatr Neurol.* 1997;17(2):155–157.
407. Leuzzi V, Bianchi MC, Tosetti M, et al. Brain creatine depletion: guanidinoacetate methyltransferase deficiency (improving with creatine supplementation). *Neurology.* 2000;55(9):1407–1409.
408. Mercimek-Mahmutoglu S, Stoeckler-Ipsiroglu S, Adami A, et al. GAMT deficiency: features, treatment, and outcome in an inborn error of creatine synthesis. *Neurology.* 2006;67(3):480–484.
409. Schulze A, Bachert P, Schlemmer H, et al. Lack of creatine in muscle and brain in an adult with GAMT deficiency. *Ann Neurol.* 2003;53(2):248–251.
410. Dhar SU, Scaglia F, Li FY, et al. Expanded clinical and molecular spectrum of guanidinoacetate methyltransferase (GAMT) deficiency. *Mol Genet Metab.* 2009;96(1):38–43.
411. Stockler S, Schutz PW, Salomons GS. Cerebral creatine deficiency syndromes: clinical aspects, treatment and pathophysiology. *Subcell Biochem.* 2007;46:149–166.
412. Schulze A, Ebinger F, Rating D, Mayatepek E. Improving treatment of guanidinoacetate methyltransferase deficiency: reduction of guanidinoacetic acid in body fluids by arginine restriction and ornithine supplementation. *Mol Genet Metab.* 2001;74(4):413–419.
413. Bianchi MC, Tosetti M, Fornai F, et al. Reversible brain creatine deficiency in two sisters with normal blood creatine level. *Ann Neurol.* 2000;47(4):511–513.
414. Battini R, Leuzzi V, Carducci C, et al. Creatine depletion in a new case with AGAT deficiency: clinical and genetic study in a large pedigree. *Mol Genet Metab.* 2002;77(4):326–331.

415. Schulze A, Battini R. Pre-symptomatic treatment of creatine biosynthesis defects. *Subcell Biochem*. 2007;46:167–181.

416. Item CB, Stockler-Ipsiroglu S, Stromberger C, et al. Arginine:glycine amidinotransferase deficiency: the third inborn error of creatine metabolism in humans. *Am J Hum Genet*. 2001;69(5):1127–1133.

417. Hahn KA, Salomons GS, Tackels-Horne D, et al. X-linked mental retardation with seizures and carrier manifestations is caused by a mutation in the creatine-transporter gene (SLC6A8) located in Xq28. *Am J Hum Genet*. 2002;70(5):1349–1356.

418. deGrauw TJ, Cecil KM, Byars AW, Salomons GS, Ball WS, Jakobs C. The clinical syndrome of creatine transporter deficiency. *Mol Cell Biochem*. 2003;244(1-2):45–48.

419. Ardon O, Amat di San Filippo C, Salomons GS, Longo N. Creatine transporter deficiency in two half-brothers. *Am J Med Genet A*. 2010;152a(8):1979–1983.

420. Jaeken J. Congenital disorders of glycosylation. *Handb Clin Neurol*. 2013;113:1737–1743.

421. Freeze HH, Chong JX, Bamshad MJ, Ng BG. Solving glycosylation disorders: fundamental approaches reveal complicated pathways. *Am J Hum Genet*. 2014;94(2):161–175.

422. Freeze HH. Update and perspectives on congenital disorders of glycosylation. *Glycobiology*. 2001;11(12):129R–143R.

423. Marquardt T, Denecke J. Congenital disorders of glycosylation: review of their molecular bases, clinical presentations and specific therapies. *Eur J Pediatr*. 2003;162(6):359–379.

424. Wolfe LA, Krasnewich D. Congenital disorders of glycosylation and intellectual disability. *Dev Disabil Res Rev*. 2013;17(3):211–225.

425. Scott K, Gadomski T, Kozicz T, Morava E. Congenital disorders of glycosylation: new defects and still counting. *J Inherit Metab Dis*. 2014;37(4):609–617.

426. Miossec-Chauvet E, Mikaeloff Y, Heron D, et al. Neurological presentation in pediatric patients with congenital disorders of glycosylation type Ia. *Neuropediatrics*. 2003;34(1):1–6.

427. Grunewald S. Congenital disorders of glycosylation: rapidly enlarging group of (neuro)metabolic disorders. *Early Hum Dev*. 2007;83(12):825–830.

428. Lacey JM, Bergen HR, Magera MJ, Naylor S, O'Brien JF. Rapid determination of transferrin isoforms by immunoaffinity liquid chromatography and electrospray mass spectrometry. *Clin Chem*. 2001;47(3):513–518.

429. Sparks SE, Krasnewich DM. Congenital Disorders of N-linked Glycosylation Pathway Overview All rights reserved. In: Pagon RA, Adam MP, Ardinger HH, eds. *GeneReviews(R)*. Seattle: Seattle (WA): University of Washington, Seattle University of Washington; 1993.

430. Leroy JG. Congenital disorders of N-glycosylation including diseases associated with O- as well as N-glycosylation defects. *Pediatr Res*. 2006;60(6):643–656.

431. Janssen MC, de Kleine RH, van den Berg AP, et al. Successful liver transplantation and long-term follow-up in a patient with MPI-CDG. *Pediatrics*. 2014;134(1):e279–283.

432. Johnson JL, Rajagopalan KV, Wadman SK. Human molybdenum cofactor deficiency. *Adv Exp Med Biol*. 1993;338:373–378.

433. Graf WD, Oleinik OE, Jack RM, Weiss AH, Johnson JL. Ahomocysteinemia in molybdenum cofactor deficiency. *Neurology*. 1998;51(3):860–862.

434. Basheer SN, Waters PJ, Lam CW, et al. Isolated sulfite oxidase deficiency in the newborn: lactic acidaemia and leukoencephalopathy. *Neuropediatrics*. 2007;38(1):38–41.

435. Boles RG, Ment LR, Meyn MS, Horwich AL, Kratz LE, Rinaldo P. Short-term response to dietary therapy in molybdenum cofactor deficiency. *Ann Neurol*. 1993;34(5):742–744.

436. Ramaekers V, Sequeira JM, Quadros EV. Clinical recognition and aspects of the cerebral folate deficiency syndromes. *Clin Chem Lab Med*. 2013;51(3):497–511.

437. Bonkowsky JL, Ramaekers VT, Quadros EV, Lloyd M. Progressive encephalopathy in a child with cerebral folate deficiency syndrome. *J Child Neurol*. 2008;23(12):1460–1463.

438. Ramaekers VT, Sequeira JM, Blau N, Quadros EV. A milk-free diet downregulates folate receptor autoimmunity in cerebral folate deficiency syndrome. *Dev Med Child Neurol*. 2008;50(5):346–352.

439. Steinfeld R, Grapp M, Kraetzner R, et al. Folate receptor alpha defect causes cerebral folate transport deficiency: a treatable neurodegenerative disorder associated with disturbed myelin metabolism. *Am J Hum Genet*. 2009;85(3):354–363.

440. Mangold S, Blau N, Opladen T, et al. Cerebral folate deficiency: a neurometabolic syndrome? *Mol Genet Metab*. 2011;104(3):369–372.

441. Alfadhel M, Almuntashri M, Jadah RH, et al. Biotin-responsive basal ganglia disease should be renamed biotin-thiamine-responsive basal ganglia disease: a retrospective review of the clinical, radiological and molecular findings of 18 new cases. *Orphanet J Rare Dis.* 2013;8:83.

442. Bindu PS, Noone ML, Nalini A, Muthane UB, Kovoor JM. Biotin-responsive basal ganglia disease: a treatable and reversible neurological disorder of childhood. *J Child Neurol.* 2009;24(6):750–752.

443. Debs R, Depienne C, Rastetter A, et al. Biotin-responsive basal ganglia disease in ethnic Europeans with novel SLC19A3 mutations. *Arch Neurol.* 2010;67(1):126–130.

444. De Vivo DC, Trifiletti RR, Jacobson RI, Ronen GM, Behmand RA, Harik SI. Defective glucose transport across the blood-brain barrier as a cause of persistent hypoglycorrhachia, seizures, and developmental delay. *N Engl J Med.* 1991;325(10):703–709.

445. Wang D, Pascual JM, Yang H, et al. Glut-1 deficiency syndrome: clinical, genetic, and therapeutic aspects. *Ann Neurol.* 2005;57(1):111–118.

446. Klepper J, Leiendecker B. GLUT1 deficiency syndrome--2007 update. *Dev Med Child Neurol.* 2007;49(9):707–716.

447. De Giorgis V, Veggiotti P. GLUT1 deficiency syndrome 2013: current state of the art. *Seizure.* 2013;22(10):803–811.

448. Zorzi G, Castellotti B, Zibordi F, Gellera C, Nardocci N. Paroxysmal movement disorders in GLUT1 deficiency syndrome. *Neurology.* 2008;71(2):146–148.

449. Anand G, Padeniya A, Hanrahan D, et al. Milder phenotypes of glucose transporter type 1 deficiency syndrome. *Dev Med Child Neurol.* 2011;53(7):664–668.

450. Pons R, Collins A, Rotstein M, Engelstad K, De Vivo DC. The spectrum of movement disorders in Glut-1 deficiency. *Mov Disord.* 2010;25(3):275–281.

451. Brockmann K. The expanding phenotype of GLUT1-deficiency syndrome. *Brain Dev.* 2009;31(7):545–552.

452. Weber YG, Kamm C, Suls A, et al. Paroxysmal choreoathetosis/spasticity (DYT9) is caused by a GLUT1 defect. *Neurology.* 2011;77(10):959–964.

453. Schneider SA, Paisan-Ruiz C, Garcia-Gorostiaga I, et al. GLUT1 gene mutations cause sporadic paroxysmal exercise-induced dyskinesias. *Mov Disord.* 2009;24(11):1684–1688.

454. Pascual JM, Van Heertum RL, Wang D, Engelstad K, De Vivo DC. Imaging the metabolic footprint of Glut1 deficiency on the brain. *Ann Neurol.* 2002;52(4):458–464.

455. Leen WG, Wevers RA, Kamsteeg EJ, Scheffer H, Verbeek MM, Willemsen MA. Cerebrospinal fluid analysis in the workup of GLUT1 deficiency syndrome: a systematic review. *JAMA neurology.* 2013;70(11):1440–1444.

456. Yang H, Wang D, Engelstad K, et al. Glut1 deficiency syndrome and erythrocyte glucose uptake assay. *Ann Neurol.* 2011;70(6):996–1005.

457. Klepper J. Absence of SLC2A1 mutations does not exclude Glut1 deficiency syndrome. *Neuropediatrics.* 2013;44(4):235–236.

458. Suls A, Dedeken P, Goffin K, et al. Paroxysmal exercise-induced dyskinesia and epilepsy is due to mutations in SLC2A1, encoding the glucose transporter GLUT1. *Brain.* 2008;131(Pt 7):1831–1844.

459. Pascual JM, Liu P, Mao D, et al. Triheptanoin for glucose transporter type I deficiency (G1D): modulation of human ictogenesis, cerebral metabolic rate, and cognitive indices by a food supplement. *JAMA neurology.* 2014;71(10):1255–1265.

460. Jung HH, Danek A, Walker RH. Neuroacanthocytosis syndromes. *Orphanet J Rare Dis.* 2011;6:68.

461. Walker RH, Jung HH, Danek A. Neuroacanthocytosis. *Handb Clin Neurol.* 2011;100:141–151.

462. Dobson-Stone C, Velayos-Baeza A, Filippone LA, et al. Chorein detection for the diagnosis of chorea-acanthocytosis. *Ann Neurol.* 2004;56(2):299–302.

463. Kurano Y, Nakamura M, Ichiba M, et al. In vivo distribution and localization of chorein. *Biochem Biophys Res Commun.* 2007;353(2):431–435.

464. Walterfang M, Yucel M, Walker R, et al. Adolescent obsessive compulsive disorder heralding chorea-acanthocytosis. *Mov Disord.* 2008;23(3):422–425.

465. Hardie RJ, Pullon HW, Harding AE, et al. Neuroacanthocytosis. A clinical, haematological and pathological study of 19 cases. *Brain.* 1991;114(Pt 1A):13–49.

466. Limos LC, Ohnishi A, Sakai T, Fujii N, Goto I, Kuroiwa Y. "Myopathic" changes in chorea-acanthocytosis. Clinical and histopathological studies. *J Neurol Sci.* 1982;55(1):49–58.

467. Ishida C, Makifuchi T, Saiki S, Hirose G, Yamada M. A neuropathological study of autosomal-dominant chorea-acanthocytosis with a mutation of VPS13A. *Acta Neuropathol.* 2008.

468. Tanaka M, Hirai S, Kondo S, et al. Cerebral hypoperfusion and hypometabolism with altered striatal signal intensity in chorea-acanthocytosis: a combined PET and MRI study. *Mov Disord*. 1998;13(1):100–107.

469. Sorrentino G, De Renzo A, Miniello S, Nori O, Bonavita V. Late appearance of acanthocytes during the course of chorea-acanthocytosis. *J Neurol Sci*. 1999;163(2):175–178.

470. Henkel K, Danek A, Grafman J, Butman J, Kassubek J. Head of the caudate nucleus is most vulnerable in chorea-acanthocytosis: a voxel-based morphometry study. *Mov Disord*. 2006;21(10):1728–1731.

471. Dubinsky RM, Hallett M, Levey R, Di Chiro G. Regional brain glucose metabolism in neuroacanthocytosis. *Neurology*. 1989;39(9):1253–1255.

472. Brooks DJ, Ibanez V, Playford ED, et al. Presynaptic and postsynaptic striatal dopaminergic function in neuroacanthocytosis: a positron emission tomographic study. *Ann Neurol*. 1991;30(2):166–171.

473. Rodrigues GR, Walker RH, Bader B, Danek A, Marques Jr. W, Tumas V. Chorea-acanthocytosis: Report of two Brazilian cases. *Mov Disord*. 2008.

474. Ho M, Chelly J, Carter N, Danek A, Crocker P, Monaco AP. Isolation of the gene for McLeod syndrome that encodes a novel membrane transport protein. *Cell*. 1994;77(6):869–880.

475. Jung HH, Danek A, Frey BM. McLeod syndrome: a neurohaematological disorder. *Vox Sang*. 2007;93(2):112–121.

476. Danek A, Tison F, Rubio J, Oechsner M, Kalckreuth W, Monaco AP. The chorea of McLeod syndrome. *Mov Disord*. 2001;16(5):882–889.

477. Miranda M, Jung HH, Danek A, Walker RH. The chorea of McLeod syndrome: progression to hypokinesia. *Mov Disord*. 2012;27(13):1701–1702.

478. Danek A, Uttner I, Vogl T, Tatsch K, Witt TN. Cerebral involvement in McLeod syndrome. *Neurology*. 1994;44(1):117–120.

479. Oechsner M, Buchert R, Beyer W, Danek A. Reduction of striatal glucose metabolism in McLeod choreoacanthocytosis. *J Neurol Neurosurg Psychiatry*. 2001;70(4):517–520.

480. Bassen FA, Kornzweig AL. Malformation of the erythrocytes in a case of atypical retinitis pigmentosa. *Blood*. 1950;5:381–387.

481. Kane JP, Havel RJ. Disorders of the biogenesis and secretion of lipoproteins containing the B apolipoproteins. In: Scriver CR, Beaudet AL, Sly WS, Valle D, eds. *The metabolic basis of inherited disease*. 7th ed. New York: McGraw-Hill; 1995:1853–1885.

482. Zamel R, Khan R, Pollex RL, Hegele RA. Abetalipoproteinemia: two case reports and literature review. *Orphanet J Rare Dis*. 2008;3:19.

483. Shoulders CC, Brett DJ, Bayliss JD, et al. Abetalipoproteinemia is caused by defects of the gene encoding the 97 kDa subunit of a microsomal triglyceride transfer protein. *Hum Mol Genet*. 1993;2(12):2109–2116.

484. Berriot-Varoqueaux N, Aggerbeck LP, Samson-Bouma M, Wetterau JR. The role of the microsomal triglyceride transfer protein in abetalipoproteinemia. *Annu Rev Nutr*. 2000;20:663–697.

485. Muller DP, Lloyd JK, Wolff OH. The role of vitamin E in the treatment of the neurological features of abetalipoproteinaemia and other disorders of fat absorption. *J Inherit Metab Dis*. 1985;8(Suppl 1):88–92.

486. Crow YJ. Aicardi-Goutieres syndrome. *Handb Clin Neurol*. 2013;113:1629–1635.

487. Vanderver A, Prust M, Kadom N, et al. Early-Onset Aicardi-Goutieres Syndrome: Magnetic Resonance Imaging (MRI) Pattern Recognition. *J Child Neurol*. 2014.

488. Dale RC, Gornall H, Singh-Grewal D, Alcausin M, Rice GI, Crow YJ. Familial Aicardi-Goutieres syndrome due to SAMHD1 mutations is associated with chronic arthropathy and contractures. *Am J Med Genet A*. 2010;152a(4):938–942.

489. Crow YJ, Livingston JH. Aicardi-Goutieres syndrome: an important Mendelian mimic of congenital infection. *Dev Med Child Neurol*. 2008;50(6):410–416.

490. D'Arrigo S, Riva D, Bulgheroni S, et al. Aicardi-Goutieres syndrome: description of a late onset case. *Dev Med Child Neurol*. 2008;50(8):631–634.

491. Stephenson JB. Aicardi-Goutieres syndrome (AGS). *Eur J Paediatr Neurol*. 2008;12(5):355–358.

492. Rice G, Patrick T, Parmar R, et al. Clinical and molecular phenotype of Aicardi-Goutieres syndrome. *Am J Hum Genet*. 2007;81(4):713–725.

493. Orcesi S, Pessagno A, Biancheri R, et al. Aicardi-Goutieres syndrome presenting atypically as a sub-acute leukoencephalopathy. *Eur J Paediatr Neurol*. 2008;12(5):408–411.

18

Movement Disorders in Autoimmune Diseases

Harvey S. Singer[1], Jonathan W. Mink[2],
Donald L. Gilbert[3] and Joseph Jankovic[4]

[1]Department of Neurology, Johns Hopkins Hospital, Baltimore, MD, USA;
[2]Division of Child Neurology, University of Rochester Medical Center,
Rochester, NY, USA; [3]Division of Neurology, Cincinnati Children's Hospital
Medical Center, Cincinnati, OH, USA; [4]Department of Neurology, Baylor
College of Medicine, Houston, TX, USA

O U T L I N E

Movement Disorders in Childhood, Second Edition.
DOI: http://dx.doi.org/10.1016/B978-0-12-411573-6.00018-8

Autoimmune disorders are complex, multifactorial entities with underlying genetic and environmental factors.[1] In this chapter, autoimmune disorders occurring in children and presenting with associated movement disorders have been divided into five major topics (see Table 18.1). As will be discussed, for many of the proposed autoimmune disorders the pathophysiological mechanism remains undetermined. The initiating triggers for many autoimmune processes (e.g., tumor, infection, other) are often external to the brain itself, leading to the question of how immune cells enter this structure. While the precise answer remains unclear, possibilities include: the presence of activated lymphocytes which are capable of crossing the blood brain barrier (BBB) and targeting self-antigens[2,3]; a compromised BBB that allows antibody entrance into brain parenchyma; and a BBB that is more actively involved in the transfer of molecules and proteins.[4]

Several important basic principles are essential to recognize when considering a potential pathophysiological role for a particular antibody.[5,6] First, antibodies that bind to intracellular proteins, especially if measured using techniques with denatured intracellular antigens (e.g., homogenized tissue), may be valuable biomarkers, but are usually not pathogenic. Second, antibodies that bind to cell surface markers are more likely to be associated with clinical symptoms, but it is essential to confirm that there is binding to the protein in its conformational state (i.e., using assays that express the suspected antigen) at the cell surface of live eukaryotic cells.

TABLE 18.1   Childhood Autoimmune Movement Disorders

1. Complication of a systemic autoimmune disorder
     Systemic lupus erythematosus (SLE)
     Antiphospholipid syndrome
     Hashimoto's encephalopathy
2. Post-streptococcal infections
     Sydenham's chorea
     PANDAS (hypothesized)
     Post-streptococcal acute disseminated encephalomyelitis and others
3. Autoimmune basal ganglia encephalitis
4. Autoimmune encephalopathies
     NMDAR encephalitis
     LGI1, Caspr2, GABAaR, GABAbR
     Progressive encephalomyelitis with rigidity and myoclonus (PERM)
5. Other paraneoplastic disorders
     Opsoclonus myoclonus syndrome

COMPLICATION OF A SYSTEMIC AUTOIMMUNE DISORDER

Systemic Lupus Erythematosus (SLE)

SLE is a common chronic rheumatic illness in children, with a female predominance. In approximately 25% of cases the disorder presents before age 19 years and in 3.5% before age 10 years. Affected individuals have multiorgan involvement and diagnostic criteria have been published.[7] Chorea is the most common movement disorder in SLE, occurring in about 5% of affected children, with onset often preceding the clinical diagnosis.[8] Lupus chorea is frequently the initial neurological symptom and about one-half of the children develop other CNS manifestations including seizures and neuropsychiatric problems. In adult cases, in addition to chorea, reported movement disorders are parkinsonism,[9,10] isolated tremor,[11] blepharospasm,[12] stiff person syndrome,[13–15] and cervical dystonia.[16] Laboratory findings include low complement C3 and C4 levels and the following antibodies: Anti-Smith (Sm), Anti-double stranded DNA (dsDNA), Antinuclear antibody (ANA), Anti-RNP, Anti-SS-A (also called Ro), and Anti-SS-B (also La). Pediatric case reports have shown a correlation between disease and anticardiolipins.[17]

The precise mechanism(s) underlying the pathogenesis of movement abnormalities in SLE remains unclear. In many patients with documented CNS lupus, evidence of immune-mediated abnormalities cannot be found. Imaging studies are typically normal or have non-specific findings.[18] PET studies with [18F] deoxyglucose have shown evidence of hypermetabolism in the contralateral striatum in patients with asymmetric lupus chorea.[19] Potential supporting evidence for an immune mechanism includes elevated CSF IgG, IgG/albumin ratio, IgG index, and the presence of oligoclonal bands, anti-double–stranded DNA complexes, and anticardiolipins. Clinical improvement of chorea has been reported with valproic acid, haloperidol, tetrabenazine, clonidine, corticosteroids, anticoagulants, aspirin, and dopamine receptor antagonists.[20] IVIG and plasmapheresis have been beneficial in treating refractory chorea.[21]

Antiphospholipid syndrome (APL)

Antiphospholipid syndrome (APL) is typically defined by a hypercoagulable state leading to the presence of arterial, venous, or small vessel thrombosis. Symptoms are associated with persistently positive APL antibodies (aPL). aPL antibodies are a heterogeneous population of antibodies directed against phospholipid binding proteins, phospholipids, and other proteins.[22] More specifically, they consist of three separate antibodies including lupus anticoagulant (LA; directed against prothrombin and $\beta2$ glycoproteinI), anticardiolipin (aCL; directed against anti-$\beta2$ glycoproteinI), and anti-$\beta2$ glycoproteinI (anti-B2 GPI) antibodies. Binding to the $\beta2$ glycoproteinI has been suggested as the primary abnormality.[23] In females, the disorder is associated with spontaneous abortions and increased morbidity during pregnancy. Chorea is the most common movement disorder in APL, although its prevalence is only 1.3%.[24] Other neurological manifestations include migraine, epilepsy, myelopathy, and dementia.[25] Additional movement abnormalities have been associated with ischemic changes in various brain regions.[25]

Investigators have long noted overlapping neurological symptoms and immune findings in APL and SLE. Chorea in APL has a waxing and waning nature and does not appear to be associated with vessel thrombosis in the basal ganglia.[26] It has therefore been suggested that aPL antibodies bind to phospholipid rich areas in the basal ganglia leading to depolarization or neuronal injury. 18-FDG PET studies have shown increased uptake in the striatum contralateral to the side with involuntary movements.[27] Low and non-pathogenic titers of aPL are present in 1–5% of healthy individuals.[28] In animal models receiving either the passive transfer of aPL or immunization against the $\beta2$ glycoprotein, changes have been identified in motor behaviors and antineuronal antibody binding.[29–31] A genetic predisposition has been reported[32] and various environmental factors may trigger the appearance of antibodies.[22]

Therapeutically, individuals with recurrent arterio-thromboembolic events should be treated with anticoagulation therapy. Some authors have suggested discontinuing potential triggers, e.g., estroprogesterone therapy, and using anticoagulant therapy as the first step for treating chorea.[22,33] Others, in contrast, noting a lack of association between thrombosis and chorea do not recommend the use of anticoagulants.[34] Corticosteroids and dopamine receptor antagonists have been beneficial in treating patients with chorea.[25]

Hashimoto's Encephalopathy (HE)

Despite its initial description in 1966,[134] Hashimoto's encephalopathy remains an ill-defined disorder with some investigators suggesting the term "encephalopathy associated with auto-immune thyroid disease".[35] The disorder is characterized by the acute or subacute onset of seizures, myoclonus, ataxia, tremor, sleep, behavioral alterations, and an altered level of consciousness.[135] Relatively few cases have been described, most occurring in mid-adulthood, although about one-fifth (<40 cases) were present in childhood. HE is usually defined by the presence of thyroid peroxidase antibodies (anti-TPO), the aforementioned symptoms, and a therapeutic response to corticosteroids. The CSF is abnormal in most cases with an elevated protein and in some a lymphocytic pleocytosis and/or oligoclonal bands. Anti-TPO and thyroglobulin have been present in the CSF of some, but not all patients.[36] The majority are euthyroid at the time of diagnosis, despite having anti-TPO antibodies. The EEG is typically abnormal with a wide range of non-specific activity or focal spike and spike-wave discharges.[37] About one-half of adult cases have diffuse white matter changes and meningeal enhancement, although this is seen less commonly in children.[38]

Therapeutically, despite the required defining response to corticosteroids, the effect of treatment is variable. In 25 pediatric patients, mostly girls, only 55% had complete recovery.[39] Cases have responded to plasmapheresis, although a recent case report showed no correlation between the reduction in anti-TPO antibodies and clinical outcome.[40]

The pathophysiology of HE is poorly understood. Anti-TPO antibodies occur in about 10% of healthy children.[41] The reported binding of anti-TPO antibodies to cerebellar astrocytes expressing glial fibrillary acid protein[42] is considered controversial. In addition, investigators have raised the possibility of misdiagnoses, based on the co-presence of antibodies associated with other autoimmune encephalitis such as GABAb, LGI1, and NMDAR.[35] Other proposed mechanisms include a vascular, demyelinating, or immune-complex-mediated process. Autopsy studies in a small number of adults showed CNS lymphocytic infiltration.[43] As in other disorders, anti-TPO antibodies should be considered a marker of autoimmunity rather than the specific mechanism.

POST-STREPTOCOCCAL INFECTIONS

Sydenham's Chorea

Sydenham's chorea (SC) is the most common form of acute, isolated chorea in children. It is also one of the major criteria for the diagnosis of acute rheumatic fever. Pathophysiologically, it is often hypothesized that chorea arises from an alteration within the basal ganglia; more specifically an underactive indirect pathway.[44] Nevertheless, a recent study, using transcranial magnetic stimulation to evaluate motor cortex hyperexcitability, suggested a decrease in the excitability of the axons synapsing onto cortical motor neurons.[45,46]

SC is defined by the presence of generalized chorea (hemichorea in about 20–35%).[47,48] The usual age of onset of SC is 5–15 years with females > males, although some have developed chorea in their third decade of life. Symptoms of SC typically develop 4–8 weeks after an episode of group A beta-hemolytic streptococci (GABHS) pharyngitis and SC is present in about 10–20% of patients with rheumatic fever. Chorea is often predated by the appearance of neuropsychiatric symptoms including obsessive compulsive behaviors (20–70%), personality changes, emotional lability, distractibility, anxiety, age-regressed behaviors, and anorexia. Other clinical symptoms include motor impersistence (tongue darting, milkmaid, and pronator signs), hypometric saccades, reduced muscle tone, tics, grimacing, clumsiness, dysarthria, and weakness. Cardiac involvement, especially affecting the mitral valve, is present in 60–70%, and arthritis is less common (about 30%). Most symptoms resolve in 1–6 months, although persistent active chorea for more than 2 years has been reported in one-quarter to one-half of patients.[48] Recurrences occur in about one-third; triggers including GABHS or other infections, oral contraceptive agents, pregnancy, and unknown.

Laboratory studies assist in eliminating alternative causes of chorea, but do not confirm the diagnosis of SC. Throat cultures may identify a preceding GABHS infection, but cultures are positive in only a minority of cases. Acute-phase reactants (erythrocyte sedimentation rate and C-reactive protein) are usually normal in SC, since the interval between the GABHS infection and onset of chorea is relatively long. The percentage of patients with elevated antistreptococcal titers has ranged from about 15–80%.[47] Imaging is primarily recommended to rule out other causes of chorea. MRI studies are usually normal in SC, but have been shown to have basal ganglia enlargement and increased T2 intensity during the acute phase. Positron emission tomography and single-photon emission computed tomography have identified transient increases in basal ganglia metabolism. Electroencephalographic changes are seen in about 30–85% of patients, but are nonspecific.

The pathophysiological mechanism in SC is a GABHS-induced autoimmune disorder secondary to polyreactive antibodies against streptococci that also recognize neuronal extracellular surface or intracellular antigens. Through the process of molecular mimicry, clinical symptoms may be secondary to altered cell signaling, cellular toxicity, or other mechanisms. Evidence supporting an autoimmune etiology for SC includes a characteristic syndrome, a proven role for GABHS, and a beneficial effect of immune therapy. An immune mechanism is further supported by the finding of IgG reactivity to neuronal cytoplasm from human caudate and subthalamic nuclei that appeared to correlate with the severity and duration of clinical attacks.[49] Other investigators have proposed that anti-D1 and D2 receptor antibodies are the primary factors,[50–52] although cross reactive antibodies are also present against lysoganglioside-GM1,[53] and the cytoskeletal protein tubulin.[54] The presence of D2R antibodies have been confirmed in cell based assays: 10 of 30 SC patients showed reactivity to surface D2R long antigens transfected in HEK293 cells[55] and 4/4 had binding to FLAG epitope tagged D2R long antigen transfected in HEK293 cells. The mechanism causing neurological symptomatology is hypothesized to involve the alteration of neuronal cell signal transduction via calcium calmodulin dependent protein kinase II (CaMKII) activation.[53,56] In animal models, rats immunized with GABHS developed antibodies against D1 and D2 receptors and clinically showed compulsive-like behaviors[52] and passively transferred serum obtained from GABHS-immunized mice caused behavioral disturbances.[57]

Therapeutically, it is generally recommended that penicillin therapy be given, despite the fact that most patients do not have active GABHS infections. Several studies have suggested that valproate, pimozide, risperidone, haloperidol, tiapride, tetrabenazine, and carbamazepine may be effective for the symptomatic treatment of chorea. Selective serotonin reuptake inhibitors are effective for obsessive-compulsive behaviors, benzodiazepines are used for anxiety, and in some patients antidepressants are required. Once the patient has become symptom free for at least 1 month, consideration should be given to gradually reducing the dosage. Recognizing the autoimmune nature of SC, intravenous immunoglobulin (IVIG), plasma exchange, and oral prednisone have been used in small studies and shown to accelerate recovery.[58,59] The current recommendation is to reserve autoimmune therapies for patients with refractory chorea, i.e., have been unsuccessfully treated with other anti-chorea medications. The recommendation of the World Health Organization is the regular use of secondary prophylaxis with penicillin G benzathine (1.2 million units IM every 21 days). Allergic patients are treated with oral sulfur drugs, such as sulfadiazine, 500 mg every 6 h.

Pediatric Autoimmune Neuropsychiatric Disorder Associated with a Streptococcal Infection (PANDAS)

PANDAS, modeled upon Sydenham's chorea, is proposed to be a Group A β-hemolytic streptococcal induced autoimmune disorder. The formal diagnosis requires the affected individual to meet five specific criteria: prepubertal onset, obsessive compulsive disorder (OCD) and/or a tic disorder, the dramatic sudden explosive onset of symptoms, a relapsing and remitting course of symptoms that are temporally associated with GABHS infections, and the presence of other neuropsychiatric abnormalities (hyperactivity, emotional lability, anxiety, or piano-playing choreiform movements).[60] Historically, several reports, some published under the heading PITANDS (pediatric infection triggered autoimmune neuropsychiatric disorders), suggested that a variety of infectious agents could cause acute neuropsychiatric symptoms including *Borrelia burgdorferi*, herpes simplex virus, varicella zoster virus, human immunodeficiency virus, *Mycoplasma pneumoniae*, and the common cold. Nevertheless, because of a suggested link between OCD and Sydenham's chorea, the major diagnostic criterion for PANDAS remains its temporal association with GABHS.

The PANDAS hypothesis remains controversial on both clinical grounds and the failure to confirm an immune process. Clinically, there are many concerns about its defining features and proposed criteria.[61] In many individuals the diagnosis is based on incomplete criteria,[62,63] family histories are similar to individuals with standard tic disorders,[64] neuropsychological functioning is similar to subjects without an infectious background,[65] and missed diagnoses are likely.[66] The essence of PANDAS is its hypothesized temporal association between the onset and exacerbation of tic or OCD symptoms and a GABHS infection. Correlation of the initial episode of symptoms with GABHS may be difficult, especially if similar to SC, the appearance may lag behind the inciting infection by many months. In contrast to the initial event, however, recurrences of symptoms should occur within several weeks of a new infection. Problematic laboratory support for an association with GABHS has included the use of single-point-in-time assessments of anti-streptococcal antibodies, conflicting data as to whether children with OCD, tic disorder, or TS were more likely to have had a streptococcal infection in the 3 months or year prior to the onset of neuropsychiatric symptoms,[67–70] and findings in two longitudinal studies showing that there was little association between clinical exacerbations and a new GABHS infection.[71,72] Further in the original PANDAS cohort, no individual had "overt chorea," but all except one had choreiform movements and 50% had "marked choreiform" movements. Some investigators have responded to the aforementioned by suggesting that the proper diagnosis was likely Sydenham's chorea; a possibility enhanced by the finding of overlapping biomarkers for SC in children with PANDAS having choreiform movements.[50–53]

Ongoing attempts to confirm an immune-mediated process as the underlying mechanism in PANDAS have been equivocal depending on the study group. Serum antibody reactivity in children against antigens at 60, 45, and 40 kDa in postmortem basal ganglia (later defined as pyruvate kinase M1, neuron-specific and non-neuronal enolase, and aldolase C) have been reported,[73,74] but could not be duplicated.[75] No correlation was identified between exacerbation of symptoms and changes in anti-neuronal antibodies against caudate, putamen, or frontal cortex (BA 10),[76] and the results of immunofluorescent histochemical studies on brain tissues have been variable.[77,78] Several reports have suggested that individuals with PANDAS possessing choreiform ("piano-playing") movements have similar anti-neuronal antibodies to those identified in SC, including anti-D1R, anti-D2R,[50,53] and anti-lysoganglioside-GM1,[79] as well as antibodies that activate CaMKII activity.[53,56,79] Nevertheless, antibody binding to transfected D1 and D2 receptors in PANDAS has been variable depending on the cell line and clinical presence of choreiform movements.[50,55] Further, binding was not increased in differentiated SH-SY5Y cells.[80] Several longitudinal studies in children with PANDAS-chronic tics and OCD have failed to identify a temporal association between symptom exacerbation and an elevation of anti-D1R, anti-D2R, anti-lysoganglioside-GM1, or anti-tubulin antibodies.[81,82] In addition, when data from this cohort was compared to a combined control population from four institutions ($n=70$) and to a published ($n=15$) group, there were no significant differences for antibody titers against D2R and tubulin. For anti-lysoganglioside-GM1 and D1R measurements, values differed from a small published control group, but not from the larger multi-institutional controls.[82] In two cell based assays, no binding was identified to surface D2R long antigens transfected in HEK293 cells.[50,55]

In order to circumvent the issue of "associated with streptococci", authors have proposed terms such as CANS (children with acute neuropsychiatric symptoms)[61] or PANS (pediatric autoimmune neuropsychiatric symptoms).[83] In the latter, the presence of tics has been de-emphasized. A comprehensive investigation should be performed to identify the proper diagnosis in children presenting with CANS/PANS/PANDAS. A small treatment study for PANDAS showed IVIG therapy improved OCD symptoms, but not tics, and plasma exchange improved both.[84] Standard symptomatic therapy is recommended for treating tics and OCD symptoms; whereas prophylactic antibiotics and immunotherapy remain unproven.

Post-streptococcal Acute Disseminated Encephalomyelitis and Others

Ten children (mean age 4.2 years) have been reported with a post streptococcal acute disseminated encephalomyelitis (PSADEM).[85] Symptoms occurred a mean of 18 days following the infection, and consisted of behavioral disturbances (emotional lability, inappropriate laughter, somnolence, and coma) and an extrapyramidal movement disorder (dystonic posturing, axial and limb rigidity, and tremor). Basal ganglia T2 hyperintense lesions were identified in 9/10 patients (caudate 50%, putamen 60%, and globus pallidus 40%) and/or the thalamus (60%). In contrast, basal ganglia lesions were only apparent in 18% of ADEM controls. Clinical improvement was rapid and eight children made a complete recovery. Antibasal ganglia antibody assays against human basal ganglia included ELISA (elevated serum IgG antibodies), Western immunoblotting (showed reactivity to three dominant bands at 60, 67, and 80 kDa), and immunohistochemistry (demonstrated specific binding to large striatal neurons). Antibodies to similar proteins were not demonstrated in patients with PANDAS and chronic tics and OCD.[75,76]

Two children have been reported with a post-streptococcal dystonia associated with isolated bilateral striatal necrosis. Both individuals had reactive antibodies against basal ganglia constituents at 40 kDa.[86] In another child, a post-streptococcal etiology was proposed for frequent, brief episodes of paroxysmal dystonic choreoathetosis. The MRI was normal and antibodies were present against basal ganglia antigens at 80 and 95 kDa.[87] Lastly, 20 patients have been reported with a post pharyngitis encephalitis lethargica like-syndrome (sleep disorder, basal ganglia signs, and neuropsychiatric sequelae). MRIs were abnormal in about 40%, ASO titers were elevated in 65%, and antibodies were reactive against basal ganglia antigens at 40, 45, 60, and 98 kDa.[88] In a subsequent manuscript, 10/20 of these affected individuals were shown to have NMDAR antibodies, indicating that they had NMDAR encephalitis.[89] Additional studies on non-NMDA positive patients with an encephalitis lethargica like-syndrome are presented in the next section.

AUTOIMMUNE BASAL GANGLIA ENCEPHALITIS

Movement disorders associated with encephalitis can be the direct result of inflammation or in some cases secondary to a subsequent autoimmune process. For example, infection-related movement disorders have been reported after a variety of infections including enterovirus, Epstein-Barr virus, Mycoplasma pneumonia, and Japanese B encephalitis. In contrast, investigators have proposed a diagnosis of "autoimmune basal ganglia encephalitis (BGE)" for a group of patients with an encephalitis lethargica like-syndrome, but lacking NMDAR antibodies.[5,55] More specifically, 17 patients (9 males/8 females) were clinically characterized by the presence of extrapyramidal movement disorders, sleep disturbances (hypersomnolence, sleep-wake cycle alterations), dysautonomia, and a neuropsychiatric sequelae following an infectious prodrome (EBV, respiratory viruses).[5,55] Movement abnormalities included dystonia ($n = 10$), parkinsonism, namely, bradykinesia/akinesia, rigidity, and a resting tremor ($n = 7$), chorea ($n = 4$), tics and ocular flutter ($n = 1$ each). Eight patients had T2 hyperintense lesions in the basal ganglia, seven EEG compatible with encephalitis, and six CSF pleocytosis. In the majority, the disorder was monophasic, and three cases relapsed. In 12/17 patients, serum D2 receptor (D2R) antibodies were detected using a cell-based assay expressing D2R at the cell surface. In contrast, antibodies were absent against surface D1R, D3R, D5R, and the dopamine transporter.[55] Recovery was hastened by the use of intravenous steroids and IVIG. A high rate of motor fluctuations and dyskinesias was noted in association with prescribed dopaminergic therapy for parkinsonian symptoms. In conclusion, D2R antibodies may prove to be an important diagnostic biomarker. In a subsequent comparison of movement disorder phenomenology in BGE, NMDAR encephalitis, and SC, the BGE group was characterized by more frequent akinesia and tremor and the absence of stereotypies or perseveration.[90]

AUTOIMMUNE ENCEPHALOPATHIES

Historically, prior to 2005, the only cell-surface antibodies associated with limbic encephalitis were believed to be the Kv1.1 and Kv1.2 subunits of the voltage-gated potassium channels (VGKC). After much controversy, these were later shown to be associated with the leucine-rich glioma inactivated 1 (LGI1) and contactin-associated protein-like 2 (Caspr 2) antigens. Clearly, however, the major breakthrough came with the identification of antibodies to the N-methyl-D-aspartate receptor (NMDAR) in adults with encephalitis, who responded to immunotherapy, and had associated tumors.[91] Subsequent to this time, the field has dramatically expanded and the list of antibodies targeting cell surface receptors or synaptic proteins involved with synaptic neurotransmission and plasticity is rapidly growing (see Table 18.2). In contrast to intracellular antigens, extracellular antibodies are directed against conformational epitopes and reactivity is lost when the antigen is denatured. Hence, the detection of antibodies targeting cell surface antigens requires either the use of live neuronal cultures, immunohistochemical protocols using cell surface antigens, or cell-based arrays, in which recombinant antigens are expressed in mammalian cells.[92] In the remainder of this section, the focus will be on those disorders reported in children and associated with movement abnormalities.

Anti-N-methyl-D-aspartate (NMDA) Receptor Encephalitis

Anti-NMDA receptor encephalitis is now considered one of the most common immune mediated encephalitides. Anti-NMDAR antibodies target the NR1 subunit of the receptor, primarily the N-terminus. Antibody binding causes receptor internalization and diminished synaptic NMDAR-mediated currents.[93,94] Ovarian teratomas can express neuronal tissues thereby providing immunologic cross reactivity. In cases following a viral infection, antibody synthesis may occur via molecular mimicry, with expansion of the process in the CNS.[5]

Initially characterized in young women with ovarian teratomas, anti-NMDAR encephalitis has been shown to occur in all age groups and to be associated with infection in younger children. The typical presentation includes psychiatric symptoms (changes in mood, behavior, personality, hallucinations, agitation, insomnia, mutism) followed by seizures, fever, altered consciousness, dyskinesias, catatonia, autonomic instability, hypoventilation, and coma (Video 18.1).

TABLE 18.2   Antibodies Targeting Extracellular Receptors or Other Cell Surface Proteins

Antigen	Clinical symptoms	Tumor
NMDAR	Anti-NMDA encephalitis	
	Children < 12 years: Seizures, abnormal movements, autonomic symptoms	usually none
	Adults: Psychiatric symptoms, seizures, fever, altered consciousness, dyskinesias, catatonia, autonomic instability, hypoventilation, and coma	ovarian teratoma/ testicular tumor
LGI1	Rare in childhood: Limbic encephalitis, faciobrachial dystonic seizures, myoclonus, chorea, sleep disorders	<10% thymoma
Caspr2	*Adults*: Encephalitis, neuromyotonia, Morvan's syndrome	thymoma 20–40%
GlyR	*Children*: PERM-like symptoms, stiff person	infrequent, lung,
	Adults: Stiff person, PERM, limbic encephalitis, CB degen, optic neuritis	lymphoma, thymoma
D2R	*Children*: Basal ganglia encephalitis; movement disorders, sleep disturbances, dysautonomia, and neuropsychiatric sequelae	none
AMPAR	*Adults*: limbic encephalitis, atypical psychosis	70%, small cell lung/ breast cancer
GABAbR	*Adults*: limbic encephalitis, prominent seizures	50%; small cell lung
GABAaR	Refractory seizures, status epilepticus, epilepsy partialis continuans, stiff person, opsoclonus	infrequent
mGluR5	*Teens and adults*: Ophelia syndrome—psychiatric symptoms, cognitive and memory impairments	Hodgkin lymphoma
DPPX	*Adults*: Encephalitis, agitation, myoclonus, seizures, tremor, PERM-like symptoms, ataxia, hyperekplexia, nystagmus	none

Abbreviations: N-methyl-D-aspartate receptor (NMDAR); leucine-rich glioma inactivated 1 (LGI1); contactin-associated protein-related 2 (Caspr 2); glycine receptor (GlyR); dopamine 2 receptor (D2R); α-amino-3-hydroxy-5 methyl-4 isoxazolepropionic acid receptor (AMPAR); γ-aminobutyric acid receptors (GABAaR and GABAbR); metabotropic glutamate receptor 5 (mGluR5), dipeptyl-peptidase-like protein-6 (DPPX); progressive encephalomyelitis with rigidity and myoclonus (PERM.).

Initial symptoms in children less than 12 years tend to be seizures, abnormal movements, and autonomic symptoms whereas in individuals greater than 18 years, psychosis is predominant. Typical movements in children may include chorea, dystonia, myorhythmia (slow rest and postural movements), orolingual dyskinesia, or stereotypic movements (cycling, picking, self-injurious behaviors), with some displaying multiple and mixed abnormal movements.[5,95] The presence of stereotypies and perseverations were the major factors distinguishing NMDAR encephalitis from SC and BGE.[90] Children may also have a stormy generalized hyperkinetic movement disorder with agitation, muscle rigidity, rhythmic abdominal contractions, kicking movements, and intermittent dystonic or opistotonic posturing.[5,96] In adults, movements involving the face and body such as orobuccolingual movements including jaw opening and closing, facial grimacing, tongue protrusion, kissing, pouting, and frowning were present in about 80% of cases.[93,97,98]

The most common alteration on brain MRI, occurring in only about one-half of patients, is a mild T2/FLAIR signal hyperintensity in various brain regions.[91] A case with reversible caudate MRI and PET abnormalities has been reported.[99] EEGs are usually slow and disorganized.[100] The CSF may show pleocytosis, elevated protein levels, and in some positive oligoclonal bands. Individuals should be screened for the presence of tumors: ovarian teratomas are common in adult women, present in about one-third of teenage girls, and infrequent in those younger than age 14. Testicular tumors have been reported in adult males but are infrequent in boys.[34] Screening for anti-NMDAR antibodies should include CSF, since serum cell-based assays may be falsely negative. Several studies have reported the presence of anti-NMDAR antibodies in patients who developed movement disorders weeks after the diagnosis of herpes simplex encephalitis.[101–103] These findings confirm the hypothesis that certain viral infections can trigger brain autoimmunity.

Most patients with anti-NMDAR encephalitis have full or substantial neurological recovery. Factors for a good outcome include early initiation of therapy, low disease severity within 4 weeks of onset, and the absence of an intensive care unit admission.[104] Treatment consists of tumor removal, if present, and immunotherapy (corticosteroids, IVIG, or plasmapheresis). Individuals refractory to these treatments have responded to rituximab or cyclophosphamide. CSF levels of the B-cell attracting C-X-C motif chemokine 13 (CXCL13) may be a potential biomarker of treatment response and outcome.[105] Symptoms may relapse in up to one-quarter of patients, especially in those without a tumor or in those who received suboptimal treatment. Symptomatic treatment has been used for movement disorders and psychiatric symptoms.[106,107]

Antibodies to LGI1, Caspr2, GABAaR, and GABAbR

For several years, voltage-gated potassium channel (VGKC) antibodies were considered the abnormality in non-paraneoplastic limbic encephalitis, neuromyotonia, and Morvan's syndrome. Subsequently, however, it was identified that the two specific targets of these antibodies (Kv1.1 and Kv1.2) were actually leucine-rich glioma inactivated 1 (LGI1) and contactin-associated protein-related 2 (Caspr 2).[108] The identification of these antigens has clarified, in part, the diversity of symptoms previously attributed to VGKC. Antibodies to LGI1 cause limbic encephalitis, hyponatremia, and facio-brachial dystonic seizures.[109] Facio-brachial dystonic seizures consist of unilateral upper limb jerking and ipsilateral facial grimacing, the absence of an cortical electrographic correlate, poor response to anticonvulsants, but rapid improvement with corticosteroids.[110] Whether the movements are actually epileptic in origin is controversial.[111] LGI1 is typically non-paraneoplastic and highly responsive to corticosteroid therapy. Movement disorders are uncommon but have included chorea, parkinsonism, and tremor.[112,113] A steroid-responsive, isolated case of chorea associated with LGI1 has been reported.[114] Antibodies to CASPR2 cause Morvan's syndrome, characterized by symptoms of encephalitis (amnesia, hallucinations, sleep and autonomic dysregulation) and neuromyotonia.

The GABAa receptor is a ligand-gated ion channel that modulates fast inhibitory synaptic transmission in the brain. High serum and CSF titers of antibodies against the GABAaR have been identified in patients with a severe form of encephalitis with seizures and refractory status.[115] The complexity of autoimmune encephalopathies is highlighted by the coexistence of GABAaR and LGI1 antibodies in an adult with autoimmune encephalitis and thymoma.[116] The GABAb receptor is a G-protein-coupled receptor. In two series of more than 35 adult patients with GABAbR antibodies, the most common symptoms were limbic encephalitis, seizures, ataxia, and opsoclonus myoclonus.[117,118] About one-half of the cases were paraneoplastic in origin, with small cell lung cancer being the most commonly identified neoplasm. In possibly the first pediatric case, a 3-year-old previously healthy child, presented with a 1-day history of confusion and lethargy.[119] His initial examination showed opsoclonus, dystonic movements of the tongue, ataxia and chorea of the limbs and trunk. Within 24h, he developed frequent partial seizures, CSF showed a lymphocytic pleocytosis, and there were ultimately T2 hyperintensities in the basal ganglia. There was little response to treatment with high-dose corticosteroids/IVIG and the patient died 4 weeks after initial presentation.

Progressive Encephalomyelitis with Rigidity and Myoclonus (PERM)

Progressive encephalomyelitis with rigidity and myoclonus (PERM) results from an immune-related dysfunction of the brainstem and spinal cord. One underlying abnormality is the presence of antibodies targeting the α1-subunit of the glycine receptor (GlyR).[120,121] Most patients do not have associated tumors. In a retrospective study, the median age was 50 years, but four individuals were younger than 15 years.[122] Individuals were differentiated from the stiff person syndrome (associated with GAD65 antibodies, see Video 18.2) by the presence of encephalopathy, brainstem dysfunction, cranial neuropathies, and autonomic dysregulation. Hyperekplexia was a common finding. In the first pediatric case, 5 days after a cold, a 14-month-old developed startle-induced episodes of generalized rigidity and myoclonus, axial hyperextension, and trismus without loss of consciousness.[123] Imaging and CSF were normal and GlyR alpha 1 antibodies were found in serum and CSF. The specificity of anti-GlyR has been questioned and in some patients antibodies overlap with GAD65.[124,125] Another neuronal cell-surface autoantigen associated with PERM is dipeptyl-peptidase-like protein-6 (DPPX). DPPX is a cell surface auxillary subunit of the Kv4.2 Shal potassium channel family. In three cases with PERM, ages 16, 26, and 27 years, all had prominent hyperekplexia, cerebellar-ocular movement abnormalities, ataxia, muscle stiffness and spasms.[126] CSF showed a mild pleocytosis, MRI was normal, DPPX titers were detected in serum and CSF, and response to immunotherapy was good.

OTHER PARANEOPLASTIC SYNDROMES

Paraneoplastic syndromes represent a remote effect of cancer that is not related to metastases, cancer treatment, infection, or nutritional problems. Overall, these syndromes are uncommon, occur more frequently in adulthood, and develop before the underlying tumor is recognized.[34,127] Tumors commonly involved in paraneoplastic syndromes contain neuronal tissue (teratoma), express neuroendocrine proteins (neuroblastoma, small cell lung cancer), or have immunoregulatory properties (thymoma). In the past, more classical paraneoplastic syndromes were associated with a variety of intracellular onconeuronal antigens including Hu, CRMP5, Ri, Yo, Ma2, and amphiphysin. More recently, however, as described above, paraneoplastic syndromes can also include antibodies targeting extracellular receptors or other cell surface proteins. In general, intracellular antibodies provide valuable biomarkers for the identification of an underlying tumor, but, in contrast to extracellular targeted antibodies, are usually not pathogenic.

Opsoclonus Myoclonus Syndrome (OMS)

In children, the major paraneoplastic syndrome associated with a movement abnormality is the opsoclonus myoclonus syndrome (aka Kinsbourne syndrome). Clinical symptoms include opsoclonus, diffuse myoclonus often misdiagnosed as cerebellar ataxia, speech problems, drooling, hypotonia, and sleep disturbances.[128] When paraneoplastic, OMS is associated with an occult neuroblastoma; found in as many as 50% of children with OMS.[127] In children with neuroblastoma, immunotherapies are useful, although the best treatment remains unknown. Although symptoms improve following therapy with ACTH, steroids or IVIG, residual behavioral, language, and cognitive problems are common.[129,130] Support for a possible cerebellar cognitive affective syndrome[131] is derived from imaging studies showing that the cerebellar vermis and flocculonodular lobes are preferentially affected.[132] Several intracellular and surface protein antibodies have been identified that bind to and damage cerebellar Purkinje and granule cells, but their specificity is unclear.[133] A role for B-cell involvement has been postulated.[127]

References

1. Goodnow CC. Multistep pathogenesis of autoimmune disease. *Cell*. 2007;130(1):25–35.
2. Hickey WF. Basic principles of immunological surveillance of the normal central nervous system. *Glia*. 2001;36(2):118–124.
3. Knopf PM, Harling-Berg CJ, Cserr HF, et al. Antigen-dependent intrathecal antibody synthesis in the normal rat brain: tissue entry and local retention of antigen-specific B cells. *J Immunol*. 1998;161(2):692–701.
4. Neuwelt EA, Bauer B, Fahlke C, et al. Engaging neuroscience to advance translational research in brain barrier biology. *Nat Rev Neurosci*. 2011;12(3):169–182.
5. Mohammad SS, Ramanathan S, Brilot F, Dale RC. Autoantibody-associated movement disorders. *Neuropediatrics*. 2013;44(6):336–345.
6. Martino D, Dale RC, Gilbert DL, Giovannoni G, Leckman JF. Immunopathogenic mechanisms in Tourette syndrome: A critical review. *Mov Disord*. 2009;24(9):1267–1279.
7. Petri M, Purvey S, Fang H, Magder LS. Predictors of organ damage in systemic lupus erythematosus: the Hopkins Lupus Cohort. *Arthritis Rheum*. 2012;64(12):4021–4028.
8. Nordal EB, Nielsen J, Marhaug G. Chorea in juvenile primary antiphospholipid syndrome. Reversible decreased circulation in the basal ganglia visualised by single photon emission computed tomography. *Scand J Rheumatol*. 1999;28(5):324–327.
9. Tan EK, Chan LL, Auchus AP. Reversible parkinsonism in systemic lupus erythematosus. *J Neurol Sci*. 2001;193(1):53–57.
10. Joseph FG, Lammie GA, Scolding NJ. CNS lupus: a study of 41 patients. *Neurology*. 2007;69(7):644–654.
11. Robert M, Sunitha R, Thulaseedharan NK. Neuropsychiatric manifestations systemic lupus erythematosus: a study from South India. *Neurology India*. 2006;54(1):75–77.
12. Jankovic J, Patten BM. Blepharospasm and autoimmune diseases. *Mov Disord*. 1987;2(3):159–163.
13. Munhoz RP, Fameli H, Teive HA. Stiff person syndrome as the initial manifestation of systemic lupus erythematosus. *Mov Disord*. 2010;25(4):516–517.

14. Fekete R, Jankovic J. Childhood stiff-person syndrome improved with rituximab. *Case reports in neurology.* 2012;4(2):92–96.
15. Baizabal-Carvallo JF, Jankovic J. Stiff-person syndrome: insights into a complex autoimmune disorder. *J Neurol Neurosurg Psychiatry.* 2014
16. Rajagopalan N, Humphrey PR, Bucknall RC. Torticollis and blepharospasm in systemic lupus erythematosus. *Mov Disord.* 1989;4(4):345–348.
17. von Scheven E, Athreya BH, Rose CD, Goldsmith DP, Morton L. Clinical characteristics of antiphospholipid antibody syndrome in children. *J Pediatr.* 1996;129(3):339–345.
18. Galanaud D, Dormont D, Marsault C, Wechsler B, Piette JC. Brain MRI in patients with past lupus-associated chorea. *Stroke.* 2000;31(12):3079–3083.
19. Krakauer M, Law I. FDG PET brain imaging in neuropsychiatric systemic lupus erythematosis with choreic symptoms. *Clin Nucl Med.* 2009;34(2):122–123.
20. Baizabal-Carvallo JF, Jankovic J. Movement disorders in autoimmune diseases. *Mov Disord.* 2012;27(8):935–946.
21. Lazurova I, Macejova Z, Benhatchi K, et al. Efficacy of intravenous immunoglobulin treatment in lupus erythematosus chorea. *Clin Rheumatol.* 2007;26(12):2145–2147.
22. Peluso S, Antenora A, De Rosa A, et al. Antiphospholipid-related chorea. *Front Neurol.* 2012;3:150.
23. Meroni PL, Borghi MO, Raschi E, Tedesco F. Pathogenesis of antiphospholipid syndrome: understanding the antibodies. *Nat Rev Rheumatol.* 2011;7(6):330–339.
24. Abreu MM, Danowski A, Wahl DG, et al. The relevance of "non-criteria" clinical manifestations of antiphospholipid syndrome: 14th International Congress on Antiphospholipid Antibodies Technical Task Force Report on Antiphospholipid Syndrome Clinical Features. *Autoimmun Rev.* 2015.
25. Baizabal-Carvallo JF, Bonnet C, Jankovic J. Movement disorders in systemic lupus erythematosus and the antiphospholipid syndrome. *J Neural Transm.* 2013;120(11):1579–1589.
26. Orzechowski NM, Wolanskyj AP, Ahlskog JE, Kumar N, Moder KG. Antiphospholipid antibody-associated chorea. *J Rheumatol.* 2008;35(11):2165–2170.
27. Wu RM, Shan DE, Sun CM, et al. Clinical, 18F-dopa PET, and genetic analysis of an ethnic Chinese kindred with early-onset parkinsonism and parkin gene mutations. *Mov Disord.* 2002;17(4):670–675.
28. Petri M. Epidemiology of the antiphospholipid antibody syndrome. *J Autoimmun.* 2000;15(2):145–151.
29. Shoenfeld Y. Systemic antiphospholipid syndrome. *Lupus.* 2003;12(7):497–498.
30. Katzav A, Pick CG, Korczyn AD, et al. Hyperactivity in a mouse model of the antiphospholipid syndrome. *Lupus.* 2001;10(7):496–499.
31. Tanne D, Katzav A, Beilin O, et al. Interaction of inflammation, thrombosis, aspirin and enoxaparin in CNS experimental antiphospholipid syndrome. *Neurobiol Dis.* 2008;30(1):56–64.
32. Domenico Sebastiani G, Minisola G, Galeazzi M. HLA class II alleles and genetic predisposition to the antiphospholipid syndrome. *Autoimmun Rev.* 2003;2(6):387–394.
33. Reiner P, Galanaud D, Leroux G, et al. Long-term outcome of 32 patients with chorea and systemic lupus erythematosus or antiphospholipid antibodies. *Mov Disord.* 2011;26(13):2422–2427.
34. Panzer J, Dalmau J. Movement disorders in paraneoplastic and autoimmune disease. *Curr Opin Neurol.* 2011;24(4):346–353.
35. Shaw PJ, Walls TJ, Newman PK, Cleland PG, Cartlidge NE. Hashimoto's encephalopathy: a steroid-responsive disorder associated with high anti-thyroid antibody titers--report of 5 cases. *Neurology.* 1991;41(2 (Pt 1)):228–233.
36. Rodriguez AJ, Jicha GA, Steeves TD, Benarroch EE, Westmoreland BF. EEG changes in a patient with steroid-responsive encephalopathy associated with antibodies to thyroperoxidase (SREAT, Hashimoto's encephalopathy). *J Clin Neurophysiol.* 2006;23(4):371–373.
37. Nguyen TP, El-Hakam LM. Clinical reasoning: a 9-year-old girl with seizures and encephalopathy. *Neurology.* 2010;74(22):e97–e100.
38. Alink J, de Vries TW. Unexplained seizures, confusion or hallucinations: think Hashimoto encephalopathy. *Acta Paediatr.* 2008;97(4):451–453.
39. Cook MK, Malkin M, Karafin MS. The use of plasma exchange in Hashimoto's encephalopathy: A case report and review of the literature. *J Clin Apher.* 2014
40. Zois C, Stavrou I, Kalogera C, et al. High prevalence of autoimmune thyroiditis in schoolchildren after elimination of iodine deficiency in northwestern Greece. *Thyroid.* 2003;13(5):485–489.

41. Blanchin S, Coffin C, Viader F, et al. Anti-thyroperoxidase antibodies from patients with Hashimoto's encephalopathy bind to cerebellar astrocytes. *J Neuroimmunol*. 2007;192(1-2):13–20.

42. Armangue T, Petit-Pedrol M, Dalmau J. Autoimmune encephalitis in children. *J Child Neurol*. 2012;27(11):1460–1469.

43. Paulus W, Nolte KW. Neuropathology of Hashimoto's encephalopathy. *J Neurol Neurosurg Psychiatry*. 2003;74(7):1009. author reply 1009.

44. DeLong MR. Primate models of movement disorders of basal ganglia origin. *Trends Neurosci*. 1990;13(7):281–285.

45. Khedr EM, Ahmed MA, Ali AM, Badry R, Rothwell JC. Changes in motor cortical excitability in patients with Sydenham's chorea. *Mov Disord*. 2015;30(2):259–262.

46. Hallett M, Obeso J. Where does chorea come from? Cortical excitability findings challenge classic pathophysiological concepts. *Mov Disord*. 2015;30(2):169–170.

47. Oosterveer DM, Overweg-Plandsoen WC, Roos RA. Sydenham's chorea: a practical overview of the current literature. *Pediatr Neurol*. 2010;43(1):1–6.

48. Cardoso F. Sydenham's chorea *Handb Clin Neurol*, Vol. 100. Amsterdam, The Netherlands: Elsevier B.V; 2011.

49. Husby G, van de Rijn I, Zabriskie JB, Abdin ZH, Williams Jr. RC. Antibodies reacting with cytoplasm of subthalamic and caudate nuclei neurons in chorea and acute rheumatic fever. *J Exp Med*. 1976;144(4):1094–1110.

50. Cox CJ, Sharma M, Leckman JF, et al. Brain Human Monoclonal Autoantibody from Sydenham Chorea Targets Dopaminergic Neurons in Transgenic Mice and Signals Dopamine D2 Receptor: Implications in Human Disease. *The Journal of Immunology*. 2013;191(11):5524–5541.

51. Ben-Pazi H, Stoner JA, Cunningham MW. Dopamine Receptor Autoantibodies Correlate with Symptoms in Sydenham's Chorea. *PLoS One*. 2013;8(9):e73516.

52. Brimberg L, Benhar I, Mascaro-Blanco A, et al. Behavioral, pharmacological, and immunological abnormalities after streptococcal exposure: a novel rat model of sydenham chorea and related neuropsychiatric disorders. *Neuropsychopharmacology*. 2012;37(9):2076–2087.

53. Kirvan CA, Swedo SE, Heuser JS, Cunningham MW. Mimicry and autoantibody-mediated neuronal cell signaling in Sydenham chorea. *Nat Med*. 2003;9(7):914–920.

54. Kirvan CA, Cox CJ, Swedo SE, Cunningham MW. Tubulin is a neuronal target of autoantibodies in Sydenham's chorea. *J Immunol*. 2007;178(11):7412–7421.

55. Dale RC, Merheb V, Pillai S, et al. Antibodies to surface dopamine-2 receptor in autoimmune movement and psychiatric disorders. *Brain*. 2012:aws256.

56. Kirvan CA, Swedo SE, Kurahara D, Cunningham MW. Streptococcal mimicry and antibody-mediated cell signaling in the pathogenesis of Sydenham's chorea. *Autoimmunity*. 2006;39(1):21–29.

57. Yaddanapudi K, Hornig M, Serge R, et al. Passive transfer of streptococcus-induced antibodies reproduces behavioral disturbances in a mouse model of pediatric autoimmune neuropsychiatric disorders associated with streptococcal infection. *Mol Psychiatry*. 2010;15(7):712–726.

58. Walker K, Brink A, Lawrenson J, Mathiassen W, Wilmshurst JM. Treatment of sydenham chorea with intravenous immunoglobulin. *J Child Neurol*. 2012;27(2):147–155.

59. Fusco C, Ucchino V, Frattini D, Pisani F, Della Giustina E. Acute and chronic corticosteroid treatment of ten patients with paralytic form of Sydenham's chorea. *Eur J Paediatr Neurol*. 2012;16(4):373–378.

60. Swedo SE, Leonard HL, Garvey M, et al. Pediatric autoimmune neuropsychiatric disorders associated with streptococcal infections: clinical description of the first 50 cases. *Am J Psychiatry*. 1998;155(2):264–271.

61. Singer HS, Gilbert DL, Wolf DS, Mink JW, Kurlan R. Moving from PANDAS to CANS. *J Pediatr*. 2012;160(5):725–731.

62. Gabbay V, Coffey BJ, Babb JS, et al. Pediatric autoimmune neuropsychiatric disorders associated with streptococcus: comparison of diagnosis and treatment in the community and at a specialty clinic. *Pediatrics*. 2008;122(2):273–278.

63. Shet A, Kaplan EL. Clinical use and interpretation of group A streptococcal antibody tests: a practical approach for the pediatrician or primary care physician. *Pediatr Infect Dis J*. 2002;21(5):420–426.

64. Lougee L, Perlmutter SJ, Nicolson R, Garvey MA, Swedo SE. Psychiatric disorders in first-degree relatives of children with pediatric autoimmune neuropsychiatric disorders associated with streptococcal infections (PANDAS). *J Am Acad Child Adolesc Psychiatry*. 2000;39(9):1120–1126.

65. Hirschtritt ME, Hammond CJ, Luckenbaugh D, et al. Executive and Attention Functioning Among Children in the PANDAS Subgroup. *Child Neuropsychol*. 2008:1–16.

V. SELECTED SECONDARY MOVEMENT DISORDERS

66. Kurlan R. The PANDAS hypothesis: losing its bite? *Mov Disord.* 2004;19(4):371–374.
67. Mell LK, Davis RL, Owens D. Association between streptococcal infection and obsessive-compulsive disorder, Tourette's syndrome, and tic disorder. *Pediatrics.* 2005;116(1):56–60.
68. Schrag A, Gilbert R, Giovannoni G, Robertson MM, Metcalfe C, Ben-Shlomo Y. Streptococcal infection, Tourette syndrome, and OCD: is there a connection? *Neurology.* 2009;73(16):1256–1263.
69. Perrin EM, Murphy ML, Casey JR, et al. Does group A beta-hemolytic streptococcal infection increase risk for behavioral and neuropsychiatric symptoms in children? *Arch Pediatr Adolesc Med.* 2004;158(9):848–856.
70. Leslie DL, Kozma L, Martin A, et al. Neuropsychiatric disorders associated with streptococcal infection: a case-control study among privately insured children. *J Am Acad Child Adolesc Psychiatry.* 2008;47(10):1166–1172.
71. Kurlan R, Johnson D, Kaplan EL, Group TSS Streptococcal infection and exacerbations of childhood tics and obsessive-compulsive symptoms: a prospective blinded cohort study. *Pediatrics.* 2008;121(6):1188–1197.
72. Leckman JF, King RA, Gilbert DL, et al. *J Am Acad Child Adolesc Psychiatry.* 2011
73. Dale RC, Candler PM, Church AJ, Wait R, Pocock JM, Giovannoni G. Neuronal surface glycolytic enzymes are autoantigen targets in post-streptococcal autoimmune CNS disease. *J Neuroimmunol.* 2005;172(1-2):187–197.
74. Church AJ, Dale RC, Lees AJ, Giovannoni G, Robertson MM. Tourette's syndrome: a cross sectional study to examine the PANDAS hypothesis. *J Neurol Neurosurg Psychiatry.* 2003;74(5):602–607.
75. Singer HS, Hong JJ, Yoon DY, Williams PN. Serum autoantibodies do not differentiate PANDAS and Tourette syndrome from controls. *Neurology.* 2005;65:1701–1707.
76. Singer HS, Gause C, Morris C, Lopez P. Serial immune markers do not correlate with clinical exacerbations in pediatric autoimmune neuropsychiatric disorders associated with streptococcal infections. *Pediatrics.* 2008;121(6):1198–1205.
77. Pavone P, Bianchini R, Parano E, et al. Anti-brain antibodies in PANDAS versus uncomplicated streptococcal infection. *Pediatr Neurol.* 2004;30(2):107–110.
78. Morris CM, Pardo-Villamizar C, Gause CD, Singer HS. Serum autoantibodies measured by immunofluorescence confirm a failure to differentiate PANDAS and Tourette syndrome from controls. *J Neurol Sci.* 2009;276:45–48.
79. Kirvan CA, Swedo SE, Snider LA, Cunningham MW. Antibody-mediated neuronal cell signaling in behavior and movement disorders. *J Neuroimmunol.* 2006;179(1-2):173–179.
80. Brilot F, Merheb V, Ding A, Murphy T, Dale RC. Antibody binding to neuronal surface in Sydenham chorea, but not in PANDAS or Tourette syndrome. *Neurology.* 2011;76(17):1508–1513.
81. Morris-Berry C, Pollard M, Gao S, Thompson C, Singer H. Anti-streptococcal, tubulin, and dopamine receptor 2 antibodies in children with PANDAS and Tourette syndrome: Single-point and longitudinal assessments. *Journal of Neuroimmunology.* 2013;264(1):106–113.
82. Singer H, Mascaro-Blanco A, Alvarez K, et al. Neuronal antibody biomarkers for Sydenham's chorea identify a new group of children with chronic recurrent episodic acute exacerbations of tic and obsessive compulsive symptoms following a streptococcal infection. *PLoS One.* 2015
83. Swedo SE, Leckman J, Rose NR. From Research Subgroup to Clinical Syndrome: Modifying the PANDAS Criteria to Describe PANS (Pediatric Acute-onset Neuropsychiatric Syndrome). *Pediatr Therapeut.* 2012;2(2):113–122.
84. Perlmutter SJ, Leitman SF, Garvey MA, et al. Therapeutic plasma exchange and intravenous immunoglobulin for obsessive-compulsive disorder and tic disorders in childhood. *Lancet.* 1999;354(9185):1153–1158.
85. Dale RC, Church AJ, Cardoso F, et al. Poststreptococcal acute disseminated encephalomyelitis with basal ganglia involvement and auto-reactive antibasal ganglia antibodies. *Ann Neurol.* 2001;50(5):588–595.
86. Dale RC, Church AJ, Benton S, et al. Post-streptococcal autoimmune dystonia with isolated bilateral striatal necrosis. *Dev Med Child Neurol.* 2002;44(7):485–489.
87. Dale RC, Church AJ, Surtees RA, Thompson EJ, Giovannoni G, Neville BG. Post-Streptococcal Autoimmune Neuropsychiatric Disease Presenting as Paroxysmal Dystonic Choreoathetosis. *Mov Disord.* 2002;17(4):817–820.
88. Dale RC, Church AJ, Surtees RA, et al. Encephalitis lethargica syndrome: 20 new cases and evidence of basal ganglia autoimmunity. *Brain.* 2004;127(Pt 1):21–33.
89. Dale RC, Irani SR, Brilot F, et al. N-methyl-D-aspartate receptor antibodies in pediatric dyskinetic encephalitis lethargica. *Ann Neurol.* 2009;66(5):704–709.
90. Mohammad SS, Fung VS, Grattan-Smith P, et al. Movement disorders in children with anti-NMDAR encephalitis and other autoimmune encephalopathies. *Mov Disord.* 2014;29(12):1539–1542.

91. Dalmau J, Tuzun E, Wu HY, et al. Paraneoplastic anti-N-methyl-D-aspartate receptor encephalitis associated with ovarian teratoma. *Ann Neurol.* 2007;61(1):25–36.

92. Rosenfeld MR, Titulaer MJ, Dalmau J. Paraneoplastic syndromes and autoimmune encephalitis: Five new things. *Neurology. Clinical practice.* 2012;2(3):215–223.

93. Dalmau J, Gleichman AJ, Hughes EG, et al. Anti-NMDA-receptor encephalitis: case series and analysis of the effects of antibodies. *Lancet Neurol.* 2008;7(12):1091–1098.

94. Hughes EG, Peng X, Gleichman AJ, et al. Cellular and synaptic mechanisms of anti-NMDA receptor encephalitis. *J Neurosci.* 2010;30(17):5866–5875.

95. Baizabal-Carvallo JF, Jankovic J. The clinical features of psychogenic movement disorders resembling tics. *Journal of Neurology, Neurosurgery & Psychiatry.* 2013 jnnp-2013-305594.

96. Lebas A, Husson B, Didelot A, Honnorat J, Tardieu M. Expanding spectrum of encephalitis with NMDA receptor antibodies in young children. *J Child Neurol.* 2010;25(6):742–745.

97. Poewe W, Djamshidian-Tehrani A. Movement disorders in systemic diseases. *Neurol Clin.* 2015;33(1):269–297.

98. Kleinig TJ, Thompson PD, Matar W, et al. The distinctive movement disorder of ovarian teratoma-associated encephalitis. *Mov Disord.* 2008;23(9):1256–1261.

99. Tobin WO, Strand EA, Clark HM, Lowe VJ, Robertson CE, Pittock SJ. NMDA receptor encephalitis causing reversible caudate changes on MRI and PET imaging. *Neurology. Clinical practice.* 2014;4(6):470–473.

100. Florance NR, Davis RL, Lam C, et al. Anti-N-methyl-D-aspartate receptor (NMDAR) encephalitis in children and adolescents. *Ann Neurol.* 2009;66(1):11–18.

101. Pruss H, Finke C, Holtje M, et al. N-methyl-D-aspartate receptor antibodies in herpes simplex encephalitis. *Ann Neurol.* 2012;72(6):902–911.

102. Armangue T, Titulaer MJ, Malaga I, et al. Pediatric anti-N-methyl-D-aspartate receptor encephalitis-clinical analysis and novel findings in a series of 20 patients. *J Pediatr.* 2013;162(4)

103. Yushvayev-Cavalier Y, Nichter C, Ramirez-Zamora A. Possible Autoimmune Association Between Herpes Simplex Virus Infection and Subsequent Anti-N-Methyl-d-Aspartate Receptor Encephalitis: A Pediatric Patient With Abnormal Movements. *Pediatr Neurol.* 2014

104. Titulaer MJ, McCracken L, Gabilondo I, et al. Treatment and prognostic factors for long-term outcome in patients with anti-NMDA receptor encephalitis: an observational cohort study. *Lancet Neurol.* 2013;12(2):157–165.

105. Leypoldt F, Hoftberger R, Titulaer MJ, et al. Investigations on CXCL13 in Anti-N-Methyl-D-Aspartate Receptor Encephalitis: A Potential Biomarker of Treatment Response. *JAMA neurology.* 2015;72(2):180–186.

106. Baizabal-Carvallo JF, Stocco A, Muscal E, Jankovic J. The spectrum of movement disorders in children with anti-NMDA receptor encephalitis. *Mov Disord.* 2013;28(4):543–547.

107. Maat P, de Graaff E, van Beveren NM, et al. Psychiatric phenomena as initial manifestation of encephalitis by anti-NMDAR antibodies. *Acta neuropsychiatrica.* 2013;25(3):128–136.

108. Lai M, Huijbers MG, Lancaster E, et al. Investigation of LGI1 as the antigen in limbic encephalitis previously attributed to potassium channels: a case series. *Lancet Neurol.* 2010;9(8):776–785.

109. Irani SR, Michell AW, Lang B, et al. Faciobrachial dystonic seizures precede Lgi1 antibody limbic encephalitis. *Ann Neurol.* 2011;69(5):892–900.

110. Irani SR, Stagg CJ, Schott JM, et al. Faciobrachial dystonic seizures: the influence of immunotherapy on seizure control and prevention of cognitive impairment in a broadening phenotype. *Brain.* 2013;136(Pt 10):3151–3162.

111. Chang BS. The Face (and Arm) of Treatment for Seizures in VGKC/LGI1 Antibody-Associated Limbic Encephalitis. *Epilepsy Curr.* 2014;14(4):180–182.

112. Tan TM, Caputo C, Medici F, et al. MELAS syndrome, diabetes and thyroid disease: the role of mitochondrial oxidative stress. *Clin Endocrinol (Oxf).* 2008

113. Tofaris GK, Irani SR, Cheeran BJ, Baker IW, Cader ZM, Vincent A. Immunotherapy-responsive chorea as the presenting feature of LGI1-antibody encephalitis. *Neurology.* 2012;79(2):195–196.

114. Ramdhani RA, Frucht SJ. Isolated Chorea Associated with LGI1 Antibody. *Tremor and other hyperkinetic movements (New York, N.Y.).* 2014:4.

115. Petit-Pedrol M, Armangue T, Peng X, et al. Encephalitis with refractory seizures, status epilepticus, and antibodies to the GABAA receptor: a case series, characterisation of the antigen, and analysis of the effects of antibodies. *Lancet Neurol.* 2014;13(3):276–286.

V. SELECTED SECONDARY MOVEMENT DISORDERS

116. Simabukuro MM, Petit-Pedrol M, Castro LH, et al. GABAA receptor and LGI1 antibody encephalitis in a patient with thymoma. *Neurol Neuroimmunol Neuroinflamm*. 2015;2(2):e73.

117. Hoftberger R, Titulaer MJ, Sabater L, et al. Encephalitis and GABAB receptor antibodies: novel findings in a new case series of 20 patients. *Neurology*. 2013;81(17):1500–1506.

118. Jeffery OJ, Lennon VA, Pittock SJ, Gregory JK, Britton JW, McKeon A. GABAB receptor autoantibody frequency in service serologic evaluation. *Neurology*. 2013;81(10):882–887.

119. Kruer MC, Hoeftberger R, Lim KY, et al. Aggressive course in encephalitis with opsoclonus, ataxia, chorea, and seizures: the first pediatric case of gamma-aminobutyric acid type B receptor autoimmunity. *JAMA neurology*. 2014;71(5):620–623.

120. Hutchinson M, Waters P, McHugh J, et al. Progressive encephalomyelitis, rigidity, and myoclonus: a novel glycine receptor antibody. *Neurology*. 2008;71(16):1291–1292.

121. Mas N, Saiz A, Leite MI, et al. Antiglycine-receptor encephalomyelitis with rigidity. *J Neurol Neurosurg Psychiatry*. 2011;82(12):1399–1401.

122. Carvajal-Gonzalez A, Leite MI, Waters P, et al. Glycine receptor antibodies in PERM and related syndromes: characteristics, clinical features and outcomes. *Brain*. 2014;137(Pt 8):2178–2192.

123. Damasio J, Leite MI, Coutinho E, et al. Progressive encephalomyelitis with rigidity and myoclonus: the first pediatric case with glycine receptor antibodies. *JAMA neurology*. 2013;70(4):498–501.

124. Clardy SL, Lennon VA, Dalmau J, et al. Childhood onset of stiff-man syndrome. *JAMA neurology*. 2013;70(12):1531–1536.

125. McKeon A, Martinez-Hernandez E, Lancaster E, et al. Glycine receptor autoimmune spectrum with stiff-man syndrome phenotype. *JAMA neurology*. 2013;70(1):44–50.

126. Balint B, Jarius S, Nagel S, et al. Progressive encephalomyelitis with rigidity and myoclonus: a new variant with DPPX antibodies. *Neurology*. 2014;82(17):1521–1528.

127. Wells EM, Dalmau J. Paraneoplastic neurologic disorders in children. *Curr Neurol Neurosci Rep*. 2011;11(2):187–194.

128. Gorman MP. Update on diagnosis, treatment, and prognosis in opsoclonus-myoclonus-ataxia syndrome. *Curr Opin Pediatr*. 2010;22(6):745–750.

129. Turkel SB, Brumm VL, Mitchell WG, Tavare CJ. Mood and behavioral dysfunction with opsoclonus-myoclonus ataxia. *J Neuropsychiatry Clin Neurosci*. 2006;18(2):239–241.

130. De Grandis E, Parodi S, Conte M, et al. Long-term follow-up of neuroblastoma-associated opsoclonus-myoclonus-ataxia syndrome. *Neuropediatrics*. 2009;40(3):103–111.

131. Wells EM, Walsh KS, Khademian ZP, Keating RF, Packer RJ. The cerebellar mutism syndrome and its relation to cerebellar cognitive function and the cerebellar cognitive affective disorder. *Dev Disabil Res Rev*. 2008;14(3):221–228.

132. Anand G, Bridge H, Rackstraw P, et al. Cerebellar and cortical abnormalities in paediatric opsoclonus-myoclonus syndrome. *Dev Med Child Neurol*. 2015;57(3):265–272.

133. Fuhlhuber V, Bick S, Kirsten A, et al. Elevated B-cell activating factor BAFF, but not APRIL, correlates with CSF cerebellar autoantibodies in pediatric opsoclonus-myoclonus syndrome. *J Neuroimmunol*. 2009;210(1-2):87–91.

134. Brain L, Jellinek EH, Ball K, et al. Hashimoto's disease and encephalopathy. *Lancet*. 1966;2(7462):512–514.

135. Nandi-Munshi D, Taplin CE. Thyroid-related neurological disorders and complications in children. *Pediatr Neurol*. 2015;52(4):373–382.

Movements that Occur in Sleep

Harvey S. Singer[1], Jonathan W. Mink[2],
Donald L. Gilbert[3] and Joseph Jankovic[4]

[1]Department of Neurology, Johns Hopkins Hospital, Baltimore, MD, USA;
[2]Division of Child Neurology, University of Rochester Medical Center,
Rochester, NY, USA; [3]Division of Neurology, Cincinnati Children's Hospital
Medical Center, Cincinnati, OH, USA; [4]Department of Neurology, Baylor
College of Medicine, Houston, TX, USA

OUTLINE

Movement Disorders in Childhood, Second Edition.
DOI: http://dx.doi.org/10.1016/B978-0-12-411573-6.00019-X

Sleep is a universal experience; infants spend more than half of their time sleeping and adults about one-third of the day asleep. Sleep is an active process, frequently filled with various movements, some of which are normal whereas others might have a more pathologic basis. Pediatric neurologists are frequently confronted with interpreting descriptions of movements that occur during sleep. Is the described movement abnormal, a component of a sleep-related disorder, an extension of a preexisting movement disorder, or a seizure? Physicians have long known that sleep disturbances could represent a sign of disease, but the recognition of the existence of primary sleep disorders first occurred in the 1950s. The discovery of rapid eye movement (REM) sleep and subsequently the nightly repetitive cycles of non-rapid eye movement (NREM) and REM sleep led to the recognition that sleep is an active process with distinct neurophysiologic abnormalities. This chapter reviews various movements that occur as part of primary sleep disorders, movements that are present during the day and persist in sleep, and nocturnal seizures. Since the categorization of involuntary movements that occur around the time of sleep requires a working knowledge of sleep–wake cycles, a brief review of sleep physiology is provided.

OVERVIEW OF SLEEP PHYSIOLOGY

The sleep–wake cycle is subdivided into three states: wake, NREM, and REM sleep. NREM sleep (stages N1–N3) cyclically alternates with REM sleep throughout the sleep period. This normal transition from wake to sleep is defined by electroencephalogram (EEG) scalp recordings showing a typical progression, i.e., shift from alpha (8–12 Hz) to an increase in theta (4–7 Hz) activity. NREM sleep typically initiates sleep, i.e., drowsiness merges with sleep. NREM is divided into three stages: stage N1 (drowsy and physically relaxed) has the loss of the posterior dominant rhythm, mild slowing of the background activity, and the appearance of vertex sharp waves; stage N2 (true sleep) has distinctive features of sleep spindles (7–14 Hz) or K complexes; and stage 3 (slow-wave sleep) has the presence of large amplitude slow (0.5–4 Hz) delta frequency waves. REM sleep is characterized by distinct intermittent rapid eye movements, a low-amplitude mixed-frequency pattern on EEG, the absence of muscle tone in voluntary muscles, and behavioral quiescence.

Normal sleep architecture in older children and adults consists of progressive cycles throughout the night. At the onset of sleep, the individual moves from drowsiness into the NREM phase stage N1, then progresses to stage N2, and subsequently into delta or

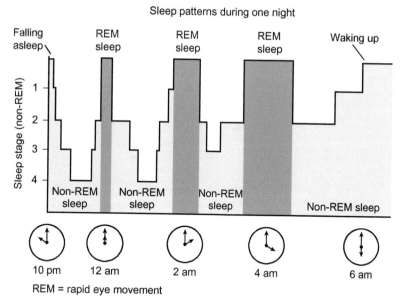

FIGURE 19.1   In adults, about one half of the sleep period is spent in stage 2 sleep, 20% in stage 3 and 4, and 25% in REM sleep. Non-REM is darker gray, REM is lighter gray.

slow-wave sleep (stage N3). After about 80–90 min, the first period of REM sleep occurs, lasting about 5–10 min. The individual then typically returns to stage N1 or N2 sleep before again entering delta sleep. The next episode of REM sleep occurs in about 60–90 min. As the night progresses, NREM–REM cycles continue with fewer stages of N3 sleep. In the early-morning hours, cycles alternate between stages N1–N2 and REM. Most delta sleep occurs during the first third of the night and most REM sleep occurs in the last third. Developmentally, sleep systems in children mature rapidly: in the first year of life, REM sleep predominates, but in the preschool and school-age years NREM stage 3 predominates, with longer periods of deeper stages of sleep. Normal sleep movements, such as position shifts, are common in infants and decrease with age.[1] Infants also lack the typical REM motor inhibition seen in older children and adults.[2] In adults, about one half of the sleep period is spent in stage N2 sleep, 20% in N3, and 25% in REM sleep (Figure 19.1).

Mechanisms for the induction and maintenance of normal sleep and the control of both circadian (24-h) and ultradian (90–120 min cycles of NREM/REM) rhythm generation is complex involving coordination of neuronal activity among the hypothalamus, brainstem, thalamus, and cortex.[3] Simplistically, "wake regions" consist of the brainstem reticular activating system that includes the pedunculopontine nucleus (acetylcholine), lateral dorsal tegmentum (acetylcholine), locus coeruleus (norepinephrine), dorsal and median raphe nuclei (serotonin), subcoeruleus complex (glutamate), and ventral periaqueductal gray (dopamine) (see Figure 19.2). The hypothalamus is widely recognized to have primary regulation over the aforementioned sleep–wake cycle systems. Several areas in the hypothalamus, including orexin-containing cells in the lateral hypothalamus (LH) and

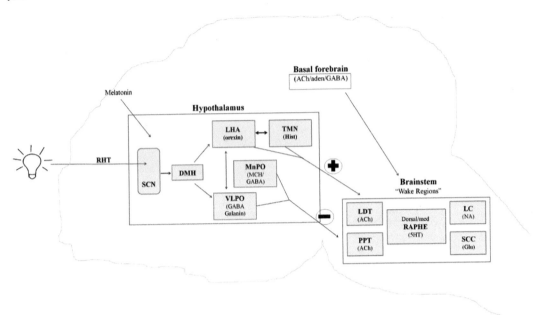

FIGURE 19.2 Pathways involved in sleep–wake cycle. Abbreviations: DMH, dorsomedial hypothalamic nucleus; GABA, gamma-amino butyric acid; LHA, lateral hypothalamic area; LDT, laterodorsal tegmental; PPT, peduncular pontine tegmentum; LC, locus coeruleus; MnPO, median preoptic nucleus; MCH, melanin concentrating hormone; RAPHE, dorsal and median raphe nuclei; RHT, retino-hypothalamic tract; SCC, subcoerulear complex; SCN, suprachiasmatic nucleus; TMN, tuberomammillary nucleus; VLPO, ventrolateral preoptic area; 5HT, serotonin; ACh, acetylcholine; Aden, adenosine; Glu, glutamate; Hist, histamine; NA, noradrenaline.

histaminergic neurons in the tuberomammillary nucleus, have a major role in the induction and maintenance of the waking state. In contrast, outputs from the ventrolateral preoptic area (VLPO) using GABA and galanin, and cells in the median preoptic area (MnPO), possessing melanin concentrating hormone (MCH) and GABA, have inhibitory influences on these "wake regions." Hence, the preoptic area of the hypothalamus appears to be a major sleep-promoting area with neurons in this region inhibiting neurons in the brainstem that are involved with arousal, i.e., neurons in the pedunculopontine, lateral dorsal tegmental nuclei, locus coeruleus, and dorsal raphe.[4] Other regions playing a role in sleep induction include the basal forebrain, via its acetylcholine and adenosine secreting neurons, and melatonin released from the pineal gland. Regulation of sleep–wake cycles by the circadian system is related to, but separate from, the promotion of sleep. The suprachiasmatic nucleus (SCN), located in the anterior hypothalamus is the recipient of information on light via the retinohypothalamic tract, is believed to be the major circadian pacemaker (oscillator) for motor activity.[5] Other factors mediating the SCN include humoral factors,[6] mTOR signaling,[205] pathway mediators located in the subparaventricular zone of the hypothalamus,[7] and "clock genes" such as the period gene rPer2.7.[8] Body temperature regulation, controlled by the hypothalamus, can also influence sleep; increases in body temperature generally lead to postponement of sleep. It is also recognized that thalamo-cortical interactions are important in generating the sleep rhythms recorded on scalp electrodes.[3]

CLASSIFICATION OF MOVEMENTS IN SLEEP

Movements that occur in sleep, in general, can be classified on the basis of whether they are

I. Sleep-related movement disorders (involuntary movements that occur around the time of sleep)
  A. Myoclonus
  B. Movements associated with dyssomnias
    1. Cataplexy
    2. Periodic limb movements of sleep
  C. Movements associated with parasomnias
    1. NREM disorders of arousal
    2. Sleep–wake transition disorders
    3. REM disorders
  D. Other
II. Hyperkinetic movement disorders that are present during the daytime and persist during sleep
III. Seizures in and around the time of sleep
IV. Related to other factors: sleep apnea, gastrointestinal reflux, and panic attacks.

SLEEP-RELATED MOVEMENT DISORDERS

Sleep-Related Myoclonic Disorders

Hypnic Jerks (Sleep Starts; Hypnagogic Jerks)

The transition between periods of wakefulness and NREM sleep may feature sleep starts or hypnic jerks. These movements, often accompanied by an illusion of falling, a vivid dream, or some other sensation, are a sudden, abrupt myoclonic jerk of all or parts of the body, which occasionally may wake the patient. Unless frequent,[9] these movements are benign and associated with a normal prognosis. Excessive sleep starts have been reported in children with migraine[10] and in neurologically impaired children.[11] Hypnic jerks occur in approximately 70% of people and are believed to represent a release phenomenon generated at the level of the brainstem or spinal cord due to a brief loss of suprasegmental descending inhibitory inputs.[12] The electromyogram (EMG) shows brief (less than 250 ms) complexes that may be simultaneous or sequential. No treatment is necessary. Sensory (acoustic) sleep starts are usually benign, although one case has been associated with a brainstem lesion.[13]

Benign Neonatal Sleep Myoclonus

In benign neonatal sleep myoclonus, movements are intermittent, repetitive, unilateral or bilateral, and largely confined to sleep.[14–16] Onset is usually in the first month of life and myoclonus persists for several months, but rarely into early childhood. Jerks may be triggered by noise and usually occur in brief clusters for several minutes before stopping spontaneously. The frequency of movement is about 1 per second with burst duration of 40–300 ms in clusters of four to five. Although clusters may last for up to an hour,[15] they typically do not arouse or wake the infant, and cease with awakening.[17,18] The jerks occur during all stages of sleep, most in NREM sleep. Neurologic examination is normal, and there is no association with developmental delay or seizures. Recognition of this condition is important, since it can avoid unnecessary and costly EEGs and neuroimaging testing. Anticonvulsants are not necessary or effective and may actually worsen the myoclonus.[15]

Propriospinal Myoclonus

Myoclonic jerks involving primarily the trunk, with possible extension into the limbs, occur in a small number of patients during the transition between wakefulness and drowsiness.[19,20] In some patients, jerks may be confined to abdominal muscles or spread to involve muscles of the legs and neck, and occur during wakefulness.[21] In others it may only be evident when the individual is drowsy, relaxed, or recumbent.[22,23] Movements may produce difficulty with sleep induction but are abolished by light sleep. The mechanism appears to involve excitatory impulses that travel through relatively slowly conducting intersegmental propriospinal pathways.

Excessive Fragmentary Myoclonus in NREM Sleep

Fragmentary myoclonus, brief, asymmetric, focal jerks of the face and limbs, usually appears in NREM sleep,[24] but can also occur in REM sleep.[25] Fragmentary myoclonus may be associated with a variety of sleep disorders or occur in isolation.[26,27] It is unclear whether this represents an inadequate inhibitory drive failing to block descending activation or a condition of excessive activation.

Idiopathic Myoclonus in the Oromandibular Region during Sleep (Nocturnal Faciomandibular Myoclonus)

This disorder consists of isolated or short runs of shock-like jaw movements. It occurs predominantly in stages 1 and 2 NREM sleep and may be confused with bruxism.[26,28,29] A mother and son have been reported with tongue biting and bleeding during sleep attributed to faciomandibular myoclonus.[26]

Isolated Sleep Paralysis

Transient inability to move while falling asleep or immediately upon arousing from sleep has been reported most commonly in adolescents and young adults.[30] The individual is aware of the surroundings and hallucinations are common. Sleep deprivation and anxiety can be triggers.[31]

Movements Associated with Dyssomnias

Dyssomnias are disorders that are characterized by excessive daytime sleepiness (EDS) or complaints of difficulty initiating or maintaining sleep.

Narcolepsy

CLINICAL FEATURES

The classic tetrad of symptoms, including EDS, cataplexy (sudden episode of muscle weakness provoked by laughter, fright or surprise, without loss of consciousness), sleep hallucinations, and sleep paralysis, occurs in only 15% of narcoleptics.[32] *EDS* is required for the diagnosis and consists of a continuous, irresistible sleepiness that fluctuates and often includes involuntary naps or "sleep attacks" while driving, walking, talking, and eating. Sleep attacks and episodes of decreased vigilance may be mistaken for syncope or seizures. *Cataplexy*, often involving antigravity muscles, can occur in various forms, including a simple buckling of the knees, head nodding, facial muscle flickering, weakness in the arms, or collapsing to the floor.[33] In children, knees, head, and jaw are the most compromised body regions with about one-third having a semipermanent state of eyelid and jaw weakness on which there is a superimposed cataplectic attack.[34] Events may occur daily and their duration tends to be brief, lasting seconds to a minute. Laughing is the most frequent emotional trigger, but excitement, surprise, tickling, fear, or anger can also be precipitants. In children, typical triggers may be absent and cataplectic attacks may occur spontaneously.[34] The cataplectic muscle weakness is associated with muscle hypotonia, absence of muscle stretch reflexes, and preservation of consciousness. *Sleep hallucinations*, or dream-like experiences, may occur while the individual is falling asleep (hypnagogic hallucinations) or while awakening (hypnopompic hallucinations). Hallucinations can be simple or complex and tend to be visual, but can include auditory, olfactory, gustatory, or somatosensory sensations. They are reported in 15–66% of patients with narcolepsy. *Sleep paralysis* is the inability to move during REM sleep, sleep onset (hypnagogic sleep paralysis), or awakening (hypnopompic sleep paralysis). Muscle atonia and paralysis last for less than 10 min. Sleep paralysis is reported by 17–80% of narcoleptic patients, but it also occurs in normal individuals.[32]

Narcolepsy is rare, with a prevalence of 20–30 per 100,000 persons. About 34% of all narcoleptic subjects have onset of symptoms before the age of 15 years and about 16% of narcoleptics have their onset before age 10 years.[35] In children, cataplexy is present in 15–80% of cases and may be the first symptom in 3–9%.[34,36] Children with narcolepsy can have difficulties with concentration, attention, educational difficulties, conduct, and emotional problems.[37–39] The etiology of narcolepsy is unclear.[40] There is experimental support for an autoimmune etiology and symptomatic cases in children have been reported in association with Niemann–Pick disease type C, Norrie's disease, Prader–Willi syndrome, tumors, trauma, and brainstem lesions.[35,41,42] Anecdotal studies have linked narcolepsy-cataplexy to obesity and becoming overweight.[43]

PATHOPHYSIOLOGY

The hypocretin (orexin) neuronal system is involved in narcolepsy.[44,45] Hypocretins are peptides synthesized in a few thousand cell bodies located within the lateral region of the hypothalamus. These neurons project widely in the central nervous system (CNS), including to the limbic system, intrahypothalamic nuclei, periventricular areas, and monoaminergic cell groups (locus ceruleus, raphe nuclei, ventral tegmental area, substantia nigra, and tuberomamillary nuclei).[46–48] The potential role of hypocretin in the regulation of normal sleep continues to be defined.[49] In studies of patients with narcolepsy-cataplexy, reduced levels of cerebrospinal fluid (CSF) hypocretin-1, less than 110 pg/mL, have been diagnostic.[44,50–51] Cataplexy, which is accompanied by reduced EMG tone and areflexia, is proposed to be the result of disinhibition of a ponto-medullary-spinal pathway.[52]

DIAGNOSIS

Narcolepsy is a clinical diagnosis comprised of two distinct disorders, both with marked daytime sleepiness; narcolepsy with cataplexy (narcolepsy/hypocretin deficiency disorder) and narcolepsy without cateplexsy.[53] Narcolepsy is defined in the sleep laboratory by a short sleep latency and two or more sleep-onset REM periods during multiple sleep latency tests (MSLTs) in which individuals are given four to five standardized nap opportunities. In the narcolepsy with cataplexy group, the combination of a history of cataplexy and more than two abnormal REM transitions during the MSLT is typical for the diagnosis. Other diagnostic approaches include the presence of the HLA markers DQB1*0602 found in over 90% of cases, and the specific and sensitive measure of a low level of CSF hypocretin-1 (orexin) (e.g., less than 100 pg/mL).[50,54]

TREATMENT

Treatment of narcolepsy includes education, good sleep habits, daytime naps, counseling, and pharmacotherapy. The child should observe regular sleep onset and morning arising times, avoid alcohol, and exercise regularly. Modafinil and stimulant medications (methylphenidate, amphetamines) are effective for EDS.[55] Frequent or severe cataplexy is treated with tricyclic antidepressants (imipramine, clomipramine) or serotonin-specific reuptake inhibitors (fluoxetine, paroxetine), venlafaxine, or sodium oxybate.[56,57] Sodium oxybate is a formulation of gamma hydroxybutyrate that has been shown to be highly effective in reducing cataplexy and at high doses reduce daytime sleepiness.[58,59] Experimental treatments are focusing on hypocretin (orexin) replacement, gene therapy, and cell transplantation.[60]

Restless Legs Syndrome

CLINICAL FEATURES AND DIAGNOSIS

Restless legs syndrome (RLS), also known as Willis–Ekbom disease (WED) is a neurological, sensorimotor disorder that affects both adults and children. The disorder was first described by Thomas Willis in 1685 and formal criteria were established by Karl-Axel Ekbom in 1945.[61,62] Criteria for this disorder have been recently revised and include a fifth essential criterion, the addition of specifiers to delineate clinical significance of a classification as either chronic-persistent or intermittent, and a merging of pediatric with adult criteria.[63,64] RLS is now characterized by the following essential criteria:

1. "An urge to move the legs usually, but not always accompanied by, or felt to be caused by, uncomfortable and unpleasant sensations in the legs."
   Affected individuals have an irresistible desire to move the extremities, particularly the lower extremities, accompanied by an uncomfortable, deep, distressing, crawling, creeping, jumping, or jittery sensation localized in the body part with akathisia. These movements typically involve the legs, but can be more generalized during the time of RLS symptoms.

2. "The urge to move the legs and any accompanying unpleasant sensations begin or worsen during rest or inactivity such as lying down or sitting."
3. "The urge to move the legs and any accompanying unpleasant sensations are partially or totally relieved by movement, such as walking or stretching, at least as long as the activity continues."
4. "The urge to move the legs and any accompanying unpleasant sensations during rest or inactivity only occur or are worse in the evening or night than during the day."
5. "The occurrence of the above features is not solely accounted for as symptoms primary to another medical behavior condition (e.g., myalgia, venous stasis, leg edema, arthritis, leg cramps, positional discomfort, habitual foot tapping)."

Specifiers:

a. For clinical course of RLS: Does not apply for pediatric cases.
b. For clinical significance of RLS/WED: The symptoms of RLS cause significant distress or impairment in social, occupational, educational, or other important areas of functioning by their impact on sleep, energy/vitality, daily activities, behavior, cognition, or mood.

RLS is primarily a disorder of middle-aged and older adults, but it has been reported in children with a prevalence ranging from 2% to 5%.[65,66] Definitive diagnostic criteria for RLS in children include meeting all five essential adult criteria *with* a description of these symptoms in the child's own words. Rather than "urge," more age-appropriate terms such as "need to move," "want to move," and "got to kick" are expected. Most children report both the urge and discomfort. Supportive clinical features include: (a) polysomnography documenting a periodic limb movements of sleep (PLMS) index of greater than 5 per hour of sleep; (b) a family history of RLS among first-degree relatives; (c) family history of PLMS >5 per hour; (d) family history of periodic limb movement disorder (PLMD) among first-degree relatives.[63] In pediatric RLS, a clinical sleep disorder (trouble falling or staying asleep) often precedes the diagnosis. Common comorbidities include parasomnias, attention-deficit/hyperactivity disorder (ADHD), anxiety, depression, and PLMS, plus a history of "growing pains" is common.[63,67–71] The basis for these relationships is unknown. The PLMS index is abnormal in about two-thirds of cases.[72] Family history is often positive in children with RLS and is more common in parents of children with ADHD as compared with those of control children.[67–70] Serum ferritin (iron-storing protein) levels are low in most children with RLS. Renal failure can be a potentially aggravating factor.[70,73] Research diagnostic criteria for probable and possible pediatric RLS is presented in Table 19.1.

TABLE 19.1 Research Diagnostic Criteria for Probable and Possible Pediatric RLS

Probable RLS	The child meets all five essential criteria for RLS, except criterion 4 (occurrence only or worsening in the evening or night)
Possible RLS	The child is observed to have behavior manifestations of lower extremity discomfort when sitting or lying, accompanied by motor movement of the affected limbs. The discomfort is characterized by RLS criteria 2–5 (is worse during rest and inactivity, relieved by movement, worse in the evening or night, and is not solely accounted for as primary to another medical or a behavioral condition)

From Picchietti et al.[63]

V. SELECTED SECONDARY MOVEMENT DISORDERS

Although there may be remissions, a progressive course is most common. Akathisia, induced by neuroleptics or associated with Parkinsonism, can be distinguished from RLS by its generation from an inner sense of restlessness, failure to be relieved by activity, lack of localization to the extremities, and lack of diurnal fluctuation.[74] Neurologic examination in the idiopathic or familial forms of RLS is normal, but a peripheral neuropathy or radiculopathy may be present in "secondary" forms. Secondary (symptomatic) RLS has been found in individuals with renal insufficiency or failure, and symptoms may be exacerbated by deficiencies of iron, vitamin B_{12}, or folate, and pregnancy.[75–77]

PATHOPHYSIOLOGY

The primary form of RLS is believed to be genetic and at least six risk factor genes have been identified through genome-wide association studies.[78] The pathophysiology of RLS is unclear and the location of the specific lesion is uncertain. CNS iron insufficiency and alterations in the dopamine, glutamate, and opioid systems have been hypothesized.[79] CSF ferritin is low in RLS cases, iron stores are reduced in the striatum and red nucleus, the substantia nigra has reduced iron echogenicity, and postmortem brain studies show reduced ferritin receptors.[80–84] The primary implicating factor for a CNS dopaminergic abnormality in RLS is the positive therapeutic response to dopaminergic agents. Iron is a cofactor for tyrosine hydroxylase and iron is a component of the D2 receptor. Opioids may also be involved based on a therapeutic response to narcotics and reduced beta-endorphin and Met-enkephalin positive cells.[85]

TREATMENT

All pharmacotherapy, with the exception of iron, is symptomatic and the treatment of pediatric RLS has not been well studied. Aggressive iron treatment is strongly recommended[78] Levodopa plus a decarboxylase inhibitor has improved dysesthesias, PLMS, quality of sleep, and life quality measures.[86] Based on adult studies, long-term use, however, may be complicated by rebound augmentation of symptoms.[87] Other dopamine agonists (pramipexole, ropinirole, and rotigotine patches) have been effective in improving RLS symptoms. Gabapentin and pregabalin, with affinity for the alpha-2-(delta) subunit of the sodium channel, have improved RLS symptoms in large multicenter trials in adults[55,88,89] and there is anecdotal evidence for use in children. Opioids have been reserved for individuals who have failed dopamine agonists because of insufficient effect, adverse events, or the development of tolerance.[78]

Periodic Limb Movements of Sleep (PLMS; Nocturnal Myoclonus, Periodic Limb Movement Disorder)

CLINICAL FEATURES AND DIAGNOSIS

PLMS is a broad term used to include both periodic stereotypic leg movements and the rare periodic arm movements of sleep. The typical triple flexion-like leg movements consist of a rapid partial flexion of the foot at the ankle, dorsiflexion of the big toe with fanning of small toes, and partial flexion of the knee and hip followed by a slow recovery of the extended posture. The movements last from 0.5 to 5 s (too slow to be called myoclonus), with a periodicity of 20–40 s in a stereotyped fashion; clusters may be present for minutes to hours or can last throughout the entire sleep period.[90–92] PLMS are confirmed by surface

TABLE 19.2   Criteria for the Diagnosis of Pediatric Periodic Limb Movements during Sleep

1. Polysomnography shows repetitive stereotyped limb movements that are:
   a. 0.5–10s in duration,
   b. minimum amplitude of 8 μV above resting EMG,
   c. in a sequence of four or more movements,
   d. separated by an interval of more than 5s (from limb movement onset to limb movement onset) and less than 90s (intermovement intervals often are short and variable in children).
2. The PLMS index exceeds 5/h in pediatric cases.
3. The PLMS cause clinically significant sleep disturbance or impairment in mental, physical, social, occupational, educational, behavioral, or other important areas of functioning.
4. The PLMS are not better explained by another current sleep disorder, medical or neurologic disorder, mental disorder, medication use, or substance use disorder (e.g., exclude from PLMS counts the movements at the termination of cyclically occurring apneas).

From Picchietti et al.[63]
Abbreviations: s, seconds; EMG, electromyogram; PLMS, periodic limb movements during sleep.

EMG recordings from both anterior tibialis muscles and scored according to established criteria. They occur most frequently during stages 1 and 2 of NREM sleep or even during the wake state and less frequently during deep sleep stage N3.[93,94] The occurrence of PLMS in repetitive periodic patterns is in distinct contrast to seizure activity. The periodic repetitive nature and exacerbation in light NREM sleep are important components of PLMS. The term *periodic limb movement disorder* is used when PLMS are accompanied by fragmented sleep, insomnia, and EDS (Table 19.2).[95]

PLMS has a prevalence of 4–11% in the general population, typically appears in middle age, and is more common in the elderly.[96] In a large sample of pediatric polysomnographies, the prevalence in childhood was 7.8%.[97] Episodes can occur without any sleep disturbance as an isolated condition or can be associated with sleep arousals, which can lead to EDS. In addition to RLS,[98] PLMS may be associated with other sleep disorders (e.g., narcolepsy, REM sleep behavioral disorder (RBD)),[99,100] with various neurologic disorders (e.g., dopa-responsive dystonia, Tourette syndrome, Huntington's disease, Parkinson's disease, stiff-person syndrome, hyperekplexia, ADHD, and Williams syndrome),[68,69,71,101–105] with other medical conditions (childhood leukemia, uremia),[106,107] and with the use of antidepressants and antipsychotics.[108,109]

PATHOPHYSIOLOGY

Little is known about the pathophysiology of PLMS and, similar to RLS, a role for ferritin has been hypothesized.[97,110] Cerebral generator abnormalities have been proposed for the periodic limb movements seen in RLS based on functional magnetic resonance imaging (fMRI) activation of the red nucleus and brainstem.[111]

TREATMENT

The treatment of PLMS, especially in patients with RLS, includes pharmacotherapy with dopaminergic agonists, benzodiazepines, and opioids. Clonazepam is generally the initial medication, and long-acting benzodiazepines are not recommended because they may cause excessive sedation.[112–114]

Movements Associated with Parasomnias

Parasomnias are undesirable physical phenomena (motor, verbal, or behavioral) that occur during sleep but are not associated with complaints of EDS (hypersomnia) or insomnia.[115,116] These events can occur at the transition to sleep, during REM sleep, or when shifting from N3 sleep into N2/N1 sleep.[12] They are thought to represent activation of central pattern generators located in either the brainstem or spinal cord. Parasomnias can be divided into several subgroups: (1) arousal disorders; (2) sleep–wake transition disorders; (3) disorders associated with REM sleep; and (4) others that could occur in either REM or NREM sleep. Nocturnal seizures, with origin from over the frontal or temporal regions, can mimic parasomnias but clues to their identification include: random occurrence throughout the night; brief duration (lasting 30s to a few minutes); multiple events in a single night; and the presence of daytime seizures. Mild daytime sleepiness is also more commonly seen in patients with nocturnal seizures.[117] A 16-channel EEG montage should be incorporated into the polysomnogram if one is suspecting that nocturnal events may be seizures.

Disorders of Arousal

Arousal disorders are the most common childhood movement disorders in sleep; they tend to occur during the first third of the night, and arise during attempted transition from N3 into N2/N1 sleep. These entities (sleepwalking, sleep terrors, and confusional arousals) are grouped together, because they possess common aspects including immaturity of arousal mechanisms, automatic behavior, altered perception of the environment, and varying degrees of amnesia. Differences among the three types of parasomnias reflect varying degrees of emotional, autonomic, and motor activation. There is no known specific pathophysiologic mechanism, and psychotropic medication and physiologic sleep disruptions have provoked episodes. Disorders of arousal are also seen as symptoms in individuals with obstructive sleep apnea syndrome, upper airway resistance syndrome, RLS, and PLMS.[118] Confusional arousals are seen most often in toddlers whereas sleepwalking and sleep terrors occur throughout the first decade. Peak prevalence is between 4 and 8 years; episodes are infrequent and may last for minutes. Most disorders of arousal improve when children reach preadolescence and disappear after puberty or early adulthood.[119,120] If present, treatment of obstructive sleep apnea, gastroesophageal reflux, anxiety, RLS, or PLMS lessen arousals, and help in resolution of the parasomnias.[55] Although rarely indicated, benzodiazepines (clonazepam and diazepam) can prevent recurrences. These medications reduce slow-wave sleep, but their effectiveness may be due to a blunting of motor or autonomic susceptibility to arousal stimuli. Treating associated sleep disorders (RLS/PLMS) may also remove triggers for sleepwalking or sleep terrors.[118]

Sleepwalking (Somnambulism)

CLINICAL FEATURES

The prevalence of sleepwalking is up to 15% in children age 5–12 years.[119,121] There is no gender preference. Onset typically appears 1–2h after sleep. The child suddenly sits up, gets out of bed, and walks for 5s to 30min. During the event, the child is difficult to arouse, and afterward, he usually has no recall of the event. Sleepwalking events can be elaborate and include leaving the house, dressing, opening locks, cooking, eating, and cleaning. Injuries may occur during this activity,[122] but generally the individual can negotiate around the house. Some individuals have been injured by unconsciously carrying out dangerous behaviors or suffering hypothermia from walking out into the cold. Sleepwalking has a heritable predisposition, a higher concordance in monozygotic than dizygotic twins, and a positive correlation with the HLA-DQB1*05 subtype.[123–125] Symptoms usually begin between ages 4 and 12 years and lessen during and after the teenage years.[124] Factors that may serve as precipitants include fatigue, sleep deprivation, concurrent illnesses, and medications (sedatives, desipramine, lithium, paroxetine, olanzepine, thioridazine, and others). An inability of the brain to awaken fully from slow-wave sleep (disordered arousal mechanism) is thought to cause this disorder.[126] A laboratory method has been developed to trigger somnambulistic behaviors by combining sleep deprivation and acoustic stimuli.[127]

TREATMENT

Therapy includes parent reassurance and safeguarding the environment. Scheduled awakenings, i.e., routinely awakening the child after several hours of sleep and just before the usual time of occurrence, have been moderately successful.[128] Environmental safety measures, such as door locks, may be necessary in patients with habitual sleepwalking. Other treatment includes avoiding precipitating events and, if indicated, low-dose clonazepam at bedtime or serotonin-reuptake inhibitors.[129,130]

Sleep Terrors (Night Terrors, Pavor Nocturnus)

Sleep terrors are more common in boys and the prevalence rate may be up to 3.5% of children.[121] They consist of the sudden arousal from deep sleep with autonomic activation. Onset typically appears 1–2h after sleep, the child abruptly screams out or cries piercingly, and develops intense motor symptoms. Patients are agitated with a sense of intense terror and have a significant autonomic response (tachycardia, tachypnea, diaphoresis, hypertension, and mydriasis). The individual is difficult to arouse, appears not to recognize parents, and is inconsolable. The event may last for more than 30min. Symptoms usually begin between ages 18 months and 12 years with the peak onset between 5 and 7 years. Most individuals have a gradual, spontaneous resolution over months to years. They are typically differentiated from nightmares by the child's inability to recall a dream and lack of memory of the event, although some children report vague recollections of threatening situations.[118] Events may also occur as symptoms of obstructive sleep apnea and PLMS, with or without RLS. Many patients also have sleepwalking. Precipitating factors are similar to those causing somnambulism and treatment is similar to that for other arousal disorders.

Confusional Arousals

Symptoms may occur in up to 25% of children, usually begin before age 5, and may persist into adulthood. These events typically occur in the first half of the night, at the time of transition from slow-wave sleep (N3) to a lighter state of sleep. They usually begin less dramatically than sleep terrors, with moaning sounds gradually progressing to crying, sitting, and thrashing as if having a temper tantrum. The child may sit up in bed, moan, whimper, or utter words like "no" or "go away," appear frightened, confused, or disoriented, but there are no autonomic responses. Duration may be from 5 to 30 min, after which the child goes back to sleep, and has no recognition in the morning. Picking up the child is generally not beneficial. EEG may show generalized, high-amplitude rhythmic delta or theta activity. Confusional arousals are more common when the individual is overtired, there has been a disruption of the routine schedule, or after the use of alcohol.[131] Occasional events require no treatment, but when frequent, small doses of benzodiazepines at bedtime have been beneficial.[132]

Sleep–Wake Transition Disorders

RHYTHMIC MOVEMENT DISORDERS

CLINICAL FEATURES Rhythmic movement disorders (RMDs) are characterized by repetitive stereotyped movements that define the clinical pattern, e.g., head banging, head rolling, body rocking, or leg banging.[133] Head banging, or jactatio capitis nocturna, refers to vigorous anteroposterior movements of the head usually onto the pillow or an adjacent object. Head rolling, in contrast, has lateral rotation or rolling of the head and neck. In body rocking, the child rocks back and forth while on hands and knees. Children do not recall the events and are unresponsive during the attack. Less common RMDs include leg banging, kicking, and body rolling. Vocalizations, such as humming or moaning, may accompany these activities. RMD is common in the first year of life and seldom begins after 18 months.[134] Prevalence in a Swedish population followed longitudinally ranged from 66% at 9 months to 6% at 5 years of age.[135] There is a male predominance. Movements typically occur in clusters, usually at a frequency of 0.5–2 Hz, and last up to 15 min, although they can persist for hours. RMD usually resolves between 2 and 5 years of age, but in a small number of individuals may persist into adolescence or rarely into adulthood.[136,137] Rhythmic movements are seen in idiopathic REM sleep behavior disorder.[138] Polysomnographic studies have shown that these behaviors arise most commonly in transition from drowsiness to N1, during NREM sleep and in REM sleep. On only rare occasions does RMD result in a serious injury.[134,139,140]

PATHOPHYSIOLOGY The etiology of RMD is unknown. Most affected children are healthy, but RMD does occur in developmentally delayed individuals.[134] The etiology of this condition is unknown but postulated to represent a release phenomenon with activation of a central pattern generator following a brief diminution of descending supraseg-mental inhibitory input.[141] Higher anxiety scores have been found in children with RMD as compared to children without this disorder,[137] but any association remains unproven.

DIAGNOSIS The diagnosis of RMD is clinical, based on history. Polysomnography has been suggested for diagnosis when the clinical history is insufficient to provide a definitive diagnosis or movements are atypical or violent.[142,143]

TREATMENT Reassurance generally is all that is needed. Helmets, padding the sides of the crib, behavior modification, and aggressive management of neuropsychologic difficulties may be beneficial. There is no good treatment for RMD, and short-acting benzodiazepines, such as oxazepam and triazolam, or the tricyclic antidepressant imipramine may transiently reduce rhythmic movements.[144–146] Controlled sleep restriction with hypnotic administration has been recommended.[147]

REM Sleep Disorders (Second Half of Night)

NIGHTMARES (DREAM ANXIETY ATTACKS)

Nightmares are frightening vivid dreams that are typically visual but sometimes auditory. They usually begin between 3 and 6 years of age, occur in more than 50% of children, are more common in female adults (no gender predilection in children), and are present during REM sleep. The individual is fully alert upon awakening and has intact recall of the dream. About one-third of adults with recurrent nightmares had their onset during childhood.[148] Autonomic manifestations tend to be mild and body movement tends to be rare, since the event occurs during REM sleep. Nightmares can be secondary to pharmacotherapy, especially with beta-blockers, anticholinergics, and dopamine agonists.

REM SLEEP BEHAVIORAL DISORDER

RBD is characterized by varied and violent behaviors that occur during REM sleep.[149] Patients may punch, kick, leap, or run while actively participating in a dream. For example, persons enacting dreams about sporting events have run into their bedroom wall or while dreaming about a physical encounter, persons may actually punch their bedmate. The dream precipitating RBD is readily recalled, in marked contrast to the lack of memory with sleep terrors. This disorder usually affects middle-aged or older men, but has been reported in children,[150–153] including some with combined RBD and narcolepsy-cataplexy,[154] and others with congenital or degenerative disturbances of the brainstem.[12] RBD can occur as an idiopathic disease or appear as an early manifestation of a group of neurodegenerative diseases (synucleinopathies) such as Parkinson's disease, multiple systems atrophy, or dementia with Lewy bodies.[155–157] Transient forms have been precipitated by withdrawal from REM-suppressing medications (benzodiazepines), by withdrawal from drugs (fluoxetine, alcohol), or by intoxication with tricyclic antidepressants. RBD is also common in patients with narcolepsy.[151] The minimal diagnostic criteria for RBD include a polysomnographic abnormality during REM sleep (intermittent or complete loss of REM sleep, muscle atonia, and excessive phasic EMG activity), documentation of abnormal REM sleep behaviors, the history of injurious disruptive sleep behaviors, and the absence of EEG epileptiform activity during REM sleep. The long-term outcome of RBD in children is unknown.

An unusual feature of RBD is the absence of the classic REM-associated skeletal muscle atonia that keeps individuals from acting out their dreams.[158] The absence of typical REM atonia is believed due to a failure of inhibition of skeletal muscle activity by the medullary nucleus recticularis gigantocellularis. The nocturnal polysomnogram shows increased phasic EMG activity during REM sleep. Magnetic resonance spectroscopy has failed, however, to demonstrate in REM patients either marked neuronal loss or metabolic problems within the upper brainstem.[159] Further, the loss of REM atonia alone is not sufficient to generate RBD. Reductions of dopaminergic terminals in the striatum[160] and diminished dopamine transporter binding[161] have suggested the presence of a presynaptic dopaminergic defect in this disorder. Treatment with clonazepam or melatonin at bedtime may be effective in preventing most REM parasomnias.[55]

Other Disorders

Paroxysmal Hypnogenic Dyskinesia (Nocturnal Paroxysmal Dystonia)

Paroxysmal hypnogenic dyskinesia (nocturnal paroxysmal dystonia) includes violent, dystonic stiffening, choreoathetoid, or hemiballismic movements occurring primarily during NREM sleep. Movements last for seconds to hours and events are sometimes associated with somnambulism. There is no postevent confusion and the affected person usually returns to sleep. Attacks of different duration have been described: short-lasting attacks are often variants of frontal lobe epilepsy, whereas longer attacks represent a paroxysmal movement disorder occurring during non-REM sleep. Ictal single-photon emission computed tomography in a patient with epileptic seizures manifesting as nocturnal paroxysmal dystonia showed hyperperfusion in the anterior part of the cingulate gyrus.[162] Persons of all ages may be affected.

Delayed Sleep Phase Disorder

Delayed sleep phase disorder is a common circadian rhythm sleep disorder in which the patient is unable to fall asleep before the early morning hours. Often confused with insomnia, the disorder can have medical, psychological, and social consequences.[163] The disorder typically has onset in adolescence, occurs more in males, and has a genetic predisposition. Studies have suggested an alteration in the SCN and an association with the expression of *Period* (1–3) and *Cryptochrome* genes.[164] This disorder should be differentiated in adolescents with delinquent and anti-social behavior attempting to avoid school. Bright light therapy has been used to advance sleep-onset time to an earlier hour.[165]

Sleep Bruxism (Nocturnal Tooth Grinding)

CLINICAL FEATURES

This disorder is characterized by frequent and intense grinding or clenching of the teeth during sleep.[166] Bruxism often produces an unpleasant sound that is disturbing to others, but usually not to the initiator. In severe cases, it causes damage to the teeth, periodontal tissue, or jaw.[167] Masseter muscle hypertrophy, morning muscle discomfort, temporomandidular soreness, and temporal headache may also be present. Teeth grinding may occur at any age and has been observed in up to 20% of children.[137,168] There is no difference in gender and the prevalence decreases with age. Most of the oromotor activity associated with sleep bruxism appears during stages 1 and 2 of sleep.[169]

Although observed in children with mental retardation, sleep bruxism clearly occurs in normal individuals, and a familial tendency has been noted.[170] Multiple causal factors have been suggested, including malocclusion, psychological, or developmental factors, but no pathologic lesion has been identified. Others have suggested that sleep bruxism represents an extreme manifestation of normal masticatory muscle activity associated with sleep microarousal.[171,172] Its presence has also been reported in individuals treated with selective serotonin-reuptake inhibitors and certain street drugs such as ecstasy.[173] Studies on the effect of dopamine agonists and antagonists have suggested a central role for dopamine in cases of pharmacologically induced bruxism.[174] Bruxism should be distinguished from oromandibular dystonia or idiopathic myoclonus in the oromandibular region during sleep.

TREATMENT

Treatment is indicated when the condition affects the integrity of teeth. A variety of approaches have been advocated, ranging from stress management and hypnosis[175] to the use of muscle relaxants (diazepam and centrally acting methocarbamol) and injections of botulinum toxin into the masseter muscles.[176–178] Dental mouth guards have also been recommended to prevent the unpleasant sound and tooth destruction.[179] There was no effect of sleep hygiene measures together with progressive relaxation techniques on sleep bruxism or sleep over a 4-week observation period.[180] Further, there is insufficient evidence on the effectiveness of pharmacotherapy for the treatment of sleep bruxism.[181]

HYPERKINETIC MOVEMENT DISORDERS THAT ARE PRESENT DURING THE DAYTIME AND PERSIST DURING SLEEP

Although it is often stated that most movement disorders are abolished by sleep, some movements typically persist whereas others may involve brief remnants of abnormal activity, especially in transitions to light sleep or wakefulness. One must also recognize that affected individuals can have co-occurring sleep fragmentation, high arousal rates, parasomnias, periodic limb movements, and increased general sleep movements.[182,183] Movement disorders that typically persist during sleep include myoclonus associated with lesions in the lower brainstem or spinal cord,[184] palatal tremor due to lesions in the Mollaret triangle,[185] and individuals with hemifacial spasm. Tics seen in Tourette syndrome can persist in both REM and non-REM sleep in up to 80% of cases, although typically in a reduced form as compared to those seen during the daytime.[186–188] Chorea, dystonia, hemiballismus, and Parkinsonian tremor are typically reduced during sleep, but studies have shown characteristic movements during sleep.[186,187] Patients with dopa-responsive dystonia (Segawa's disease) often have excessive movements and periodic limb movements while sleeping.[189] In Huntington's disease, sleep fragmentation is common and increases with the severity of the disease.[186] Only a few movement disorders, including tardive dyskinesias and essential palatal tremor, show complete cessation of movements in sleep.[190,191] Tremors are uncommon during sleep, but two reports have described infantile tremors related to sleep onset.[192] Geniospasm is an inherited paroxysmal tremulous movement of the mentalis muscle that begins in childhood and may be induced by emotional stress.[193] A patient with paroxysmal rhythmic movements of the chin during N2 that ceased with onset of REM has been described.[194]

SEIZURES IN AND AROUND THE TIME OF SLEEP

Movement abnormalities occurring during sleep can be a manifestation of epilepsy and their differentiation from a sleep disorder is essential for appropriate evaluation and treatment.[195,196] Several epilepsy syndromes occur predominantly during NREM sleep, a finding attributed to NREM sleep being a period during which there is a coordination of synaptic activity that enhances the recruitment of a critical mass of neurons necessary to initiate and propagate a seizure.[197] Some investigators have noted that seizures are more common in N1 and N2, despite N3 having the greatest activating influence on interictal epileptiform discharges.[198,199]

Several clinical characteristics are helpful in distinguishing seizures from a sleep movement abnormality. These typically include a stereotyped appearance, random occurrence, brief duration, presence of gaze deviation, incontinence, and a postictal period of confusion.[145] Although nocturnal seizures may often be readily identifiable, at times a video EEG polysomnographic recording may be required for clarification. Seizures also have a direct effect on sleep by causing a shift to a lighter stage of sleep or awakening the individual. For example, patients with primary or secondary generalized tonic-clonic seizures had reduced total sleep time, reduced REM sleep periods, increased wake time after sleep onset, and an increased proportion of stage N2 sleep on nights when seizures occurred as compared to seizure-free nights.[200]

Nocturnal frontal lobe epilepsy is associated with an epileptic focus located in the mesial and orbital regions of the frontal cortex and comprises a wide spectrum of motor features that may be misdiagnosed as parasomnias, dystonia, or other movement disorders.[201,202] They are typified by their recurrence in early stages of sleep, frequency, presence of stereotyped behaviors that have a bizarre complex motor character (running, struggling, wanderings, dyskinetic or dystonic movements), vocalizations (yelling, cursing), brief duration (usually less than 1 min), stable to increasing course, presence of gaze deviation, incontinence, and a postictal period of confusion.[145,203,204] Scalp EEGs may not detect an abnormality that can be recorded with depth electrodes. In contrast to frontal lobe seizures, parasomnias tend to occur at a younger age, lack a specific stereotyped movement pattern, last longer than a minute, are less frequent, and improve over time.

References

1. De Koninck J, Lorrain D, Gagnon P. Sleep positions and position shifts in five age groups: an ontogenetic picture. *Sleep*. 1992;15(2):143–149.
2. Kohyama J, Ohsawa Y, Shimohira M, Iwakawa Y. Phasic motor activity reduction occurring with horizontal rapid eye movements during REM sleep is disturbed in infantile spasms. *J Neurol Sci*. 1996;138(1–2):82–87.
3. Larson-Prior LJ, Ju Y-E, Galvin JE. Cortical–subcortical interactions in hypersomnia disorders: mechanisms underlying cognitive and behavioral aspects of the sleep–wake cycle. *Front Neurol*. 2014;5:165.
4. Saper CB, Chou TC, Scammell TE. The sleep switch: hypothalamic control of sleep and wakefulness. *Trends Neurosci*. 2001;24(12):726–731.
5. Moore R. Circadian timing. In: Squire L, Roberts J, Spitzer N, Zigmond M, McConnell S, Bloom F, eds. *Fundamental Neuroscience*. 2nd ed. San Diego, CA: Academic Press; 2002:1067–1084.
6. LeSauter J, Silver R. Output signals of the SCN. *Chronobiol Int*. 1998;15(5):535–550.
7. Sakamoto K, Nagase T, Fukui H, et al. Multitissue circadian expression of rat period homolog (rPer2) mRNA is governed by the mammalian circadian clock, the suprachiasmatic nucleus in the brain. *J Biol Chem*. 1998;273(42):27039–27042.
8. Franken P, Dijk DJ. Circadian clock genes and sleep homeostasis. *Eur J Neurosci*. 2009;29(9):1820–1829.
9. Broughton R, Valley V, Aguirre M, Roberts J, Suwalski W, Dunham W. Excessive daytime sleepiness and the pathophysiology of narcolepsy: a laboratory perspective. *Sleep*. 1986;9:205–215.
10. Bruni O, Galli F, Guidetti V. Sleep hygiene and migraine in children and adolescents. *Cephalalgia*. 1999;19(suppl 25):57–59.
11. Fusco L, Pachatz C, Cusmai R, Vigevano F. Repetitive sleep starts in neurologically impaired children: an unusual non-epileptic manifestation in otherwise epileptic subjects. *Epileptic Disord*. 1999;1(1):63–67.

12. Kotagal S. Parasomnias in childhood. *Sleep Med Rev.* 2009;13(2):157–168.

13. Salih F, Klingebiel R, Zschenderlein R, Grosse P. Acoustic sleep starts with sleep-onset insomnia related to a brainstem lesion. *Neurology.* 2008;70(20):1935–1937.

14. Alfonso I, Papazian O, Aicardi J, Jeffries HE. A simple maneuver to provoke benign neonatal sleep myoclonus. *Pediatrics.* 1995;96(6):1161–1163.

15. Daoust-Roy J, Seshia SS. Benign neonatal sleep myoclonus. A differential diagnosis of neonatal seizures. *Am J Dis Child.* 1992;146(10):1236–1241.

16. Di Capua M, Fusco L, Ricci S, Vigevano F. Benign neonatal sleep myoclonus: clinical features and video-poly-graphic recordings. *Mov Disord.* 1993;8(2):191–194.

17. Ramelli GP, Sozzo AB, Vella S, Bianchetti MG. Benign neonatal sleep myoclonus: an under-recognized, non-epileptic condition. *Acta Paediatr.* 2005;94(7):962–963.

18. Walters AS. Clinical identification of the simple sleep-related movement disorders. *Chest J.* 2007;131(4):1260–1266.

19. Brown P, Rothwell JC, Thompson PD, Marsden CD. Propriospinal myoclonus: evidence for spinal "pattern" generators in humans. *Mov Disord.* 1994;9(5):571–576.

20. Chokroverty S. Propriospinal myoclonus. *Clin Neurosci.* 1995;3(4):219–222.

21. Vetrugno R, Provini F, Plazzi G, et al. Focal myoclonus and propriospinal propagation. *Clin Neurophysiol.* 2000;111(12):2175–2179.

22. Montagna P, Provini F, Plazzi G, Liguori R, Lugaresi E. Propriospinal myoclonus upon relaxation and drowsi-ness: a cause of severe insomnia. *Mov Disord.* 1997;12(1):66–72.

23. Tison F, Arne P, Dousset V, Paty J, Henry P. Propriospinal myoclonus induced by relaxation and drowsiness. *Rev Neurol (Paris).* 1998;154(5):423–425.

24. Broughton R, Tolentino MA, Krelina M. Excessive fragmentary myoclonus in NREM sleep: a report of 38 cases. *Electroencephalogr Clin Neurophysiol.* 1985;61(2):123–133.

25. Lins O, Castonguay M, Dunham W, Nevsimalova S, Broughton R. Excessive fragmentary myoclonus: time of night and sleep stage distributions. *Can J Neurol Sci.* 1993;20(2):142–146.

26. Vetrugno R, Provini F, Plazzi G, et al. Familial nocturnal facio-mandibular myoclonus mimicking sleep bruxism. *Neurology.* 2002;58(4):644–647.

27. Broughton RJ, Fleming JA, George CF, et al. Randomized, double-blind, placebo-controlled crossover trial of modafinil in the treatment of excessive daytime sleepiness in narcolepsy. *Neurology.* 1997;49(2):444–451.

28. Loi D, Provini F, Vetrugno R, D'Angelo R, Zaniboni A, Montagna P. Sleep-related faciomandibular myoclonus: a sleep-related movement disorder different from bruxism. *Mov Disord.* 2007;22(12):1819–1822.

29. Kato T, Montplaisir JY, Blanchet PJ, Lund JP, Lavigne GJ. Idiopathic myoclonus in the oromandibular region during sleep: a possible source of confusion in sleep bruxism diagnosis. *Mov Disord.* 1999;14(5):865–871.

30. Sharpless BA, Grom JL. Isolated sleep paralysis: fear, prevention, and disruption. *Behav Sleep Med.* 2014; 14 October:1–6. [Epub ahead of print], Doi: http://dx.doi.org/10.1080/15402002.2014.963583.

31. McCarty DE, Chesson Jr AL. A case of sleep paralysis with hypnopompic hallucinations. *J Clin Sleep Med.* 2009;5(1):83.

32. Bassetti C, Aldrich MS. Narcolepsy. *Neurol Clin.* 1996;14(3):545–571.

33. Dauvilliers Y, Siegel JM, Lopez R, Torontali ZA, Peever JH. Cataplexy—clinical aspects, pathophysiology and management strategy. *Nat Rev Neurol.* 2014;10(7):386–395.

34. Serra L, Montagna P, Mignot E, Lugaresi E, Plazzi G. Cataplexy features in childhood narcolepsy. *Mov Disord.* 2008;23(6):858–865.

35. Challamel MJ, Mazzola ME, Nevsimalova S, Cannard C, Louis J, Revol M. Narcolepsy in children. *Sleep.* 1994;17(8 suppl):S17–S20.

36. Vendrame M, Havaligi N, Matadeen-Ali C, Adams R, Kothare SV. Narcolepsy in children: a single-center clini-cal experience. *Pediatr Neurol.* 2008;38(5):314–320.

37. Naumann A, Bellebaum C, Daum I. Cognitive deficits in narcolepsy. *J Sleep Res.* 2006;15(3):329–338.

38. Rieger M, Mayer G, Gauggel S. Attention deficits in patients with narcolepsy. *Sleep.* 2003;26(1):36–43.

39. Bayard S, Langenier MC, De Cock VC, Scholz S, Dauvilliers Y. Executive control of attention in narcolepsy. *PLoS One.* 2012;7(4):e33525.

40. Kumar S, Sagili H. Etiopathogenesis and neurobiology of narcolepsy: a review. *J Clin Diagn Res.* 2014;8(2):190.

41. Stahl SM, Layzer RB, Aminoff MJ, Townsend JJ, Feldon S. Continuous cataplexy in a patient with a midbrain tumor: the limp man syndrome. *Neurology.* 1980;30(10):1115–1118.

42. D'Cruz OF, Vaughn BV, Gold SH, Greenwood RS. Symptomatic cataplexy in pontomedullary lesions. *Neurology*. 1994;44(11):2189–2191.

43. Kotagal S, Kumar S. Childhood onset narcolepsy cataplexy—more than just a sleep disorder. *Sleep*. 2013;36(2):161.

44. Nishino S, Ripley B, Overeem S, Lammers GJ, Mignot E. Hypocretin (orexin) deficiency in human narcolepsy. *Lancet*. 2000;355(9197):39–40.

45. Nishino S, Ripley B, Overeem S, et al. Low cerebrospinal fluid hypocretin (Orexin) and altered energy homeostasis in human narcolepsy. *Ann Neurol*. 2001;50(3):381–388.

46. Nambu T, Sakurai T, Mizukami K, Hosoya Y, Yanagisawa M, Goto K. Distribution of orexin neurons in the adult rat brain. *Brain Res*. 1999;827(1–2):243–260.

47. Peyron C, Tighe DK, van den Pol AN, et al. Neurons containing hypocretin (orexin) project to multiple neuronal systems. *J Neurosci*. 1998;18(23):9996–10015.

48. Saper CB. Staying awake for dinner: hypothalamic integration of sleep, feeding, and circadian rhythms. *Prog Brain Res*. 2006;153:243–252.

49. Nishino S. Narcolepsy: pathophysiology and pharmacology. *J Clin Psychiatry*. 2007;68(suppl 13):9–15.

50. Mignot E, Lammers GJ, Ripley B, et al. The role of cerebrospinal fluid hypocretin measurement in the diagnosis of narcolepsy and other hypersomnias. *Arch Neurol*. 2002;59(10):1553–1562.

51. Nishino S, Tafti M, Reid MS, et al. Muscle atonia is triggered by cholinergic stimulation of the basal forebrain: implication for the pathophysiology of canine narcolepsy. *J Neurosci*. 1995;15(7 Pt 1):4806–4814.

52. Bassetti C, Aldrich MS. Narcolepsy. *Neurol Clin*. 1996;14(3):545–571.

53. American Psychiatric Association *The Diagnostic and Statistical Manual of Mental Disorders: DSM 5*. Arlington, VA: American Psychiatric Association; 2013.

54. Nishino S, Okuro M, Kotorii N, et al. Hypocretin/orexin and narcolepsy: new basic and clinical insights. *Acta Physiologica*. 2009;198(3):209–222.

55. Kotagal S. Treatment of dyssomnias and parasomnias in childhood. *Curr Treat Options Neurol*. 2012;14(6):630–649.

56. Moller LR, Ostergaard JR. Treatment with venlafaxine in six cases of children with narcolepsy and with cataplexy and hypnagogic hallucinations. *J Child Adolesc Psychopharmacol*. 2009;19(2):197–201.

57. Thorpy M. Current concepts in the etiology, diagnosis and treatment of narcolepsy. *Sleep Med*. 2001;2(1):5–17.

58. Mansukhani MP, Kotagal S. Sodium oxybate in the treatment of childhood narcolepsy–cataplexy: a retrospective study. *Sleep Med*. 2012;13(6):606–610.

59. Robinson DM, Keating GM. Sodium oxybate: a review of its use in the management of narcolepsy. *CNS Drugs*. 2007;21(4):337–354.

60. Ritchie C, Okuro M, Kanbayashi T, Nishino S. Hypocretin ligand deficiency in narcolepsy: recent basic and clinical insights. *Curr Neurol Neurosci Rep*. 2010;10(3):180–189.

61. Willis T. *The London Practice of Physick*. London: Dring, Harper and Crook Basset; 1685.

62. Ekbom K-A. Restless legs syndrome. *Neurology*. 1960;10(9):868–873.

63. Picchietti DL, Bruni O, de Weerd A, et al. Pediatric restless legs syndrome diagnostic criteria: an update by the International Restless Legs Syndrome Study Group. *Sleep Med*. 2013;14(12):1253–1259.

64. Allen RP, Picchietti DL, Garcia-Borreguero D, et al. Restless legs syndrome/Willis–Ekbom disease diagnostic criteria: updated International Restless Legs Syndrome Study Group (IRLSSG) consensus criteria—history, rationale, description, and significance. *Sleep Med*. 2014;15(8):860–873.

65. Picchietti D, Allen RP, Walters AS, Davidson JE, Myers A, Ferini-Strambi L. Restless legs syndrome: prevalence and impact in children and adolescents—the Peds REST study. *Pediatrics*. 2007;120(2):253–266.

66. Picchietti DL, Stevens HE. Early manifestations of restless legs syndrome in childhood and adolescence. *Sleep Med*. 2007;9(7):770–781.

67. Muhle H, Neumann A, Lohmann-Hedrich K, et al. Childhood-onset restless legs syndrome: clinical and genetic features of 22 families. *Mov Disord*. 2008;23(8):1113–1121.

68. Picchietti DL, England SJ, Walters AS, Willis K, Verrico T. Periodic limb movement disorder and restless legs syndrome in children with attention-deficit hyperactivity disorder. *J Child Neurol*. 1998;13(12):588–594.

69. Picchietti DL, Underwood DJ, Farris WA, et al. Further studies on periodic limb movement disorder and restless legs syndrome in children with attention-deficit hyperactivity disorder. *Mov Disord*. 1999;14(6):1000–1007.

70. Picchietti MA, Picchietti DL. Restless legs syndrome and periodic limb movement disorder in children and adolescents. *Semin Pediatr Neurol*. 2008;15(2):91–99.

71. Chervin RD, Archbold KH, Dillon JE, et al. Associations between symptoms of inattention, hyperactivity, restless legs, and periodic leg movements. *Sleep*. 2002;25(2):213–218.
72. Kotagal S, Silber MH. Childhood-onset restless legs syndrome. *Ann Neurol*. 2004;56(6):803–807.
73. Applebee GA, Guillot AP, Schuman CC, Teddy S, Attarian HP. Restless legs syndrome in pediatric patients with chronic kidney disease. *Pediatr Nephrol*. 2009;24(3):545–548.
74. Walters AS, Hening W, Rubinstein M, Chokroverty S. A clinical and polysomnographic comparison of neuroleptic-induced akathisia and the idiopathic restless legs syndrome. *Sleep*. 1991;14(4):339–345.
75. McParland P, Pearce JM. Restless legs syndrome in pregnancy. Case reports. *Clin Exp Obstet Gynecol*. 1990;17(1):5–6.
76. Ondo W, Jankovic J. Restless legs syndrome. Clinicoetiologic correlates. *Neurology*. 1996;47(6):1435–1441.
77. Allen RP, Earley CJ. Restless legs syndrome: a review of clinical and pathophysiologic features. *J Clin Neurophysiol*. 2001;18(2):128–147.
78. Ondo WG. Restless legs syndrome: pathophysiology and treatment. *Curr Treat Options Neurol*. 2014;16(11):1–17.
79. Allen RP, Earley CJ. The role of iron in restless legs syndrome. *Mov Disord*. 2007;22(S18):S440–S448.
80. Allen R, Barker P, Wehrl F, Song H, Earley C. MRI measurement of brain iron in patients with restless legs syndrome. *Neurology*. 2001;56(2):263–265.
81. Connor J, Wang X, Patton S, et al. Decreased transferrin receptor expression by neuromelanin cells in restless legs syndrome. *Neurology*. 2004;62(9):1563–1567.
82. Connors SL, Crowell DE, Eberhart CG, et al. Beta2-adrenergic receptor activation and genetic polymorphisms in autism: data from dizygotic twins. *J Child Neurol*. 2005;20(11):876–884.
83. Earley CJ, Connor JR, Beard JL, Malecki EA, Epstein DK, Allen RP. Abnormalities in CSF concentrations of ferritin and transferrin in restless legs syndrome. *Neurology*. 2000;54(8):1698–1700.
84. Godau J, Klose U, Di Santo A, Schweitzer K, Berg D. Multiregional brain iron deficiency in restless legs syndrome. *Mov Disord*. 2008;23(8):1184–1187.
85. Walters AS, Ondo WG, Zhu W, Le W. Does the endogenous opiate system play a role in the restless legs syndrome?: a pilot post-mortem study. *J Neurol Sci*. 2009;279(1):62–65.
86. England SJ, Picchietti DL, Couvadelli BV, Fisher BC, Siddiqui F, Wagner ML, et al. L-Dopa improves restless legs syndrome and periodic limb movements in sleep but not attention-deficit-hyperactivity disorder in a double-blind trial in children. *Sleep Med*. 2011;12(5):471–477.
87. Allen RP, Earley CJ. Augmentation of the restless legs syndrome with carbidopa/levodopa. *Sleep*. 1996;19(3):205–213.
88. Van Meter SA, Kavanagh ST, Warren S, Barrett RW. Dose response of gabapentin Enacarbil versus placebo in subjects with moderate-to-severe primary restless legs syndrome. *CNS Drugs*. 2012;26(9):773–780.
89. Allen RP, Stillman P, Myers AJ. Physician-diagnosed restless legs syndrome in a large sample of primary medical care patients in western Europe: prevalence and characteristics. *Sleep Med*. 2010;11(1):31–37.
90. Lugaresi E, Cirignotta F, Coccagna G, Montagna P. Nocturnal myoclonus and restless legs syndrome. *Adv Neurol*. 1986;43:295–307.
91. Trenkwalder C, Walters AS, Hening W. Periodic limb movements and restless legs syndrome. *Neurol Clin*. 1996;14(3):629–650.
92. Coleman RM, Pollak CP, Weitzman ED. Periodic movements in sleep (nocturnal myoclonus): relation to sleep disorders. *Ann Neurol*. 1980;8(4):416–421.
93. Pollmacher T, Schulz H. Periodic leg movements (PLM): their relationship to sleep stages. *Sleep*. 1993;16(6):572–577.
94. Gingras JL, Gaultney JF, Picchietti DL. Pediatric periodic limb movement disorder: sleep symptom and polysomnographic correlates compared to obstructive sleep apnea. *J Clin Sleep Med*. 2011;7(6):603.
95. Picchietti DL, Walters AS. Moderate to severe periodic limb movement disorder in childhood and adolescence. *Sleep*. 1999;22(3):297–300.
96. Hornyak M, Trenkwalder C. Restless legs syndrome and periodic limb movement disorder in the elderly. *J Psychosom Res*. 2004;56(5):543–548.
97. Bokkala S, Napalinga K, Pin ninti N, et al. Correlates of periodic limb movements of sleep in the pediatric population. *Pediatr Neurol*. 2008;39(1):33–39.
98. Winkelman JW. Periodic limb movements in sleep—endophenotype for restless legs syndrome? *N Engl J Med*. 2007;357(7):703–705.

99. Warnes H, Dinner DS, Kotagal P, Burgess RC. Periodic limb movements and sleep apnoea. *J Sleep Res*. 1993;2(1):38–44.

100. Fantini ML, Michaud M, Gosselin N, Lavigne G, Montplaisir J. Periodic leg movements in REM sleep behavior disorder and related autonomic and EEG activation. *Neurology*. 2002;59(12):1889–1894.

101. Martinelli P, Pazzaglia P, Montagna P, et al. Stiff-man syndrome associated with nocturnal myoclonus and epilepsy. *J Neurol Neurosurg Psychiatry*. 1978;41(5):458–462.

102. Voderholzer U, Muller N, Haag C, Riemann D, Straube A. Periodic limb movements during sleep are a frequent finding in patients with Gilles de la Tourette's syndrome. *J Neurol*. 1997;244(8):521–526.

103. Wetter TC, Collado-Seidel V, Pollmacher T, Yassouridis A, Trenkwalder C. Sleep and periodic leg movement patterns in drug-free patients with Parkinson's disease and multiple system atrophy. *Sleep*. 2000;23(3):361–367.

104. Yokota T, Hirose K, Tanabe H, Tsukagoshi H. Sleep-related periodic leg movements (nocturnal myoclonus) due to spinal cord lesion. *J Neurol Sci*. 1991;104(1):13–18.

105. Gadoth N, Costeff H, Harel S, Lavie P. Motor abnormalities during sleep in patients with childhood hereditary progressive dystonia, and their unaffected family members. *Sleep*. 1989;12(3):233–238.

106. Walker SL, Fine A, Kryger MH. L-DOPA/carbidopa for nocturnal movement disorders in uremia. *Sleep*. 1996;19(3):214–218.

107. Kotagal S, Rathnow SR, Chu JY, O'Connor DM, Cross J, Sterneck RL. Nocturnal myoclonus—a sleep disturbance in children with leukemia. *Dev Med Child Neurol*. 1985;27(1):124–126.

108. Salin-Pascual RJ, Galicia-Polo L, Drucker-Colin R. Sleep changes after 4 consecutive days of venlafaxine administration in normal volunteers. *J Clin Psychiatry*. 1997;58(8):348–350.

109. Dorsey CM, Lukas SE, Cunningham SL. Fluoxetine-induced sleep disturbance in depressed patients. *Neuropsychopharmacology*. 1996;14(6):437–442.

110. Beard JL. Iron status and periodic limb movements of sleep in children: a causal relationship? *Sleep Med*. 2004;5(1):89–90.

111. Bucher SF, Seelos KC, Dodel RC, Reiser M, Oertel WH. Activation mapping in essential tremor with functional magnetic resonance imaging. *Ann Neurol*. 1997;41(1):32–40.

112. Montplaisir J, Lapierre O, Warnes H, Pelletier G. The treatment of the restless leg syndrome with or without periodic leg movements in sleep. *Sleep*. 1992;15(5):391–395.

113. Saletu M, Anderer P, Saletu-Zyhlarz G, et al. Restless legs syndrome (RLS) and periodic limb movement disorder (PLMD): acute placebo-controlled sleep laboratory studies with clonazepam. *Eur Neuropsychopharmacol*. 2001;11(2):153–161.

114. Kaplan PW, Allen RP, Buchholz DW, Walters JK. A double-blind, placebo-controlled study of the treatment of periodic limb movements in sleep using carbidopa/levodopa and propoxyphene. *Sleep*. 1993;16(8):717–723.

115. Mahowald MW, Bornemann MC, Schenck CH. Parasomnias. *Semin Neurol*. 2004;24(3):283–292.

116. Mason II TB, Pack AI. Pediatric parasomnias. *Sleep*. 2007;30(2):141–151.

117. Kotagal S. Training issues pertaining to sleep medicine and child neurology *Seminars in Pediatric Neurology*. Philadelphia, PA: WB Saunders; 2011: 139–141.

118. Guilleminault C, Palombini L, Pelayo R, Chervin RD. Sleepwalking and sleep terrors in prepubertal children: what triggers them? *Pediatrics*. 2003;111(1):e17–e25.

119. Cirignotta F, Zucconi M, Mondini S, Lenzi PL, Lugaresi E. Enuresis, sleepwalking, and nightmares: an epidemiological survey in the Republic of San Marino. In: Guilleminault C, Lugaresi E, eds. *Sleep/Wake Disorders: Natural History, Epidemiology, and Long-Term Evolution*. New York, NY: Raven Press; 1983:237–241.

120. Hublin C, Kaprio J, Partinen M, Heikkila K, Koskenvuo M. Prevalence and genetics of sleepwalking: a population-based twin study. *Neurology*. 1997;48(1):177–181.

121. Klackenberg G. Somnambulism in childhood—prevalence, course and behavioral correlations. A prospective longitudinal study (6–16 years). *Acta Paediatr Scand*. 1982;71(3):495–499.

122. Stores G. Dramatic parasomnias. *J R Soc Med*. 2001;94(4):173–176.

123. Lecendreux M, Bassetti C, Dauvilliers Y, Mayer G, Neidhart E, Tafti M. HLA and genetic susceptibility to sleepwalking. *Mol Psychiatry*. 2003;8(1):114–117.

124. Hublin C, Kaprio J, Partinen M, Koskenvu M. Parasomnias: co-occurrence and genetics. *Psychiatr Genet*. 2001;11(2):65–70.

125. Kales A, Soldatos CR, Bixler EO, et al. Hereditary factors in sleepwalking and night terrors. *Br J Psychiatry*. 1980;137:111–118.

126. Broughton RJ. Sleep disorders: disorders of arousal? Enuresis, somnambulism, and nightmares occur in confusional states of arousal, not in "dreaming sleep". *Science.* 1968;159(819):1070–1078.

127. Pilon M, Montplaisir J, Zadra A. Precipitating factors of somnambulism: impact of sleep deprivation and forced arousals. *Neurology.* 2008;70(24):2284–2290.

128. Frank NC, Spirito A, Stark L, Owens-Stively J. The use of scheduled awakenings to eliminate childhood sleepwalking. *J Pediatr Psychol.* 1997;22(3):345–353.

129. Schenck CH, Mahowald MW. Long-term, nightly benzodiazepine treatment of injurious parasomnias and other disorders of disrupted nocturnal sleep in 170 adults. *Am J Med.* 1996;100(3):333–337.

130. Crisp AH. The sleepwalking/night terrors syndrome in adults. *Postgrad Med J.* 1996;72(852):599–604.

131. Roth B, Nevsimalova S, Rechtschaffen A. Hypersomnia with "sleep drunkenness". *Arch Gen Psychiatry.* 1972;26(5):456–462.

132. Rosen G, Mahowald MW, Ferber R. Sleepwalking, confusional arousals, and sleep terrors in the child. In: Ferber R, Kryger MH, eds. *Principles and Practice of Sleep Medicine in the Child.* Philadelphia, PA: WB Saunders; 1995:99.

133. Sallustro F, Atwell CW. Body rocking, head banging, and head rolling in normal children. *J Pediatr.* 1978;93(4):704–708.

134. Thorpy MJ, Glovinsky PB. Parasomnias. *Psychiatr Clin North Am.* 1987;10(4):623–639.

135. Klackenberg G. A prospective longitudinal study of children. Data on psychic health and development up to 8 years of age. *Acta Paediatr Scand Suppl.* 1971;224:1–239.

136. Chisholm T, Morehouse RL. Adult headbanging: sleep studies and treatment. *Sleep.* 1996;19(4):343–346.

137. Laberge L, Tremblay RE, Vitaro F, Montplaisir J. Development of parasomnias from childhood to early adolescence. *Pediatrics.* 2000;106(1 Pt 1):67–74.

138. Manni R, Terzaghi M. Rhythmic movements in idiopathic REM sleep behavior disorder. *Mov Disord.* 2007;22(12):1797–1800.

139. Mackenzie JM. "Headbanging" and fatal subdural haemorrhage. *Lancet.* 1991;338(8780):1457–1458.

140. Bemporad JR, Sours JA, Spalter HF. Cataracts following chronic headbanging: a report of two cases. *Am J Psychiatry.* 1968;125(2):245–249.

141. Manni R, Terzaghi M. Rhythmic movements during sleep: a physiological and pathological profile. *Neurol Sci.* 2005;26(suppl 3):s181–s185.

142. Hoban TF. Rhythmic movement disorder in children. *CNS Spectr.* 2003;8(2):135–138.

143. Kohyama J, Matsukura F, Kimura K, Tachibana N. Rhythmic movement disorder: polysomnographic study and summary of reported cases. *Brain Dev.* 2002;24(1):33–38.

144. Thorpy MJ. Classification of sleep disorders. *J Clin Neurophysiol.* 1990;7(1):67–81.

145. Ambrogetti A, Olson LG, Saunders NA. Disorders of movement and behaviour during sleep. *Med J Aust.* 1991;155(5):336–340.

146. Alves RS, Aloe F, Silva AB, Tavares SM. Jactatio capitis nocturna with persistence in adulthood. Case report. *Arq Neuropsiquiatr.* 1998;56(3B):655–657.

147. Etzioni T, Katz N, Hering E, Ravid S, Pillar G. Controlled sleep restriction for rhythmic movement disorder. *J Pediatr.* 2005;147(3):393–395.

148. Bixler EO, Kales A, Soldatos CR, Kales JD, Healey S. Prevalence of sleep disorders in the Los Angeles metropolitan area. *Am J Psychiatry.* 1979;136(10):1257–1262.

149. Lloyd R, Tippmann-Peikert M, Slocumb N, Kotagal S. Characteristics of REM sleep behavior disorder in childhood. *J Clin Sleep Med.* 2012;8(2):127.

150. Schenck CH, Bundlie SR, Ettinger MG, Mahowald MW. Chronic behavioral disorders of human REM sleep: a new category of parasomnia. *Sleep.* 1986;9(2):293–308.

151. Schenck CH, Mahowald MW. Motor dyscontrol in narcolepsy: rapid-eye-movement (REM) sleep without atonia and REM sleep behavior disorder. *Ann Neurol.* 1992;32(1):3–10.

152. Sheldon SH, Jacobsen J. REM-sleep motor disorder in children. *J Child Neurol.* 1998;13(6):257–260.

153. Herman JH, Blaw ME, Steinberg JB. REM behavior disorder in a two-year old male with evidence of brainstem pathology. *Sleep Res.* 1989;18:242.

154. Nevsimalova S, Prihodova I, Kemlink D, Lin L, Mignot E. REM behavior disorder (RBD) can be one of the first symptoms of childhood narcolepsy. *Sleep Med.* 2007;8(7):784–786.

155. Postuma RB, Lang AE, Massicotte-Marquez J, Montplaisir J. Potential early markers of Parkinson disease in idiopathic REM sleep behavior disorder. *Neurology.* 2006;66(6):845–851.

V. SELECTED SECONDARY MOVEMENT DISORDERS

156. Boeve BF, Silber MH, Ferman TJ, Lucas JA, Parisi JE. Association of REM sleep behavior disorder and neurodegenerative disease may reflect an underlying synucleinopathy. *Mov Disord.* 2001;16(4):622–630.

157. Boeve BF, Silber MH, Parisi JE, et al. Synucleinopathy pathology and REM sleep behavior disorder plus dementia or parkinsonism. *Neurology.* 2003;61(1):40–45.

158. Schenck CH, Mahowald MW. Polysomnographic, neurologic, psychiatric, and clinical outcome report on 70 consecutive cases, with the REM sleep behavior disorders (RBD): sustained clonazepam efficacy in 89.5% of 57 treated patients. *Clev Clin J Med.* 1990;57:S10–S24.

159. Iranzo A, Santamaria J, Pujol J, Moreno A, Deus J, Tolosa E. Brainstem proton magnetic resonance spectroscopy in idiopathic REM sleep behavior disorder. *Sleep.* 2002;25(8):867–870.

160. Albin RL, Koeppe RA, Chervin RD, et al. Decreased striatal dopaminergic innervation in REM sleep behavior disorder. *Neurology.* 2000;55(9):1410–1412.

161. Eisensehr I, Linke R, Noachtar S, Schwarz J, Gildehaus FJ, Tatsch K. Reduced striatal dopamine transporters in idiopathic rapid eye movement sleep behaviour disorder. Comparison with Parkinson's disease and controls. *Brain.* 2000;123(Pt 6):1155–1160.

162. Schindler K, Gast H, Bassetti C, et al. Hyperperfusion of anterior cingulate gyrus in a case of paroxysmal nocturnal dystonia. *Neurology.* 2001;57(5):917–920.

163. Kim KB, Cabanillas ME, Lazar AJ, et al. Clinical responses to vemurafenib in patients with metastatic papillary thyroid cancer harboring BRAF(V600E) mutation. *Thyroid.* 2013;23(10):1277–1283.

164. Wulff K, Porcheret K, Cussans E, Foster RG. Sleep and circadian rhythm disturbances: multiple genes and multiple phenotypes. *Curr Opin Genet Dev.* 2009;19(3):237–246.

165. Cole RJ, Smith JS, Alcal YC, Elliott JA, Kripke DF. Bright-light mask treatment of delayed sleep phase syndrome. *J Biol Rhythms.* 2002;17(1):89–101.

166. Lavigne GJ, Rompre PH, Poirier G, Huard H, Kato T, Montplaisir JY. Rhythmic masticatory muscle activity during sleep in humans. *J Dent Res.* 2001;80(2):443–448.

167. Bader G, Lavigne G. Sleep bruxism; an overview of an oromandibular sleep movement disorder—review article. *Sleep Med Rev.* 2000;4(1):27–43.

168. Widmalm SE, Christiansen RL, Gunn SM, Hawley LM. Prevalence of signs and symptoms of craniomandibular disorders and orofacial parafunction in 4–6-year-old African-American and Caucasian children. *J Oral Rehabil.* 1995;22(2):87–93.

169. Lavigne GJ, Rompre PH, Montplaisir JY. Sleep bruxism: validity of clinical research diagnostic criteria in a controlled polysomnographic study. *J Dent Res.* 1996;75(1):546–552.

170. Hublin C, Kaprio J, Partinen M, Koskenvuo M. Sleep bruxism based on self-report in a nationwide twin cohort. *J Sleep Res.* 1998;7(1):61–67.

171. Kato T, Montplaisir JY, Guitard F, Sessle BJ, Lund JP, Lavigne GJ. Evidence that experimentally induced sleep bruxism is a consequence of transient arousal. *J Dent Res.* 2003;82(4):284–288.

172. Lavigne GJ, Kato T, Kolta A, Sessle BJ. Neurobiological mechanisms involved in sleep bruxism. *Crit Rev Oral Biol Med.* 2003;14(1):30–46.

173. Ellison JM, Stanziani P. SSRI-associated nocturnal bruxism in four patients. *J Clin Psychiatry.* 1993;54(11):432–434.

174. Falisi G, Rastelli C, Panti F, Maglione H, Quezada Arcega R. Psychotropic drugs and bruxism. *Expert Opin Drug Saf.* 2014;13(10):1319–1326.

175. Clarke JH, Reynolds PJ. Suggestive hypnotherapy for nocturnal bruxism: a pilot study. *Am J Clin Hypn.* 1991;33(4):248–253.

176. Tan E, Jankovic J. Treating severe bruxism with botulinum toxin. *J Am Dent Assoc.* 2000;131(2):211–216.

177. Chasins AI. Methocarbamol (robaxin) as an adjunct in the treatment of bruxism. *J Dent Med.* 1959;14:166–169.

178. Lavigne GJ, Montplaisir JV. Bruxism: epidemiology, diagnosis, pathophysiology, and pharmacology. In: Friction JR, Dubner R, eds. *Orofacial Pain and Temporomandibular Disorders.* New York, NY: Raven Press; 1995:387–404.

179. Dao TT, Lavigne GJ. Oral splints: the crutches for temporomandibular disorders and bruxism? *Crit Rev Oral Biol Med.* 1998;9(3):345–361.

180. Valiente López M, Selms M, Zaag J, Hamburger H, Lobbezoo F. Do sleep hygiene measures and progressive muscle relaxation influence sleep bruxism? Report of a randomised controlled trial. *J Oral Rehabil.* 2014;42(4):259–265.

181. Macedo CR, Macedo EC, Torloni MR, Silva AB, Prado GF. Pharmacotherapy for sleep bruxism. *Cochrane Database Syst Rev.* 2014;10:CD005578.

182. Mahowald MW, Schenck CH. REM sleep parasomnias. In: Kryger MH, Roth T, Dement WC, eds. *Principles and Practice of Sleep Medicine.* Philadelphia, PA: WB Saunders; 2000:724–741.

183. Rothenberger A, Kostanecka T, Kinkelbur J, Cohrs S, Woerner W, Hajak G. Sleep and Tourette syndrome. *Adv Neurol.* 2001;85:245–259.

184. Mano T, Shiozawa Z, Sobue I. Extrapyramidal involuntary movements during sleep. *Electroencephalogr Clin Neurophysiol Suppl.* 1982;35:431–442.

185. Chokroverty S, Barron KD. Palatal myoclonus and rhythmic ocular movements: a polygraphic study. *Neurology.* 1969;19(10):975–982.

186. Cohrs S, Rasch T, Altmeyer S, et al. Decreased sleep quality and increased sleep related movements in patients with Tourette's syndrome. *J Neurol Neurosurg Psychiatry.* 2001;70(2):192–197.

187. Fish DR, Sawyers D, Allen PJ, Blackie JD, Lees AJ, Marsden CD. The effect of sleep on the dyskinetic movements of Parkinson's disease, Gilles de la Tourette syndrome, Huntington's disease, and torsion dystonia. *Arch Neurol.* 1991;48(2):210–214.

188. Glaze DG, Frost Jr. JD, Jankovic J. Sleep in Gilles de la Tourette's syndrome: disorder of arousal. *Neurology.* 1983;33(5):586–592.

189. Van Hove JL, Steyaert J, Matthijs G, et al. Expanded motor and psychiatric phenotype in autosomal dominant Segawa syndrome due to GTP cyclohydrolase deficiency. *J Neurol Neurosurg Psychiatry.* 2006;77(1):18–23.

190. Baca-Garcia E, Stanilla JK, Buchel C, Gattaz WF, de Leon J. Diurnal variability of orofacial dyskinetic movements. *Pharmacopsychiatry.* 1999;32(2):73–75.

191. Yokota T, Atsumi Y, Uchiyama M, Fukukawa T, Tsukagoshi H. Electroencephalographic activity related to palatal myoclonus in REM sleep. *J Neurol.* 1990;237(5):290–294.

192. Singh K. Sleep related infantile tremors. *Indian Pediatr.* 2001;38(10):1197–1198.

193. Jarman PR, Wood NW, Davis MT, et al. Hereditary geniospasm: linkage to chromosome 9q13-q21 and evidence for genetic heterogeneity. *Am J Hum Genet.* 1997;61(4):928–933.

194. Kharraz B, Reilich P, Noachtar S, Danek A. An episode of geniospasm in sleep: toward new insights into pathophysiology? *Mov Disord.* 2008;23(2):274–276.

195. Malow BA, Vaughn BV. Treatment of sleep disorders in epilepsy. *Epilepsy Behav.* 2002;3(5S):35–37.

196. Zucconi M, Ferini-Strambi L. NREM parasomnias: arousal disorders and differentiation from nocturnal frontal lobe epilepsy. *Clin Neurophysiol.* 2000;111(suppl 2):S129–S135.

197. Steriade M, McCormick DA, Sejnowski TJ. Thalamocortical oscillations in the sleeping and aroused brain. *Science.* 1993;262(5134):679–685.

198. Malow BA, Lin X, Kushwaha R, Aldrich MS. Interictal spiking increases with sleep depth in temporal lobe epilepsy. *Epilepsia.* 1998;39(12):1309–1316.

199. Minecan D, Natarajan A, Marzec M, Malow B. Relationship of epileptic seizures to sleep stage and sleep depth. *Sleep.* 2002;25(8):899–904.

200. Touchon J, Baldy-Moulinier M, Billiard M, Besset A, Cadilhac J. Sleep organization and epilepsy. In: Degen R, Rodin EA, eds. *Epilepsy, Sleep and Sleep Deprivation (Epilepsy Research Supplement).* 2nd ed. Amsterdam: Elsevier Science Ltd; 1991:286.

201. Nobili L. Nocturnal frontal lobe epilepsy and non-rapid eye movement sleep parasomnias: differences and similarities. *Sleep Med Rev.* 2007;11(4):251–254.

202. Tinuper P, Provini F, Bisulli F, et al. Movement disorders in sleep: guidelines for differentiating epileptic from non-epileptic motor phenomena arising from sleep. *Sleep Med Rev.* 2007;11(4):255–267.

203. Provini F, Montagna P, Plazzi G, Lugaresi E. Nocturnal frontal lobe epilepsy: a wide spectrum of seizures. *Mov Disord.* 2000;15(6):1264.

204. Provini F, Plazzi G, Lugaresi E. From nocturnal paroxysmal dystonia to nocturnal frontal lobe epilepsy. *Clin Neurophysiol.* 2000;111:S2–S8.

205. Cao R, Obrietan K. mTOR Signaling and entrainment of the mammalian circadian clock. *Mol Cell Pharmacol.* 2010;2(4):125–130.

Cerebral Palsy

Harvey S. Singer[1], Jonathan W. Mink[2],
Donald L. Gilbert[3] and Joseph Jankovic[4]

[1]Department of Neurology, Johns Hopkins Hospital, Baltimore, MD, USA;
[2]Division of Child Neurology, University of Rochester Medical Center,
Rochester, NY, USA; [3]Division of Neurology, Cincinnati Children's Hospital
Medical Center, Cincinnati, OH, USA; [4]Department of Neurology, Baylor
College of Medicine, Houston, TX, USA

O U T L I N E

Movement Disorders in Childhood, Second Edition.
DOI: http://dx.doi.org/10.1016/B978-0-12-411573-6.00020-6

INTRODUCTION

Use of the term *cerebral palsy* has been controversial, considered by some to be a nonspecific "wastebasket" and by others a valuable diagnostic tool.[1] The diagnosis, which rests solely upon the presence of motor disability and a nonprogressive course, provides individuals with greater access to medical care, rehabilitation, educational, and social services. Historically, the initial association among prematurity, birth injury, and perinatal asphyxia with cerebral palsy (CP) is attributed to Dr William John Little in a lecture presented to the Obstetric Society of London.[2] Subsequent major contributions were made by William Osler, who introduced the phrase "cerebral palsy" to describe this nonprogressive disorder,[3] and Sigmund Freud, who extended Little's observations to include factors in early pregnancy, as well as emphasizing the cerebral abnormality in spastic diplegia.[4,5] Despite these early seminal contributions and the efforts of multiple other investigators, the definition of cerebral palsy continues to evolve, a widely accepted classifications system remains a goal, the epidemiology of this disorder continues to be augmented, and its therapy remains a challenge.

A recent definition by an international executive committee proposed, "cerebral palsy describes a group of permanent disorders of the development of movement and posture, causing activity limitation, that are attributed to non-progressive disturbances that occurred in the developing fetal or infant brain. The motor disorders of cerebral palsy are often accompanied by disturbances of sensation, perception, cognition, communication and behavior, by epilepsy, and by secondary musculoskeletal problems."[6] Whether this broad definition will be widely endorsed remains unknown. For example, despite requirements of nonprogressive disturbances, motor abnormalities, especially tone and posture, are not always fixed even in the presence of underlying static brain lesions.[7–9] Further, there is no consensus for a required etiology, leading to the inclusion of subjects under this rubric who have diverse etiologies ranging from developmental malformations to metabolic disorders. Proposed classifications for this clinical syndrome have included the anatomical site of the lesion (cortex, basal ganglia, cerebellum), type of movement (chorea, dystonia, ataxic, and mixed) or presence of spasticity, type of tone abnormality (hypotonia or hypertonia), involvement of extremities (hemiplegia, diplegia, quadriplegia), and causation and timing of the insult (prepartum, intrapartum, postnatal). In the future, it is likely that the umbrella term CP will be classified based on causal factors with a description of physical alterations and functional impairments.

EPIDEMIOLOGY

The overall prevalence of CP is about 2.0 to 3.5/1000 live births. The prevalence is greater in low birth weight infants (90/1000 weighing less than 1000 g versus 1.5/1000 in those weighing 2500 g or more).[6,10–12] Term infants represent more than half of all cases with CP.[13] Compared with singletons, the relative risk of CP in twins is 5.6 and in triplets is 12.6.[6] The death in utero of a co-twin places the surviving twin at high risk for developmental problems. Improvements in obstetric and neonatal care have reduced the incidence of CP in prematures,[14,15] but the overall prevalence has not changed due to a stable rate in term infants, greater survival in preterm, and extended longevity.[16] Most cases of CP have no relationship to prematurity or asphyxia.[17] The full extent of the motor disability may not be evident until 3–4 years of age. The majority of children affected with CP survive into adulthood, but life expectancy is negatively affected by the presence of severe quadriplegia, profound retardation, visual impairments, and lack of appropriate medical care. In addition to the defining motor disabilities, individuals with CP have a variety of non-movement problems, including intellectual disability (40–70%), epilepsy (35–94%), speech and language disorders (50–60%), chronic sleep disorders, and disorders of vision or hearing (10–30%).[18–26] Children with CP also have more psychological difficulties than do children in the general population.[27,28] The association between socioeconomic status (SES) and CP is controversial; with some evidence suggesting that the effect of SES goes beyond just mediating factors affecting preterm birth, low birth weight, and postnatal trauma.[28]

ETIOLOGY

The etiology of CP is extensive, ranging from prenatal and perinatal events to postnatal insults (Table 20.1).[16,17,29–31] Hypoxic-ischemic encephalopathy (HIE) represents only a small category within the neonatal encephalopathies and an even smaller contributor to the causes of CP. Non-hypoxia/asphyxia causes of CP are numerous and include cerebral dysgenesis, intra-uterine infection,[32] intrauterine growth restriction,[33] preterm birth,[34,35] coagulation disorders, antepartum hemorrhage,[35] multiple pregnancies, abnormal presentations, neurometabolic diseases,[36,37] chromosomal anomalies,[37] selected polymorphisms,[38,39] congenital abnormalities, and many others affecting either the mother or child.[16] Neonatal stroke (ischemic perinatal infarction or sinovenous thrombosis) is an important cause of CP. It has been emphasized that treatable inborn errors of metabolism can present as cerebral palsy mimics.[36]

An ongoing challenge in children presenting with motor delays or impairment early in life is to identify those that are due to neurogenetic disorders masquerading as CP.[40] The possibility of identifying a treatable genetic or metabolic etiology emphasizes the need for identifying the underlying etiology. Clinical and imaging indicators that suggest a need to consider additional evaluation for an impersonator or "masquerader" for CP include: a normal MRI; abnormal imaging restricted to the globus pallidus; severe symptoms in the absence of a history of perinatal insult; a positive family history; progressive worsening of symptomatology or neurodevelopmental regression; and physical findings of isolated muscle hypotonia, rigidity, and paraplegia.[40] Despite the extensive list of potential etiologies, it is not unusual to fail to identify a clear etiology.

Criteria supporting an acute intrapartum hypoxic event sufficient to cause a CP event are presented in Tables 20.2 and 20.3.[41,42]

DIFFERENTIATING HYPERTONIA IN CHILDREN

Hypertonia is defined as an abnormally increased resistance, perceived by the examiner, to an externally imposed movement about a joint, while the patient is attempting to maintain a relaxed state of muscle activity. A National Institutes of Health (NIH)–sponsored task force has established a classification and definition of disorders causing hypertonia in children (Table 20.4).[43]

TABLE 20.1   Etiological Factors in CP

Maternal	Child
History of fetal loss	Prematurity
Unusual menstrual periods	Low birth weight
Thyroid disease	Multiple birth
Estrogen administration	Death in utero of a co-twin
Febrile urinary tract infections	Abnormal presentations
Thrombophilic disorders	Growth retardation
Hemorrhage (placental separation)	Nuchal cord
Toxic ingestion	Chorioamnionitis
Toxemia	Infections (uterine and neonatal)
Low socioeconomic status	Developmental brain malformations
	Thrombophilic disorders (neonatal stroke)
	Vascular malformations
	Congenital heart disease
	Chromosomal abnormalities
	Neonatal encephalopathy (hypoxic ischemic)
	Metabolic abnormalities
	Endocrine abnormalities
	Trauma
	Kernicterus
	Intraventricular hemorrhage
	Intracranial hemorrhage

TABLE 20.2   Four Essential Criteria Required to Define an Acute Intrapartum Hypoxic Event Sufficient to Cause CP

1. Evidence of metabolic acidosis in fetal umbilical arterial cord blood obtained at delivery (e.g., pH <7 and base deficit $\geq 12\,mmol/L$)
2. Early onset of severe or moderate neonatal encephalopathy in infants born at 34 or more weeks of gestation
3. CP of the spastic quadriplegic or dyskinetic type
4. Exclusion of other identifiable etiologies (e.g., trauma, coagulation defects, infectious conditions, or genetic abnormalities)

Adapted from Ref. [42].

TABLE 20.3   Other Criteria Suggesting Intrapartum Timing for the Occurrence of the Injury

1. A sentinel (signal) hypoxic event occurring immediately before or during labor
2. A sudden sustained fetal bradycardia or the absence of fetal heart rate variability in the presence of persistent late or persistent variable decelerations, usually after a hypoxic sentinel event when the pattern was previously normal
3. Apgar scores of 0 to 3 beyond 5 min
4. Onset of multisystem involvement within 72 h after birth
5. An early imaging study showing evidence of acute nonfocal cerebral edema

Adapted from Ref. [42].

TABLE 20.4   Differentiating Childhood Hypertonia

	Spasticity	Dystonia	Rigidity
Summary	Velocity-dependent resistance	Sustained or intermittent muscle contractions	Independent of both speed and posture
Effect of increasing speed of passive movement on resistance	Increases	No effect	No effect
Effect of rapid reversal of direction on resistance	Delayed	Immediate	Immediate
Presence of a fixed posture	Only in severe cases	Yes	No
Effect of behavioral and emotional state on pattern of activated muscles	Minimal	Yes	Minimal
Direction	Unidirectional	Bidirectional	Bidirectional
Presence of upper motor neuron findings (clonus, hyperreflexia, +Babinski)	Yes	No	No

Adapted in part from Ref. [43].

A valid and reliable "Hypertonia Assessment Tool" (HAT) has been developed to assist in distinguishing among these forms of hypertonia.[177,178] The major causes for hypertonia include the following:

Spasticity

Hypertonia in which one or both of the following signs are present:
1. Resistance to externally imposed movement increases with increasing speed of stretch and varies with the direction of joint movement.
2. Resistance to externally imposed movement rises rapidly above a threshold speed or joint angle. *Note:* Spasticity is defined only in terms of properties of the joint being examined. It does not depend on the presence of other positive (clonus, Babinski sign, hyperactive reflexes) or negative (weakness, poor coordination, loss of control) features, although these are frequently present.[43]

Dystonia

Dystonia is a movement disorder characterized by sustained or intermittent muscle contractions causing abnormal, often repetitive, movements, postures, or both. Dystonic movements are typically patterned, twisting, and may be tremulous (see Chapter 3).

Note: Dystonia causes hypertonia only when there is co-contraction. Not all dystonia is hypertonic!

Rigidity

Hypertonia with all of the following:

1. The resistance to externally imposed joint movement is present at very low speeds of movement, does not depend on imposed speed, and does not exhibit a speed or angle threshold.
2. Simultaneous co-contraction of agonists and antagonists may occur, and this is reflected in an immediate resistance to a reversal of the direction of movement about a joint.
3. The limb does not tend to return toward a particular fixed posture or extreme joint angle.
4. Voluntary activity in distant muscle groups does not lead to involuntary movements about the rigid joints, although rigidity may worsen.

CEREBRAL PALSY SYNDROMES

Cerebral palsy is usually evident in the first 12–18 months of life. The typical presentation is a delay in attaining motor milestones, or findings of asymmetric motor function or abnormalities of muscle tone. Serial neurodevelopmental evaluations are often required for proper classification of the subtype, because findings on examination may be affected by the state of alertness, emotional stress, and irritability. Additionally, neurologic findings that are considered abnormal in adults may be physiologic during the first months of life (e.g., ankle clonus, brisk reflexes, and extensor plantar responses). Several early indicators of the presence of significant motor disability include delay in the appearance of motor milestones, early hand preference, and exaggerated or persistent primitive reflexes.[45,46] Classification systems with prognostic implications for development and provisions for comparisons between centers have been published.[47,48] Gross motor function tends to improve in most children up to the age of 6–7 years which then tends to remain stable at least until early adolescence.[47] Conventionally CP has been classified by the (i) predominant motor disability: *spastic* (about 50%); *dyskinetic* (about 20%); *ataxic* (about 10%); and *mixed* (about 20%). In actuality most CP patients are mixed in type to some degree, e.g., mild dyskinetic signs are often present in subtypes of spastic CP and (ii) the topographic involvement (hemiplegia, diplegia, and quadriplegia). Although these classifications continue to have clinical utility, in terms of prognosis they are not very reliable or predictable.

Spastic Type

The spastic type of CP is further divided into several subtypes on the basis of distribution of impairment: *hemiplegia*, with homolateral involvement of the arm and leg; *quadriplegia*, with severe impairment of all four extremities, usually the lower more than the upper; *tetraplegia*, with involvement of all four extremities, usually the upper greater than the lower; and *diplegia*, with milder impairment of all four extremities, but with the arms relatively spared. Although the frequency of types varies in different populations, a Scandinavian study reported that 33% of cases were hemiplegic, 6% quadriplegic, and 44% diplegic.[49] All subtypes of spastic CP are associated with increased resistance to passive joint extension (hypertonia), hyperreflexia, clonus, and abnormal plantar responses. Many infants with CP, however, pass through an initial hypotonic phase. In general, neurologic abnormalities indicating spasticity are present during quiet periods and sleep and do not change significantly with activity or emotional stress. Pseudobulbar palsy, indicated by expressionless facies and clonus, may be seen in both spastic and dyskinetic forms. The child with spastic CP is typically prone to develop earlier contractures and have more frequent orthopedic problems than does a child with choreoathetotic CP.

The *hemiplegic* form has findings localized to one extremity, usually with the upper extremity more involved than the lower. Hemiplegia tends to be obvious in the second year of life, but maybe missed in the first 3–5 months of life. For unknown reasons, the left hemisphere is affected in two-thirds of children.[50] The appearance of hemiplegic CP in full-term infants is usually associated with prenatal circulatory disturbances (stroke) or, less commonly, cerebral dysgenesis (schizencephaly).[51,52] The etiologies of vascular occlusions include thrombophilic disorders (e.g., deficiencies of factor V Leiden, protein C or S, and the presence of anticardiolipin antibodies), an infectious process, venous sinus thrombosis, or congenital heart disease. Children with hemiplegic CP typically learn to walk by approximately age 2 years. The incidence of seizures approaches 70%, but cognitive capabilities are generally spared.

The *diplegic* subtype has spasticity greater in the legs than in the arms. This form typically appears in infants born prematurely and is associated with destruction of cerebral white matter adjacent to the lateral ventricles, i.e., periventricular leukomalacia (PVL). Preferential involvement of the corticostriatal fibers adjacent to the ventricle, which carry inputs to the lower extremities, explains the clinical presentation. More than half of the children learn to walk, usually by age 3 years, but assisted devices are often required. Retardation of linear growth of the lower limb is often present.

The neurobiological mechanism of PVL in the premature infant involves several interacting factors.[53,54] Predisposing conditions for involvement of the cerebral white matter include immature development of the vascular supply to this region and a maturation-dependent impairment of regulation of cerebral blood flow. Another major factor is the vulnerability of the oligodendroglial precursor cell (pre-OL) to attack by free radicals and glutamate generated by ischemia-reperfusion. The pre-OL, in turn, undergoes an apoptotic death.[55] Severity of white matter injury correlates with the distribution of pre-OL.[56] Other factors besides ischemia-reperfusion and excitotoxic agents may also be involved in causing damage to the immature oligodendrocyte. For example, maternal or fetal infection, inflammation, cytokines, and hyaluronic acid have been hypothesized to play important contributory roles through their effect on either vascular hemodynamics, generation of reactive oxygen species, direct toxicity, or ability to block remyelination. Others suggest an additional role for nutritional and hormonal deprivation.[57] A study demonstrating distinct differences in inflammatory response and cytokine expression in postmortem neonatal brains with and without PVL provides support for involvement of an inflammatory cytokine-mediated hypothesis.[58] Hyaluronic acid blocks pre-OL differentiation into mature oligodendroglia

TABLE 20.5   Neurogenetic Disorders Impersonating Spasticity CP

Developmental brain abnormalities: Holoprosencephaly; schizencephaly; lissencephaly; hemimegancephaly; polymicrogyria; agenesis of the corpus callosum; X-linked hydrocephalus with aqueductal stenosis; Aicardi Goutières syndrome.

Dysmyelinating disorders: Krabbe disease, Alexander disease, Pelizaeus Merzbacher disease, hereditary spastic paraplegias.

Aminoacids: Arginase deficiency, homocystinuria

Mitochondria: Mitochondrial DNA depletion syndrome

Cofactors: Sulfite oxidase/molybdenum cofactor deficiency

Others: Hyperekplexia

and, in turn, remyelination.[59] The greater predilection for PVL in the presence of interventricular hemorrhage may be related to local increases in iron concentration. Cystic PVL and concurrent grade 3 germinal matrix hemorrhages are associated with more severe CP.[60]

The *quadriplegic* subtype is the most severe form, with all four limbs significantly involved and considerable compromise of motor function. These children have the early onset of motor delays and are at greater risk for severe mental retardation, epilepsy, dysarthria, microcephaly, and strabismus.[61] Approximately one-quarter require total care and one-third walk after age 3 years. Intellectual dysfunction and involvement of bulbar musculature are major life limiting problems.

Spastic quadriplegia in the premature infant may be the result of severe PVL and in the full-term infant may be caused by prenatal insults, such as severe PVL, developmental brain malformations (e.g., holoprosencephaly, lissencephaly, and pachygyria), destructive brain lesions (e.g., intrauterine infections, infarction, hydrocephalus), perinatal asphyxia, or other neurogenetic disorders (see Table 20.5). Neonatal hypoxic-ischemic injury affects a variety of brain regions in the prenatal and perinatal brain through multiple mechanisms including energy depletion, release of excitatory amino acids, accumulation of reactive oxygen species, and initiation of apoptosis.[62,63] Ischemic cell death is initiated by the decline of cerebral microcirculation and inhibition of oxidative phosphorylation, which in turn causes a cascade of disturbances of intracellular homeostasis, e.g., decreased pH, decreased adenosine triphosphate (ATP), increased mitochondrial free radical production via the mitochondrial redox chain, diminished function of the Na^+-K^+ ATPase pump with increased intracellular sodium and subsequently water, and membrane depolarization.[64,65] These primary events, in turn, lead to a secondary cascade including the release of excitatory amino acids (e.g., glutamate), activation of NMDA receptors, influx of calcium, the formation of more reactive ion species that cause oxidative damage to lipids, proteins, and other cell constituents, and ultimately to cell death.[66]

Dyskinetic (Choreoathetoid; Extrapyramidal) Type

Dyskinetic CP syndromes are characterized by the presence of the involuntary movements of chorea, athetosis, and dystonia (Video 20.1). These movements typically begin after the second year of life, may progress slowly for several years, and persist into adulthood.

TABLE 20.6   Neurogenetic Disorders Impersonating Dyskinetic CP

Pediatric Neurotransmitter disorders: Aromatic acid decarboxylase deficiency; dopa-responsive dystonia; dopamine transporter deficiency; brain dopamine-serotonin vesicular transport disease; succinic semialdehyde dehydrogenase deficiency

Mineral accumulation: Pantothenate kinase–associated neurodegeneration; Wilson's disease

Neuronal storage disorders: Infantile GM2 gangliosidosis; Neimann–Pich type A; Infantile neuronal ceroid lipofuscinosis

Aminoacids: Non-ketotic hyperglycinemia; Maple syrup urine disease

Organic acids: Glutaric aciduria; proprionic aciduria; methylmalonic aciduria

Mitochondria: Leigh syndrome

Purine metabolism: Lesch-Nyhan disease

Glycolysis: Triose phosphate isomerase deficiency

Creatine metabolism: Creatine deficiency syndrome

Cofactor disorders: Molybdenum cofactor (sulfite oxidase) deficiency

Others: Glucose transporter 1 deficiency; congenital disorders of glycosylation; pontocerebellar hypoplasia type 2

The time delay in the onset of dystonia following perinatal asphyxia has ranged from 1–32 years.[67] Abnormal movements usually involve all four extremities with the upper usually being functionally more involved than the lower extremities. Dyskinetic CP is often misdiagnosed as a spastic form because of the misinterpretation of clinical signs, e.g., spontaneous extensor plantar responses may represent dystonic posturing, rather than a traditional Babinski sign. Furthermore, extrapyramidal hypertonicity is present throughout flexion and extension of an extremity (lead pipe rigidity). Cogwheel rigidity is unusual in young children with CP. Oral motor dysfunction and tongue thrusting are common symptoms. Extrapyramidal movements show marked variability depending on the state of the individual; they are decreased during relaxation and sleep and increased by anxiety and stress. Dyskinetic forms of CP, especially those associated with athetosis, tend to occur in term infants with severe perinatal asphyxia. Pathophysiologically, extrapyramidal CP has been localized within the basal ganglia (neostriatum and/or globus pallidus) and/or thalamus, although more precise localization is lacking.[68] Lesions in these regions often appear at the end of a term gestation, usually after acute near total asphyxia.[69]

Since the etiology for dyskinetic CP may be heterogeneous and include metabolic or genetic components, it is important to follow the patient for progressive changes and to consider a broader diagnostic evaluation. Other disorders to consider include kernicterus, mitochondrial abnormalities, dopa-responsive dystonia, organic acidurias, Krebs cycle defects, creatine deficiency, succinic semialdehyde dehydrogenase deficiency, Lesch-Nyhan syndrome, ataxia telangiectasia, and female carriers of ornithine transcarbamylase deficiency.[70–77] (see Table 20.6 and Chapter 17).

Ataxic (Cerebellar) Type

The cerebellar or ataxic form represents a clinically and etiologically heterogeneous group.[78] Classic associated findings include hypotonia, truncal titubation, dysmetria, cerebellar eye movements, and an ataxic gait. Children with ataxic syndromes usually have a prenatal etiology (e.g., developmental malformations of the cerebellum), but this can also be of heterogeneous origin (e.g., mitochondrial disorder, carbohydrate deficient glycoprotein

TABLE 20.7 Neurogenetic Disorders Impersonating Ataxic CP

Developmental brain abnormalities: Dandy–Walker malformation; Joubert syndrome; rhombencephalosynapsis
Dysmyelinating disorders: Vanishing white matter disease; hypomyelination with congenital cataract; metachromatic leukodystrophy; peroxisome biogenesis disorders; Canavan disease
Lysosomal storage: Neimann–Pick type C; GM1 and GM2 gangliosidoses; neuronal ceroid lipofuscinosis; infantile sialic acid storage disorder; Gaucher disease type II and III
Aminoacids: Phenylketonuria
Organic acids: L-2-hydroxyglutaric aciduria; methylmalonic aciduria
Glycolosis, pyruvate metabolism, and TCA cycle: Pyruvate dehydrogenase deficiency; fumerase deficiency; galactosemia
Mitochondria: MELAS; coenzyme Q10 deficiency
Purine metabolism: Lesch–Nyhan disease
Creatine metabolism: Creatine deficiency syndromes
Cofactors: Vitamin E deficiency; thiamine transporter deficiency; biotinidase deficiency; abetalipoproteinemia
Others: Angelman syndrome; ataxia-telangiectasia; MECP2 duplication syndrome; Rett syndrome; infantile neuroaxonal dystrophy; 4-H syndrome; congenital disorders of glycosylation
Muscle disorders: Merosin-deficient muscular dystrophy; Duchenne muscular dystrophy

disorder, Joubert syndrome) (see Table 20.7 and Chapter 17). Children with this type are generally born after a full-term gestation and asphyxia is generally not a major factor.

Mixed Type

Children with a combination of spastic and dyskinetic types are labeled as having a mixed type.

DIAGNOSTIC TESTS

A useful algorithm for the evaluation of the child with CP has been published and is modified below (Table 20.8).

Neuroimaging

CP is a clinical diagnosis and a careful history and examination is necessary both to confirm the diagnosis and to determine an etiology. A practice parameter on the diagnostic assessment of the child with CP has recommended that the evaluation include neuroimaging, preferably magnetic resonance imaging (MRI), because of its sensitivity in identifying acquired lesions, PVL, and congenital brain anomalies.[79] MRI has demonstrated abnormal brain findings in about 89% of individuals with CP[13,80–84] The scan is helpful in determining the timing of the injury and in some instances can provide important etiologic and prognostic clues.[85,86] Identification of a radiographic abnormality may not, however, clarify the etiology of the motor deficit, e.g., delayed myelination or cortical atrophy. Equally important is the presence of a normal MRI in the presence of a child with spasticity or dystonia but lacking a history of a perinatal brain injury. The later suggests the need for screening catecholamine metabolites.[87]

TABLE 20.8   Evaluation of the Child with CP

Evaluation of the Child with CP

1.   Confirm that the history does not suggest a progressive or degenerative central nervous system disorder.
2.   Assure that features suggestive of progressive or degenerative disease are not present on examination.
3.   Further investigation if there are severe symptoms in the absence of a history of perinatal injury.
4.   Classify the type of CP.
5.   Screen for associated conditions including:
    a)   Developmental delay/mental retardation
    b)   Ophthalmologic/hearing impairments
    c)   Speech and language delay
    d)   Feeding/swallowing dysfunction
    e)   If history of suspected seizures, obtain an EEG

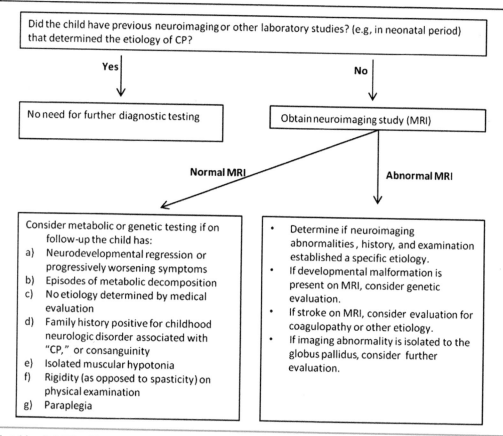

Did the child have previous neuroimaging or other laboratory studies? (e.g, in neonatal period) that determined the etiology of CP?

Yes → No need for further diagnostic testing

No → Obtain neuroimaging study (MRI)

Normal MRI

Consider metabolic or genetic testing if on follow-up the child has:
a)   Neurodevelopmental regression or progressively worsening symptoms
b)   Episodes of metabolic decomposition
c)   No etiology determined by medical evaluation
d)   Family history positive for childhood neurologic disorder associated with "CP," or consanguinity
e)   Isolated muscular hypotonia
f)   Rigidity (as opposed to spasticity) on physical examination
g)   Paraplegia

Abnormal MRI

• Determine if neuroimaging abnormalities, history, and examination established a specific etiology.
• If developmental malformation is present on MRI, consider genetic evaluation.
• If stroke on MRI, consider evaluation for coagulopathy or other etiology.
• If imaging abnormality is isolated to the globus pallidus, consider further evaluation.

Adapted from Refs [40] and [79].

In term and near-term infants with CP, HIE, perinatal stroke with focal arterial infarction, and brain malformation are the most common abnormalities.[88,89] In HIE, the brain insult is predominantly located in the basal ganglia (posterior putamen), ventrolateral thalamus, and peri-Rolandic motor strip.[90] In preterm infants, PVL and germinal matrix hemorrhage are common forms of brain injury. Abnormalities in the periventricular region (T2-weighted scans), however, are not specific for PVL and may occur in disorders masquerading as CP such as neuronal ceroid lipofuscinosis, Krabbe disease, or metachromatic leukodystrophy. In PVL, the periventricular gliotic scarring is most prominent in the posterior ventricular system, tends to be permanent, and shows either moderate ventricular enlargement or a "squared-off" ventricular enlargement. Diminished cortical and subcortical gray matter is not uncommon in the preterm infant.[91] Abnormal findings on MRI, measured at term equivalent in very preterm infants, strongly predict adverse neurodevelopmental outcome at 2 years of age.[85] Others have reported that the extent of motor and cognitive impairment in children with PVL correlates with the degree of ventricular enlargement.[92] In children with dyskinetic CP, the MRI often shows lesions in the basal ganglia or thalamus.[93,94] Lesions in both of these areas in term neonates have been identified as indicators of a hypoxic-ischemic sentinel event.[95] Neuroimaging in ataxic CP may be normal or show either biparietal or infratentorial lesions.[78] Several studies show cerebellar injury in the extremely premature infant.[96,97] Ultrasound evaluations in low and extremely low birth weight infants have a poor predictive value, being normal in infants who developed adverse neurodevelopmental outcomes.[98]

Newer neuroimaging techniques have been applied to CP, including techniques that demonstrate fiber tracts, areas of cortical activation, and concentrations of neurometabolites. Diffusion tensor imaging (DTI) is a magnetic imaging technique that enables evaluation of white matter tracts in the brain and provides quantitative data on their physical integrity.[99] DTI in preterm infants has demonstrated disruption of thalamocortical connections and descending corticospinal pathways.[100] In one study, the degree of restricted water movement (fractional anisotropy) was useful in predicting those cases with PVL who would develop significant motor disabilities.[101] Functional magnetic resonance imaging (fMRI), which identifies activated brain regions, has shown that those with hemiplegia may have differences in sensory and motor organization.[102] Studies with magnetic resonance spectroscopy have been limited, but an analysis of the basal ganglia in children with CP showed that results failed to correlate with clinical severity.[102]

Other Laboratory Tests

The diagnostic yields from metabolic and genetic evaluations are small, but testing should be considered in appropriate cases with dyskinetic and ataxic CP, and in those individuals with specific brain developmental malformations, e.g., migrational defects, that are associated with specific chromosomal abnormalities. An electroencephalogram is not recommended unless seizures are part of the clinical picture.

Chromosomal microarray, especially single nucleotide polymorphism (SNP) based platforms, which detect both copy number variation and copy neutral loss of heterozygosity due to uniparental disomy or parental consanguinity, are recommended when further evaluation is required. Whole exome sequencing (WES) analyzes the protein coding regions (exons) of more than 20,000 genes in the human genome whereas whole genome sequencing analyzes coding and non-coding regions. WES and WGS are not of standard diagnostic practice at this time.

Assessment Scales

Several instruments are available to monitor the development of motor function in children with CP, including the Gross Motor Function Classification System (GMFCS) for Cerebral Palsy,[103] Child Health Questionnaire,[6,104–113] the Manual Ability Classification System,[114] the Gross Motor Function Measure,[108] the Functional Mobility Scale,[112] the Pediatric Evaluation of Disability Inventory (PEDI),[115] the Gillette Functional Assessment Questionnaire,[105] the Drooling Impact Scale,[107] and the Viking Speech Scale.[106] Some scales focus narrowly on the physical impairment rather than functional consequence, some evaluate capability rather than actual performance of functional activities, and others miss important items, or include unimportant information.[104] The GMFCS, a 5-level ordinal rating scale based on the severity of motor disability, has good reliability and good prognostic utility.[47,116] In brief, children in the GMFCS level I have some difficulty with speed, balance and coordination, but do all activities; level II do well on flat surfaces but need support on stairs or uneven surfaces; level III are independent walkers, but require a cane, crutch, or walker; level IV are non-ambulatory, but can weight bear for transfers and use a walker; and level V are non-ambulatory with no functional weight-bearing and are totally dependent.

MANAGEMENT OF CEREBRAL PALSY

Neuroprotection

Neonatal neuroprotection focuses on minimizing brain damage in babies at high risk for a perinatal hypoxic-ischemic event. In term infants, the mechanism for brain injury after an asphyxia insult is thought to involve a series of events within the "excito-oxidative cascade."[113] This cascade involves early activation of excitatory glutamate receptors, especially NMDA, followed by oxidative stress associated with deteriorating mitochondrial dysfunction and failure. Several randomized controlled trials have shown that hypothermia has reduced the risk for of death and disability.[117–119] Further research is required to understand the neuroprotective effect of hypothermia and to identify adjuvant treatments. Several anticonvulsant, anti-excitatory, and anti-inflammatory agents are under investigation including phenobarbital, topiramate, levetiracetam, memantine, inhaled xenon, allopurinol, and melatonin. Meta-analyses of clinical trials suggest that maternal magnesium sulfate therapy is associated with a reduced risk of CP and gross motor dysfunction after premature birth, but has no effect on death or disability.[111] Erythropoietin has also been shown to have a protective effect against HIE injury acting via stimulating neurogenesis and through anti-inflammatory, anti-oxidative, anti-apoptotic, and neurotrophic mechanisms.[110,120] Individuals with CP usually have a variety of comorbidities including epilepsy, feeding and swallowing issues, abnormal bowel motility, poor nutrition and growth, increased infections, vision and hearing difficulties, and psychological issues.[6] Hence, the management of CP requires close surveillance and a comprehensive multidisciplinary team approach that can deal with the numerous psychological, behavioral, and physical needs of the child and family. Appropriate interventions are dictated by the child's functional ability, severity, motor disability, associated pain, and age. Treatment should begin as early as possible, with the goal of therapy formulated to improve care, optimize motor function, prevent orthopedic deformities, and address associated impairments. Rehabilitative programs have direct benefit on parent–child relationships, socioemotional status, confidence, and self-esteem.[121]

Physical Therapy

An important component of rehabilitation is occupational and physical therapy. It is unclear, however, what type of therapy should be initiated, since proof of efficacy is often lacking. Traditionally, physical therapy is designed to use passive positioning to inhibit the impact of primitive reflexes, to facilitate the acquisition of gross and fine motor skills, and to prevent contractures,[122] but its effectiveness on functional motor outcome is controversial.[123,124] Similarly, the use of neurodevelopmental treatments that emphasize specific handling techniques (Bobath method) or conductive educational approaches has been questioned.[125–127] Neuromuscular electrical stimulation has been claimed to improve muscle strength, but the approach remains controversial.[128–130] Constraint-induced movement therapy involves physical constraint of the uninvolved or less affected extremity.[131,132] Evidence for its beneficial effect is increasing, but additional studies are necessary to provide further support of efficacy and developmental appropriateness.[133,134] Muscle strengthening with the Adeli suit, which provides resistance to some movements, is claimed to improve sensory feedback during movement and subsequent mechanical efficiency.[135] Horseback riding therapy, also known as hippotherapy, has also been shown to be beneficial.[136] One debate is whether outcomes of therapy should be based on improvement from a baseline impairment level or evidence-based improvement of functional capabilities and societal participation.[137]

Spastic CP: Pharmacotherapy and Surgical Approaches

Spasticity can affect function, compromise comfort and hygiene, and lead to musculoskeletal complications, including contractures, subluxation, and pain. A variety of antispasticity interventions are available for the treatment of children with CP, including physical therapy, oral medications, neurolytic blocking agents, intrathecal baclofen pumps, tendon-lengthening procedures, and selective dorsal rhizotomy.[133,138,139]

Oral Medications

Oral therapy is usually of greater relevance for individuals with diplegic or quadriplegic CP. Several agents have been used with some benefit, including benzodiazepines, dantrolene, baclofen, and alpha-2-adrenergic-agonists.[140] In general, these approaches help to reduce spasticity, but have little beneficial effect on signs of weakness and incoordination.

Benzodiazepines (diazepam) are commonly used for short- or long-term treatment of spasticity in children. The benefit of diazepam, however, is limited by side effects, including sedation, weakness, memory disturbances, excess drooling, and a state of dependency.[141]

Dantrolene sodium improves tone, range of motion, and reflexes, but its effectiveness is restricted by side effects such as weakness, drowsiness, lethargy, gastrointestinal disturbances, and liver damage.[142] Dantrolene reduces muscle contractions by inhibiting the release of calcium ions from the sarcoplasmic reticulum.

Baclofen, an analog of gamma-aminobutyric acid (GABA), binds to GABA receptors and impedes the release of the excitatory neurotransmitters glutamate and aspartate. Its efficacy in treating spasticity is probably based on its action at bicuculline-insensitive GABA type B receptors located within the spinal cord. Oral baclofen does have a mild effect on cerebral spasticity but its use is limited by both poor lipid solubility and side effects.[143] Dose-dependent side effects include sedation, hypoventilation, and increased seizures.

Tizanidine is a central acting alpha-2-receptor agonist that primarily reduces polysynaptic spinal stretch reflexes.[144] Its use in the treatment of spasticity has been largely focused on adult patients with multiple sclerosis and spinal cord injury.[145] In a combined clinical analysis of control trials, it was suggested that tizanidine was similar in efficacy to baclofen and diazepam.[144] Common side effects include dry mouth, somnolence, asthenia, and dizziness.

Neurolytic Agents

Neuromuscular blocking agents, including alcohol, aqueous phenol, local anesthetics, and botulinum A toxin, have been used to improve the balance between overly spastic agonist muscles and weakened antagonist muscles.[146] Botulinum A toxin (BTX-A), the most widely used agent in this category, acts by blocking acetylcholine release at the neuromuscular junction. Typically, the peak effect occurs at 2–4 weeks and reinjection is necessary at 12–14 weeks. Side effects include weakness or pain/bruising at the injection site. Several studies in patients with CP have demonstrated the value of BTX-A for equinus positioning of the foot while walking[147–149] or improved upper limb movement and function.[150] A Cochrane Database review suggested that data were insufficient to indicate its use to treat leg spasticity,[104,151] however, subsequent reviews have confirmed its effectiveness.[104,152] A randomized double-masked placebo-controlled study in children with spastic diplegia receiving 12 units/kg of BTX-A showed an excellent safety profile, physiologic and mechanical benefits, but no significant differences from control in performance goals achieved, energy expended, or Ashworth score.[153] Both a subcommittee of the American Academy of Neurology and European guidelines have recommended that botulinum neurotoxin be offered as a treatment option in children with spasticity.[154,155] The combination of BTX-A and serial casting has been used effectively in the management of equinus in children with CP.[152,156] The long-term effects or benefits of BTX-A in terms of improved muscle growth, mobility, and function remain unclear.[104,157]

Intrathecal Baclofen Pump

Continuous intrathecal baclofen infusion through indwelling catheters and a programmable pump has been shown to reduce spasticity in the upper and lower extremities and improve function and activities of daily living.[158–160] Complications include infections, problems with the catheter (kinking, migration), headaches, nausea, and unresponsiveness or profound hypotonia caused by overdosing.[161,162] Intrathecal baclofen has been shown to be beneficial in dystonic CP, but not in other dyskinetic forms.[163] Typical candidates for this therapy include children with moderate to severe spastic quadriplegia who have failed oral therapy, respond to a screening bolus of medication, and have adequate body size for placement of the subcutaneous pump.

Orthopedic Surgery

The role of the orthopedic surgeon is to maintain or enhance motor abilities and to prevent deformities through procedures such as tendonotomies, muscle transfers, osteotomies, and arthrodeses. Monitoring for hip joint displacement, scoliosis, and contractures are essential. Aggressive use of BTX-A, physical therapy, casting, and orthotics has effectively delayed the timing of surgical intervention to later ages in childhood. There is also an increasing trend toward "single-event multilevel surgery," i.e., addressing all deformities simultaneously rather than sequential, more piecemeal approaches.[104] Computerized gait analysis for preoperative planning may be beneficial, but it remains an area of controversy among pediatric orthopedic surgeons.[104]

One surgical procedure for spastic diplegia and quadriplegia, which has recently been revived, is selective functional dorsal (posterior) rhizotomy. In this procedure the posterior branches of the spinal nerves producing spasticity are sectioned in an attempt to alter the modulating influence of the interneuron pool, which in turn controls the reactivity of alpha motor neurons. The use of intraoperative nerve stimulation to determine which rootlets to cut is controversial. In carefully selected patients with spastic diplegia this procedure has reduced spasticity, changed gait patterns, and improved the patient's ability to deal with the environment or tasks of daily care.[164] A comparative analysis and meta-analysis of three randomized clinical trials suggested that selective dorsal rhizotomy plus physiotherapy reduced spasticity in children with spastic diplegia and had a small effect on gross motor function.[165] A second meta-analysis confirmed a reduction, but whether this reduction led to improved long-term functional goals is controversial.[166] Other reports, however, have suggested that there is no benefit from rhizotomy when compared with intensive physical therapy and there is only limited evidence that it reduces the need for orthopedic surgery.[167] Hence, since this is a major operative procedure, it remains controversial whether the functional outcomes outweigh potential intraoperative and postoperative complications or are cost-effective.

Dyskinetic CP: Pharmacotherapy and Surgical Approaches

Oral Therapy

The treatment of dyskinetic CP is complicated, because most individuals have mixed degrees of chorea, athetosis, and dystonia. The general approach to therapy in the child with CP is to target the dyskinetic movement that is causing the greatest difficulty. Therapeutic trials are largely empirical, and responses are often individualized.[140] When the symptom is primarily chorea or athetosis, benzodiazepines, valproate, carbamazepine, tetrabenazine, and neuroleptics are often prescribed. In contrast, therapy for dystonic CP includes trials with anticholinergic medications (trihexyphenidyl),[168] baclofen, anticonvulsants (carbamazepine, clonazepam), antiparkinsonian medications (levodopa/carbidopa), and botulinum toxin. Oral baclofen may be more effective as an anti-dystonic agent in children than in adults.[169] A therapeutic trial with levodopa should be considered in all patients in whom dystonia has developed in childhood or early life.[170,171] This recommendation is proposed for several reasons, including a potential response to levodopa in children with symptomatic dystonia[171–173] and the knowledge that dopa-responsive dystonia has clinical patterns that simulate CP.[174] Levodopa has also been used successfully in patients with athetoid CP.[172,173,175]

Intrathecal Baclofen Pump

Intrathecal baclofen has been beneficial in a small number of patients with severe generalized dystonia or choreoathetosis.[161,163,176] A test bolus of baclofen given via a lumbar puncture is not thought to be accurate in predicting the ultimate response to infusion therapy.[163,172,173]

Deep Brain Stimulation

Preliminary studies have suggested that deep brain stimulation may be effective in selected patients with dystonia and possibly choreoathetosis.[172,173] Insufficient studies, however, have been done to determine long-term clinical outcome.

References

1. Sanger TD. Is cerebral palsy a wastebasket diagnosis? *J Child Neurol*. 2008;23(7):726–728.
2. Little WJ. On the influence of abnormal parturition, difficult labours, premature birth and asphyxia neonatorum on the mental and physical condition of the child, especially in relation to deformity. *Trans Obstet Soc London*. 1861;3:293.
3. Osler W. *The Cerebral Palsies of Children: A Clinical Study from the Infirmary for Nervous Diseases*. Philadelphia, PA: P. Blakiston; 1889.
4. Accardo PJ. Freud on diplegia. Commentary and translation. *Am J Dis Child*. 1982;136(5):452–456.
5. Longo LD, Ashwal S. William Osler, Sigmund Freud and the evolution of ideas concerning cerebral palsy. *J Hist Neurosci*. 1993;2(4):255–282.
6. Colver A, Rapp M, Eisemann N, Ehlinger V, Thyen U, Dickinson HO, et al. Self-reported quality of life of adolescents with cerebral palsy: a cross-sectional and longitudinal analysis. *Lancet*. 2014.
7. Saint Hilaire MH, Burke RE, Bressman SB, Brin MF, Fahn S. Delayed-onset dystonia due to perinatal or early childhood asphyxia. *Neurology*. 1991;41(2 (Pt 1)):216–222.
8. Scott BL, Jankovic J. Delayed-onset progressive movement disorders after static brain lesions. *Neurology*. 1996;46(1):68–74.
9. Smithers-Sheedy H, Badawi N, Blair E, Cans C, Himmelmann K, Krägeloh-Mann I, et al. What constitutes cerebral palsy in the twenty-first century? *Dev Med Child Neurol*. 2014;56(4):323–328.
10. Hagberg B, Hagberg G, Olow I, van Wendt L. The changing panorama of cerebral palsy in Sweden. VII. Prevalence and origin in the birth year period 1987-90. *Acta Paediatr*. 1996;85(8):954–960.
11. Ancel P-Y, Livinec F, Larroque B, Marret S, Arnaud C, Pierrat V, et al. Cerebral palsy among very preterm children in relation to gestational age and neonatal ultrasound abnormalities: the EPIPAGE cohort study. *Pediatrics*. 2006;117(3):828–835.
12. Kuban KC, Leviton A. Cerebral palsy. *N Engl J Med*. 1994;330(3):188–195.
13. Bax M, Tydeman C, Flodmark O. Clinical and MRI correlates of cerebral palsy: the European Cerebral Palsy Study. *JAMA*. 2006;296(13):1602–1608.
14. Doyle LW, Anderson PJ, Group VICS Improved neurosensory outcome at 8 years of age of extremely low birthweight children born in Victoria over three distinct eras. *Arch Dis Child Fetal Neonatal Ed*. 2005;90:F484–F488.
15. Himmelmann K, Hagberg G, Beckung E, Hagberg B, Uvebrant P. The changing panorama of cerebral palsy in Sweden. IX. Prevalence and origin in the birth-year period 1995-1998. *Acta Paediatr*. 2005;94(3):287–294.
16. Keogh JM, Badawi N. The origins of cerebral palsy. *Curr Opin Neurol*. 2006;19(2):129–134.
17. Nelson KB. The epidemiology of cerebral palsy in term infants. *Ment Retard Dev Disabil Res Rev*. 2002;8(3):146–150.
18. Newman CJ, O'Regan M, Hensey O. Sleep disorders in children with cerebral palsy. *Dev Med Child Neurol*. 2006;48(7):564–568.
19. Odding E, Roebroeck ME, Stam HJ. The epidemiology of cerebral palsy: incidence, impairments and risk factors. *Disabil Rehabil*. 2006;28(4):183–191.
20. Singhi P, Jagirdar S, Khandelwal N, Malhi P. Epilepsy in children with cerebral palsy. *J Child Neurol*. 2003;18(3):174–179.

21. von Wendt L, Rantakallio P, Saukkonen AL, Tuisku M, Makinen H. Cerebral palsy and additional handicaps in a 1-year birth cohort from northern Finland—a prospective follow-up study to the age of 14 years. *Ann Clin Res*. 1985;17(4):156–161.

22. Borg E. Perinatal asphyxia, hypoxia, ischemia and hearing loss. An overview. *Scand Audiol*. 1997;26(2):77–91.

23. Carlsson M, Hagberg G, Olsson I. Clinical and aetiological aspects of epilepsy in children with cerebral palsy. *Dev Med Child Neurol*. 2003;45(6):371–376.

24. Evans P, Elliot M, Alberman E, Evans S. Prevalence and disabilities in 4- to 8-year-olds with cerebral palsy. *Arch Dis Child*. 1985;60:940–945.

25. Guzzetta A, Mercuri E, Cioni G. Visual disorders in children with brain lesions: 2. Visual impairment associated with cerebral palsy. *Eur J Paediatr Neurol*. 2001;5(3):115–119.

26. Hundozi-Hysenaj H, Boshnjaku-Dallku I. Epilepsy in children with cerebral palsy. *J Pediatr Neurol*. 2008;6(1):43–46.

27. Sigurdardottir S, Vik T. Speech, expressive language, and verbal cognition of preschool children with cerebral palsy in Iceland. *Dev Med Child Neurol*. 2011;53(1):74–80.

28. Solaski M, Majnemer A, Oskoui M. Contribution of socio-economic status on the prevalence of cerebral palsy: a systematic search and review. *Dev Med Child Neurol*. 2014;56(11):1043–1051.

29. Miller G, Clark GD. *The Cerebral Palsies: Causes, Consequences, and Management*. Boston: Butterworth–Heinemann; 1998.

30. Mutch L, Alberman E, Hagberg B, Kodama K, Perat MV. Cerebral palsy epidemiology: where are we now and where are we going? *Dev Med Child Neurol*. 1992;34(6):547–551.

31. O'Shea TM. Cerebral palsy in very preterm infants: new epidemiological insights. *Ment Retard Dev Disabil Res Rev*. 2002;8(3):135–145.

32. Hermansen MC, Hermansen MG. Perinatal infections and cerebral palsy. *Clin Perinatol*. 2006;33(2):315–333.

33. Jarvis S, Glinianaia SV, Blair E. Cerebral palsy and intrauterine growth. *Clin Perinatol*. 2006;33(2):285–300.

34. Msall ME. The panorama of cerebral palsy after very and extremely preterm birth: evidence and challenges. *Clin Perinatol*. 2006;33(2):269–284.

35. Pharoah PO. Risk of cerebral palsy in multiple pregnancies. *Clin Perinatol*. 2006;33(2):301–313.

36. Leach E, Shevell M, Bowden K, et al. Treatable inborn errors of metabolism presenting as cerebral palsy mimics: systematic literature review. *Orphanet J Rare Dis*. 2014;9:197.

37. Menkes JH, Flores-Sarnat L. Cerebral palsy due to chromosomal anomalies and continuous gene syndromes. *Clin Perinatol*. 2006;33(2):481–501.

38. Nelson KB, Dambrosia JM, Iovannisci DM, Cheng S, Grether JK, Lammer E. Genetic polymorphisms and cerebral palsy in very preterm infants. *Pediatr Res*. 2005;57(4):494–499.

39. Costeff H. Estimated frequency of genetic and nongenetic causes of congenital idiopathic cerebral palsy in west Sweden. *Ann Hum Genet*. 2004;68(Pt 5):515–520.

40. Lee RW, Poretti A, Cohen JS, Levey E, Gwynn H, Johnston MV, et al. A diagnostic approach for cerebral palsy in the genomic era. *Neuromol Med*. 2014;16(4):821–844.

41. Adamo R, Acog *Neonatal Encephalopathy and Cerebral Palsy: Defining the Pathogenesis and Pathophysiology: A Report*. Washington, D.C.: American College of Obstetricians and Gynecologists; 2003.

42. MacLennan A. A template for defining a causal relation between acute intrapartum events and cerebral palsy: international consensus statement. *BMJ*. 1999;319(7216):1054–1059.

43. Sanger TD, Delgado MR, Gaebler-Spira D, Hallett M, Mink JW. Classification and definition of disorders causing hypertonia in childhood. *Pediatrics*. 2003;111(1):e89–e97.

44. Sanger TD. Toward a definition of childhood dystonia. *Curr Opin Pediatr*. 2004;16(6):623–627.

45. Capute AJ. Identifying cerebral palsy in infancy through study of primative reflex profiles. *Pediatr Ann*. 1979;8:589–595.

46. Capute AJ, Palmer FB, Shapiro BK, Wachtel RC, Ross A, Accardo PJ. Primitive reflex profile: a quantitation of primitive reflexes in infancy. *Dev Med Child Neurol*. 1984;26(3):375–383.

47. Rosenbaum PL, Walter SD, Hanna SE, Palisano RJ, Russell DJ, Raina P, et al. Prognosis for gross motor function in cerebral palsy: creation of motor development curves. *JAMA*. 2002;288(11):1357–1363.

48. Kuban KC, Allred EN, O'Shea M, Paneth N, Pagano M, Leviton A. An algorithm for identifying and classifying cerebral palsy in young children. *J Pediatr*. 2008;153(4):466–472.

49. Hagberg B, Hagberg G, Beckung E, Uvebrant P. Changing panorama of cerebral palsy in Sweden. VIII. Prevalence and origin in the birth year period 1991-94. *Acta Paediatr*. 2001;90(3):271–277.

50. Nelson KB, Lynch JK. Stroke in newborn infants. *Lancet Neurol*. 2004;3(3):150–158.

51. Scher MS, Belfar H, Martin J, Painter MJ. Destructive brain lesions of presumed fetal onset: antepartum causes of cerebral palsy. *Pediatrics*. 1991;88(5):898–906.

52. Hayashi N, Tsutsumi Y, Barkovich AJ. Morphological features and associated anomalies of schizencephaly in the clinical population: detailed analysis of Mr images. *Neuroradiology*. 2002;44(5):418–427.

53. Volpe JJ. Neurobiology of periventricular leukomalacia in the premature infant. *Pediatr Res*. 2001;50(5):553–562.

54. Folkerth RD. Neuropathologic substrate of cerebral palsy. *J Child Neurol*. 2005;20(12):940–949.

55. Ness JK, Romanko MJ, Rothstein RP, Wood TL, Levison SW. Perinatal hypoxia-ischemia induces apoptotic and excitotoxic death of periventricular white matter oligodendrocyte progenitors. *Dev Neurosci*. 2001;23(3):203–208.

56. Back SA, Luo NL, Mallinson RA, O'Malley JP, Wallen LD, Frei B, et al. Selective vulnerability of preterm white matter to oxidative damage defined by F2-isoprostanes. *Ann Neurol*. 2005;58(1):108–120.

57. Elitt C, Rosenberg P. The challenge of understanding cerebral white matter injury in the premature infant. *Neuroscience*. 2014;276:216–238.

58. Kadhim H, Tabarki B, Verellen G, De Prez C, Rona AM, Sebire G. Inflammatory cytokines in the pathogenesis of periventricular leukomalacia. *Neurology*. 2001;56(10):1278–1284.

59. Back SA, Tuohy TM, Chen H, Wallingford N, Craig A, Struve J, et al. Hyaluronan accumulates in demyelinated lesions and inhibits oligodendrocyte progenitor maturation. *Nat Med*. 2005;11(9):966–972.

60. Roze E, Kerstjens JM, Maathuis CG, ter Horst HJ, Bos AF. Risk factors for adverse outcome in preterm infants with periventricular hemorrhagic infarction. *Pediatrics*. 2008;122(1):e46–e52.

61. Shevell MI, Dagenais L, Hall N. The relationship of cerebral palsy subtype and functional motor impairment: a population-based study. *Dev Med Child Neurol*. 2009;51(11):872–877.

62. Vexler ZS, Ferriero DM. Molecular and biochemical mechanisms of perinatal brain injury. *Semin Neonatol*. 2001;6(2):99–108.

63. Johnston MV, Trescher WH, Ishida A, Nakajima W. Neurobiology of hypoxic-ischemic injury in the developing brain. *Pediatr Res*. 2001;49(6):735–741.

64. Lee JM, Grabb MC, Zipfel GJ, Choi DW. Brain tissue responses to ischemia. *J Clin Invest*. 2000;106(6):723–731.

65. Lipton P. Ischemic cell death in brain neurons. *Physiol Rev*. 1999;79(4):1431–1568.

66. Dirnagl U, Iadecola C, Moskowitz MA. Pathobiology of ischaemic stroke: an integrated view. *Trends Neurosci*. 1999;22(9):391–397.

67. Cerovac N, Petrovic I, Klein C, Kostic VS. Delayed-onset dystonia due to perinatal asphyxia: A prospective study. *Mov Disord*. 2007;22(16):2426–2429.

68. Filloux FM. Neuropathophysiology of movement disorders in cerebral palsy. *J Child Neurol*. 1996;11(Suppl 1):S5–12.

69. Johnston MV, Hoon AH. Excitotoxicity and patterns of brain injury from fetal or perinatal asphyxia. In: Maulik D, ed. *Asphyxia and fetal brain damage*. New York: Wiley-Liss; 1998:113–125.

70. Mitchell G, McInnes RR. Differential diagnosis of cerebral palsy: Lesch-Nyhan syndrome without self-mutilation. *Can Med Assoc J*. 1984;130(10):1323–1324.

71. Pantaleoni C, D'Arrigo S, D'Incerti L, Rimoldi M, Riva D. A case of 3-methylglutaconic aciduria misdiagnosed as cerebral palsy. *Pediatr Neurol*. 2000;23(5):442–444.

72. Prasad AN, Breen JC, Ampola MG, Rosman NP. Argininemia: a treatable genetic cause of progressive spastic diplegia simulating cerebral palsy: case reports and literature review. *J Child Neurol*. 1997;12(5):301–309.

73. Straussberg R, Brand N, Gadoth N. 3-Methyl glutaconic aciduria in Iraqi Jewish children may be misdiagnosed as cerebral palsy. *Neuropediatrics*. 1998;29(1):54–56.

74. Willis TA, Davidson J, Gray RG, Poulton K, Ramani P, Whitehouse W. Cytochrome oxidase deficiency presenting as birth asphyxia. *Dev Med Child Neurol*. 2000;42(6):414–417.

75. Christodoulou J, Qureshi IA, McInnes RR, Clarke JT. Ornithine transcarbamylase deficiency presenting with strokelike episodes. *J Pediatr*. 1993;122(3):423–425.

76. Gibson KM, Christensen E, Jakobs C, Fowler B, Clarke MA, Hammersen G, et al. The clinical phenotype of succinic semialdehyde dehydrogenase deficiency (4-hydroxybutyric aciduria): case reports of 23 new patients. *Pediatrics*. 1997;99(4):567–574.

77. Lissens W, Vreken P, Barth PG, Wijburg FA, Ruitenbeek W, Wanders RJ, et al. Cerebral palsy and pyruvate dehydrogenase deficiency: identification of two new mutations in the E1alpha gene. *Eur J Pediatr*. 1999;158(10):853–857.

78. Miller G, Cala LA. Ataxic cerebral palsy—clinico-radiologic correlations. *Neuropediatrics*. 1989;20(2):84–89.

79. Ashwal S, Russman B, Blasco P, Miller G, Sandler A, Shevell M, et al. Practice parameter: diagnostic assessment of the child with cerebral palsy report of the quality standards subcommittee of the American Academy of Neurology and the Practice Committee of the Child Neurology Society. *Neurology*. 2004;62(6):851–863.

V. SELECTED SECONDARY MOVEMENT DISORDERS

80. Sugimoto T, Woo M, Nishida N, Araki A, Hara T, Yasuhara A, et al. When do brain abnormalities in cerebral palsy occur? An MRI study. *Dev Med Child Neurol.* 1995;37(4):285–292.

81. Yin R, Reddihough D, Ditchfield M, Collins K. Magnetic resonance imaging findings in cerebral palsy. *J Paediatr Child Health.* 2000;36(2):139–144.

82. Candy EJ, Hoon AH, Capute AJ, Bryan RN. MRI in motor delay: important adjunct to classification of cerebral palsy. *Pediatr Neurol.* 1993;9(6):421–429.

83. Cioni G, Sales B, Paolicelli PB, Petacchi E, Scusa MF, Canapicchi R. MRI and clinical characteristics of children with hemiplegic cerebral palsy. *Neuropediatrics.* 1999;30(5):249–255.

84. Krageloh-Mann I, Petersen D, Hagberg G, Vollmer B, Hagberg B, Michaelis R. Bilateral spastic cerebral palsy—MRI pathology and origin. Analysis from a representative series of 56 cases. *Dev Med Child Neurol.* 1995;37(5):379–397.

85. Woodward LJ, Anderson PJ, Austin NC, Howard K, Inder TE. Neonatal MRI to predict neurodevelopmental outcomes in preterm infants. *N Engl J Med.* 2006;355(7):685–694.

86. Zimmerman RA, Bilaniuk LT. Neuroimaging evaluation of cerebral palsy. *Clin Perinatol.* 2006;33(2):517–544.

87. Friedman J, Roze E, Abdenur JE, Chang R, Gasperini S, Saletti V, et al. Sepiapterin reductase deficiency: a treatable mimic of cerebral palsy. *Ann Neurol.* 2012;71(4):520–530.

88. Nelson KB, Chang T. Is cerebral palsy preventable? *Curr Opin Neurol.* 2008;21(2):129–135.

89. Wu YW, Croen LA, Shah SJ, Newman TB, Najjar DV. Cerebral palsy in a term population: risk factors and neuroimaging findings. *Pediatrics.* 2006;118(2):690–697.

90. Przekop A, Sanger T. Birth-related syndromes of athetosis and kernicterus. *Handb Clin Neurol.* 2011;100:387–395.

91. Inder TE, Warfield SK, Wang H, Huppi PS, Volpe JJ. Abnormal cerebral structure is present at term in premature infants. *Pediatrics.* 2005;115(2):286–294.

92. Melhem ER, Hoon Jr. AH, Ferrucci Jr. JT, Quinn CB, Reinhardt EM, Demetrides SW, et al. Periventricular leukomalacia: relationship between lateral ventricular volume on brain Mr images and severity of cognitive and motor impairment. *Radiology.* 2000;214(1):199–204.

93. Pasternak JF, Gorey MT. The syndrome of acute near-total intrauterine asphyxia in the term infant. *Pediatr Neurol.* 1998;18(5):391–398.

94. Menkes JH, Curran J. Clinical and Mr correlates in children with extrapyramidal cerebral palsy. *AJNR Am J Neuroradiol.* 1994;15(3):451–457.

95. Okereafor A, Allsop J, Counsell SJ, Fitzpatrick J, Azzopardi D, Rutherford MA, et al. Patterns of brain injury in neonates exposed to perinatal sentinel events. *Pediatrics.* 2008;121(5):906–914.

96. Bodensteiner JB, Johnsen SD. Cerebellar injury in the extremely premature infant: newly recognized but relatively common outcome. *J Child Neurol.* 2005;20(2):139–142.

97. Johnsen SD, Bodensteiner JB, Lotze TE. Frequency and nature of cerebellar injury in the extremely premature survivor with cerebral palsy. *J Child Neurol.* 2005;20(1):60–64.

98. Laptook AR, O'Shea TM, Shankaran S, Bhaskar B. Adverse neurodevelopmental outcomes among extremely low birth weight infants with a normal head ultrasound: prevalence and antecedents. *Pediatrics.* 2005;115(3):673–680.

99. Nagae LM, Hoon Jr. AH, Stashinko E, Lin D, Zhang W, Levey E, et al. Diffusion tensor imaging in children with periventricular leukomalacia: variability of injuries to white matter tracts. *AJNR Am J Neuroradiol.* 2007;28(7):1213–1222.

100. Hoon AJ, Stashinko EE, Nagae LM, Lin DD, Keller J, Bastian A, et al. Sensory and motor deficits in children with cerebral palsy born preterm correlate with diffusion tensor imaging abnormalities in thalamocortical pathways. *Dev Med Child Neurol.* 2009;51(9):697–704.

101. Murakami A, Morimoto M, Yamada K, Kizu O, Nishimura A, Nishimura T, et al. Fiber-tracking techniques can predict the degree of neurologic impairment for periventricular leukomalacia. *Pediatrics.* 2008;122(3):500–506.

102. Thickbroom GW, Byrnes ML, Archer SA, Nagarajan L, Mastaglia FL. Differences in sensory and motor cortical organization following brain injury early in life. *Ann Neurol.* 2001;49(3):320–327.

103. Palisano RJ, Cameron D, Rosenbaum PL, Walter SD, Russell D. Stability of the gross motor function classification system. *Dev Med Child Neurol.* 2006;48(6):424–428.

104. Narayanan UG. Management of children with ambulatory cerebral palsy: an evidence-based review. *J Pediatr Orthop.* 2012;32:S172–S181.

105. Novacheck TF, Stout JL, Tervo R. Reliability and validity of the Gillette Functional Assessment Questionnaire as an outcome measure in children with walking disabilities. *J Pediatr Orthop.* 2000;20(1):75.

106. Pennington L, Virella D, Mjøen T, da Graça Andrada M, Murray J, Colver A, et al. Development of The Viking Speech Scale to classify the speech of children with cerebral palsy. *Res Dev Disabil.* 2013;34(10):3202–3210.

107. Reid SM, Johnson HM, Reddihough DS. The Drooling Impact Scale: a measure of the impact of drooling in children with developmental disabilities. *Dev Med Child Neurol.* 2010;52(2):e23–e28.

108. Russell DJ, Avery LM, Rosenbaum PL, Raina PS, Walter SD, Palisano RJ. Improved scaling of the gross motor function measure for children with cerebral palsy: evidence of reliability and validity. *Phys Ther.* 2000;80(9):873–885.

109. Vargus-Adams J. Longitudinal use of the Child Health Questionnaire in childhood cerebral palsy. *Dev Med Child Neurol.* 2006;48(5):343–347.

110. Fan X, Heijnen CJ, van der Kooij MA, Groenendaal F, van Bel F. Beneficial effect of erythropoietin on sensorimotor function and white matter after hypoxia-ischemia in neonatal mice. *Pediatr Res.* 2011;69(1):56–61.

111. Galinsky R, Bennet L, Groenendaal F, Lear CA, Tan S, van Bel F, et al. Magnesium is not consistently neuroprotective for perinatal hypoxia-ischemia in term-equivalent models in preclinical studies: a systematic review. *Dev Neurosci.* 2014;36(2):73–82.

112. Graham HK, Harvey A, Rodda J, Nattrass GR, Pirpiris M. The functional mobility scale (FMS). *J Pediatr Orthop.* 2004;24(5):514–520.

113. Johnston MV, Fatemi A, Wilson MA, Northington F. Treatment advances in neonatal neuroprotection and neurointensive care. *Lancet Neurol.* 2011;10(4):372–382.

114. Eliasson AC, Krumlinde-Sundholm L, Rosblad B, Beckung E, Arner M, Ohrvall AM, et al. The Manual Ability Classification System (MACS) for children with cerebral palsy: scale development and evidence of validity and reliability. *Dev Med Child Neurol.* 2006;48(7):549–554.

115. Ostensjø S, Carlberg EB, Vøllestad NK. Motor impairments in young children with cerebral palsy: relationship to gross motor function and everyday activities. *Dev Med Child Neurol.* 2004;46(9):580–589.

116. Wood E, Rosenbaum P. The gross motor function classification system for cerebral palsy: a study of reliability and stability over time. *Dev Med Child Neurol.* 2000;42(5):292–296.

117. Shah PS. Hypothermia: a systematic review and meta-analysis of clinical trials. *Semin Fetal Neonatal Med.* 2010;15(5):238–246.

118. Shankaran S. Outcomes of hypoxic-ischemic encephalopathy in neonates treated with hypothermia. *Clin Perinatol.* 2014;41(1):149–159.

119. Edwards AD, Brocklehurst P, Gunn AJ, Halliday H, Juszczak E, Levene M, et al. Neurological outcomes at 18 months of age after moderate hypothermia for perinatal hypoxic ischaemic encephalopathy: synthesis and meta-analysis of trial data. *BMJ.* 2010;340:c363.

120. Wang H, Zhang L, Jin Y. A meta-analysis of the protective effect of recombinant human erythropoietin (rhEPO) for neurodevelopment in preterm infants. *Cell Biochem Biophys.* 2014;71(2):795–802.

121. Parry TS. The effectiveness of early intervention: a critical review. *J Paediatr Child Health.* 1992;28(5):343–346.

122. Barry MJ. Physical therapy interventions for patients with movement disorders due to cerebral palsy. *J Child Neurol.* 1996;11(Suppl 1):S51–S60.

123. Palmer FB, Shapiro BK, Wachtel RC, Allen MC, Hiller JE, Harryman SE, et al. The effects of physical therapy on cerebral palsy. A controlled trial in infants with spastic diplegia. *N Engl J Med.* 1988;318(13):803–808.

124. Turnbull JD. Early intervention for children with or at risk of cerebral palsy. *Am J Dis Child.* 1993;147(1):54–59.

125. Odman PE, Oberg BE. Effectiveness and expectations of intensive training: a comparison between child and youth rehabilitation and conductive education. *Disabil Rehabil.* 2006;28(9):561–570.

126. Butler C, Darrah J. Effects of neurodevelopmental treatment (NDT) for cerebral palsy: an AACPDM evidence report. *Dev Med Child Neurol.* 2001;43(11):778–790.

127. Darrah J, Watkins B, Chen L, Bonin C. Conductive education intervention for children with cerebral palsy: an AACPDM evidence report. *Dev Med Child Neurol.* 2004;46(3):187–203.

128. Ozer K, Chesher SP, Scheker LR. Neuromuscular electrical stimulation and dynamic bracing for the management of upper-extremity spasticity in children with cerebral palsy. *Dev Med Child Neurol.* 2006;48(7):559–563.

129. Stackhouse SK, Binder-Macleod SA, Stackhouse CA, McCarthy JJ, Prosser LA, Lee SCK. Neuromuscular electrical stimulation versus volitional isometric strength training in children with spastic diplegic cerebral palsy: a preliminary study. *Neurorehabil Neural Repair.* 2007;21:475–485.

V. SELECTED SECONDARY MOVEMENT DISORDERS

130. Kerr C, McDowell B, Cosgrove A, Walsh D, Bradbury I, McDonough S. Electrical stimulation in cerebral palsy: a randomized controlled trial. *Dev Med Child Neurol.* 2006;48(11):870–876.

131. Naylor CE, Bower E. Modified constraint-induced movement therapy for young children with hemiplegic cerebral palsy: a pilot study. *Dev Med Child Neurol.* 2005;47(6):365–369.

132. Charles JR, Wolf SL, Schneider JA, Gordon AM. Efficacy of a child-friendly form of constraint-induced movement therapy in hemiplegic cerebral palsy: a randomized control trial. *Dev Med Child Neurol.* 2006;48(8):635–642.

133. Papavasiliou AS. Management of motor problems in cerebral palsy: a critical update for the clinician. *Eur J Paediatr Neurol.* 2009;13(5):387–396.

134. Chen Y-p, Pope S, Tyler D, Warren GL. Effectiveness of constraint-induced movement therapy on upper-extremity function in children with cerebral palsy: a systematic review and meta-analysis of randomized controlled trials. *Clin Rehabil.* 2014. http://dx.doi.org/10.1177/0269215514544982.

135. Bar-Haim S, Harries N, Belokopytov M, Frank A, Copeliovitch L, Kaplanski J, et al. Comparison of efficacy of Adeli suit and neurodevelopmental treatments in children with cerebral palsy. *Dev Med Child Neurol.* 2006;48(5):325–330.

136. Sterba JA. Does horseback riding therapy or therapist-directed hippotherapy rehabilitate children with cerebral palsy? *Dev Med Child Neurol.* 2007;49(1):68–73.

137. Mayston M. Evidence-based physical therapy for the management of children with cerebral palsy. *Dev Med Child Neurol.* 2005;47(12):795.

138. Sanger TD. Hypertonia in children: how and when to treat. *Curr Treat Options Neurol.* 2005;7(6):427–439.

139. Verrotti A, Greco R, Spalice A, Chiarelli F, Iannetti P. Pharmacotherapy of spasticity in children with cerebral palsy. *Pediatr Neurol.* 2006;34(1):1–6.

140. Pranzatelli MR. Oral pharmacotherapy for the movement disorders of cerebral palsy. *J Child Neurol.* 1996;11(Suppl 1):S13–S22.

141. Denhoff E. Cerebral palsy—a pharmacologic approach. *Clin Pharmacol Ther.* 1964;5(6):947–954.

142. Glenn M, Whyte J, eds. *The Practical Management of Spasticity in Children and Adults.* Philadelphia: Lea & Febiger; 1990.

143. Scheinberg A, Hall K, Lam LT, O'Flaherty S. Oral baclofen in children with cerebral palsy: a double-blind cross-over pilot study. *J Paediatr Child Health.* 2006;42(11):715–720.

144. Wallace JD. Summary of combined clinical analysis of controlled clinical trials with tizanidine. *Neurology.* 1994;44(11 Suppl 9) S60-8; discussion S8-9.

145. Lataste X, Emre M, Davis C, Groves L. Comparative profile of tizanidine in the management of spasticity. *Neurology.* 1994;44(11 Suppl 9):S53–S59.

146. Koman LA, Mooney 3rd JF, Smith BP. Neuromuscular blockade in the management of cerebral palsy. *J Child Neurol.* 1996;11(Suppl 1):S23–S28.

147. Molenaers G, Fagard K, Van Campenhout A, Desloovere K. Botulinum toxin A treatment of the lower extremities in children with cerebral palsy. *J Child Orthop.* 2013;7(5):383–387.

148. Baker R, Jasinski M, Maciag-Tymecka I, Michalowska-Mrozek J, Bonikowski M, Carr L, et al. Botulinum toxin treatment of spasticity in diplegic cerebral palsy: a randomized, double-blind, placebo-controlled, dose-ranging study. *Dev Med Child Neurol.* 2002;44(10):666–675.

149. Reddihough DS, King JA, Coleman GJ, Fosang A, McCoy AT, Thomason P, et al. Functional outcome of botulinum toxin A injections to the lower limbs in cerebral palsy. *Dev Med Child Neurol.* 2002;44(12):820–827.

150. Lowe K, Novak I, Cusick A. Low-dose/high-concentration localized botulinum toxin A improves upper limb movement and function in children with hemiplegic cerebral palsy. *Dev Med Child Neurol.* 2006;48(3):170–175.

151. Ade-Hall RA, Moore AP. Botulinum toxin type A in the treatment of lower limb spasticity in cerebral palsy. *Cochrane Database Syst Rev.* 2000;(2):CD001408.

152. Ackman JD, Russman BS, Thomas SS, Buckon CE, Sussman MD, Masso P, et al. Comparing botulinum toxin A with casting for treatment of dynamic equinus in children with cerebral palsy. *Dev Med Child Neurol.* 2005;47(9):620–627.

153. Bjornson K, Hays R, Graubert C, Price R, Won F, McLaughlin JF, et al. Botulinum toxin for spasticity in children with cerebral palsy: a comprehensive evaluation. *Pediatrics.* 2007;120(1):49–58.

154. Simpson DM, Blitzer A, Brashear A, Comella C, Dubinsky R, Hallett M, et al. Assessment: Botulinum neurotoxin for the treatment of movement disorders (an evidence-based review): report of the Therapeutics and Technology Assessment Subcommittee of the American Academy of Neurology. *Neurology.* 2008;70(19):1699–1706.

155. Heinen F, Desloovere K, Schroeder AS, Berweck S, Borggraefe I, van Campenhout A, et al. The updated European Consensus 2009 on the use of Botulinum toxin for children with cerebral palsy. *Eur J Paediatr Neurol.* 2010;14(1):45–66.

156. Flett PJ, Stern LM, Waddy H, Connell TM, Seeger JD, Gibson SK. Botulinum toxin A versus fixed cast stretching for dynamic calf tightness in cerebral palsy. *J Paediatr Child Health.* 1999;35(1):71–77.

157. Gough M, Fairhurst C, Shortland A. Botulinum toxin and cerebral palsy: time for reflection? *Dev Med Child Neurol.* 2005;47(10):709–712.

158. Dan B, Motta F, Vles JS, Vloeberghs M, Becher JG, Eunson P, et al. Consensus on the appropriate use of intrathecal baclofen (ITB) therapy in paediatric spasticity. *Eur J Paediatr Neurol.* 2010;14(1):19–28.

159. Gilmartin R, Bruce D, Storrs BB, Abbott R, Krach L, Ward J, et al. Intrathecal baclofen for management of spastic cerebral palsy: multicenter trial. *J Child Neurol.* 2000;15(2):71–77.

160. Latash ML, Penn RD. Changes in voluntary motor control induced by intrathecal baclofen in patients with spasticity of different etiology. *Physiother Res Int.* 1996;1(4):229–246.

161. Butler C, Campbell S. Evidence of the effects of intrathecal baclofen for spastic and dystonic cerebral palsy. AACPDM Treatment Outcomes Committee Review Panel. *Dev Med Child Neurol.* 2000;42(9):634–645.

162. Anderson KJ, Farmer JP, Brown K. Reversible coma in children after improper baclofen pump insertion. *Paediatr Anaesth.* 2002;12(5):454–460.

163. Albright AL. Intrathecal baclofen in cerebral palsy movement disorders. *J Child Neurol.* 1996;11 (Suppl 1):S29–S35.

164. Steinbok P. Outcomes after selective dorsal rhizotomy for spastic cerebral palsy. *Childs Nerv Syst.* 2001;17(1–2):1–18.

165. McLaughlin J, Bjornson K, Temkin N, Steinbok P, Wright V, Reiner A, et al. Selective dorsal rhizotomy: meta-analysis of three randomized controlled trials. *Dev Med Child Neurol.* 2002;44(1):17–25.

166. Grunt S, Becher JG, Vermeulen RJ. Long-term outcome and adverse effects of selective dorsal rhizotomy in children with cerebral palsy: a systematic review. *Dev Med Child Neurol.* 2011;53(6):490–498.

167. Hägglund G, Andersson S, Düppe H, Pedertsen HL, Nordmark E, Westbom L. Prevention of severe contractures might replace multilevel surgery in cerebral palsy: results of a population-based health care programme and new techniques to reduce spasticity. *J Pediatr Orthop B.* 2005;14(4):269–273.

168. Hoon Jr. AH, Freese PO, Reinhardt EM, Wilson MA, Lawrie Jr. WT, Harryman SE, et al. Age-dependent effects of trihexyphenidyl in extrapyramidal cerebral palsy. *Pediatr Neurol.* 2001;25(1):55–58.

169. Greene P. Baclofen in the treatment of dystonia. *Clin Neuropharmacol.* 1992;15(4):276–288.

170. Brunstrom JE, Bastian AJ, Wong M, Mink JW. Motor benefit from levodopa in spastic quadriplegic cerebral palsy. *Ann Neurol.* 2000;47(5):662–665.

171. Fletcher NA, Thompson PD, Scadding JW, Marsden CD. Successful treatment of childhood onset symptomatic dystonia with levodopa. *J Neurol Neurosurg Psychiatry.* 1993;56(8):865–867.

172. Keen JR, Przekop A, Olaya JE, Zouros A, Hsu FP. Deep brain stimulation for the treatment of childhood dystonic cerebral palsy: Clinical article. *J Neurosurg Pediatr.* 2014;14(6):585–593.

173. Koy A, Hellmich M, Pauls KAM, Marks W, Lin JP, Fricke O, et al. Effects of deep brain stimulation in dyskinetic cerebral palsy: a meta-analysis. *Mov Disord.* 2013;28(5):647–654.

174. Nygaard TG, Waran SP, Levine RA, Naini AB, Chutorian AM. Dopa-responsive dystonia simulating cerebral palsy. *Pediatr Neurol.* 1994;11(3):236–240.

175. Rosenthal RK, McDowell FH, Cooper W. Levodopa therapy in athetoid cerebral palsy. A preliminary report. *Neurology.* 1972;22(1):1–11.

176. Gottlob I, Wizov SS, Reinecke RD. Spasmus nutans. A long-term follow-up. *Invest Ophthalmol Vis Sci.* 1995;36(13):2768–2771.

177. Knights S, Datoo N, Kawamura A, Switzer L, Fehlings D. Further evaluation of the scoring, reliability, and validity of the Hypertonia Assessment Tool (HAT). *J Child Neurol.* 2014;29(4):500–504.

178. Jethwa A, Mink J, Macarthur C, Knights S, Fehlings T, Fehlings D. Development of the Hypertonia Assessment Tool (HAT): a discriminative tool for hypertonia in children. *Dev Med Child Neurol.* 2010;52(5):e83–e87.

Movement Disorders and Neuropsychiatric Conditions

Harvey S. Singer[1], Jonathan W. Mink[2],
Donald L. Gilbert[3] and Joseph Jankovic[4]

[1]Department of Neurology, Johns Hopkins Hospital, Baltimore, MD, USA;
[2]Division of Child Neurology, University of Rochester Medical Center,
Rochester, NY, USA; [3]Division of Neurology, Cincinnati Children's Hospital
Medical Center, Cincinnati, OH, USA; [4]Department of Neurology, Baylor
College of Medicine, Houston, TX, USA

O U T L I N E

Movement Disorders in Childhood, Second Edition.
DOI: http://dx.doi.org/10.1016/B978-0-12-411573-6.00021-8

Caring for children with movement disorders involves substantial exposure to psychiatric diagnoses. Subthreshold symptoms as well as overt psychiatric diagnoses commonly co-occur with many pediatric movement disorders (as well as with other symptomatic and genetic conditions involving cerebral cortex, basal ganglia, and cerebellum). To give just a few examples, in the case of Tourette syndrome, the majority of affected children seen in clinical settings have Obsessive Compulsive Disorder (OCD), Attention Deficit Hyperactivity Disorder (ADHD), some combination of these, or other psychiatric diagnoses.[1] In Wilson's disease, psychiatric symptoms may precede the neurological presentation.[2] In persons with DYT1 dystonia, as well as non-manifesting family members carrying the Tor1A mutation, recurring major depression,[3] but not OCD,[4] occurs more commonly. Increased risks of OCD and alcohol dependence are linked to myoclonus dystonia (DYT11).[5,6] These and other neurology/psychiatry associations are described in phenomenology chapters in more detail.

The common co-occurrence of psychiatric diagnoses and neurological diagnoses has important implications. First, with regard to patient care, the neurologist diagnosing and managing pediatric movement disorders may need to think systematically about how to provide needed services to children with these diagnoses,[1,7] as these may cause more impairment than the primary movement disorder.[8] Second, prominent psychiatric symptoms could obscure neurological symptoms or delay neurological diagnoses.[2] Third, medications used to treat neurological symptoms may induce, unmask, or exacerbate psychiatric symptoms and, conversely, psychiatric medications may induce, unmask, or exacerbate movement disorders. Finally, and most pertinent to this chapter, subtle neurological signs are often identified during clinical encounters with children with a variety of developmental or psychiatric conditions. In the absence of known structural lesions in the brain, these findings are referred to as "neurological soft signs."

The purpose of this chapter is to review common movement disorders and subtle neurological findings that are more prevalent in children with developmental psychiatric disorders. This chapter will focus on the three most common developmental and psychiatric conditions likely to be seen in a pediatric movement disorder clinic: ADHD, OCD, and Autism Spectrum Disorder (ASD). The focus will be idiopathic conditions, with a few pertinent references to rarer genetic and acquired ones. Referrals to neurology for these children may come from pediatricians, mental health providers, geneticists, and other clinicians. While no group of motor findings is specific enough for clinical diagnosis, understanding these trends or patterns has a number of potential clinical and research applications. In some children, difficulties with coordination, in the absence of another known neurological disorder such as ataxia, may interfere significantly with performance of everyday tasks. A diagnosis of Developmental Coordination Disorder may be appropriate in this setting.

From a purely clinical standpoint, neurological soft signs can be seen during a routine, detailed neurological examination. Documenting these in the electronic patient record is useful, for example, if the child presents at a later time for evaluation of a possible drug-induced dyskinesia. From a research standpoint, formal assessment batteries include the Physical and Neurological Examination for Soft Signs (PANESS) scale[9] and the Cambridge Neurological Inventory.[10] Domains evaluated include motor and sensory function, development, and maturation. Ratings are based on presence of preserved primitive reflexes, coordination and timing in performance of repeated and sequential finger movements, presence of/failure to inhibit mirror movements, and higher cortical sensory perception such as stereognosis and graphesthesia.

Uses of these motor assessment scales for soft neurological signs have several rationales. A typical study design involves evaluation of cases and controls, where children with a clinical categorical diagnosis are compared as a group with age and sex matched typically developing peers. Test batteries are scored in total, by domain, and by body side (right/left). Investigators test hypotheses about group differences to attempt to understand what structural and functional abnormalities, as indicated by differences in the motor system, may be present in a parallel fashion in circuits forming the substrate for emotional and cognitive dysfunction.[11] Correlational analyses with clinical symptom severity rating scales and correspondence with other assessments such as IQ scores provide additional support for utility of these motor batteries. A further aim is to use the scales' findings to identify predictors of responses to standard pharmacological or behavioral interventions. Corroborating the results with functional or connectivity imaging or quantitative neurophysiological findings could also provide a foundation for testing noninvasive[12–14] or invasive[15] brain stimulation at specific circuit nodes.

ATTENTION DEFICIT HYPERACTIVITY DISORDER

In the *Diagnostic and Statistical Manual of Mental Disorders*, fifth edition (DSM-5), ADHD, combined type, is defined based on the presence of at least six of nine symptoms from inattention criteria and at least six of nine from hyperactivity and impulsivity criteria. The hyperactivity in children with ADHD involves motor restlessness and an increase in typical motor activity, rather than tics, chorea, stereotypies, myoclonus, or dystonia. These symptoms must be present and cause difficulties in multiple settings, and onset must be present prior to age 12 years. Five of nine symptoms are sufficient at ages 17 years.[16] The prevalence of ADHD in the United States in childhood is estimated to be 9.0%.[17] While often considered a disorder of childhood, ADHD symptoms may persist into adulthood.[18]

Motor Deficits and Subtle Neurological Signs in ADHD

Motor impairments in children with ADHD have been recognized for decades, dating back to the era where it was referred to as "Minimal Brain Dysfunction."[19,20] These clinical observations have been validated through identification of underlying differences in brain structure and development.[21–24] While clinically ADHD is defined in terms of inattention, hyperactive motor behavior, and impulsivity, it is recognized that a core neuropsychological feature is impaired executive function. Executive function and motor control develop together through maturation of frontal/subcortical and cerebellar networks. In children with ADHD, this development of motor control is delayed. As a group, ADHD children manifest below average scores on timed repetitive and sequential movements as well as exhibit excess motor overflow and other neurological soft signs.[25–28] This suggests an impaired capacity to inhibit unwanted movements, paralleling impaired capacity to inhibit socially inappropriate behaviors. These observations are supported by physiological studies showing reduced inhibition[29] and GABA levels[30] in motor cortex as well as larger network studies mapping intrinsic brain connectivity.[31]

Common and Rare Movement Disorders in ADHD

Tics in ADHD

The high prevalence of ADHD, OCD, and other psychiatric disorders in Tourette syndrome is well established, although there is some variability in clinical (higher burden of co-morbidity) versus community (lower burden) based samples.[32–34] The prevalence of tic disorders is higher in children with ADHD than in the general population, with recent estimates among children with ADHD ranging from 1.3% to 2.3% in community based samples.[35,36] The patterned motor behavior and urge driven nature of tics distinguishes them from the more general motor hyperactivity in ADHD. Unusual dystonic tics have been associated with ADHD.[37] Treatment of ADHD with both stimulant and non-stimulant medications in some cases reduces tics as well.[38–40]

Stereotypies in ADHD

The prevalence of stereotypies in ADHD is not well characterized. In cohorts of children with complex motor stereotypies (see Chapter 8), recruited from movement disorder clinics, ADHD is seen in approximately one-third of cases.[41,42] In ASD, there are some interesting and surprising overlaps between motor development, stereotypic movements and behaviors, and ADHD. Genetic correlations have been identified between repetitive, restricted behaviors and ADHD symptoms.[43] In addition, children with combined type ADHD and motor coordination disorder also are more likely to show autistic traits.[41,42,44]

Chorea in ADHD

Choreiform movements have long been described in children with ADHD symptoms both clinically[45] and as part of more formal assessments of neurological soft signs.[25,46] ADHD has been described in studies of benign hereditary chorea due to mutations in the *TITF1/NKX2-1* gene.[47] ADHD appears to be a risk factor,[48] an acute symptom,[49] and possibly a consequence of auto-immune, Sydenham's chorea.[50,51] Treatment of ADHD with stimulant medication can induce or exacerbate choreic movements.[52,53]

OBSESSIVE COMPULSIVE DISORDER

In the *Diagnostic and Statistical Manual of Mental Disorders*, fifth edition (DSM-5), OCD is grouped in the category of Obsessive Compulsive and Related Disorders.[16] A number of other idiopathic conditions are included based on their similarity in phenomenology but which are also sufficiently different that they are considered distinct: body dysmorphic disorder, trichotillomania (hair-pulling disorder), hoarding disorder, and excoriation disorder. OCD is diagnosed based on the presence of obsessions and compulsions. *Obsessions* are defined as recurrent and persistent thoughts, urges, or images that are experienced as intrusive and unwanted, and that cause marked anxiety and distress. The individual should on at least some occasions attempt to suppress or ignore such thoughts, impulses, or images or to neutralize them with some other thought or action, although young children may fail to do so. *Compulsions* are defined as repetitive behaviors (e.g., hand washing, ordering, checking) or mental acts (e.g., praying, counting, repeating words silently) in response to an obsession or according to rules that must be applied rigidly. These behaviors or mental acts should aim at a goal of reducing distress related to the obsession. The relationship between the compulsive behavior and a likely outcome may be like a superstition—not based in facts or realistic probabilities. In other cases, the behavioral may be reasonable, like washing to remove contamination, but done to excess in unnecessary situations. Note that young children with OCD may not have insight or be able to describe obsessions accompanying compulsions.

In Western nations, prevalence estimates of OCD range from 0.25% to 2%, with peaks of onset in both pre-adolescent children and in young adult life.[54,55]

Motor Deficits and Subtle Neurological Signs in OCD

Over 25 years, a number of small case-control studies of heterogeneous groups of OCD patients have been evaluated using motor scales, with mixed results.[56–60] The largest study and meta-analysis was performed in adults. This study evaluated 85 adults with OCD and 88 matched controls at sites in Spain and the United Kingdom.[61] The authors also performed a meta-analysis of 20 studies, 15 of which used structured assessments, involving 498 OCD patients and 520 controls.[61] In the primary analysis, the OCD patients from the United Kingdom had modestly higher (worse) primitive reflex and total soft-sign scores. The Spanish investigators found that their OCD cohort had substantially and statistically significantly worse score in primitive reflexes, motor coordination, and sensory integration. In the meta-analysis, the total scores for neurological soft signs had a large, statistically significant positive effect size of 1.27. Effect sizes for both left (0.72) and right (0.68) soft sign scores were comparably elevated. Effect sizes for subscores for primitive reflexes (0.81), sensory integration (0.67), and motor coordination (0.61) were each statistically significant as well.[61] Small studies in children have demonstrated links between neurological soft signs, developmental coordination disorder, and OCD.[62,63] As in adults, studies in a large sample of children with OCD might provide more precise estimates of effect sizes. Clustering children based on a motor score profile could be considered for imaging, treatment, or prognostic research.

Common and Rare Movement Disorders in OCD

Tics in OCD

OCD is common in Tourette syndrome,[32,34] and the pairing of obsessions and compulsions in OCD phenomenologically resemble the pairings of premonitory urges and tics, although premonitory urges generally correlate poorly or not at all with other symptom rating scale scores.[64] As neither OCD nor tic disorders have a biomarker, it was reasonable to query whether OCD with tics or Tourette Syndrome is distinct from OCD with more minor tics or OCD in the absence of tics. Small observational studies suggest there may be differences. For example, the diagnosis of ADHD is more common in OCD patients with Tourette Syndrome. Tics in OCD also segregate with a higher probability of obsessions about symmetry and compulsive evening, touching, blinking, staring, and counting.[65] Several adult studies have compared OCD patients with and without tics to Tourette patients with and without OCD. Results suggested that OCD and Tourette with OCD are distinct from one another. Further, analysis of symptom domains suggest that OCD patients with tics, while "intermediate" with regard to obsessive compulsive themes and behaviors, overall mostly resemble OCD patients.[66–68] In children and adolescents with OCD, those with tics were found to have less compulsive ordering, hoarding, and washing.[69] Pediatric OCD patients with tics have a less robust response to selective serotonin uptake inhibitors but not to cognitive behavioral therapy.[70]

An implication for neurologists who manage children and adolescents with Tourette syndrome is that there is a group of OCD patients who may present for evaluation with acute or chronic tics. If tics are mild and criteria for ADHD are not met, the overall phenotype of such patients may be most similar to OCD without tics. The neurologist may consider providing reassurance and referral to psychology for cognitive behavioral therapy for OCD or to a psychiatrist for further treatment.

OCD with Stereotypy

Data on prevalence of stereotypies in children and adolescents with OCD are limited. Stereotypies are less prevalent than tics in the general population, and many clinicians may fail to accurately distinguish these.[71,72] Complex motor stereotypies may occur in children with and without ASD. A clinic-based study of non-autistic children with motor stereotypies found that 10% of children met criteria for OCD,[41] but that ADHD and tics were more common. It is not known whether OCD with stereotypies represents any specific or clinically meaningful subtype.

OCD with Chorea

Chorea and obsessive compulsive symptoms may co-occur due to pathology in overlapping and parallel cortical-striatal circuits. Mild choreic movements are considered to be neurological soft signs and maybe seen in persons with OCD. Examining children and adolescents with OCD, it is not uncommon to find mild distal hand "spooning" (hyperextension of the metacarpophalangeal joints), or small amplitude, adventitious finger movements, best seen with both arms fully extended and hands palms down with fingers spread. If the choreic soft signs are mild but seem excessive, close clinical follow-up is warranted. In the presence of a subacute history, particularly if there is a systolic heart murmur, a diagnostic evaluation for Sydenham's Chorea may be indicated. If the chorea is clearly more than mild or if it is getting worse, a thorough diagnostic evaluation for auto-immune and other causes is warranted. Differential diagnosis includes auto-immune, rheumatic (Sydenham's) chorea,[51] vasculitides, drug-induced chorea, and psychogenic chorea. In chronic progressive chorea or in the presence of other concerning findings, neuroimaging is generally warranted. In addition to the association to myoclonus dystonia (DYT11),[5] OCD and chorea have been described in chorea acanthocytosis[73] and Wilson's disease.[74] OCD may also occur in benign hereditary chorea.[75]

AUTISM SPECTRUM DISORDER

Autism is a developmental disorder characterized by social deficits, impaired expressive prosody and language, and the presence of restricted, repetitive behaviors. In the latest revision of the DSM (DSM-5 criteria), in order to be diagnosed with autistic spectrum disorder

(ASD), the individual must have (i) Social and Communication deficits that include: problems reciprocating social or emotional interaction; severe problems maintaining relationships; and nonverbal communication problems and (ii) Repetitive and Restrictive Behaviors displaying at least two of the following: extreme attachment to routines and patterns with resistance to changes in routines; repetitive speech or movements; intense and restrictive interests; difficulty integrating sensory information or strong seeking or avoiding behavior toward sensory stimuli. Symptoms should start in early childhood and must impair the individual's ability to function in day-to-day life. The four separate disorders (autistic disorder, Asperger's disorder, childhood disintegrative disorder, pervasive developmental disorder not otherwise specified), allowed under DSM-IV, have been merged in the DSM-5 into a single entity with continuum of symptoms ranging from mild to severe.

The Centers for Disease Control and Prevention (CDC) estimate that the prevalence rate of autism is 1 in 68 births, or 14.7 children per 1000.[76] The onset of symptoms usually occurs before age 3 years. Phenotypic overlap exists between ASDs and other neurodevelopmental disorders such as Tourette syndrome, ADHD, and motor coordination disorders. The precise underlying biological reason for this connection is unknown, although some investigators have suggested a convergence of genes toward a core set of dysregulated processes.[77]

Motor Deficits and Subtle Neurological Signs in ASD

Leo Kanner, in an early description of autism, commented on a variety of motor deficits associated with this disorder. Although some difficulties are noted in the first 6 months of life, typically from the toddler years on a variety of disabilities are noted in children with autism including stereotypies, toe-walking, clumsiness, gait abnormalities, unusual postures, and hypotonia.[78,79] In a study comparing children with ASD and age-matched normally developing children, the former had greater joint mobility, more gait abnormalities, and walked 1.6 months later than their non-autistic peers.[80] More than twice as many ASD children have hypotonia with preserved muscle strength and tendon reflexes. Toe-walking, considered to be a marker for developmental delay,[81] has been reported in almost two-thirds of children with ASD.[82] Gait abnormalities, including descriptions of wide-based, clumsy, and variable stride length are common.[80,83] Others have suggested that motor skill deficits may not be pervasive in autism, but more apparent in activities involving balance or complex interceptive actions (catching a ball).[84] In a study comparing children with autism and Asperger syndrome, both had deficits in coordination, ambulation, and Romberg testing, but measures of cerebellar functioning were less impaired in the Asperger group.[85] In a kinematic study of adults with autism, individuals moved with atypical kinematics (did not minimize jerk) and moved with greater acceleration and velocity.[86]

The substrate for abnormal motor control in ASD may involve cerebellum and cerebellar circuits, as supported by structural[87–91] and functional[92–94] imaging studies. Inconsistencies across studies support the continuation of studies in larger clinical research networks incorporating careful phenotyping, genetics, and imaging.[95] With the development of more sophisticated animal models based on genetic findings in autism, putative mechanisms involving cerebellar structure[96] and Purkinje cell plasticity[97] have been identified. Taken together, these studies suggest careful studies of motor function in children with ASD might provide insights into the core clinical features.

Sleep Disorders in ASD

Patients with ASD are at high risk for having sleep disorders and dysregulation of the sleep–wake cycle.[98] For example up to 60% have sleep disturbances including sleep fragmentation, periodic limb movements of sleep (PLMS), and frequent night time arousals.[99,100] In a polysomnographic study,[101] the prevalence of PLMS in children with ASD was three times higher than non-autistic peers. Forty-two percent of ASD patients had sleep fragmentation, with more girls having alpha intrusions and lower sleep efficiency than boys. There is no association between the severity of cognitive impairment or the subtype of ASD and the prevalence of sleep abnormalities.[100,102] In contrast, the presence of anxiety and/or depression in children with ASD is more common in poor versus good sleepers. In addition, the success of early developmental and behavioral intervention in ASD has been shown to be influenced by the child getting adequate sleep.

Pathophysiologically, abnormally low levels of melatonin and ferritin have been documented in autistic subjects, and polymorphisms have been identified in time-keeping period 1 genes. Supplemental iron treatment in ASD has reduced restless sleep and increased ferritin levels.[103] Behavioral measures for sleep disorders include a consistent sleeping environment and routine, avoiding exciting and stimulating activities in the hours before bedtime, extra quiet time, weighted blankets, and behavioral extinction therapy.[98] Melatonin administered at bedtime improved sleep in individuals with neurodevelopmental disabilities.[104,105]

Movement Disorders in ASD

Tics and Stereotypies in ASD

The prevalence of tics disorders in children with autism is as high as 20–25% in some cohorts,[106] with more frequent tics also identified in children with Fragile X Syndrome and their siblings.[107] Stereotypies are a cardinal repetitive behavior often seen in children with ASDs. Sensory processing differences may predict the likelihood of repetitive, stereotyped movements in children with autism.[108]

Catatonia in ASD

Although not considered a movement disorder, catatonia should be considered in any individual with ASD who has a marked deterioration in movement.[109,110] Common features of catatonia-like deterioration are slowness and difficulty initiating movements unless prompted, odd gait, odd stiff postures, freezing during actions, reductions in speech, and mutism. A variety of pharmacological agents, infections, metabolic dysfunctions, endocrine, neurological, and autoimmune disorders have been associated with catatonia.[111] Lorazepam is recommended therapy.

CONCLUSION

Anomalous motor development as well as movement disorders are common in the heterogeneous developmental diagnoses of ADHD, OCD, and ASD. Detailed clinical, imaging, and animal model studies are providing new insights into the neural substrate of typical childhood development as well as the pathophysiology of anomalous development in these conditions. These insights may provide a better basis for identifying both common and diverging mechanisms for producing the core impairments in children with these diagnoses, and ultimately point the way to more effective treatments.

References

1. Bitsko RH, Danielson M, King M, Visser SN, Scahill L, Perou R. Health care needs of children with Tourette syndrome. *J Child Neurol*. 2013;28(12):1626–1636.
2. Walshe JM, Yealland M. Wilson's disease: the problem of delayed diagnosis. *J Neurol Neurosurg Psychiatry*. 1992;55(8):692–696.
3. Heiman GA, Ottman R, Saunders-Pullman RJ, Ozelius LJ, Risch NJ, Bressman SB. Increased risk for recurrent major depression in DYT1 dystonia mutation carriers. *Neurology*. 2004;63(4):631–637.
4. Heiman GA, Ottman R, Saunders-Pullman RJ, Ozelius LJ, Risch NJ, Bressman SB. Obsessive-compulsive disorder is not a clinical manifestation of the DYT1 dystonia gene. *Am J Med Genet B Neuropsychiatr Genet*. 2007;144B(3):361–364.
5. Hess CW, Raymond D, Aguiar Pde C, et al. Myoclonus-dystonia, obsessive-compulsive disorder, and alcohol dependence in SGCE mutation carriers. *Neurology*. 2007;68(7):522–524.
6. Bonello M, Larner AJ, Alusi SH. Myoclonus-dystonia (DYT11) with novel SGCE mutation misdiagnosed as a primary psychiatric disorder. *J Neurol Sci*. 2014;346(1-2):356–357.
7. Gilbert DL. Treatment of children and adolescents with tics and Tourette syndrome. *J Child Neurol*. 2006;21:690–700.
8. Eddy CM, Cavanna AE, Gulisano M, et al. Clinical correlates of quality of life in Tourette syndrome. *Mov Disord*. 2011;26(4):735–738.
9. Holden EW, Tarnowski KJ, Prinz RJ. Reliability of neurological soft signs in children: reevaluation of the PANESS. *J Abnorm Child Psychol*. 1982;10(2):163–172.
10. Chen EY, Shapleske J, Luque R, et al. The Cambridge Neurological Inventory: a clinical instrument for assessment of soft neurological signs in psychiatric patients. *Psychiatry Res*. 1995;56(2):183–204.
11. Alexander GE, DeLong MR, Strick PL. Parallel organization of functionally segregated circuits linking basal ganglia and cortex. *Annu Rev Neurosci*. 1986;9:357–381.
12. Wu SW, Maloney T, Gilbert DL, et al. Functional MRI-navigated repetitive transcranial magnetic stimulation over supplementary motor area in chronic tic disorders. *Brain Stimul*. 2014;7(2):212–218.
13. Narayanaswamy JC, Jose D, Chhabra H, et al. Successful Application of Add-on Transcranial Direct Current Stimulation (tDCS) for Treatment of SSRI Resistant OCD. *Brain Stimul*. 2015;8(3):655–657.
14. Enticott PG, Fitzgibbon BM, Kennedy HA, et al. A double-blind, randomized trial of deep repetitive transcranial magnetic stimulation (rTMS) for autism spectrum disorder. *Brain Stimul*. 2014;7(2):206–211.
15. Lipsman N, Giacobbe P, Lozano AM. Deep brain stimulation in obsessive-compulsive disorder: neurocircuitry and clinical experience. *Handb Clin Neurol*. 2013;116:245–250.
16. American Psychological Association. *Diagnostic and Statistical Manual of Mental Disorders, (DSM-5®)*. Washington, DC: American Psychiatric Publishing; 2013.
17. Akinbami LJ, Liu X, Pastor PN, Reuben CA. Attention deficit hyperactivity disorder among children aged 5-17 years in the United States, 1998-2009. *NCHS Data Brief*. 2011;70.
18. Volkow ND, Swanson JM. Clinical practice: adult attention deficit-hyperactivity disorder. *N Engl J Med*. 2013;369(20):1935–1944.
19. Seger EY, Hallum G. Methylphenidate in children with minimal brain dysfunction: effects on attention span, visual-motor skills, and behavior. *Curr Ther Res Clin Exp*. 1974;16(6):635–641.
20. Levy HB. Minimal brain dysfunction/specific learning disability: a clinical approach for the primary physician. *South Med J*. 1976;69(5):642–653.
21. Shaw P, Gilliam M, Liverpool M, et al. Cortical development in typically developing children with symptoms of hyperactivity and impulsivity: support for a dimensional view of attention deficit hyperactivity disorder. *Am J Psychiatry*. 2011;168(2):143–151.

22. Shaw P, Malek M, Watson B, Sharp W, Evans A, Greenstein D. Development of cortical surface area and gyrification in attention-deficit/hyperactivity disorder. *Biol Psychiatry*. 2012;72(3):191–197.

23. Shaw P, Malek M, Watson B, Greenstein D, de Rossi P, Sharp W. Trajectories of cerebral cortical development in childhood and adolescence and adult attention-deficit/hyperactivity disorder. *Biol Psychiatry*. 2013; 74(8):599–606.

24. Shaw P, De Rossi P, Watson B, et al. Mapping the development of the basal ganglia in children with attention-deficit/hyperactivity disorder. *J Am Acad Child Adolesc Psychiatry*. 2014;53(7):780–789 e711.

25. Denckla MB, Rudel RG. Anomalies of motor development in hyperactive boys. *Ann Neurol*. 1978;3(3):231–233.

26. Mostofsky SH, Rimrodt SL, Schafer JG, et al. Atypical motor and sensory cortex activation in attention-deficit/hyperactivity disorder: a functional magnetic resonance imaging study of simple sequential finger tapping. *Biol Psychiatry*. 2006;59(1):48–56.

27. Macneil LK, Xavier P, Garvey MA, et al. Quantifying excessive mirror overflow in children with attention-deficit/hyperactivity disorder. *Neurology*. 2011;76(7):622–628.

28. Chan RC, McAlonan GM, Yang B, Lin L, Shum D, Manschreck TC. Prevalence of neurological soft signs and their neuropsychological correlates in typically developing Chinese children and Chinese children with ADHD. *Dev Neuropsychol*. 2010;35(6):698–711.

29. Gilbert DL, Isaacs KM, Augusta M, Macneil LK, Mostofsky SH. Motor cortex inhibition: a marker of ADHD behavior and motor development in children. *Neurology*. 2011;76(7):615–621.

30. Edden RA, Crocetti D, Zhu H, Gilbert DL, Mostofsky SH. Reduced GABA concentration in attention-deficit/hyperactivity disorder. *Arch Gen Psychiatry*. 2012;69(7):750–753.

31. Castellanos FX, Proal E. Large-scale brain systems in ADHD: beyond the prefrontal-striatal model. *Trends Cogn Sci*. 2012;16(1):17–26.

32. Hirschtritt ME, Lee PC, Pauls DL, et al. Lifetime prevalence, age of risk, and genetic relationships of comorbid psychiatric disorders in Tourette syndrome. *JAMA Psychiatry*. 2015;72(4):325–333.

33. Scharf JM, Miller LL, Mathews CA, Ben-Shlomo Y. Prevalence of Tourette syndrome and chronic tics in the population-based Avon longitudinal study of parents and children cohort. *J Am Acad Child Adolesc Psychiatry*. 2012;51(2):192–201 e195.

34. Robertson MM, Cavanna AE, Eapen V. Gilles de la Tourette syndrome and disruptive behavior disorders: prevalence, associations, and explanation of the relationships. *J Neuropsychiatry Clin Neurosci*. 2015;27(1):33–41.

35. Schlander M, Schwarz O, Rothenberger A, Roessner V. Tic disorders: administrative prevalence and co-occurrence with attention-deficit/hyperactivity disorder in a German community sample. *Eur Psychiatry*. 2011;26(6):370–374.

36. Larson K, Russ SA, Kahn RS, Halfon N. Patterns of comorbidity, functioning, and service use for US children with ADHD, 2007. *Pediatrics*. 2011;127(3):462–470.

37. Jankovic J, Stone L. Dystonic tics in patients with Tourette's syndrome. *Mov Disord*. 1991;6(3):248–252.

38. Tourette's Syndrome Study G. Treatment of ADHD in children with tics: a randomized controlled trial. *Neurology*. 2002;58(4):527–536.

39. Allen AJ, Kurlan RM, Gilbert DL, et al. Atomoxetine treatment in children and adolescents with ADHD and comorbid tic disorders. *Neurology*. 2005;65(12):1941–1949.

40. Scahill L, Chappell PB, Kim YS, et al. A placebo-controlled study of guanfacine in the treatment of children with tic disorders and attention deficit hyperactivity disorder. *Am J Psychiatry*. 2001;158(7):1067–1074.

41. Harris KM, Mahone EM, Singer HS. Nonautistic motor stereotypies: clinical features and longitudinal follow-up. *Pediatr Neurol*. 2008;38(4):267–272.

42. Oakley C, Mahone EM, Morris-Berry C, Kline T, Singer HS. Primary complex motor stereotypies in older children and adolescents: clinical features and longitudinal follow-up. *Pediatr Neurol*. 2015;52(4):398–403 e391.

43. Polderman TJ, Hoekstra RA, Posthuma D, Larsson H. The co-occurrence of autistic and ADHD dimensions in adults: an etiological study in 17,770 twins. *Transl Psychiatry*. 2014;4:e435.

44. Reiersen AM, Constantino JN, Todd RD. Co-occurrence of motor problems and autistic symptoms in attention-deficit/hyperactivity disorder. *J Am Acad Child Adolesc Psychiatry*. 2008;47(6):662–672.

45. Debray-Ritzen P, Messerschmitt P, Madelin C, Fallet M. [Minimal brain dysfunction. Our investigation of choreiform syndrome in children with MBD (author's transl)]. *Sem Hop*. 1978;54(37–40):1165–1166.

46. Cole WR, Mostofsky SH, Larson JC, Denckla MB, Mahone EM. Age-related changes in motor subtle signs among girls and boys with ADHD. *Neurology*. 2008;71(19):1514–1520.

47. Gras D, Jonard L, Roze E, et al. Benign hereditary chorea: phenotype, prognosis, therapeutic outcome and long term follow-up in a large series with new mutations in the TITF1/NKX2-1 gene. *J Neurol Neurosurg Psychiatry.* 2012;83(10):956–962.

48. Mercadante MT, Busatto GF, Lombroso PJ, et al. The psychiatric symptoms of rheumatic fever. *Am J Psychiatry.* 2000;157(12):2036–2038.

49. Freeman JM, Aron AM, Collard JE, Mackay MC. The emotional correlates of Sydenham's chorea. *Pediatrics.* 1965;35:42–49.

50. Ridel KR, Lipps TD, Gilbert DL. The prevalence of neuropsychiatric disorders in Sydenham's chorea. *Pediatr Neurol.* 2010;42(4):243–248.

51. Maia DP, Teixeira Jr. AL, Quintao Cunningham MC, Cardoso F. Obsessive compulsive behavior, hyperactivity, and attention deficit disorder in Sydenham chorea. *Neurology.* 2005;64(10):1799–1801.

52. Ford JB, Albertson TE, Owen KP, Sutter ME, McKinney WB. Acute, sustained chorea in children after suprathreapeutic dosing of amphetamine-derived medications. *Pediatr Neurol.* 2012;47(3):216–218.

53. Weiner WJ, Nausieda PA, Klawans HL. Methylphenidate-induced chorea: case report and pharmacologic implications. *Neurology.* 1978;28(10):1041–1044.

54. Flament MF, Whitaker A, Rapoport JL, et al. Obsessive compulsive disorder in adolescence: an epidemiological study. *J Am Acad Child Adolesc Psychiatry.* 1988;27(6):764–771.

55. Heyman I, Fombonne E, Simmons H, Ford T, Meltzer H, Goodman R. Prevalence of obsessive-compulsive disorder in the British nationwide survey of child mental health. *Int Rev Psychiatry.* 2003;15(1–2):178–184.

56. Guz H, Aygun D. Neurological soft signs in obsessive-compulsive disorder. *Neurol India.* 2004;52(1):72–75.

57. Hollander E, Schiffman E, Cohen B, et al. Signs of central nervous system dysfunction in obsessive-compulsive disorder. *Arch Gen Psychiatry.* 1990;47(1):27–32.

58. Flament MF, Koby E, Rapoport JL, et al. Childhood obsessive-compulsive disorder: a prospective follow-up study. *J Child Psychol Psychiatry.* 1990;31(3):363–380.

59. Bihari K, Pato MT, Hill JL, Murphy DL. Neurologic soft signs in obsessive-compulsive disorder. *Arch Gen Psychiatry.* 1991;48(3):278–279.

60. Jaafari N, Baup N, Bourdel MC, et al. Neurological soft signs in OCD patients with early age at onset, versus patients with schizophrenia and healthy subjects. *J Neuropsychiatry Clin Neurosci.* 2011;23(4):409–416.

61. Jaafari N, Fernandez de la Cruz L, Grau M, et al. Neurological soft signs in obsessive-compulsive disorder: two empirical studies and meta-analysis. *Psychol Med.* 2013;43(5):1069–1079.

62. Pine D, Shaffer D, Schonfeld IS. Persistent emotional disorder in children with neurological soft signs. *J Am Acad Child Adolesc Psychiatry.* 1993;32(6):1229–1236.

63. Pratt ML, Hill EL. Anxiety profiles in children with and without developmental coordination disorder. *Res Dev Disabil.* 2011;32(4):1253–1259.

64. Reese HE, Scahill L, Peterson AL, et al. The premonitory urge to tic: measurement, characteristics, and correlates in older adolescents and adults. *Behav Ther.* 2014;45(2):177–186.

65. Petter T, Richter MA, Sandor P. Clinical features distinguishing patients with Tourette's syndrome and obsessive-compulsive disorder from patients with obsessive-compulsive disorder without tics. *J Clin Psychiatry.* 1998;59(9):456–459.

66. Cath DC, Spinhoven P, Hoogduin CA, et al. Repetitive behaviors in Tourette's syndrome and OCD with and without tics: what are the differences? *Psychiatry Res.* 2001;101(2):171–185.

67. Cath DC, Spinhoven P, van Woerkom TC, et al. Gilles de la Tourette's syndrome with and without obsessive-compulsive disorder compared with obsessive-compulsive disorder without tics: which symptoms discriminate? *J Nerv Ment Dis.* 2001;189(4):219–228.

68. Diniz JB, Rosario-Campos MC, Hounie AG, et al. Chronic tics and Tourette syndrome in patients with obsessive-compulsive disorder. *J Psychiatr Res.* 2006;40(6):487–493.

69. Hanna GL, Piacentini J, Cantwell DP, Fischer DJ, Himle JA, Van Etten M. Obsessive-compulsive disorder with and without tics in a clinical sample of children and adolescents. *Depress Anxiety.* 2002;16(2):59–63.

70. March JS, Franklin ME, Leonard H, et al. Tics moderate treatment outcome with sertraline but not cognitive-behavior therapy in pediatric obsessive-compulsive disorder. *Biol Psychiatry.* 2007;61(3):344–347.

71. Freeman RD, Soltanifar A, Baer S. Stereotypic movement disorder: easily missed. *Dev Med Child Neurol.* 2010;52(8):733–738.

72. Zinner SH, Mink JW. Movement disorders I: tics and stereotypies. *Pediatr Rev.* 2010;31(6):223–233.

V. SELECTED SECONDARY MOVEMENT DISORDERS

73. Walterfang M, Yucel M, Walker R, et al. Adolescent obsessive compulsive disorder heralding chorea-acanthocytosis. *Mov Disord*. 2008;23(3):422–425.

74. Kumawat BL, Sharma CM, Tripathi G, Ralot T, Dixit S. Wilson's disease presenting as isolated obsessive-compulsive disorder. *Indian J Med Sci*. 2007;61(11):607–610.

75. Peall KJ, Lumsden D, Kneen R, et al. Benign hereditary chorea related to NKX2.1: expansion of the genotypic and phenotypic spectrum. *Dev Med Child Neurol*. 2014;56(7):642–648.

76. Falco M. Autism rates now 1 in 68 U.S. children: CDC. *CNN*2014.

77. Eapen V, Clarke RA. Autism spectrum disorders: from genotypes to phenotypes. *Front Hum Neurosci*. 2014:8.

78. Tsai LY. Brief report: comorbid psychiatric disorders of autistic disorder. *J Autism Dev Disord*. 1996;26(2):159–163.

79. Goldman S, Wang C, Salgado MW, Greene PE, Kim M, Rapin I. Motor stereotypies in children with autism and other developmental disorders. *Dev Med Child Neurol*. 2009;51(1):30–38.

80. Shetreat-Klein M, Shinnar S, Rapin I. Abnormalities of joint mobility and gait in children with autism spectrum disorders. *Brain Dev*. 2014;36(2):91–96.

81. Shulman LH, Sala DA, Chu MLY, McCaul PR, Sandler BJ. Developmental implications of idiopathic toe walking. *J Pediatr*. 1997;130(4):541–546.

82. Accardo P, Whitman B. Toe walking. A marker for language disorders in the developmentally disabled. *Clin Pediatr*. 1989;28(8):347–350.

83. Rinehart NJ, Tonge BJ, Bradshaw JL, Iansek R, Enticott PG, Johnson KA. Movement-related potentials in high-functioning autism and Asperger's disorder. *Dev Med Child Neurol*. 2006;48(4):272–277.

84. Whyatt CP, Craig CM. Motor skills in children aged 7-10 years, diagnosed with autism spectrum disorder. *J Autism Dev Disord*. 2012;42(9):1799–1809.

85. Behere A, Shahani L, Noggle CA, Dean R. Motor functioning in autistic spectrum disorders: a preliminary analysis. *J Neuropsychiatry Clin Neurosci*. 2012;24(1):87–94.

86. Cook JL, Blakemore SJ, Press C. Atypical basic movement kinematics in autism spectrum conditions. *Brain*. 2013;136(Pt 9):2816–2824.

87. Holttum JR, Minshew NJ, Sanders RS, Phillips NE. Magnetic resonance imaging of the posterior fossa in autism. *Biol Psychiatry*. 1992;32(12):1091–1101.

88. Courchesne E, Townsend J, Saitoh O. The brain in infantile autism: posterior fossa structures are abnormal. *Neurology*. 1994;44(2):214–223.

89. Mitchell SR, Reiss AL, Tatusko DH, et al. Neuroanatomic alterations and social and communication deficits in monozygotic twins discordant for autism disorder. *Am J Psychiatry*. 2009;166(8):917–925.

90. Scott JA, Schumann CM, Goodlin-Jones BL, Amaral DG. A comprehensive volumetric analysis of the cerebellum in children and adolescents with autism spectrum disorder. *Autism Res*. 2009;2(5):246–257.

91. Ameis SH, Fan J, Rockel C, et al. Impaired structural connectivity of socio-emotional circuits in autism spectrum disorders: a diffusion tensor imaging study. *PLoS One*. 2011;6(11):e28044.

92. Murphy CM, Christakou A, Daly EM, et al. Abnormal functional activation and maturation of fronto-striato-temporal and cerebellar regions during sustained attention in autism spectrum disorder. *Am J Psychiatry*. 2014;171(10):1107–1116.

93. Nair A, Treiber JM, Shukla DK, Shih P, Muller RA. Impaired thalamocortical connectivity in autism spectrum disorder: a study of functional and anatomical connectivity. *Brain*. 2013;136(Pt 6):1942–1955.

94. Thakkar KN, Polli FE, Joseph RM, et al. Response monitoring, repetitive behaviour and anterior cingulate abnormalities in autism spectrum disorders (ASD). *Brain*. 2008;131(Pt 9):2464–2478.

95. Hernandez LM, Rudie JD, Green SA, Bookheimer S, Dapretto M. Neural signatures of autism spectrum disorders: insights into brain network dynamics. *Neuropsychopharmacology*. 2015;40(1):171–189.

96. Steadman PE, Ellegood J, Szulc KU, et al. Genetic effects on cerebellar structure across mouse models of autism using a magnetic resonance imaging atlas. *Autism Res*. 2014;7(1):124–137.

97. Piochon C, Kloth AD, Grasselli G, et al. Cerebellar plasticity and motor learning deficits in a copy-number variation mouse model of autism. *Nat Commun*. 2014;5:5586.

98. Kotagal S, Broomall E. Sleep in children with autism spectrum disorder. *Pediatr Neurol*. 2012;47(4):242–251.

99. Cortesi F, Giannotti F, Ivanenko A, Johnson K. Sleep in children with autistic spectrum disorder. *Sleep Med*. 2010;11(7):659–664.

100. Richdale AL, Schreck KA. Sleep problems in autism spectrum disorders: prevalence, nature, & possible biopsychosocial aetiologies. *Sleep Med Rev.* 2009;13(6):403–411.

101. Youssef J, Singh K, Huntington N, Becker R, Kothare SV. Relationship of serum ferritin levels to sleep fragmentation and periodic limb movements of sleep on polysomnography in autism spectrum disorders. *Pediatr Neurol.* 2013;49(4):274–278.

102. Polimeni MA, Richdale AL, Francis AJ. A survey of sleep problems in autism, Asperger's disorder and typically developing children. *J Intellect Disabil Res.* 2005;49(Pt 4):260–268.

103. Dosman CF, Brian JA, Drmic IE, et al. Children with autism: effect of iron supplementation on sleep and ferritin. *Pediatr Neurol.* 2007;36(3):152–158.

104. Johnson KP, Malow BA. Assessment and pharmacologic treatment of sleep disturbance in autism. *Child Adolesc Psychiatr Clin N Am.* 2008;17(4):773–785, viii.

105. Malow B, Adkins KW, McGrew SG, et al. Melatonin for sleep in children with autism: a controlled trial examining dose, tolerability, and outcomes. *J Autism Dev Disord.* 2012;42(8):1729–1737; author reply 1738.

106. Canitano R, Vivanti G. Tics and Tourette syndrome in autism spectrum disorders. *Autism.* 2007;11(1):19–28.

107. Gabis LV, Baruch YK, Jokel A, Raz R. Psychiatric and autistic comorbidity in fragile X syndrome across ages. *J Child Neurol.* 2011;26(8):940–948.

108. Gal E, Dyck MJ, Passmore A. Relationships between stereotyped movements and sensory processing disorders in children with and without developmental or sensory disorders. *Am J Occup Ther.* 2010;64(3):453–461.

109. Dhossche DM, Shah A, Wing L. Blueprints for the assessment, treatment, and future study of catatonia in autism spectrum disorders. *Int Rev Neurobiol.* 2006;72:267–284.

110. Wijemanne S, Jankovic J. Movement disorders in catatonia. *J Neurol Neurosurg Psychiatry,* 2015, in press. <http://dx.doi.org/10.1136/jnnp-2014-309098>.

111. Carroll B, Goforth H. Medical catatonia. In: Caroff SN, Mann SC, Francis A, eds. *Catatonia: From Psychopathology to Neurobiology.* Washington, DC: American Psychiatric Publishing; 2004:123.

22

Drug-Induced Movement Disorders in Children

Harvey S. Singer[1], Jonathan W. Mink[2],
Donald L. Gilbert[3] and Joseph Jankovic[4]

[1]Department of Neurology, Johns Hopkins Hospital, Baltimore, MD, USA;
[2]Division of Child Neurology, University of Rochester Medical Center,
Rochester, NY, USA; [3]Division of Neurology, Cincinnati Children's Hospital
Medical Center, Cincinnati, OH, USA; [4]Department of Neurology, Baylor
College of Medicine, Houston, TX, USA

Movement Disorders in Childhood, Second Edition.
DOI: http://dx.doi.org/10.1016/B978-0-12-411573-6.00022-X

491

INTRODUCTION AND OVERVIEW

Recognizing and managing drug-induced movement disorders (DIMDs) in children poses many challenges. As is the case for adults, agents that modulate dopamine are the most common causes of DIMDs. Because dopamine blocking medications are widely used in children, and are increasingly used in preschool children in the United States, these agents will receive special emphasis in this chapter.

The problem of pediatric DIMDs has received increased attention as the number of children treated with psychotropic medications has increased. Clinical trials as well as systematic reviews such as those from the Cochrane Collaboration[1] now have more pediatric data. There are studies of polypharmacy[2] as well as epidemiological studies, particularly involving children with autism.[3-5] This chapter also attempts to provide appropriate caution and discuss the limitations of what we know.

From an epidemiologic perspective, it is important to point out that increased utilization of psychiatric drugs in children in the United States over the past 20 years is well documented.[3,6-11] Of interest, the prevalence of psychotropic use in 2- to 5-year-old children in the United States, which increased from 1994 to 2005, may have plateaued at approximately 1–2%.[12,13] This still represents, collectively, an enormous exposure to psychotropic agents in the developing child. In general, the prevalence of psychotropic use outside of the United States is less.

The US Food and Drug Administration (FDA) has approved so-called atypical antipsychotics such as risperidone and aripiprazole for several pediatric indications. These include psychiatric symptoms which can be difficult to consistently define, recognize, or diagnose: irritability in autism, schizophrenia in adolescents, and manic or mixed episodes of bipolar disorder. It is important to understand that atypical does not indicate absence of risk for DIMDs. For example, risperidone has high potency for D2 receptors and can have an adverse effect profile similar to the typical antipsychotic haloperidol.[14]

Iatrogenic conditions are a sensitive topic given the bioethical principle of nonmaleficence as well as concerns about litigation and liability. In this case, some additional background is needed. First, much prescribing of medication for central nervous system (CNS) diagnoses is, necessarily, "off-label" (done outside the realm of FDA-approved indications). Second, the availability of high-quality, statistically robust clinical trial data for making clinical decisions for children is unsatisfactory, for complex reasons. These reasons include the challenges to both validity and generalizability arising from ill-defined symptom-based categorical diagnoses, inconvenience or impracticality for families of intensive clinical trials, fears about both active experimental drugs and about randomization to placebo, ethical issues of clinical trials in special populations, high costs of clinical trials, and lack of commercial interest. Third, there are inherent risks in medical treatments of all kinds, and psychiatric disorders are no different. Fourth, in many cases, even with better knowledge of iatrogenic risks than we have now, the substantial impact of psychiatric illnesses means that the benefit/risk ratio often still would favor treatment. Fifth, medication use in pediatric psychiatric disorders should be part of a comprehensive treatment plan that includes appropriate behavioral therapies. However, access to comprehensive behavioral health care for many families is limited by costs, insurance coverage, and access to providers with appropriate pediatric training.

Last, although long-term adverse neurologic or psychiatric effects of medications are unknown, in the short term, it appears that most DIMDs are reversible in children.

DEFINITION OF DIMDs

Iatrogenic movement disorders, or *DIMDs*, are conditions where the abnormal movements are related to the use of medication. Several time courses may occur, as detailed in Table 22.1.

CLINICAL CHARACTERISTICS—PHENOMENOLOGY OF DIMDS IN CHILDREN

Common DIMDs in children vary widely and include: hypokinetic/rigid syndrome (Parkinsonism), dystonia, chorea, tremor, ataxia, tics, stereotypies, and poorly specified dyskinesias. Akathisia is generally discussed as a DIMD because of the motor phenomenology of restlessness. Akathisia primarily involves uncomfortable sensations of inner restlessness, with compulsion to move secondarily. Tremor is one of the most common DIMDs and is also addressed in Chapter 13. Because the clinician generally has access, via past medical

TABLE 22.1   Temporal Classification of DIMDs

Temporal class	Time course of appearance and duration of movement disorder
Acute	Onset at treatment onset, within a short time interval, or at the time of a dose increase
Chronic	Onset early or insidiously during treatment, persistence for weeks or longer while treatment is ongoing
Tardive	Emergence gradually, after prolonged treatment with the medication
Withdrawal emergent	Onset subacutely after dose decreases or discontinuations, persistency for days or longer, or until withdrawn medication is reinitiated

history and electronic records, to information about what a child has been prescribed, this chapter will be organized according to drug class, rather than according to the phenomenology of the movement disorder.

DRUG-INDUCED MOVEMENT DISORDERS

In general, for each drug class, epidemiology, clinical features, pathophysiology, diagnostic approach, treatment, and outcome will be discussed.

DIMDs Associated with Dopamine Receptor Blockade: Typical and Atypical Antipsychotics

Epidemiology

Conventional low- and high-potency neuroleptics have been prescribed in children for decades. These agents were used to reduce aggressive behavior, particularly in children with intellectual impairment and autism.[15-18] Pimozide and haloperidol, currently approved by the US FDA for the treatment of Tourette syndrome, have been found to be effective in tic suppression, although side effects and discontinuation rates are high.[19-23] In addition, the dopamine receptor blockers metoclopramide and prochlorperazine have been used in children as antiemetics and for migraine-associated nausea for many years.

Studies of prescribing practices since the marketing of risperidone in 1993 in the United States show dramatic increases in the use of antipsychotics for behavior problems in children of all ages.[9,11,24-26] Conventional neuroleptics are still prescribed because of their effectiveness, relatively lower cost, and concerns about metabolic consequences of the atypical antipsychotics, including weight gain and increased risk of type 2 diabetes.[27] However, most of the increase in prescribing in children for the past 20 years involves atypical antipsychotics. The use of these agents for their original indications for psychotic disorders is vastly outpaced in children by use for anger, mood stabilization, aggression, and autistic spectrum disorder (ASD) behaviors. The potential relevance to public health of the practice of prescribing atypical antipsychotics as mood stabilizer is clear when placed in context of the stunning increase in the diagnosis of childhood bipolar disorder. Based on the National Medical Ambulatory Care Survey for children and youth ages 0–19 years, an estimated 25 per 100,000 office visits involved a diagnosis of bipolar disorder in 1994–1995. This skyrocketed to 1003 visits per 100,000 in 2002–2003.[28] Critics of current psychiatric practices in the United States have suggested that pharmaceutical companies' aggressive marketing has influenced both the rising prevalence of these diagnoses and the rising utilization of these medications.[29]

Many case reports describe DIMDs in children treated with neuroleptics and atypical antipsychotics used for behavior or as antiemetics.[30] Most acute DIMDs are transient and subside after withdrawal of the offending medication. Vastly different estimates of risks of acute, chronic, and tardive DIMDs are obtained depending on the sample size and study design.

It is important for neurologists to be aware of situations and groups of patients at risk for DIMDs. Table 22.2 is meant to aid in this process. Because dopamine receptor blocking agents have many short- and long-term uses outside of neurology and psychiatry, Table 22.2 shows the US FDA-labeled and non-FDA-labeled indications. It is important to

TABLE 22.2 Selected Dopamine Receptor Blocking Agents: Indications, Approvals, and Risks

Medication	FDA-labeled indications[a]	Non-FDA-labeled indications	Common adverse events: neurologic	Serious neurologic adverse events
TYPICAL NEUROLEPTICS				
Chlorpromazine	Acute intermittent porphyria	None	Akathisia, dystonia, Parkinsonism, somnolence	Ineffective thermoregulation
	Apprehension, presurgical		Tremor	Heatstroke or hypothermia
	Bipolar disorder			Neuroleptic malignant syndrome
	Hiccoughs, intractable			Seizure
	Nausea and vomiting			Tardive dyskinesia
	Problem behavior (severe)			
	Schizophrenia			
	Tetanus, adjunct			
Fluphenazine	Schizophrenia	None		
Haloperidol	Tourette syndrome, severe refractory, hyperactive behavior, problematic behavior, schizophrenia	None		Neuroleptic malignant syndrome
				Seizure
				Tardive dyskinesia
Metoclopramide	Chemotherapy-induced nausea/vomiting, prophylaxis	Administration of analgesic	Asthenia	Neuroleptic malignant syndrome
	Diabetic gastroparesis	Decreased lactation	Headache	Tardive dyskinesia
	Gastroesophageal reflux disease	Indigestion	Somnolence	
	Intestinal in tubation, small bowel	Nondiabetic gastroparesis		
	Postoperative nausea and vomiting	Pheochromocytoma, diagnosis		
	Radiography of gastrointestinal tract, adjunct	Postoperative atelectasis		
		Vomiting of pregnancy		

(Continued)

TABLE 22.2 (Continued)

Medication	FDA-labeled indications[a]	Non-FDA-labeled indications	Common adverse events: neurologic	Serious neurologic adverse events
Pimozide	Tourette syndrome	Chronic schizophrenia	Akathisia, dizziness, dystonia, Parkinsonism, somnolence Tremor	Ineffective thermoregulation, heatstroke or hypothermia, neuroleptic malignant syndrome Seizure Tardive dyskinesia
Prochlorperazine	Nausea and vomiting, severe	None	Akathisia, dizziness, dystonia Parkinsonism, somnolence Tremor	Neuroleptic malignant syndrome Tardive dyskinesia
ATYPICAL ANTIPSYCHOTICS				
Aripiprazole	Autistic disorder—agitation Bipolar disorder—agitation Bipolar I disorder, adjunctive Bipolar I disorder, manic or mixed episodes Major depressive disorder, adjunctive Schizophrenia Tourette syndrome	Borderline personality disorder	Akathisia Dystonia, headache, insomnia, somnolence Tremor	Cerebrovascular accident Seizure Tardive dyskinesia Transient ischemic attack

Drug	Approved indication (children)	Off-label/other indication	Adverse effects (common)	Adverse effects (serious)
Olanzapine	Bipolar I disorder—agitation; Bipolar disorder—manic or mixed episodes; maintenance; Depressed bipolar I disorder, adjunctive; Major depressive disorder, adjunctive; Schizophrenia	Agitation, acute—dementia; Anorexia nervosa; Nausea and vomiting, chemotherapy-induced; Delirium; Schizophrenia, refractory; Severe major depression with psychotic features	Akathisia; Asthenia; Somnolence; Tremor	Cerebrovascular disease; Dystonia; Seizure; Status epilepticus
Quetiapine	Bipolar disorder—acute mania, depressed phase, maintenance; Major depressive disorder, adjunct; Schizophrenia	Bipolar disorder, maintenance; Major depressive disorder, monotherapy	Asthenia; Dystonia; Headache; Insomnia; Somnolence; Tremor	Neuroleptic malignant syndrome; Seizure; Tardive dyskinesia
Risperidone	Autistic disorder—irritability; Bipolar I disorder; Schizophrenia	Behavioral syndrome—intellectual disability, Tourette syndrome; Autism spectrum disorder	Akathisia, Parkinsonism; Somnolence	Neuroleptic malignant syndrome, seizure; Tardive dyskinesia
Ziprasidone	Bipolar disorder—acute mania, maintenance adjunct; Schizophrenia	Schizoaffective disorder	Akathisia, anxiety; Dystonia; Headache; Psychomotor slowing; Somnolence; Spasmodic movement; Tremor	Neuroleptic malignant syndrome; Seizure; Tardive dyskinesia

aUnderlining indicates there is a US FDA indication for children. Specifics about age approval may vary, e.g., for risperidone approval the lower age limit for ASD is 5 years, for bipolar is 10 years, and for schizophrenia is 13 years. Consult Micromedex®, DrugPoint®, or other sources for details.

note that there are other uses besides those listed. Further, while pediatric indications (underlined) form only a subset of the total uses, it is common for pediatric use to follow adult approval, even in the absence of specific pediatric approval or dosing recommendations. Side effects listed are limited to neurologic. Again it is important to bear in mind that acute neurological reactions such as acute dystonic reactions can occur with any of these medications, even if not specifically listed in databases and drug package inserts. Outside of the nervous system, these medications pose risks of a variety of other common side effects, e.g., weight gain, and serious side effects, e.g., prolonged QT intervals, which are important for prescribers to be aware of but which lie outside the scope of this chapter.

Three recent systematic studies with different methods have generated widely disparate estimates of risks of DIMDs in children exposed to dopamine receptor blocking agents; however, the rates in two of the studies are remarkably close. It is worth considering each of these studies in turn, and then evaluating why the estimates differed.

The first study, a meta-analysis, identified and included 10 open-label and controlled studies of atypical antipsychotics with duration of 12 months or more, involving 783 children and adolescents, reported tardive dyskinesia in 0.4% of pediatric participants.[31] Most were studies of risperidone. Eighty percent of patients were white. Adequate data were available on fewer than half of patients. The authors reported a prevalence of DIMDs of 16%. Of the three tardive dystonia (TD) cases identified, two involved risperidone, one olanzapine. Although this study is important in providing a pediatric estimate across clinical trials, as the authors acknowledged, a number of limitations might have led to underestimates of the population prevalence of tardive dyskinesia. These include the use of different raters, different scales or no scale reported, and no consistent diagnostic criteria. In addition, it is important to remember that exclusion criteria employed, for reasons of scientific validity, in controlled clinical trials can result in nonrepresentative samples.[32]

In the second study, researchers at the Maryland Psychiatric Research Center studied a cohort of 424 pediatric psychiatry patients over a 3-year period. In 118 children ages 5–18 treated for 6 or more months with typical or atypical antipsychotics, they reported 9.3% developed TD.[33] This study represents a model for studying risks of TD and other DIMDs and can serve as a basis for future critical research in this area. Key features of this study may make the results more generalizable than the meta-analysis of clinical trial data.

Randomized controlled trials are the standard for validity in assessing treatment effects. However, in this case, the clinic-based, nonrandomized, observational study is more informative. The study methods are worth emphasizing:

- The real-world, ethnically diverse patient sample. The authors had a 90% capture rate of the children in the psychiatric facilities involved. Polypharmacy, including exposure to multiple antipsychotics, and multiple concurrent diagnoses were common.
- The use of two comparator groups: 80 neuroleptic-naïve, age- and gender-matched youths with psychiatric disorders and 35 healthy children with no psychiatric disorders.
- Standardized use of a structured and validated assessment, the Involuntary Movement Scale.[34] This scale is more anatomically specific than the Abnormal Involuntary Movement Scale (AIMS),[35] but is highly correlated with it.
- Raters using the AIMS were trained to a high inter-rater reliability (intraclass correlation coefficient) level of 0.80.

- Raters were blinded to treatment group and diagnosis.
- The AIMS-positive diagnostic threshold (cutoff for abnormal) was set based specifically on the pediatric examination, to avoid classifying age-appropriate restlessness or involuntary movements such as tics as being DIMDs.

The findings of this study are extremely important. First, over 80% of the prescriptions of antipsychotics were for youths with no documented psychotic symptoms. Most patients in both psychiatric groups were diagnosed with mood disorders and attention-deficit/hyperactivity disorder (ADHD). Second, a total of 9.3% (11 of 118) antipsychotic-treated children showed tardive DIMDs, compared to none in the antipsychotic-naïve group. This TD risk is quite high—much higher than the 0.4% risk estimate from the meta-analysis of clinical trials,[31] and higher than the 0% incidence reported in a 48-week, open-label extension of a mean 1.5 mg daily dose of risperidone.[16] Third, the TD appeared to be reversible, although long-term follow-up is still needed. Information on withdrawal dyskinesias also was not provided.

Several factors appeared to affect the risk of tardive DIMDs in this study. The risk increased with longer duration of antipsychotic treatment, ranging from 3% at 6–12 months, to 14% at greater than 2 years. Ethnicity was also important, with higher risks in African-American than European children. For type of agent, the risk was 6% (5 of 81) for atypicals only, versus 27% (11 of 37) for combined atypical and typical antipsychotics. The possibility for confounding by effects of other concomitant medications was also addressed. Over half of the antipsychotic-exposed patients were treated with mood stabilizers (75%), antidepressants (75%), and psychostimulants (68%). The rates of concurrent medications in the antipsychotic-naïve group were lower.

The methodology of the third study involved searching the medical literature from 1953 to 2009 for reports of tardive syndromes in children.[36] After removing the case reports, one study which did not specify TD, and the Maryland Study (so as not to double count), there are 50 children identified out of 540 exposed to neuroleptics, for a TD rate of 9.3%, essentially identical to the Maryland Study.

The similarity of the two estimates of children developing TD of 9.3% from the literature review[36] and the Maryland study[33] is astonishing when you consider the likely differences in case mix, comorbidities, relative use of typical and atypical antipsychotics, and concurrent medications, and variability in raters and approaches to clinical diagnosis of movement disorders. Despite the fact that both estimates may be high due to positive publication bias, their similarity supports this as a reasonable real-world estimate when skilled clinicians treat and evaluate heterogeneous groups of children over the long-term. The vastly lower 0.4% rate of TD in clinical trials of atypical antipsychotics[31] may partly reflect clinical trial selection criteria, lower treatment doses, and less polypharmacy. With regard to other types of DIMDs, studies suggest similar proportions induced by atypicals versus typicals.[37]

Clinical Features of DIMDs Induced by Dopamine Receptor Blocking Agents

As in adults, dopamine receptor blocking agents, both conventional neuroleptics and the atypical antipsychotics, are prone to induce Parkinsonism, dystonia, tics, tremor, oculogyric movements, orolingual and other dyskinesias, and akathisia.[31,33,36,38,39] Symptoms may occur at any time after treatment onset. Acute DIMDs, especially dystonia, oculogyric crises, and akathisia, are common in the first days of treatment. Chronic DIMDs occur after three or more months of treatment and may take the form of more subtle dystonia, tremor, and rigidity. Tardive DIMD phenomenologies include dyskinesias, stereotypies, tics, dystonia, and oculogyric crises. These symptoms may also develop, particularly in children, when dopamine receptor blocking agents are withdrawn or tapered down rapidly. This is termed the withdrawal emergent syndrome (WES) (Video 22.2).[36] In contrast to tardive dyskinesia in adults, which is often permanent, the involuntary movements improve and spontaneously resolve in children (Video 22.3, 22.4).[36] Development of a tardive orofacial lingual stereotypy has been described in an infant treated with metoclopramide for gastroesophageal reflux (Video 22.1).[40]

Pathophysiology

Much remains to be learned about the pathophysiology of DIMDs associated with dopamine receptor blocker use and how to predict and prevent them. Effects on striatal dopamine receptor blockade and imbalance in striatum of dopamine and acetylcholine levels play a role, but an individual's vulnerability or susceptibility to DIMDs remains an area of active research.[41]

The susceptibility to DIMDs in childhood may relate to a diathesis, or proneness to develop movement disorders, related to particular neurodevelopmental or psychiatric diagnoses treated with these agents. For example, in adults, tardive DIMDs have been reported in young adults with schizophrenia for decades.[42,43] In contrast, there are few reports of tardive dyskinesia in young adults with Tourette syndrome.[44] It is unclear biologically why this might be. A detailed overview of current theories of pathophysiology of DIMDs is based primarily on animal and adult research[41] and these factors may not apply to children. The observation that abnormal involuntary movements are more prevalent in neuroleptic-naïve adults with schizophrenia than in adults with other psychiatric disorders[45,46] may provide an insight relevant in children. Tics, stereotypies, and other movement disorders are more common in children with neurodevelopmental or psychiatric disorders, including ASDs (see Chapter 21).[47–53] Clinical experience with DIMDs in children shows that dopamine receptor blocker–related DIMDs occur more commonly in children on the autistic spectrum.

The pathophysiology of the risk for DIMDs may have an identifiable genetic component, although at this time most research is in adults identifying genetic predispositions has been difficult to confirm. A study of over 600 Europeans with schizophrenia found no evidence that dopamine D2 receptor polymorphisms influence DIMDs[54] whereas in other European cohorts evidence has been more supportive.[55] Studies of other dopamine receptors[56–58] and drug metabolizing enzymes, such as cytochrome P450,[59] do not demonstrate significant genetic prediction. Other studies suggest that genes involved in GABAergic pathways raise the risk for tardive dyskinesia.[60,61] Some studies support risk related to polymorphisms in serotonergic systems. Polymorphisms in genes encoding receptors 2A or 2C[56,62] but not 3A[63] may increase risk for DIMDs in antipsychotic-treated adults with schizophrenia. Based on views that susceptibility to oxidative stress might be important, researchers have assessed glutathione-S-transferase, glutathione peroxidase, catalase, and tumor necrosis factor alpha polymorphisms, but found no association with hyperkinetic DIMDs.[64–66] On a cellular basis, mechanisms may include long-term effects on dopamine receptor density and function, damage to GABAergic striatal neurons, and damage to cholinergic interneurons.[67] Genome-wide association studies may support other previously unsuspected pathways as well.[68,69]

Diagnosis of Acute, Chronic, Tardive, and WESs

Diagnosis of an acute DIMD is usually straightforward, when the dopamine receptor blocking medication has been prescribed as an antipsychotic or antiemetic during the appropriate antecedent timeframe and the phenomenology is characteristic. In the case of accidental ingestion, the acute onset of an involuntary movement disorder in a toddler should raise the diagnostic possibility of ingestion of a dopamine receptor blocking agent. Sources of possible exposure should be sought.

Diagnosis of a chronic or tardive DIMD in children should be considered based on the phenomenology and time course of the movement disorder. This diagnosis can be more challenging than acute DIMDs. Often, at the time of the first neurologic consultation, the baseline, pretreatment neurological examination by the primary physician or prescribing psychiatrist is not well documented. The diagnosis should be suspected when hypokinetic, rigid symptoms, stereotypic (non-tic) hyperkinetic symptoms, or dystonia occur in children prescribed antipsychotics for a period of greater than 3 months, because of the low prevalence of these symptoms on a genetic or acquired basis otherwise. Stereotypies and especially tics are less straightforward because they are common and a tendency to tic or risk for a tic disorder may have preceded drug treatment. Thus, the emergence of these symptoms later in childhood may be unrelated to medication.

When a new movement disorder occurs at the time of medication tapering or discontinuation, a WES disorder should be considered as a possibility.[70,71] However, if symptoms are mild, then the differential diagnosis includes hyperkinetic movements that may have been masked during treatment with the dopamine receptor blocker. Resuming the prior medication and dose and reducing the medication dose at a slower rate can help clarify the diagnosis.

Treatment of DIMDs Related to Use of Dopamine Receptor Blocking Agents

Few rigorous studies in adults and especially in children guide the clinician in this area.

ACUTE DIMDS

Antihistamines and anticholinergic agents such as diphenhydramine and benztropine remain the mainstay of treatment for acute DIMDs caused by dopamine receptor blockade.[72] The alpha$_2$-adrenergic agonist clonidine, anticholinergics, and beta-blockers such as propranolol may be helpful for acute akathisia.[73–75]

CHRONIC DIMDS

For chronic DIMDs that cause functionally impairing rigidity or tremor, anticholinergics are also used. In chronic and tardive DIMDs, when dyskinesias are mild, withdrawing the offending agent may be sufficient to reverse the symptoms,[31,70] although systematic data on this approach are also quite scarce.[36,76] As the major use of dopamine receptor blocking agents in children is for mood stabilization and aggression, withdrawal of these agents and substitution of other classes of medication, such as anticonvulsants, should be considered for mood stabilization when DIMDs emerge. However, ongoing collaboration with the prescribing psychiatrist is often needed because the mental illness or aggression may be severe and it may not be safe to discontinue medications in an outpatient setting.

TARDIVE MOVEMENT DISORDERS

Tardive dyskinesia, particularly in adults with schizophrenia, can become a permanent condition. Thus the primary emphasis should be given to strict and appropriate selection and management of patients by physicians with expertise in psychiatric diagnosis and treatment. Vigilance for emergence of DIMDs is important and requires regular examinations by clinicians with appropriate training. Whenever possible, the treatment duration and dose of these dopamine receptor blocking agents should be limited. When TD is diagnosed, removal of the causative drug is recommended whenever possible, via slow taper to reduce the risk of WES.

For pharmacologic treatment of TD, use of alpha-methyl-para-tyrosine (AMPT), an inhibitor of tyrosine hydroxylase, the rate-limiting enzyme in dopamine biosynthesis, has been described.[77] Reserpine, which inhibits vesicular monoamine transporters VMAT1 (peripheral) and VMAT2 (central) at the presynaptic membrane, resulting in the depletion of the synaptic pool of monoamines, may also be used. Both of these approaches may be severely limited by low availability and very high expense. Replacing the causative D2 receptor blocking agent with clozapine, a more selective D4 receptor blocker, is another option. However, this requires monitoring for white blood cell count and absolute neutrophil count due to risk of agranulocytosis. Tetrabenazine, a VMAT2 inhibitor/dopamine depletory which also blocks pre- and postsynaptic D2 receptors,[78] has been recommended for the treatment of TD.[41,79,80] Depression is sometimes noted as a side effect.[81,82] Vitamin E has been studied more extensively, based on the rationale that the pathophysiology of TD may be related to oxidative stress, but it appears to work no better than placebo. It may reduce neurologic deterioration if neuroleptic treatment is continued.[83] Calcium channel blockers are not currently considered effective.[84]

Neuroleptic Malignant Syndrome

An additional severe, and potentially life-threatening, DIMD is *neuroleptic malignant syndrome*, although it is rare in children.[85] This most commonly occurs after initiation or dose increases, has been mainly described after taking antipsychotics (including the atypicals),[86,87] but occasionally has been reported after other psychiatric medications. Neuroleptic malignant syndrome can also occur as a withdrawal phenomenon after chronic dopaminergic therapy. The main manifestations are autonomic (fever, tachycardia/tachypnea, diaphoresis), motoric (rigidity/bradykinesia with elevated rhabdomyolysis and creatine kinase), and cognitive (confusion). Treatment is emergent and may include general supportive care (hydration, fever reduction) and specific interventions (withdrawing the offending medication), and administration of the dopamine agonist bromocriptine, and the skeletal muscle relaxant dantrolene.[88]

Several other serious reactions including malignant hyperthermia (hyperpyrexia, muscle contractions due to general anesthesia) and anticholinergic or sympathomimetic poisoning are in the differential. In addition, *serotonin syndrome* may occasionally be confused. In serotonin syndrome, described later, rigidity is less prominent, but hyperreflexia, clonus, tremor, myoclonus, and shivering occur.

DIMDs Associated with ADHD Treatment

Epidemiology of Psychostimulant Use in Children

Like dopamine receptor blockers, the use of stimulants in children has increased markedly in the last 20 years in the United States.[6,89] Use of these agents among preschool children may also increase, based on results of a large randomized controlled trial.[90,91] Nonstimulant ADHD medications are also increasingly used, including atomoxetine, a selective norepinephrine reuptake inhibitor marketed for ADHD treatment[92] and the alpha-2 adrenergic agonists guanfacine[93] and clonidine.[94,95]

Clinical Features

Stimulants, prescribed at reasonably appropriate doses, rarely induce clinically significant movement disorders. Methylphenidate, dextroamphetamine products, and nonstimulants used for ADHD affect dopamine and norepinephrine and thereby the most common DIMDs, if any occur, are hyperkinetic disorders such as tics, stereotypies, chorea, or other dyskinesias.[96] The prevalence of DIMDs with stimulants is higher in children who also meet criteria for obsessive–compulsive disorder (OCD) or ASD,[97] or who display mild features of these disorders. Such children may experience new or increased repetitive behaviors, including tics, compulsions, or repetitive picking behaviors. They may also become hyperfocused or have personality changes parents describe as a "zombie" or "robot" effect.

A major clinical issue is the possibility of induction or exacerbation of tics. The concern about induction of tics on stimulant medication was based on clinician observations and case reports from the 1970s and 1980s.[98] Subsequently, FDA-mandated labeling in the United States has included the advisory that stimulant medications are contraindicated in individuals with Tourette syndrome or any family history of tics. This warning diverges from standard clinical practice by experienced clinicians as well as from recommendations of the US Tourette Association Medical Advisory Board.[99] Rigorous randomized controlled trials support that stimulants reduce ADHD symptoms for most children, irrespective of the presence of a tic disorder, and that worsening of tics is uncommon, usually transient, usually mild, and always reversible. In the case of new tics after starting stimulants, research suggests that in most cases tics would have occurred eventually, even in the absence of any psychostimulant treatment.[100–102] The most rigorous clinical assessment of the relationship between stimulants and tics is the Treatment of ADHD in Children with Tics (TACT) study.[103] In that study, children with comorbid tics and ADHD were randomized to treatment with methylphenidate, clonidine, both, or double placebo. By the end of that study, tics improved in all treated groups, compared to placebo. That is, even the group treated with methylphenidate alone had improved tics, compared to placebo. Even in cases where tics consistently worsen on stimulant medication, some individuals and families choose to continue stimulant medication if the benefits warrant.

Atomoxetine has been reported in a few cases to apparently induce tics.[104] However, in a randomized, placebo-controlled trial of atomoxetine treatment for ADHD in 148 children with tics, atomoxetine tended to reduce tic severity.[105] Other dyskinesias and tremor have been reported with atomoxetine, but this occurred in the context of rapid dose changes and polypharmacy.[106]

Pathophysiology

In cases where stimulants do induce tics, stereotypies, and chorea, there may be some preexisting susceptibility in individuals due to dopaminergic action in fronto-striatal circuits that ordinarily produce and regulate voluntary movements. Although dopamine receptors in the striatum have been considered as the likely anatomic origin for these

DIMDs, dopamine receptors in cortex may also influence hyperkinetic movement disorders.[107–109] The net effects of both stimulants and norepinephrine reuptake inhibitors on motor cortex can reduce inhibitory interneuronal function,[110] and this effect can vary related to both genetic factors and by presence of a tic disorder phenotype.[111]

The susceptibility to DIMDs may relate to a diathesis, or proneness to develop movement disorders, in individuals with neurodevelopmental or psychiatric diagnoses treated with these agents. In the absence of known diathesis, there may still be a subtle predisposition to develop hyperkinetic movements during ADHD treatment. Overflow and choreiform movements and other subtle neurologic signs are found in children with ADHD more than in typical children.[112,113] Stereotypies and tics, seen in ASD and Tourette syndrome, may be more general markers of perturbed neurodevelopment, as the prevalence of these movement disorders is increased in children with a wide variety of neurologic, developmental, and psychiatric diagnoses.[50,51,114–116]

A genetic influence on the risk of DIMDs has been suggested through genotyping data from the Preschool ADHD Treatment Study (PATS). In that study, 183 preschoolers were treated with methylphenidate at several doses or placebo. Several modestly statistically significant associations were identified, including polymorphisms in synaptosomal-associated protein 25 (SNAP25) associated with tics, buccal-lingual movements, and irritability and variants of dopamine receptor 4 (DRD4) associated with picking.[117]

Diagnosis

The diagnosis of a DIMD in a child treated for ADHD should be suspected if the movements have the typical hyperkinetic phenomenology and the onset is within a week or two of treatment onset or a dose increase. Stimulants are short acting and readily discontinued or restarted, allowing for a plan of stopping and restarting medications to clarify cause and effect.

Treatment

There are few helpful studies in this regard. It is most often not necessary to discontinue stimulants when mild tics emerge. If the stimulant dose exceeds 1 mg/kg/day, it is generally beneficial to reduce the dose, which also often helps with appetite and sleep initiation along with reducing drug-induced tics or tremor.

DIMDs Associated with Other Medications

Serotonin Reuptake Inhibitors

Selective serotonin reuptake inhibitors (SSRIs) are widely prescribed in children with mood disorders and OCD. This class of medication is generally at least somewhat effective alone or combined with cognitive behavioral therapy. The emergence of movement disorders related to use of SSRIs has been described for 20 years and can include akathisia most commonly, with Parkinsonism, dystonia, and TD-like states also described.[118] To date, SSRI-induced TD-like states have been primarily reported in adults, particularly elderly adults. Of interest, a rodent model of chronic SSRI exposure demonstrated, in adult rodents only, reduction in dopamine signaling as a possible mechanism for SSRI-induced striatal dysfunction.[119]

The most serious complication, serotonin syndrome due to excess SSRI exposure, involves neuromuscular excitation (manifest by clonus, hyperreflexia, myoclonus, tremor, shivering), autonomic stimulation (hyperthermia, diarrhea, tachycardia, diaphoresis, tremor, flushing), and changed mental state (anxiety, agitation, confusion).[120] The full syndrome is rare in children. More commonly, treatment with an SSRI results in a mild degree of hyperreflexia and tremor. The emergence of hyperreflexia in a child prescribed an SSRI is an indication that toxicity is more likely if the dose is increased or in the presence of polypharmacy. Such patients bear close clinical observation with competent repeat neurological examination. Physicians who are unaware of the SSRI-induced tremor and hyperreflexia may, after examination of a child taking an SSRI, become concerned about upper motor neuron pathology and order unnecessary brain or spine magnetic resonance imaging (MRI) scans. Similarly, physicians who fail to observe and document SSRI-induced neurological symptoms may place patients at risk of developing more severe symptoms with future dose increases or due to drug–drug interactions.

In some cases, more significant problems with Parkinsonism[121] or an exacerbation of tics[122] may occur. In a few cases, what appears to be an exacerbation of tics is actually myoclonus. The myoclonus, in distinction to tics, is involuntary and does not diminish during voluntary movements to the same degree that tics do. This is generally an indication to reduce or eliminate the SSRI. SSRIs as well as duloxetine have been reported, in rare cases, to induce dystonic reactions.[123]

The identification of SSRI-induced movement disorders in both adults[118,124] and children[125,126] supports the importance of clinician recognition and education of families about this possibility. Treatment is dose reduction, elimination of the medication, or re-evaluation of concurrent medication which may be contributing. It should be borne in mind that behavioral therapies are often an effective alternative for mood disorders,[127,128] even in children with autism,[129] and the effects of this therapy may have measurable physiological correlates.[130]

Antiseizure Medications

Antiseizure medications are used to prevent seizures and migraines, and are increasingly prescribed to stabilize mood and reduce aggression.

Numerous case reports in children describe acute and chronic DIMDs caused by antiseizure medications. The most common clinical features are acute ataxia and nystagmus.[131] Phenytoin and carbamazepine are most often identified. The pathophysiology is likely blockade of fast-firing neurons in vestibulocerebellum and spinocerebellum.

These medications are also prone to cause problems due to pharmacokinetics. Phenytoin is hydroxylated by cytochrome CYP2C9. At high levels, its metabolism saturates and becomes nonlinear, and this can contribute to induction of movement disorders.[132] Carbamazepine is subject to drug–drug interactions because its main metabolizing enzyme also metabolizes other commonly used medications, particularly macrolide antibiotics. Thus, a child on a stable dose of carbamazepine may develop ataxia or other symptoms of toxicity when a macrolide antibiotic is prescribed.[133]

Less commonly, antiseizure drugs may produce other hyperkinetic movement disorders. Phenytoin, carbamazepine, and even valproic acid have been reported to produce acute chorea,[134–137] orofacial dyskinesias,[138,139] or Tourettism.[140] Underlying brain malformations may have rendered children more susceptible in some cases. Lamotrigine has been reported to induce tics.[141,142] Tremor is also common, particularly with valproic acid. As described previously for antipsychotics and stimulants, there may be a relevant diathesis, as children at risk (based on parental diagnosis) for bipolar disorder may tend to have subnormal cerebellar function.[143]

Generally, there is no diagnostic dilemma for these children. The treatment plan is to hold or reduce the medication dose, if possible, and wait out the ataxia.

DIMDs Associated with Chemotherapeutic, Immune-Modulatory, Anti-Infectious Medications and Other Medications

Neurology consultations for oncology patients may involve a variety of neurologic symptoms, including DIMDs. Chemotherapeutic agents such as vincristine may cause a sensory ataxia, along with dysarthria and tremor.[144] Aggressive therapies such as autologous bone marrow rescue may be associated with acute neurologic symptoms such as headaches, confusion, and seizures, but may also be associated with tremor, ataxia, dysarthria, and Parkinsonism.[144]

Ifosfamide, a nitrogen mustard alkylating agent used in a number of solid tumor protocols, has a well-known CNS side effect profile, possibly related to impaired mitochondrial fatty acid oxidation and defective electron transfer.[145] In two cases of ifosfamide-associated encephalopathy, hemiballismus developed.[146] Treatment with the electron-accepting drug methylene blue may reverse or shorten the period of encephalopathy.[147]

Leukoencephalopathy and other neurological complications can occur as complications of use of immunosuppressive agents after liver transplant. Seizures are common, but tremor and acute dystonic reactions have also been observed.[148] Tacrolimus, an immunosuppressive agent utilized after organ transplant, is one of several such agents known to cause a leukoencephalopathy syndrome. Clinically, patients may present with headache, confusion, myoclonus, seizures, and disturbances in visual function.[149] High dose and intrathecal methotrexate treatment of childhood acute lymphoblastic leukemia can induce transient or persistent leukoencephalopathy in approximately 20–25% of patients. Seizures and stroke-like episodes are the most common side effects, but ataxia has also been reported. The risk for neurotoxicity may involve some genetic determinants.[150]

Metronidazole may rarely cause CNS toxicity. Most (70–80%) published cases present with cerebellar dysfunction, with lesser prevalence of seizures and altered mental status.[151] MRI findings are usually identified in cerebellum in bilateral dentate nuclei and superior olivary nuclei in the dorsal pons as well as in cerebrum, corpus callosum, midbrain, and medulla.[152]

A wide variety of other prescription medications can produce reversible, acute or chronic drug-induced tremor, typically with phenomenology of enhanced physiological tremor. Common offenders reside within neurology and psychiatry, and these include stimulants, amitriptyline, valproic acid, and lithium.[155] Medicines used for treatment of other common pediatric conditions such as beta-2 agonist bronchodilators for asthma may induce tremor well.[156] Education is generally all that is needed and if severe alternative agents may be tried.

DIMDs Associated with Vitamin Administration

In regions of the world where vitamin B12 deficiency is common, treatment with B12 can induce movement disorders.[153,154]

CONCLUSION

Children are vulnerable to the development of acute, chronic, tardive, and withdrawal DIMDs. Dopaminergic medications are common offenders, and certain children, particularly those with ASD, may be more vulnerable. Factors influencing vulnerability remain largely unknown. Clinicians need to be aware of spectrum, time course, and treatment strategies for DIMDs in children.

References

1. Brown R, Taylor MJ, Geddes J. Aripiprazole alone or in combination for acute mania. *Cochrane Database Syst Rev.* 2013;12:CD005000.
2. Zeni CP, Tramontina S, Ketzer CR, Pheula GF, Rohde LA. Methylphenidate combined with aripiprazole in children and adolescents with bipolar disorder and attention-deficit/hyperactivity disorder: a randomized crossover trial. *J Child Adolesc Psychopharmacol.* 2009;19(5):553–561.
3. Spencer D, Marshall J, Post B, et al. Psychotropic medication use and polypharmacy in children with autism spectrum disorders. *Pediatrics.* 2013;132(5):833–840.
4. Logan SL, Nicholas JS, Carpenter LA, King LB, Garrett-Mayer E, Charles JM. High prescription drug use and associated costs among Medicaid-eligible children with autism spectrum disorders identified by a population-based surveillance network. *Ann Epidemiol.* 2012;22(1):1–8.
5. Schubart JR, Camacho F, Leslie D. Psychotropic medication trends among children and adolescents with autism spectrum disorder in the Medicaid program. *Autism.* 2013;18(6):631–637.
6. Cox ER, Motheral BR, Henderson RR, Mager D. Geographic variation in the prevalence of stimulant medication use among children 5 to 14 years old: results from a commercially insured US sample. *Pediatrics.* 2003;111(2):237–243.
7. Delate T, Gelenberg AJ, Simmons VA, Motheral BR. Trends in the use of antidepressants in a national sample of commercially insured pediatric patients, 1998 to 2002. *Psychiatr Serv.* 2004;55(4):387–391.
8. Goodwin R, Gould MS, Blanco C, Olfson M. Prescription of psychotropic medications to youths in office-based practice. *Psychiatr Serv.* 2001;52(8):1081–1087.
9. Olfson M, Blanco C, Liu L, Moreno C, Laje G. National trends in the outpatient treatment of children and adolescents with antipsychotic drugs. *Arch Gen Psychiatry.* 2006;63(6):679–685.
10. Rushton JL, Whitmire JT. Pediatric stimulant and selective serotonin reuptake inhibitor prescription trends: 1992 to 1998. *Arch Pediatr Adolesc Med.* 2001;155(5):560–565.
11. Zito JM, Safer DJ, dosReis Gardner JF, Boles M, Lynch F. Trends in the prescribing of psychotropic medications to preschoolers. *JAMA.* 2000;283(8):1025–1030.
12. Chirdkiatgumchai V, Xiao H, Fredstrom BK, et al. National trends in psychotropic medication use in young children: 1994–2009. *Pediatrics.* 2013;132(4):615–623.
13. Fontanella CA, Warner LA, Phillips GS, Bridge JA, Campo JV. Trends in psychotropic polypharmacy among youths enrolled in Ohio Medicaid, 2002–2008. *Psychiatr Serv.* 2014;65(11):1332–1340.
14. Leucht S, Pitschel-Walz G, Abraham D, Kissling W. Efficacy and extrapyramidal side-effects of the new antipsychotics olanzapine, quetiapine, risperidone, and sertindole compared to conventional antipsychotics and placebo. A meta-analysis of randomized controlled trials. *Schizophr Res.* 1999;35(1):51–68.
15. Croonenberghs J, Fegert JM, Findling RL, De Smedt G, Van Dongen S, Risperidone Disruptive Behavior Study Group. Risperidone in children with disruptive behavior disorders and subaverage intelligence: a 1-year, open-label study of 504 patients. *J Am Acad Child Adolesc Psychiatry.* 2005;44(1):64–72.
16. Findling RL, Aman MG, Eerdekens M, Derivan A, Lyons B, Risperidone Disruptive Behavior Study Group. Long-term, open-label study of risperidone in children with severe disruptive behaviors and below-average IQ. *Am J Psychiatry.* 2004;161(4):677–684.
17. Findling RL, Maxwell K, Wiznitzer M. An open clinical trial of risperidone monotherapy in young children with autistic disorder. *Psychopharmacol Bull.* 1997;33(1):155–159.
18. Cunningham MA, Pillai V, Rogers WJ. Haloperidol in the treatment of children with severe behaviour disorders. *Br J Psychiatry.* 1968;114(512):845–854.

19. Bruun RD. Subtle and underrecognized side effects of neuroleptic treatment in children with Tourette's disorder. *Am J Psychiatry*. 1988;145(5):621–624.

20. Chapel JL, Brown N, Jenkins RL. Tourette's disease: symptomatic relief with haloperidol. *Am J Psychiatry*. 1964;121:608–610.

21. Sallee FR, Nesbitt L, Jackson C, Sine L, Sethuraman G. Relative efficacy of haloperidol and pimozide in children and adolescents with Tourette's disorder. *Am J Psychiatry*. 1997;154(8):1057–1062.

22. Shapiro E, Shapiro AK, Fulop G, et al. Controlled study of haloperidol, pimozide and placebo for the treatment of Gilles de la Tourette's syndrome. *Arch Gen Psychiatry*. 1989;46(8):722–730.

23. Silva RR, Munoz DM, Daniel W, Barickman J, Friedhoff AJ. Causes of haloperidol discontinuation in patients with Tourette's disorder: management and alternatives. *J Clin Psychiatry*. 1996;57(3):129–135.

24. Patel NC, Crismon ML, Hoagwood K, et al. Trends in the use of typical and atypical antipsychotics in children and adolescents. *J Am Acad Child Adolesc Psychiatry*. 2005;44(6):548–556.

25. Patel NC, Crismon ML, Shafer A. Diagnoses and antipsychotic treatment among youths in a public mental health system. *Ann Pharmacother*. 2006;40(2):205–211.

26. Safer DJ. Changing patterns of psychotropic medications prescribed by child psychiatrists in the 1990s. *J Child Adolesc Psychopharmacol*. 1997;7(4):267–274.

27. Safer DJ. A comparison of risperidone-induced weight gain across the age span. *J Clin Psychopharmacol*. 2004;24(4):429–436.

28. Moreno C, Laje G, Blanco C, Jiang H, Schmidt AB, Olfson M. National trends in the outpatient diagnosis and treatment of bipolar disorder in youth. *Arch Gen Psychiatry*. 2007;64(9):1032–1039.

29. Harris G. Psychiatrists top list in drug maker gifts. *The New York Times*. June 26, 2007, Health.

30. Derinoz O, Caglar AA. Drug-induced movement disorders in children at paediatric emergency department: "dystonia". *Emerg Med J*. 2013;30(2):130–133.

31. Correll CU, Kane JM. One-year incidence rates of tardive dyskinesia in children and adolescents treated with second-generation antipsychotics: a systematic review. *J Child Adolesc Psychopharmacol*. 2007;17(5):647–656.

32. Gilbert DL, Buncher CR. Assessment of scientific and ethical issues in two randomized clinical trial designs for patients with Tourette's syndrome: a model for studies of multiple neuropsychiatric diagnoses. *J Neuropsychiatry Clin Neurosci*. 2005;17(3):324–332.

33. Wonodi I, Reeves G, Carmichael D, et al. Tardive dyskinesia in children treated with atypical antipsychotic medications. *Mov Disord*. 2007;22(12):1777–1782.

34. Cassady SL, Thaker GK, Summerfelt A, Tamminga CA. The Maryland Psychiatric Research Center scale and the characterization of involuntary movements. *Psychiatry Res*. 1997;70(1):21–37.

35. Guy W. *ECDEU Assessment Manual for Psychopharmacology*. Rockville, MD: United States Department of Health, Education, and Welfare; 1976.

36. Mejia NI, Jankovic J. Tardive dyskinesia and withdrawal emergent syndrome in children. *Expert Rev Neurother*. 2010;10(6):893–901.

37. Woods SW, Morgenstern H, Saksa JR, et al. Incidence of tardive dyskinesia with atypical versus conventional antipsychotic medications: a prospective cohort study. *J Clin Psychiatry*. 2010;71(4):463–474.

38. Laita P, Cifuentes A, Doll A, et al. Antipsychotic-related abnormal involuntary movements and metabolic and endocrine side effects in children and adolescents. *J Child Adolesc Psychopharmacol*. 2007;17(4):487–502.

39. Peluso MJ, Lewis SW, Barnes TR, Jones PB. Extrapyramidal motor side-effects of first- and second-generation antipsychotic drugs. *Br J Psychiatry*. 2012;200(5):387–392.

40. Mejia NI, Jankovic J. Metoclopramide-induced tardive dyskinesia in an infant. *Mov Dis*. 2005;20(1):86–89.

41. Waln O, Jankovic J. An update on tardive dyskinesia: from phenomenology to treatment. *Tremor Other Hyperkinet Mov*. 2013:3.

42. Eberhard J, Lindstrom E, Levander S. Tardive dyskinesia and antipsychotics: a 5-year longitudinal study of frequency, correlates and course. *Int Clin Psychopharmacol*. 2006;21(1):35–42.

43. Jeste DV, Wyatt RJ. Changing epidemiology of tardive dyskinesia: an overview. *Am J Psychiatry*. 1981;138(3):297–309.

44. Wijemanne S, Wu LJ, Jankovic J. Long-term efficacy and safety of fluphenazine in patients with Tourette syndrome. *Mov Disord*. 2014;29(1):126–130.

45. Fenn DS, Moussaoui D, Hoffman WF, et al. Movements in never-medicated schizophrenics: a preliminary study. *Psychopharmacology*. 1996;123(2):206–210.

46. Fenton WS, Blyler CR, Wyatt RJ, McGlashan TH. Prevalence of spontaneous dyskinesia in schizophrenic and non-schizophrenic psychiatric patients [erratum appears in *Br J Psychiatry*. 1998;172:97]. *Br J Psychiatry*. 1997;171:265–268.

47. Canitano R, Vivanti G. Tics and Tourette syndrome in autism spectrum disorders. *Autism*. 2007;11(1):19–28.

48. Comings DE, Comings BG. Clinical and genetic relationships between autism-pervasive developmental disorder and Tourette syndrome: a study of 19 cases. *Am J Med Genet*. 1991;39(2):180–191.

49. Kurlan R. Hypothesis II: Tourette's syndrome is part of a clinical spectrum that includes normal brain development. *Arch Neurol*. 1994;51(11):1145–1150.

50. Kurlan R, Como PG, Miller B, et al. The behavioral spectrum of tic disorders: a community-based study. *Neurology*. 2002;59(3):414–420.

51. Kurlan R, McDermott MP, Deeley C, et al. Prevalence of tics in schoolchildren and association with placement in special education. *Neurology*. 2001;57(8):1383–1388.

52. Ringman JM, Jankovic J. Occurrence of tics in Asperger's syndrome and autistic disorder. *J Child Neurol*. 2000;15(6):394–400.

53. Rigby H, Roberts-South A, Kumar H, Cortese L, Jog M. Diagnostic challenges revealed from a neuropsychiatry movement disorders clinic. *Can J Neurol Sci*. 2012;39(6):782–788.

54. Kaiser R, Tremblay PB, Klufmoller F, Roots I, Brockmoller J. Relationship between adverse effects of antipsychotic treatment and dopamine D(2) receptor polymorphisms in patients with schizophrenia. *Mol Psychiatry*. 2002;7(7):695–705.

55. Koning JP, Vehof J, Burger H, et al. Association of two DRD2 gene polymorphisms with acute and tardive antipsychotic-induced movement disorders in young Caucasian patients. *Psychopharmacology (Berl)*. 2012;219(3):727–736.

56. Gunes A, Scordo MG, Jaanson P, Dahl M-L. Serotonin and dopamine receptor gene polymorphisms and the risk of extrapyramidal side effects in perphenazine-treated schizophrenic patients. *Psychopharmacology*. 2007;190(4):479–484.

57. Liou Y-J, Liao D-L, Chen J-Y, et al. Association analysis of the dopamine D3 receptor gene ser9gly and brain-derived neurotrophic factor gene val66met polymorphisms with antipsychotic-induced persistent tardive dyskinesia and clinical expression in Chinese schizophrenic patients. *Neuromolecular Med*. 2004;5(3):243–251.

58. Tsai HT, North KE, West SL, Poole C. The DRD3 rs6280 polymorphism and prevalence of tardive dyskinesia: a meta-analysis. *Am J Med Genet B Neuropsychiatr Genet*. 2010;153B(1):57–66.

59. Plesnicar BK, Zalar B, Breskvar K, Dolzan V. The influence of the CYP2D6 polymorphism on psychopathological and extrapyramidal symptoms in the patients on long-term antipsychotic treatment. *J Psychopharmacol*. 2006;20(6):829–833.

60. Inada T, Koga M, Ishiguro H, et al. Pathway-based association analysis of genome-wide screening data suggest that genes associated with the gamma-aminobutyric acid receptor signaling pathway are involved in neuroleptic-induced, treatment-resistant tardive dyskinesia. *Pharmacogenet Genomics*. 2008;18(4):317–323.

61. Son WY, Lee HJ, Yoon HK, et al. GABA transporter SLC6A11 gene polymorphism associated with tardive dyskinesia. *Nord J Psychiatry*. 2014;68(2):123–128.

62. Segman RH, Heresco-Levy U, Finkel B, et al. Association between the serotonin 2C receptor gene and tardive dyskinesia in chronic schizophrenia: additive contribution of 5-HT2Cser and DRD3gly alleles to susceptibility. *Psychopharmacology*. 2000;152(4):408–413.

63. Kang SG, Lee HJ, Yoon HK, Cho SN, Park YM, Kim L. There is no evidence for an association between the serotonin receptor 3A gene C178T polymorphism and tardive dyskinesia in Korean schizophrenia patients. *Nord J Psychiatry*. 2013;67(3):214–218.

64. Shinkai T, De Luca V, Hwang R, et al. Association study between a functional glutathione S-transferase (GSTP1) gene polymorphism (Ile105Val) and tardive dyskinesia. *Neurosci Lett*. 2005;388(2):116–120.

65. Boskovic M, Vovk T, Saje M, et al. Association of SOD2, GPX1, CAT, and TNF genetic polymorphisms with oxidative stress, neurochemistry, psychopathology, and extrapyramidal symptoms in schizophrenia. *Neurochem Res*. 2013;38(2):433–442.

66. Zai CC, Tiwari AK, Basile V, et al. Oxidative stress in tardive dyskinesia: genetic association study and meta-analysis of NADPH quinine oxidoreductase 1 (NQO1) and Superoxide dismutase 2 (SOD2, MnSOD) genes. *Prog Neuropsychopharmacol Biol Psychiatry*. 2010;34(1):50–56.

67. Margolese HC, Chouinard G, Kolivakis TT, Beauclair L, Miller R, Annable L. Tardive dyskinesia in the era of typical and atypical antipsychotics. Part 2: Incidence and management strategies in patients with schizophrenia. *Can J Psychiatry.* 2005;50(11):703–714.

68. Greenbaum L, Alkelai A, Rigbi A, Kohn Y, Lerer B. Evidence for association of the GLI2 gene with tardive dyskinesia in patients with chronic schizophrenia. *Mov Disord.* 2010;25(16):2809–2817.

69. Aberg K, Adkins DE, Bukszar J, et al. Genomewide association study of movement-related adverse antipsychotic effects. *Biol Psychiatry.* 2010;67(3):279–282.

70. Campbell M, Armenteros JL, Malone RP, Adams PB, Eisenberg ZW, Overall JE. Neuroleptic-related dyskinesias in autistic children: a prospective, longitudinal study. *J Am Acad Child Adolesc Psychiatry.* 1997;36(6):835–843.

71. Kumra S, Jacobsen LK, Lenane M, et al. Case series: spectrum of neuroleptic-induced movement disorders and extrapyramidal side effects in childhood-onset schizophrenia. *J Am Acad Child Adolesc Psychiatry.* 1998;37(2):221–227.

72. Tammenmaa IA, McGrath JJ, Sailas E, Soares-Weiser K. Cholinergic medication for neuroleptic-induced tardive dyskinesia [systematic review]. *Cochrane Database Syst Rev.* 2002;(3):CD000207.

73. Kurzthaler I, Hummer M, Kohl C, Miller C, Fleischhacker WW. Propranolol treatment of olanzapine-induced akathisia. *Am J Psychiatry.* 1997;154(9):1316.

74. Lipinski Jr. JF, Zubenko GS, Cohen BM, Barreira PJ. Propranolol in the treatment of neuroleptic-induced akathisia. *Am J Psychiatry.* 1984;141(3):412–415.

75. Zubenko GS, Cohen BM, Lipinski Jr. JF, Jonas JM. Use of clonidine in treating neuroleptic-induced akathisia. *Psychiatry Res.* 1984;13(3):253–259.

76. Soares-Weiser K, Rathbone J. Neuroleptic reduction and/or cessation and neuroleptics as specific treatments for tardive dyskinesia [systematic review]. *Cochrane Database Syst Rev.* 2000;(2):CD000459.

77. Ankenman R, Salvatore MF. Low dose alpha-methyl-para-tyrosine (AMPT) in the treatment of dystonia and dyskinesia. *J Neuropsychiatry Clin Neurosci.* 2007;19(1):65–69.

78. Reches A, Burke RE, Kuhn CM, Hassan MN, Jackson VR, Fahn S. Tetrabenazine, an amine-depleting drug, also blocks dopamine receptors in rat brain. *J Pharmacol Exp Ther.* 1983;225(3):515–521.

79. Kenney C, Hunter C, Jankovic J. Long-term tolerability of tetrabenazine in the treatment of hyperkinetic movement disorders. *Mov Dis.* 2007;22(2):193–197.

80. Ondo WG, Jong D, Davis A. Comparison of weight gain in treatments for Tourette syndrome: tetrabenazine versus neuroleptic drugs. *J Child Neurol.* 2008;23(4):435–437.

81. Brusa L, Orlacchio A, Moschella V, Iani C, Bernardi G, Mercuri NB. Treatment of the symptoms of Huntington's disease: preliminary results comparing aripiprazole and tetrabenazine. *Mov Disord.* 2009;24(1):126–129.

82. Kenney C, Hunter C, Mejia N, Jankovic J. Is history of depression a contraindication to treatment with tetrabenazine? *Clin Neuropharmacol.* 2006;29(5):259–264.

83. Soares KVS, McGrath JJ. Vitamin E for neuroleptic-induced tardive dyskinesia [systematic review]. *Cochrane Database Syst Rev.* 2011;(2):CD000209.

84. Soares-Weiser K, Rathbone J. Calcium channel blockers for neuroleptic-induced tardive dyskinesia [systematic review]. *Cochrane Database Syst Rev.* 2004;(1):CD000206.

85. Silva R, Mata LR, Gulbenkian S, Brito MA, Tiribelli C, Brites D. Inhibition of glutamate uptake by unconjugated bilirubin in cultured cortical rat astrocytes: role of concentration and pH. *Biochem Biophys Res Commun.* 1999;265(1):67–72.

86. Trollor JN, Chen X, Chitty K, Sachdev PS. Comparison of neuroleptic malignant syndrome induced by first- and second-generation antipsychotics. *Br J Psychiatry.* 2012;201(1):52–56.

87. Croarkin PE, Emslie GJ, Mayes TL. Neuroleptic malignant syndrome associated with atypical antipsychotics in pediatric patients: a review of published cases. *J Clin Psychiatry.* 2008;69(7):1157–1165.

88. Granato JE, Stern BJ, Ringel A, et al. Neuroleptic malignant syndrome: successful treatment with dantrolene and bromocriptine. *Ann Neurol.* 1983;14(1):89–90.

89. Zuvekas SH, Vitiello B, Norquist GS. Recent trends in stimulant medication use among U.S. children. *Am J Psychiatry.* 2006;163(4):579–585.

90. Greenhill L, Kollins S, Abikoff H, et al. Efficacy and safety of immediate-release methylphenidate treatment for preschoolers with ADHD. *J Am Acad Child Adolesc Psychiatry.* 2006;45(11):1284–1293.

91. Swanson J, Greenhill L, Wigal T, et al. Stimulant-related reductions of growth rates in the PATS. *J Am Acad Child Adolesc Psychiatry.* 2006;45(11):1304–1313.

92. Michelson D, Faries D, Wernicke J, et al. Atomoxetine in the treatment of children and adolescents with attention-deficit/hyperactivity disorder: a randomized, placebo-controlled, dose-response study. *Pediatrics*. 2001;108(5):E83.

93. Connor DF, Findling RL, Kollins SH, et al. Effects of guanfacine extended release on oppositional symptoms in children aged 6-12 years with attention-deficit hyperactivity disorder and oppositional symptoms: a randomized, double-blind, placebo-controlled trial. *CNS Drugs*. 2010;24(9):755–768.

94. Connor DF, Barkley RA, Davis HT. A pilot study of methylphenidate, clonidine, or the combination in ADHD comorbid with aggressive oppositional defiant or conduct disorder. *Clin Pediatr*. 2000;39(1):15–25.

95. Kollins SH, Jain R, Brams M, et al. Clonidine extended-release tablets as add-on therapy to psychostimulants in children and adolescents with ADHD. *Pediatrics*. 2011;127(6):e1406–1413.

96. Yilmaz AE, Donmez A, Orun E, Tas T, Isik B, Sonmez FM. Methylphenidate-induced acute orofacial and extremity dyskinesia. *J Child Neurol*. 2013;28(6):781–783.

97. Randomized, controlled, crossover trial of methylphenidate in pervasive developmental disorders with hyperactivity. *Arch Gen Psychiatry*. 2005;62(11):1266–1274.

98. Lowe TL, Cohen DJ, Detlor J, Kremenitzer MW, Shaywitz BA. Stimulant medications precipitate Tourette's syndrome. *JAMA*. 1982;247(12):1729–1731.

99. Scahill L, Erenberg G, Berlin Jr. CM, et al. Contemporary assessment and pharmacotherapy of Tourette syndrome. *NeuroRx*. 2006;3(2):192–206.

100. Castellanos FX, Giedd JN, Elia J, et al. Controlled stimulant treatment of ADHD and comorbid Tourette's syndrome: effects of stimulant and dose. *J Am Acad Child Adolesc Psychiatry*. 1997;36(5):589–596.

101. Gadow KD, Sverd J, Sprafkin J, Nolan EE, Grossman S. Long-term methylphenidate therapy in children with comorbid attention-deficit hyperactivity disorder and chronic multiple tic disorder. *Arch Gen Psychiatry*. 1999;56(4):330–336.

102. Price RA, Leckman JF, Pauls DL, Cohen DJ, Kidd KK. Gilles de la Tourette's syndrome: tics and central nervous system stimulants in twins and nontwins. *Neurology*. 1986;36(2):232–237.

103. Tourette's Syndrome Study Group. Treatment of ADHD in children with tics: a randomized controlled trial. *Neurology*. 2002;58(4):527–536.

104. Ledbetter M. Atomoxetine use associated with onset of a motor tic. *J Child Adolesc Psychopharmacol*. 2005;15(2):331–333.

105. Allen AJ, Kurlan RM, Gilbert DL, et al. Atomoxetine treatment in children and adolescents with ADHD and comorbid tic disorders. *Neurology*. 2005;65(12):1941–1949.

106. Bond GR, Garro AC, Gilbert DL. Dyskinesias associated with atomoxetine in combination with other psychoactive drugs. *Clin Toxicol*. 2007;45(2):182–185.

107. Gilbert DL, Christian BT, Gelfand MJ, Shi B, Mantil J, Sallee FR. Altered mesolimbocortical and thalamic dopamine in Tourette syndrome. *Neurology*. 2006;67(9):1695–1697.

108. Baym CL, Corbett BA, Wright SB, Bunge SA. Neural correlates of tic severity and cognitive control in children with Tourette syndrome. *Brain*. 2008;131(Pt 1):165–179.

109. Hershey T, Black KJ, Hartlein J, et al. Dopaminergic modulation of response inhibition: an fMRI study. *Brain Res Cogn Brain Res*. 2004;20(3):438–448.

110. Gilbert DL, Ridel KR, Sallee FR, Zhang J, Lipps TD, Wassermann EM. Comparison of the inhibitory and excitatory effects of ADHD medications methylphenidate and atomoxetine on motor cortex. *Neuropsychopharmacology*. 2006;31(2):442–449.

111. Gilbert DL, Wang Z, Sallee FR, et al. Dopamine transporter genotype influences the physiological response to medication in ADHD. *Brain*. 2006;129(Pt 8):2038–2046.

112. Denckla MB, Rudel RG. Anomalies of motor development in hyperactive boys. *Ann Neurol*. 1978;3(3):231–233.

113. Mostofsky SH, Newschaffer CJ, Denckla MB. Overflow movements predict impaired response inhibition in children with ADHD. *Percept Mot Skills*. 2003;97(3 Pt 2):1315–1331.

114. Bodfish JW, Newell KM, Sprague RL, Harper VN, Lewis MH. Dyskinetic movement disorder among adults with mental retardation: phenomenology and co-occurrence with stereotypy. *Am J Ment Retard*. 1996;101(2):118–129.

115. Eapen V, Robertson MM, Zeitlin H, Kurlan R. Gilles de la Tourette's syndrome in special education schools: a United Kingdom study. *J Neurol*. 1997;244(6):378–382.

116. Mahone EM, Bridges D, Prahme C, Singer HS. Repetitive arm and hand movements (complex motor stereotypies) in children. *J Pediatr*. 2004;145(3):391–395.

V. SELECTED SECONDARY MOVEMENT DISORDERS

117. McGough J, McCracken J, Swanson J, et al. Pharmacogenetics of methylphenidate response in preschoolers with ADHD. *J Am Acad Child Adolesc Psychiatry*. 2006;45(11):1314–1322.

118. Leo RJ. Movement disorders associated with the serotonin selective reuptake inhibitors. *J Clin Psychiatry*. 1996;57(10):449–454.

119. Morelli E, Moore H, Rebello TJ, et al. Chronic 5-HT transporter blockade reduces DA signaling to elicit basal ganglia dysfunction. *J Neurosci*. 2011;31(44):15742–15750.

120. Boyer EW, Shannon M. The serotonin syndrome. *N Engl J Med*. 2005;352(11):1112–1120.

121. Ak S, Anil Yagcioglu AE. Escitalopram-induced Parkinsonism. *Gen Hosp Psychiatry*. 2014;36(1):126.e121–126.e122.

122. Altindag A, Yanik M, Asoglu M. The emergence of tics during escitalopram and sertraline treatment. *Int Clin Psychopharmacol*. 2005;20(3):177–178.

123. Madhusoodanan S, Alexeenko L, Sanders R, Brenner R. Extrapyramidal symptoms associated with antidepressants—a review of the literature and an analysis of spontaneous reports. *Ann Clin Psychiatry*. 2010;22(3):148–156.

124. McKeon A, Pittock SJ, Glass GA, et al. Whole-body tremulousness: isolated generalized polymyoclonus. *Arch Neurol*. 2007;64(9):1318–1322.

125. Sokolski KN, Chicz-Demet A, Demet EM. Selective serotonin reuptake inhibitor-related extrapyramidal symptoms in autistic children: a case series [see comment]. *J Child Adolesc Psychopharmacol*. 2004;14(1):143–147.

126. Spirko BA, Wiley 2nd JF. Serotonin syndrome: a new pediatric intoxication. *Pediatr Emerg Care*. 1999;15(6):440–443.

127. Storch EA, Arnold EB, Lewin AB, et al. The effect of cognitive-behavioral therapy versus treatment as usual for anxiety in children with autism spectrum disorders: a randomized, controlled trial. *J Am Acad Child Adolesc Psychiatry*. 2013;52(2):132–142.e132.

128. Storch EA, Bussing R, Small BJ, et al. Randomized, placebo-controlled trial of cognitive-behavioral therapy alone or combined with sertraline in the treatment of pediatric obsessive-compulsive disorder. *Behav Res Ther*. 2013;51(12):823–829.

129. Sukhodolsky DG, Bloch MH, Panza KE, Reichow B. Cognitive-behavioral therapy for anxiety in children with high-functioning autism: a meta-analysis. *Pediatrics*. 2013;132(5):e1341–1350.

130. Radhu N, Daskalakis ZJ, Guglietti CL, et al. Cognitive behavioral therapy-related increases in cortical inhibition in problematic perfectionists. *Brain Stimul*. 2012;5(1):44–54.

131. Lifshitz M, Gavrilov V, Sofer S. Signs and symptoms of carbamazepine overdose in young children. *Pediatr Emerg Care*. 2000;16(1):26–27.

132. Jacobsen D, Alvik A, Bredesen JE, Brown RD. Pharmacokinetics of phenytoin in acute adult and child intoxication. *J Toxicol Clin Toxicol*. 1986;24(6):519–531.

133. Hedrick R, Williams F, Morin R, Lamb WA, Cate JC. Carbamazepine—erythromycin interaction leading to carbamazepine toxicity in four epileptic children. *Ther Drug Monit*. 1983;5(4):405–407.

134. Chalhub EG, Devivo DC, Volpe JJ. Phenytoin-induced dystonia and choreoathetosis in two retarded epileptic children. *Neurology*. 1976;26(5):494–498.

135. Koukkari MW, Vanefsky MA, Steinberg GK, Hahn JS. Phenytoin-related chorea in children with deep hemispheric vascular malformations. *J Child Neurol*. 1996;11(6):490–491.

136. Lancman ME, Asconape JJ, Penry JK. Choreiform movements associated with the use of valproate. *Arch Neurol*. 1994;51(7):702–704.

137. Weaver DF, Camfield P, Fraser A. Massive carbamazepine overdose: clinical and pharmacologic observations in five episodes. *Neurology*. 1988;38(5):755–759.

138. Garcia-Ramos R, Moreno Ramos T, Villarejo Galende A, Porta Etessam J. Phenytoin-induced acute orofacial dyskinesia. *Neurologia*. 2013;28(3):193–194.

139. Lucey BP. Teaching video neuroimages: phenytoin-induced orofacial dyskinesias. *Neurology*. 2012;79(19):e177.

140. Fountoulakis KN, Samara M, Siapera M, Iacovides A. Tardive Tourette-like syndrome: a systematic review. *Int Clin Psychopharmacol*. 2011;26(5):237–242.

141. Sotero de Menezes MA, Rho JM, Murphy P, Cheyette S. Lamotrigine-induced tic disorder: report of five pediatric cases. *Epilepsia*. 2000;41(7):862–867.

142. Thome-Souza S, Moreira B, Valente KD. Late adverse effects of the coadministration of valproate and lamotrigine. *Pediatr Neurol*. 2012;47(1):47–50.

143. Giles LL, DelBello MP, Gilbert DL, Stanford KE, Shear PK, Strakowski SM. Cerebellar ataxia in youths at risk for bipolar disorder. *Bipolar Disord*. 2008;10(6):733–737.

144. Kramer ED, Packer RJ, Ginsberg J, et al. Acute neurologic dysfunction associated with high-dose chemotherapy and autologous bone marrow rescue for primary malignant brain tumors. *Pediatr Neurosurg*. 1997;27(5):230–237.

145. Küpfer A, Aeschlimann C, Wermuth B, Cerny T. Prophylaxis and reversal of ifosfamide encephalopathy with methylene-blue. *The Lancet*. 1994;343(8900):763–764.

146. Ames B, Lewis LD, Chaffee S, Kim J, Morse R. Ifosfamide-induced encephalopathy and movement disorder. *Pediatr Blood Cancer*. 2010;54(4):624–626.

147. Pelgrims J, De Vos F, Van den Brande J, Schrijvers D, Prové A, Vermorken J. Methylene blue in the treatment and prevention of ifosfamide-induced encephalopathy: report of 12 cases and a review of the literature. *Br J Cancer*. 2000;82(2):291.

148. Erol I, Alehan F, Ozcay F, Canan O, Haberal M. Neurological complications of liver transplantation in pediatric patients: a single center experience. *Pediatr Transplant*. 2007;11(2):152–159.

149. Umeda Y, Matsuda H, Sadamori H, et al. Leukoencephalopathy syndrome after living-donor liver transplantation. *Exp Clin Transplant*. 2011;9(2):139–144.

150. Bhojwani D, Sabin ND, Pei D, et al. Methotrexate-induced neurotoxicity and leukoencephalopathy in childhood acute lymphoblastic leukemia. *J Clin Oncol*. 2014;32(9):949–959.

151. Kuriyama A, Jackson JL, Doi A, Kamiya T. Metronidazole-induced central nervous system toxicity: a systematic review. *Clin Neuropharmacol*. 2011;34(6):241–247.

152. Kim E, Na DG, Kim EY, Kim JH, Son KR, Chang KH. MR imaging of metronidazole-induced encephalopathy: lesion distribution and diffusion-weighted imaging findings. *Am J Neuroradiol*. 2007;28(9):1652–1658.

153. Ozdemir O, Baytan B, Gunes AM, Okan M. Involuntary movements during vitamin B12 treatment. *J Child Neurol*. 2010;25(2):227–230.

154. Zanus C, Alberini E, Costa P, Colonna F, Zennaro F, Carrozzi M. Involuntary movements after correction of vitamin B12 deficiency: a video-case report. *Epileptic Disord*. 2012;14(2):174–180.

155. Siegel M, Beresford CA, Bunker M, et al. Preliminary investigation of lithium for mood disorder symptoms in children and adolescents with autism spectrum disorder. *J Child Adolesc Psychopharmacol*. 2014;24(7):399–402.

156. Peters SP, Prenner BM, Mezzanotte WS, Martin P, O'Brien CD. Long-term safety and asthma control with budesonide/formoterol versus budesonide pressurized metered-dose inhaler in asthma patients. *Allergy Asthma Proc*. 2008;29(5):499–516.

Functional (Psychogenic) Movement Disorders

Harvey S. Singer[1], Jonathan W. Mink[2], Donald L. Gilbert[3] and Joseph Jankovic[4]

[1]Department of Neurology, Johns Hopkins Hospital, Baltimore, MD, USA;
[2]Division of Child Neurology, University of Rochester Medical Center,
Rochester, NY, USA; [3]Division of Neurology, Cincinnati Children's Hospital
Medical Center, Cincinnati, OH, USA; [4]Department of Neurology, Baylor
College of Medicine, Houston, TX, USA

OUTLINE

Movement Disorders in Childhood, Second Edition.
DOI: http://dx.doi.org/10.1016/B978-0-12-411573-6.00023-1

INTRODUCTION

A common problem in neurology is the existence of disorders that present with neurological symptoms, but do not have an identifiable neurological basis. Many different terms have been used to describe these disorders including "hysterical, functional, conversion disorder, and psychogenic."[1] These terms reflect the concept that the symptoms are not based on an identifiable organic disorder and that the symptoms and neurologic signs are incompatible with known anatomy and physiology. However, the historical distinction between "organic" and "psychogenic" may not be meaningful. The term "psychogenic" implies that the etiology disorder from the "mind." It has been argued that "functional" should be the preferred term because it is freer from assumptions of etiology and does not reinforce dualistic thinking.[2] Indeed, there is an emerging body of data demonstrating abnormal function of neural circuits in patients with conversion disorder.[3–5] The term "functional movement disorders" (FMDs) will be preferred in this chapter, but it should be understood that "psychogenic" and "functional" are used interchangeably in the literature and in practice.

The concept of hysteria has been present in Western medicine for over 2000 years. Briquet in the 1850s and Charcot in the 1880s are generally recognized for their early work on disorders on the border zone between neurology and psychiatry and guiding them into modern medicine.[6] The term conversion was first used by Breuer and Freud to describe the transformation of unresolved psychologic conflicts and unassimilated emotions into physical manifestations.[6] Conversion disorders fall under the broader category of "somatoform disorders" in the American Psychiatric Association's *Diagnostic and Statistical Manual of Mental Disorders, Fourth Edition – Text Revision (DSM4-TR).*[7] Diagnostic criteria for conversion disorder include the presence of symptoms affecting voluntary motor or sensory functions that suggest a neurological condition but that are judged to be caused by psychological factors. The symptoms cause impaired function, are not intentionally produced, and cannot be explained after a thorough medical evaluation.[7] Primary gain, secondary gain, or both may be present.

In the recently published DSM-5,[8] the broader category of "Somatoform Disorders" has been replaced by "Somatic Symptom and Related Disorders." This change was motivated by a need to provide greater clarity and to emphasize the prominence of somatic symptoms that cause distress in these disorders. "Conversion Disorder" remains a primary diagnosis, but the alternative name "Functional Neurological Symptom Disorder" has also been included. In the revised diagnostic criteria contained in DSM-5, there must be "evidence of incompatibility between the symptom and recognized neurological or medical conditions."

Epidemiology

Most studies of conversion disorder have focused on adult patients, and there are relatively few firm data on the prevalence of conversion disorder in children. The lack of data results from several factors including inconsistent use of terminology, lack of physician confidence in the diagnosis of conversion, and a tendency to code diagnosis by symptom. The first US description of conversion disorder in children consisted of 98 cases.[9] Despite continued study, few data exist to estimate the population prevalence of conversion disorder in children in the United States. Prevalence of conversion disorder among children has been estimated at 1–4 per 100,000.[10,11] In a study from the United Kingdom and Ireland of

204 children and adolescents with conversion disorder, the most common symptoms were motor weakness and abnormal movements.[11] Conversion disorder has been reported in children as young as 4 years, but most often presents during the peri-pubertal years.[6,12]

"Functional" disorders make up a significant percentage of referrals to neurologists. In a study of National Health Service referrals from primary care to adults neurology clinics in Scotland, 30% of patients were determined to have symptoms that were "not at all" or only "somewhat explained" by "organic disease."[13] Conversion disorder is a relatively common reason for presentation to movement disorders clinics. Among adults, estimates vary from 2% to 9% of patients.[12,14] Common FMDs include dystonia, tremor, myoclonus, tics, hemiballismus, chorea, parkinsonism, and gait disorders. Although there are few data on these disorders in children, it has been estimated that 2–5% of children presenting to movement disorders clinic have a FMD.[15–18] Twelve of fifty-two children presenting to a busy pediatric movement disorders center in Australia with an acute-onset movement disorder were diagnosed with a FMD.[19] For FMDs in children, the average age of onset is 12–14 years, with a range of 7–18 years.[15–17] No children under 7 years of age were reported in those three series. FMDs affect girls more than boys in a 3:1 to 4:1 ratio.[15–17] One report indicated a 1:1 ratio of boys to girls in children 12 years of age or younger.[15–17]

The diagnoses of conversion disorder and FMD pertain to individuals. However, in rare instances, functional signs and symptoms appear to spread rapidly among members of a cohesive group.[20] When this happens, it is called "mass psychogenic illeness." Much less is known about the biological underpinnings and clinical features of mass psychogenic illness, than is known about conversion disorder. Features of mass psychogenic illness are the occurrence of these symptoms in a cohesive group, the presence of increased anxiety, the spread of symptoms through sight, sound, or oral communication (including social media), and high female: male ratio.[20] There are many examples of mass psychogenic illness in history, most notably perhaps is the Salem "witches." A more recent example is of an outbreak of a tic-like mass psychogenic illness in Leroy, NY, in which 19 teenage students at a single high school developed symptoms over a 5-month period of time.[21]

Clinical Features of Functional Movement Disorders

Most conversion disorders in children are mono-symptomatic with a single movement disorder being present in a majority.[18] However, many patients with functional (psychogenic) disorders have a combination of complex, often bizarre, movements or gaits that are not congruous with organic movement disorders (Videos 23.1–23.5). Young children typically present after a minor injury, but older children are less likely to have a history of focal injury. In children the dominant extremities are more likely to be involved than the non-dominant extremities.[16,17,22] The typical course of conversion symptoms in children is for the symptoms to resolve within 3 months from the time of diagnosis.[23] The great majority of children have complete resolution of symptoms and recurrence of symptoms appears to be rare.[24,25] Outcome of FMDs specifically has not been studied, long-term outcome is good in the majority of cases,[16,26] but may be less good than for childhood conversion disorders more generally.[16] However, these reports from specialty clinics may reflect an ascertainment bias.

It is often possible to identify a specific precipitant for the conversion symptoms in children.[25] In a study of 47 Israeli children with conversion disorder, a specific reason for the conversion was discovered in 40.[27] Among children with FMD, antecedent history of physical or emotional stressors is common, being reported in 53–80% of the cases.[11,16,17,26] Children with FMD commonly have coexisting impairment of mood, especially anxiety, depressed mood, or irritability,[16,17] and "perfectionistic" tendencies are common.[17,25] They may also have other medically unexplained symptoms associated with their movement disorder.[18]

Pathophysiology

There is emerging evidence that conversion disorders are associated with altered brain function. All of these studies have been performed in adults, but it is reasonable to hypothesize that similar mechanisms are involved in children. One of the first studies to demonstrate this was a single photon emission computerized tomography (SPECT) study showing decreased regional cerebral blood flow in the thalamus and basal ganglia contralateral to psychogenic sensorimotor deficits in adults.[28] An important finding of that study was that the contralateral basal ganglia and thalamic hypoactivation resolved after recovery. In adult subjects with conversion hemiparesis, cerebral blood flow responses in a motor imagery task were abnormally increased in the ventromedial prefrontal cortex and superior temporal cortex despite normal task performance.[29] These studies and several other small studies using electroencephalography (EEG), structural MRI, functional MRI, PET, or SPECT have suggested that conversion disorders are associated with abnormal modulation of motor and sensory representations by affective or stress-related factors.[5,30,31]

Adult subjects with FMDs have impaired habituation to arousing stimuli and greater functional connectivity between amygdala and supplementary motor area (SMA).[32] A subsequent study of 16 subjects with FMDs showed greater activity in limbic structures (right amygdala, left anterior insula and bilateral posterior cingulate area) and decreased activity in the left SMA during a motor preparation task compared with controls.[4] These data provide strong evidence for a neurobiological basis of conversion disorders; however whether the abnormalities reflect causal mechanisms remains unknown.

Diagnosis

At first glance, some organic movement disorders may appear to be functional in origin. Historically, many physicians believed that Tourette's syndrome and task-specific focal dystonias, such as writer's cramp, were "hysterical." Some movements related to organic movement disorders can be suppressed, including: tics, tardive dyskinesia, parkinsonian rest tremor, and some choreas. Hemiballismus, brought on by brain injury or stroke, can begin precipitously and follow a static or diminishing course. Organic paroxysmal dyskinesias, by definition, occur and remit abruptly, and may be misdiagnosed as psychogenic. However, the clinical features of functional paroxysmal movement disorders allow them to be distinguished from organic paroxysmal movement disorders (Chapter 9).[33] Rapid-onset dystonia parkinsonism may have abrupt onset and reach a stable severe plateau within days.[34] Psychiatric dysfunction may be the initial presentation for diseases containing abnormal movements, such as Huntington's disease and Wilson's disease.

It is often believed that conversion disorder is a "diagnosis of exclusion" or that the diagnosis cannot be made until "everything has been ruled out." This is an incorrect view. Conversion disorder is a diagnosis that should be based on careful history, neurological and physical examination, and diagnostic criteria. Most important is for the examining physician to have sufficient knowledge of neuroanatomy and neurophysiology to determine when signs and symptoms are inconsistent with known disease processes. A thorough medical history including family history and physical examination, and in some cases diagnostic testing, is necessary to arrive at a confirmed diagnosis of a psychogenic movement disorder. Conversion disorders and organic neurological disease can coexist, most commonly in chronic relapsing diseases such as epilepsy. However, fewer than 10% of children diagnosed with conversion disorder have a preexisting physical disease.[27] In adults, once a diagnosis of a functional, nonorganic neurological disorder is made, new organic diagnoses rarely emerge, even when symptoms persist. In over 1000 adults judged by neurologists as having symptoms "unexplained by organic disease," fewer than 1% had acquired a new organic disease diagnosis 18 months later.[13]

Certain features appear to be consistent across the range of patients with FMD[12,35] and should lead to strong consideration of the diagnosis (Table 23.1).[36] These clues to making the diagnosis of a FMD may be present in the history, physical examination, or therapeutic trials. While suggestive of a FMD, the presence of these features alone does not confirm the diagnosis. Some of these features may be present in organic movement disorders, so thoughtful evaluation is required.[12]

TABLE 23.1   Useful Clues for Diagnosing Functional Movement Disorders in Children

---

HISTORICAL CLUES

---

1. Abrupt onset followed by a static course
2. Spontaneous remission or inconsistency over time
3. Remission when the child is not aware of being observed
4. Presence of secondary gain

CLINICAL CLUES

---

1. Inconsistent character of the movement (amplitude, frequency, distribution, selective disability)
2. Paroxysmal symptoms in a manner inconsistent with a known paroxysmal movement disorder
3. Movements increase with attention to the movement, or decrease with distraction
4. Ability to trigger or relieve the abnormal movements with unusual or nonphysiological interventions
5. Inconsistency of findings with known neuroanatomy and neurophysiology
6. Deliberate slowness of movements
7. Entrainment
8. Functional disability out of proportion to exam findings
9. Prominent pain out of proportion to the objective findings

---

THERAPEUTIC RESPONSES

---

1. Unresponsiveness to appropriate medications
2. Response to placebos
3. Remission with psychotherapy

V. SELECTED SECONDARY MOVEMENT DISORDERS

Diagnostic Criteria for Functional Movement Disorders

Many physicians are reluctant to make the diagnosis of a conversion disorder. This appears to be true of FMDs, too. The average time from onset of symptoms to diagnosis has been reported to range from several days to as long as 21 years.[16,17,26] Accurate diagnosis is crucial since children may undergo invasive testing and surgical procedures prior to diagnosis. In one series, 22% of children underwent unnecessary surgery prior to accurate diagnosis for symptoms related to the FMD.[17]

Aids in Diagnosing Functional Movement Disorders

Testing beyond the scope of the neurological exam can be helpful in the diagnosis of FMDs. Suggestion and placebo challenge have been used by physicians to obtain a clearer picture of a patient's symptoms, and can help distinguish organic from psychogenic disease. Placebos, including IV injections and mild skin irritants, are controversial because of the possibility of disturbing the trust implicit in the doctor–patient relationship. They are even more controversial in young children because of informed consent concerns. However, in select circumstances they may play a role in the diagnosis and treatment when used in a supportive environment as part of a comprehensive treatment plan and when the use of placebo is fully disclosed in the course of the evaluation.[37]

Diagnosis of certain FMDs may be aided by electrophysiological studies, although these are rarely used in practice. Differentiation of psychogenic jerks from myoclonus or tics may be done through electromyography (EMG). EMG bursts less than 70 ms in duration are most likely organic in nature. Longer bursts with a well-organized triphasic pattern of activation of opposing muscle groups may represent psychogenic or volitional movements. Combined application of EEG and EMG provides a more sensitive test. The post-stimulus latency of reflex or stimulus-sensitive myoclonus can be examined. Latencies greater than 100 ms from the stimulus to the onset of movement suggest that the movement is voluntary.[38]

Tremor occurring at different frequencies in different muscle groups usually indicates an organic etiology. Frequency variability can be seen in psychogenic tremor, but there is enough overlap between organic and nonorganic tremor frequency variation to prevent diagnosis based on frequency variability alone.[39] Simultaneous activity in agonists and antagonists has been associated with psychogenic tremor. Tremors faster than 11 Hz are likely beyond the upper frequency limit of voluntary tremor, and are likely of organic etiology.[38] Entrainment of tremor with voluntary rapid alternative movements of different frequencies supports the diagnosis of psychogenic tremor.

Specific Movement Disorder Types in FMDs

The most commonly reported movement disorders among children with FMD are tremor (26–65%), dystonia (39–47%), myoclonus (4–37%), and gait disorders (13–30%).[15–18] Tics may also be a manifestation of FMD.[26,40] These relative proportions are comparable to what has been reported in adults with FMDs.[41,42]

Tremor

In a report of 24 adolescent and adult patients with clinically established or documented psychogenic tremor, subjects ranged in age from 15 to 78 years with 15 women and

9 men.[43] Variability in tremor characteristics (e.g., tremor direction) was seen in greater than 90% of patients and variable tremor amplitude and frequency was observed in all patients. Unusual characteristics of these tremors included abrupt onset, bilateral involvement, distractibility, and a nonprogressive course with fluctuating severity.[44,45] These psychogenic tremors often consisted of resting, postural, and kinetic components and were associated with selective, but not task-specific, disabilities. Neurological examination often revealed other inconsistencies, and drug treatment was usually ineffective. Children with psychogenic tremor may be more likely to be diagnosed with a FMD prior based on clinical grounds and without extensive laboratory or imaging investigations.[17]

Dystonia

Fahn and Williams defined the features of psychogenic dystonia in 39 patients, who were mostly female, had symptoms lasting between 1 month to 15 years, and ranged in age between 8 and 56 years old. Eighty-five percent of these patients had movements that were incongruous or inconsistent with those of dystonia, but most had other clues including false weakness, pain, and multiple somatizations.[12] Occurring mostly in young women, these disorders occured as painful dystonias inconsistent with established organic dystonias and had associated nonanatomic sensory changes and false weakness.[46]

As noted above, organic dystonia can be misdiagnosed as psychogenic. Misdiagnosis is most likely due to the varied presentation and protean findings in dystonia. Clinical features that may appear psychogenic but are organic include varied movements (writhing, jerking, spasms, and tremors), spontaneous remission, task-specificity or action induction, normal neurological exam, relief through *geste antagoniste* (sensory trick), worsening with increased stress and relief by relaxation, and paroxysmal appearance or diurnal variation.[37] In addition, dystonias of sudden onset and remission can occur with medication ingestion, particularly dopamine blocking agents such as phenothiazines.

Myoclonus

In one report of 18 cases of psychogenic myoclonus, movements were predominantly segmental in character, occurred at rest, and were often exacerbated by voluntary movement. The psychogenic nature of these cases was suggested by "the inconsistent character of the movements, associated psychiatric symptomatology, reduction in myoclonus with distraction, exacerbation and relief with placebo and suggestion, spontaneous periods of remission, acute onset and sudden resolution, and evidence of underlying psychopathology."[47] In a series of 76 adult patients with electrophysiologically-established diagnosis of "psychogenic axial myoclonus," several factors characterized the sample.[48] The male:female ratio was 1 : 2. Forty-two percent had isolated axial myoclonus, while the rest had involvement of face or limb. In 92% of patients, the axial myoclonus was in flexion. In 42%, the jerks occurred in a nonstereotyped multifocal manner with no clear pattern. The only factor that predicted outcome was "delay of diagnosis," which portended a worse outcome.

Tics

In a study of 9 patients with "psychogenic tics," the mean age at onset was 34.1 years and the male:female ratio was 4:5.[40] Common features in that sample included lack of premonitory sensations, adult-onset of the tics, absent family history of tics, inability to suppress the movements, and coexistence with another FMD or paroxysmal nonepileptic attacks (PNEA). In a report of 19 teenagers with tics in the setting of mass psychogenic illness, all patients had sudden and dramatic onset of jerking movements usually involving one or both arms and their head and neck.[21,49] Two of the individuals had a prior diagnosis of Tourette's syndrome or chronic motor tic disorder. Eighteen of the nineteen were girls. Six also had syncope or PNEA. The tics were not preceded by premonitory urges, were not suppressible, and were not stereotyped. Thus, the movements differed from true tics in several important diagnostic features (see Chapter 7).

Treatment and Outcome

For patients with mild symptoms, a clear diagnosis and reassurance given in a nonjudgmental manner, in a way that makes sense, may be sufficient. For more significant symptoms, a multidisciplinary approach with an ongoing alliance between the neurologist and the patient is an important component of the treatment process.[50] Some patients, their families, or other physicians may be resistant to the idea of a psychiatric or psychological consultation, but in one large study 91% of families accepted a nonorganic explanation fully or partially.[11] When there is resistance, it is often helpful to emphasize the neurobiology of the disorder. It is important to validate the reality of the symptoms. It is also important to convey confidence in the diagnosis. Once the diagnosis is made, the focus should be on treatment; additional diagnostic testing should be minimized. It may be helpful to recommend that evaluation of the disorder should occur from different specialties simultaneously.[37] Identification of the precipitating stressor, which may include psychological conflict, environmental stress, or trauma, and perpetuating factors may be essential guides to treatment strategy.[51]

Physical therapy and positive reinforcement to psychotherapy appear to reduce or abolish symptoms in many cases. As discussed earlier, placebo testing may have a role in both diagnosis and treatment of symptoms, but it must be used in a supportive setting. Anxiolytics and antidepressant medications may prove useful if mood disorders appear to be playing a primary role in the etiology of the abnormal movements.[1] Biofeedback using EMG may be useful in some cases.[51]

Characteristics of patients with better prognosis include "acute onset, short duration of symptoms, healthy premorbid functioning, absence of coexisting organic psychopathology, and presence of an identifiable stressor."[1] Symptom duration of less than 2 weeks was strongly correlated with a good outcome in psychogenic disorders.[14] Of patients who had symptomatic improvement while in the hospital, 96% had good long-term outcome.[52] Conversion symptoms following mechanical trauma may have a better prognosis than those arising from severe emotional trauma. It has been postulated that mechanical trauma may provoke a simple shock reaction, while emotional trauma is more likely to elicit psychological defenses.[53]

CONCLUSION

FMDs are an important form of conversion disorder that may cause substantial morbidity and are associated with a risk of unnecessary procedures. Their incidence in movement disorders clinic has gradually been increasing as neurologists recognize typical movement disorders and refer the more atypical disorders, many of which are FMDs, to specialists. They may be difficult to distinguish from organic neurological conditions, but with careful history and neurological examination in addition to knowledge of diagnostic clues, a firm diagnosis can be made. The diagnosis should not be based on merely excluding organic causes, but on specific diagnostic criteria. There have been relatively few series of children with psychogenic movements, but those that do exist are relatively consistent across studies. Clearly, differences between adult and children with FMDs exist; however, many elements are similar. Treatment of conversion disorders, such as FMDs, often requires a multifaceted approach, including behavioral, psychological, physical, and pharmacological therapies. Children with acute onset and short duration of disease appear to have the best prognosis for recovery.

References

1. Marjama J, Troster A, Koller W. Psychogenic movement disorders. *Neurol Clin.* 1995;13:283–297.
2. Edwards MJ, Stone J, Lang AE. From psychogenic movement disorder to functional movement disorder: it's time to change the name. *Mov Disord.* 2014;29(7):849–852.
3. Bryant RA, Das P. The neural circuitry of conversion disorder and its recovery. *J Abnorm Psychol.* 2012;121(1):289–296.
4. Voon V, Brezing C, Gallea C, Hallett M. Aberrant supplementary motor complex and limbic activity during motor preparation in motor conversion disorder. *Mov Disord.* 2011;26(13):2396–2403.
5. Edwards MJ, Fotopoulou A, Pareés I. Neurobiology of functional (psychogenic) movement disorders. *Curr Opin Neurol.* 2013;26:442–447.
6. Putnam F. Conversion symptoms. In: Joseph A, Young R, eds. *Movement Disorders in Neurology and Neuropsychiatry.* Boston, MA: Blackwell Scientific Publications; 1992:430–437.
7. American Psychiatric Association. *Diagnostic and Statistical Manual of Mental Disorders.* 4th-TR ed. Washington, DC: American Psychiatric Association; 2000.
8. American Psychiatric Association. *Diagnostic and Statistical Manual of Mental Disorders.* Fifth Edition (DSM-5). 5th ed. Arlington, TX: American Psychiatric Association; 2013.
9. Sheffield HB. A contribution to the study of hysteria in childhood as it occurs in the United States of America. *NY State J Med.* 1898;68:412–436.
10. Kozlowska K, Nunn KP, Rose D, Morris A, Ouvrier RA, Varghese J. Conversion disorder in Australian pediatric practice. *J Am Acad Child Adolesc Psychiatry.* 2007;46(1):68–75.
11. Ani C, Reading R, Lynn R, Forlee S, Garralda E. Incidence and 12-month outcome of non-transient childhood conversion disorder in the U.K. and Ireland. *Br J Psychiatry.* 2013;202:413–418.
12. Williams D, Ford B, Fahn S. Phenomenology and psychopathology related to psychogenic movement disorders. *Adv Neurol.* 1995;65:231–257.
13. Stone J, Carson A, Duncan R, et al. Symptoms "unexplained by organic disease" in 1144 new neurology outpatients: how often does the diagnosis change at follow-up? *Brain.* 2009;132(Pt 10):2878–2888.
14. Lempert T, Dietrich M, Huppert D, Brandt T. Psychogenic disorders in neurology: frequency and clinical spectrum. *Acta Neurol Scand.* 1990;82:335–340.
15. Fernandez-Alvarez E. Movement disorders of functional origin (psychogenic) in children. *Rev Neurol.* 2005;40(suppl 1):S75–S77.
16. Schwingenschuh P, Pont-Sunyer C, Surtees R, Edwards MJ, Bhatia KP. Psychogenic movement disorders in children: a report of 15 cases and a review of the literature. *Mov Disord.* 2008;23:1882–1888.
17. Ferrara J, Jankovic J. Psychogenic movement disorders in children. *Mov Disord.* 2008;23:1875–1881.
18. Canavese C, Ciano C, Zibordi F, Zorzi G, Cavallera V, Nardocci N. Phenomenology of psychogenic movement disorders in children. *Mov Disord.* 2012;27(9):1153–1157.
19. Dale RC, Singh H, Troedson C, Pillai S, Gaikiwari S, Kozlowska K. A prospective study of acute movement disorders in children. *Dev Med Child Neurol.* 2010;52(8):739–748.
20. Balaratnasingam S, Janca A. Mass hysteria revisited. *Curr Opin Psychiatry.* 2006;19:171–174.
21. Mink JW. Conversion disorder and mass psychogenic illness in child neurology. *Ann NY Acad Sci.* 2013;1304:40–44.
22. Regan J, LaBarbera J. Lateralization of conversion symptoms in children and adolescents. *Am J Psychiatry.* 1984;141:1279–1280.

23. Fritz G, Fritsch S, Hagino O. Somatoform disorders in children and adolescents: a review in the past 10 years. *J Am Acad Child Adolesc Psychiatry*. 1997;36:1329–1338.

24. Turgay A. Treatment outcome for children and adolescents with conversion disorder. *Can J Psychiatry*. 1990;35(7):585–589.

25. Grattan-Smith P, Fairley M, Procopis P. Clinical features of conversion disorder. *Arch Dis Child*. 1988;63(4):408–414.

26. Ahmed MA, Martinez A, Yee A, Cahill D, Besag FM. Psychogenic and organic movement disorders in children. *Dev Med Child Neurol*. 2008;50(4):300–304.

27. Zeharia A, Mukamel M, Carel C, Weitz R, Danziger Y, Mimouni M. Conversion reaction: management by the paediatrician. *Eur J Pediatr*. 1999;158:160–164.

28. Vuilleumier P, Chicherio C, Assal F, Schwartz S, Slosman D, Landis T. Functional neuroanatomical correlates of hysterical sensorimotor loss. *Brain*. 2001;124(Pt 6):1077–1090.

29. de Lange FP, Roelofs K, Toni I. Increased self-monitoring during imagined movements in conversion paralysis. *Neuropsychologia*. 2007;45(9):2051–2058.

30. Vuilleumier P. Hysterical conversion and brain function. *Prog Brain Res*. 2005;150:309–329.

31. Labate A, Cerasa A, Mula M, et al. Neuroanatomic correlates of psychogenic nonepileptic seizures: a cortical thickness and VBM study. *Epilepsia*. 2012;53(2):377–385.

32. Voon V, Brezing C, Gallea C, et al. Emotional stimuli and motor conversion disorder. *Brain*. 2010;133(Pt 5): 1526–1536.

33. Ganos C, Aguirregomozcorta M, Batla A, et al. Psychogenic paroxysmal movement disorders – clinical features and diagnostic clues. *Parkinsonism Relat Disord*. 2014;20(1):41–46.

34. Brashear A, Dobyns WB, de Carvalho Aguiar P, et al. The phenotypic spectrum of rapid-onset dystonia-parkinsonism (RDP) and mutations in the ATP1A3 gene. *Brain*. 2007;130(Pt 3):828–835.

35. Schrag A, Lang AE. Psychogenic movement disorders. *Curr Opin Neurol*. 2005;18:399–404.

36. Kirsch DB, Mink JW. Psychogenic movement disorders in children. *Pediatr Neurol*. 2004;30(1):1–6.

37. Fahn S, Williams D. Psychogenic dystonia. *Adv Neurol*. 1988;50:431–455.

38. Brown P, Thompson P. Electrophysiological aids to the diagnosis of psychogenic jerks, spasms, and tremor. *Mov Disord*. 2001;16:595–599.

39. McAuley JH, Rothwell JC, Marsden CD, Findley LJ. Electrophysiological aids in distinguishing organic from psychogenic tremor. *Neurology*. 1998;50:1882–1884.

40. Baizabal-Carvallo JF, Jankovic J. The clinical features of psychogenic movement disorders resembling tics. *J Neurol Neurosurg Psychiatry*. 2014;85(5):573–575.

41. Factor S, Podskalny G, Molho E. Psychogenic movement disorders: frequency, clinical profile, and characteristics. *J Neurol Neurosurg Psychiatry*. 1995;59:406–412.

42. Jankovic J, Thomas M. *Psychogenic Movement Disorders*. Phildelphia, PA: Lippincott; 2005.

43. Koller W, Lang AE, Vetere-Overfield B, et al. Psychogenic tremors. *Neurology*. 1989;39:1094–1099.

44. Thenganatt MA, Jankovic J. Psychogenic tremor: a video guide to its distinguishing features. *Tremor Other Hyperkinet Mov*. 2014;4:253.

45. Kenney C, Diamond A, Mejia N, Davidson A, Hunter C, Jankovic J. Distinguishing psychogenic and essential tremor. *J Neurol Sci*. 2007;263:94–99.

46. Lang AE. Psychogenic dystonia: a review of 18 cases. *Can J Neurol Sci*. 1995;22:136–143.

47. Monday K, Jankovic J. Psychogenic myoclonus. *Neurology*. 1993;43:349–352.

48. Erro R, Edwards MJ, Bhatia KP, Esposito M, Farmer SF, Cordivari C. Psychogenic axial myoclonus: clinical features and long-term outcome. *Parkinsonism Relat Disord*. 2014;20(6):596–599.

49. McVige JW, Fritz CL, Mechtler LL. Mass psychogenic illness in Leroy High School, New York. *Ann Neurol*. 2012;72(suppl 16):S192.

50. Faust J, Soman TB. Psychogenic movement disorders in children: characteristics and predictors of outcome. *J Child Neurol*. 2012;27(5):610–614.

51. Ford C. Conversion disorder and somatoform disorder not otherwise specified. In: Gabbard G, ed. *Treatment of Psychiatric Disorders*. 3rd ed. Washington, DC: American Psychiatric Publishing; 1984:1755–1768.

52. Couprie W, Wijdicks EFM, Roojmans HGM, vanGijn J. Outcome in conversion disorder: a follow up study. *J Neurol Neurosurg Psychiatry*. 1995;58:750–752.

53. Krull F, Schifferdecker M. Inpatient treatment of conversion disorder: a clinical investigation of outcome. *Psychother Psychosom*. 1990;53:161–165.

APPENDICES

Appendix A: Drug Appendix

ACETAZOLAMIDE

Actions: A weak diuretic and carbonic anhydrase inhibitor.

Standard dose: Initial dose of 125–250 mg/day, with gradual titration as tolerated. Daily doses may range from 1000 to 2000 mg/day divided into two to four daily doses.

Contraindications: Hyponatremia, hypokalemia, hyperchloremic acidosis, adrenocortical insufficiency, a history of allergy to sulfa drugs (a sulfonamide derivative), and significant renal, or hepatic dysfunction.

Main drug interactions: Increases the serum levels of primidone, pseudoephedrine, quinidine, and lithium. Increased risk of nephrolithiasis, especially when used in combination with topiramate.

Main side effects: Drowsiness, dizziness, fatigue, paresthesias of extremities and face, tinnitus, taste changes, polyuria, muscle weakness, delirium, anorexia, nausea, vomiting, and diarrhea. Less common but potentially serious side effects include metabolic acidosis, electrolyte imbalance, nephrolithiasis, hepatotoxicity, Stevens–Johnson syndrome, bone marrow suppression, and hypersensitivity reactions.

Special points: Successful in controlling paroxysmal conditions such as periodic paralysis, episodic ataxia and vertigo in episodic ataxia types 1 and 2 and in spinocerebellar ataxia type 6 with episodic features. Treatment of paroxysmal dyskinesias has been less beneficial and only a few case reports suggest that it may help action myoclonus. Obtaining a renal ultrasound has been suggested when patients take acetazolamide for longer than 6 months. Monitor CBC and electrolyte levels.

AMANTIDINE

Actions: Antiviral agent that modestly increases dopamine release, inhibits dopamine reuptake, has N-methyl-D-aspartate receptor antagonist properties, and possibly central anticholinergic effects.

Standard dose: Children should receive about half the adult dose and increase more slowly, e.g., starting with 50 mg/day and increasing to 50 mg twice a day after 1–2 weeks, then 50 mg 2–3 times/day. Dosages in small double-blind, placebo-controlled trials in adults ranged from 200 to 400 mg/day typically administered in 100-mg increments. A liquid formulation (50 mg/5 mL) is available.

Contraindications: Hypersensitivity. Use with caution in patients with congestive heart failure. Since cleared by the kidneys, renal insufficiency will increase the risk of side effects. Relative contraindications include dementia, psychosis, enlarged prostate, neurogenic bladder, and glaucoma.

Main drug interactions: Concurrent use with anticholinergic medications may augment their side effects. Caution is advised when co-administered with CNS stimulants. Renal clearance of amantadine is reduced with the co-administration of quinine or quinidine.

Main side effects: Primarily anticholinergic-type side effects, including dry mouth, nose, and throat, blurred vision, nausea, lightheadedness, urinary frequency or retention, constipation, hypotension, headaches, sedation, disturbed sleep, memory difficulties, confusion, anxiety, psychosis, pedal edema, and livido reticularis. Abrupt withdrawal can lead to delirium.

Special points: Effective in treating symptoms of early stages of Parkinson's disease and may be effective for treating levodopa-induced dyskinesias. Refractoriness to therapy may develop, but can be restored after a brief drug holiday. The dose should be tapered over weeks to avoid inducing a neuroleptic malignant syndrome, seen with abrupt withdrawal. Limited studies exist assessing its efficacy in the treatment of movement disorders (chorea) in the pediatric population.

AMPHETAMINE

Actions: Amphetamines bind to dopamine and norepinephrine transporter molecules preventing transmitter uptake and substitute for monoamines at the level of the vesicular monoamine transporter (VMAT).

Amphetamine contains equal proportions of levo- and dextroamphetamine
Dextroamphetamine has more potent wake promoting effects.
>   *Adderall*: 3:1 ratio of D-amphetamine:L-amphetamine
>   *Dexedrine*: contains only D-amphetamine
>   *Lisdexamfetamine*: a prodrug to D-amphetamine
>   *Methamphetamine*: methyl group added to the amine of amphetamine (enables higher brain penetration)

Standard dose: Typical dosing range for amphetamine and methamphetamine is between 5–60 mg given once or twice daily. For hypersomnia, adjust dosage to its timing with usual starting dose of 10 mg twice daily upon waking up and at noon. An extended release formulation of Adderall exists.

Contraindications: Avoid in patients on monoamine oxidase inhibitors, due to risk of potentiating life-threatening hypertensive crisis. Structural heart defects, advanced heart disease, hyperthyroidism, or history of drug abuse.

Main drug interactions: Amphetamines may increase the activity of tricyclic antidepressants or sympathomimetic agents. Increases risk for serotonin syndrome.

Main side effects: Tachycardia, hypertension, palpitations, sweating, anorexia, weight loss, tremor, seizures, and increased anxiety. At high dose, amphetamines may precipitate psychosis.

Special points: Schedule II medication effective and FDA-approved for the treatment of hypersomnia in narcolepsy. Tailor to the timing of hypersomnia.

ARIPIPRAZOLE

Actions: Functions as a partial agonist at D2 and 5-HT1A receptors, and as an antagonist at the 5-HT2A receptor.

Standard dose: 10 years and older: start 2 mg every day for 3 days, then if needed 5 mg once a day. Titrate in 5 mg intervals with typical dose of 10–30 mg/day.

Contraindication: Hypersensitivity.

Drug interactions: Benzodiazepines increase risk for orthostatic hypertension and sedation. Drugs that induce CYP3A4 (e.g., carbamazepine) can cause an increase in aripiprazole clearance and lower blood levels. Inhibitors of CYP3A4 (e.g., ketoconazole) or CYP2D6 (e.g., quinidine, fluoxetine, or paroxetine) can inhibit aripiprazole elimination and cause increased blood levels.

Side effects: Suicidal ideation and behavior, worsening depression, hypotension, hyperglycemia, weight gain, dizziness, prolonged Q-T, gastrointestinal issues, akathisia, tremor, tardive dyskinesia, headache, insomnia, sedation, fatigue, anxiety, and restlessness.

Special points: Approved as a tic suppressing medication.

ATOMOXETINE

Actions: Selective norepinephrine reuptake inhibitor. Increases norepinephrine and dopamine levels in the prefrontal cortex and striatum.

Standard dose: For hypersomnia varies from 10 to 60 mg given in two divided doses. For ADHD 1 to 1.8 mg/kg/day in children.

Contraindications: Hypersensitivity, cardiac or vascular disorders, MAO inhibitor use, narrow angle glaucoma, and pheochromocytoma.

Main drug interactions: Concurrent use of albuterol may increase heart rate and blood pressure. Tricyclic antidepressants and SSRIs can increase plasma concentrations of atomoxetine.

Main side effects: Nausea, reduced appetite, weight loss, xerostomia, urinary retention, psychosis, mania, and suicide. Increased risk of suicidality in children/adolescents with major depression especially during the first month of treatment.

Special points: Need to closely monitor blood pressure and pulse.

BACLOFEN

Action: Acts at gamma-aminobutyric acid (GABA) type B receptors in the spinal cord.

Standard dosage: Start with 5–10 mg at bedtime. Titrate slowly until desired therapeutic response or side effects. Usual maintenance dose is 10–60 mg/day in three divided doses, lower dose in children ages 2–7 years. Occasionally, a maximum dose of 180 mg/day may be optimal for some children.

Contraindications: Children under 2 years. Medication may exacerbate absence seizures. Use with caution in patients with diabetes, renal insufficiency, seizure disorders, stroke, severe psychiatric disturbances, or confusional states.

Main drug interactions: Synergistic effect with other CNS depressants.

Main side effects: Sedation, dizziness, weakness, hallucinations, confusion, headache, nausea, constipation, hypotonia, paresthesias, ataxia, may increase serum glucose.

Special points: Sudden cessation can cause seizures and psychosis. Maybe helpful in dystonia.

BACLOFEN; INTRATHECAL PUMP

Action: Administered via continuous infusion via a catheter placed within the spinal dura. Treatment requires surgery for catheter placement, implantation of a small pump and reservoir in the abdomen.

Standard dosage: Variable; dose starts at about 100 μg/day; but some individuals may require as much as 1000 μg/day.

Contraindications: Infusion system should not be implanted in a child whose weight is less than 14 kg or in the presence of infection.

Main drug interactions: Synergistic effect with other CNS depressants.

Main side effects: (see Baclofen). Abrupt drug withdrawal is associated with hallucinations, seizures, and status epilepticus. Infusion system-related side effects include infection, catheter breakage, or persistent fistula.

Special points: Safety and effectiveness in children less than age 4 years has not been established. Surgery is costly and use as a treatment for generalized dystonia is controversial.

BENZTROPINE

Action: Centrally acting anticholinergic also increases dopamine effect by inhibiting presynaptic reuptake.

Standard dose: Usual dosage is 0.5–2 mg twice daily.

Contraindications: Use with caution in patients taking other drugs with anticholinergic activity, such as antihistamines, tricyclic antidepressants, or amantadine, since these medications may cause increased confusion or side effects. Benztropine can reduce plasma levels of antipsychotic medications.

Main drug interactions: Dry mouth, sedation, pupil dilatation, blurred vision, constipation, urinary hesitancy or retention, fatigue, confusion, hallucinations, weakness, tachycardia, increased intraocular pressure, precipitation of narrow angle glaucoma, impaired concentration and memory, delirium, anhidrosis, and susceptibility to hyperthermia. Other side effects include dizziness, nausea, vomiting, and anxiety. Patients may develop tolerance to some of these effects with continued low-dose treatment.

Special points: May be more effective and better tolerated in children. No evidence that one drug in this medication class (benztropine, trihexyphenidyl) is superior to another. Increase dosage very slowly to avoid side effects; relatively low doses may be helpful. Anticholinergics can exacerbate tardive dyskinesia and chorea, but may be helpful for tardive dystonia. Rapid taper can cause malignant hyperthermia, worsening dystonia, or cholinergic symptoms.

BOTULINUM TOXIN

Actions: Botulinum toxin is a neurotoxin produced by *Clostridia*. The toxin exerts its effect by inhibiting the release of acetylcholine from the presynaptic site at the muscle-nerve junction. Two serotypes, botulinum toxin type A and B are available.

Standard dose: Intramuscular dose is highly dependent on the muscle group injected and botulinum toxin serotype. Botulinum toxin A is given in dosages of 50–400 units per injection session. Botulinum toxin B is given in dosages of 5,000–25,000 units per injection session. Dosage guidance is available for individual brands.

Contraindications: Hypersensitivity to any form of botulinum toxin. Preexisting weakness due to myasthenia gravis or other neuromuscular conditions. Infection at the proposed injection site(s). Patients receiving high doses of aminoglycosides or with bleeding risks should be treated with caution.

Main drug interactions: Botox may be potentiated by aminoglycoside antibiotics or other drugs that interfere with neuromuscular transmission.

Main side effects: Excessive weakness of injected or neighboring muscles. Local side effects at the injection site include pain, erythema, ecchymosis, and rash. Generalized side effects can include malaise, headache, nausea, dysphagia, dry mouth/sore throat, and flu-like symptoms.

Special points: The onset of benefit generally takes several days; symptomatic improvement may last for as long as 2–4 months. Patients may develop antibodies to botulinum toxin, resulting in lack of efficacy of future injections. To minimize the risk of antibody formation, at least 3 months should elapse before injections are repeated. Botox injections have been used in the treatment of dystonia, blepharospasm, tremors, spasticity, and tics.

CARBAMAZEPINE

Actions: Anticonvulsant; slows the rate of recovery of inactivated sodium channels.

Standard dose: Typical pediatric dose is 10–30 mg/kg/day, divided 3 times per day. To improve tolerance, a dose of 7–10 mg/kg divided twice per day should be initiated for the first week.

Contraindications: Hypersensitivity to carbamazepine, history of bone marrow suppression or known sensitivity to tricyclic antidepressants, and use in patients who have taken an MAO inhibitor in the past 14 days.

Main drug interactions: Carbamazepine is a CYP-450-3A4 inducer. Phenytoin and phenobarbital may decrease its effect and valproic acid and erythromycin may increase its effect.

Main side effects: Dizziness, nausea, drowsiness, fatigue, unsteadiness, blurred vision, double vision, weight gain, rash, hepatotoxicity, pancreatitis, and hyponatremia. Serious side effects include bone marrow suppression and skin reactions (erythema multiforme, Stevens–Johnson syndrome, toxic epidermal necrolysis).

Special points: Paroxysmal dyskinesias typically respond to doses that are less than those necessary to control seizures. Carbamazepine may be as effective as valproic acid in managing chorea. Need to monitor sodium levels, complete blood count, and liver function tests.

CARBIDOPA/LEVODOPA

Actions: Levodopa is converted to L-dopa by dopa decarboxylase; Carbidopa is a peripheral dopa decarboxylase inhibitor which blocks the peripheral conversion of levodopa to dopamine.

Standard dose: Levodopa is commonly available in the United States as a combination of carbidopa plus levodopa (10/100, 25/100, and 25/250 mg). Initial dosage of levodopa in children is 1 mg/kg/day, divided into three doses. Dose is determined by the levodopa component and the use of 25/100 tablets are recommended in children. Medication should be gradual titrated based on efficacy or adverse effects. The target dosage of levodopa is usually 4–5 mg/kg/day, though some have suggested doses up to 10 mg/kg/day. When peripheral side effects are disturbing (nausea, vomiting, hypotension), additional carbidopa can be administered 30 min before the levodopa. Levodopa/carbidopa should be taken at least 30 min before or 60 min after meals to avoid competition with other amino acids for gastrointestinal absorption. Tablets can be crushed and dissolved in an ascorbic acid solution or in orange juice and used within 24 h.

Contraindications: Hypersensitivity, the use of monoamine oxidase inhibitors, narrow angle glaucoma, and melanoma. Use with caution in patients with orthostatic hypotension, psychosis, and asthma.

Main drug interactions: Use with caution with antihypertensive agents. Beneficial effect is reduced with simultaneous use of dopamine receptor blockers (e.g., antipsychotic agents and metoclopramide). Pyridoxine increases the peripheral metabolism of L-dopa, if it is administered in absence of carbidopa. Oral iron salts, multivitamins/minerals (with ADEK, folate, iron) and large doses of methionine may diminish the therapeutic effect of levodopa.

Main side effects: Nausea/vomiting, confusion, dizziness, somnolence, orthostatic hypotension, hallucinations, depression, impulse control, headache, dry mouth, insomnia, fatigue, muscle cramps, and constipation. Motor complications include dyskinesia, dystonia, myoclonus, and the end-of-dose wearing-off effect.

Special points: Patients with DRD show a marked response at relatively low doses of carbidopa/levodopa compared with doses used in Parkinson's disease. If dyskinesia occurs with the initiation of therapy for DRD, dose should be reduced and then gradually increased. Neuroleptic malignant syndrome has been reported upon withdrawal in patients with Parkinson's disease, especially after long-term use. Studies have suggested that L-dopa does not cause neuronal death in animal models of Parkinsonism and chronic administration of L-dopa does not exacerbate the degenerative process in Parkinson's disease. Additional carbidopa can be prescribed if nausea occurs with combined carbidopa/levodopa tablets.

CLONAZEPAM

Actions: Long-acting benzodiazepine with mechanism of action through enhancement of GABAergic transmission (primarily at the $GABA_A$ receptor) in the CNS.

Standard dose: Start with 0.25–0.5 mg at bedtime and titrate slowly as tolerated. An amount of 0.05 mg/kg per dose has been advocated (0.01 mg/kg/day in children less than age 10). Usual maintenance dose is 1–4 mg/day divided 3 times daily, although some patients require considerably more. Weekly dose escalation is recommended to allow for patients to become tolerant to the sedating effects of this medication.

Contraindications: Contraindicated in patients with significant hepatic dysfunction, respiratory depression, or acute narrow-angle glaucoma.

Main drug interactions: Central nervous system depressant action may be potentiated by other sedative hypnotic drugs (e.g., alcohol, narcotics, barbiturates, monoamine oxidase inhibitors, anxiolytic, antipsychotic, anticonvulsant, or antidepressant drugs).

Main side effects: Sedation, somnolence, fatigue, confusion, cognitive impairments, dizziness, hyperactivity, and ataxia. Serious side effects include hypotension and respiratory depression. Medication may cause a paradoxical change in behavior with increased aggression, hyperexcitability, and irritability.

Special points: Clonazepam is a controlled substance with the potential for psychological and physical dependence. Abrupt discontinuation of clonazepam may precipitate withdrawal symptoms including seizures. Tolerance is common, and dose escalation with prolonged use may be needed. Useful in treating most types of myoclonus and helpful in parasomnias of NREM and REM sleep.

CLONIDINE

Action: Alpha-adrenergic agonist.

Standard dose: Start with 0.05 mg orally at bedtime. Increase the dosage as needed, every 3–7 days by 0.05 mg/day. Use in divided doses. Twice a day dosing is often adequate for treating tics, but 3–4 times per day is required for other usages (half-life is approximately 6h). The usual maximum dosage is 0.3–0.4 mg/day. Clonidine is also available as a transdermal patch that can be used as a once weekly patch. Patches are formulated to deliver 0.1, 0.2, or 0.3 mg/day. The usual patch dose is 0.2 mg.

Contraindications: Documented hypersensitivity, pregnant and breastfeeding individuals. Use with caution if there is impaired liver or renal function.

Main drug interactions: Sedation is increased when clonidine is used in combination with CNS depressing agents. The hypotensive effects of clonidine are enhanced by narcotic analgesics and inhibited by tricyclic antidepressants. Beta-blockers may potentiate bradycardia and enhance rebound hypertension associated with abrupt withdrawal. Clonidine may enhance the CNS-depressive effects of alcohol, barbiturates, or other sedating drugs.

Main side effects: Sedation is the most common adverse effect. Other side effects include orthostatic hypotension, headache, dizziness, fatigue, bradycardia, insomnia, irritability, dysphoria, dry mouth, and nightmares. Do not discontinue suddenly because of risk of rebound hypertension and symptoms of sympathetic hyperactivity. Local dermatitis is common with the transdermal patch.

Special points: Considered first-line therapy for tics and is effective for ADHD symptoms. Combination with methylphenidate has been shown to be more effective than monotherapy for children with tics and ADHD. Tolerance can develop.

CLOZAPINE

Actions: An atypical neuroleptic that affects D_4, 5-HT_2, muscarinic, and α-1 antagonist receptors; and is a relatively weak blocker of D_2 receptors.

Standard dose: In adults, start with 25 mg/day and increase by 25 mg/day every several days according to clinical response and as tolerated. Typical dose is 50–75 mg/day.

Contraindications: Myeloproliferative disorder, previous bone marrow suppression, paralytic ileus, and uncontrolled seizure disorder.

Main drug interactions: Not to be used concomitantly with other drugs that suppress bone marrow function. May potentiate the hypotensive effect of antihypertensive drugs and enhance the atropine effect of anticholinergic drugs. Use with caution together with other drugs that prolong the QTc interval. Clozapine in combination with lithium has been reported to cause severe encephalopathy.

Main side effects: Orthostatic hypotension, sedation, dizziness, vertigo, salivation, sweating, dry mouth, constipation, tachycardia, syncope, seizures, nausea, constipation, hyperglycemia, fever, and weight gain. Rare but serious side effects of clozapine include the agranulocytosis, eosinophilia, respiratory insufficiency, cardiac arrest, myocarditis, cardiomyopathy, hyperglycemia, neuroleptic malignant syndrome, pulmonary embolism, and hepatitis. Tardive dyskinesia has been reported in clozapine-treated patients.

Special points: Because of the risk of agranulocytosis, weekly blood counts are required. Drug is available through a distribution system to assure compliance with the required leukocyte monitoring. Clozapine is generally used to treat levodopa-induced hallucinations and dyskinesias, and Parkinsonian rest tremor.

COENZYME Q10

Actions: Integral component of the mitochondrial electron transport chain.

Standard dose: *Ubiquinol* (a solubilized bioavailable form of CoQ10): 2–8 mg/kg/day in two divided doses (preferred); *Ubiquinone*: 5–30 mg/kg/day in two divided doses daily with meals; *Idebenone* (an analog of CoQ): 90–900 mg/day in divided doses with meals.

Contraindications: Hypersensitivity to CoQ10 or product component.

Main drug interactions: May reduce anticoagulant effectiveness.

Main side effects: Wakefulness, sleep disruption, gastrointestinal problems, appetite suppression, and irritability.

Special points: Ubiquinone is less potent and less well absorbed than ubiquinol. Monitor CoQ10 level in plasma and leukocytes. Idebenone has been shown to improve recovery of visual loss in Leber's hereditary optic neuropathy.

CREATINE

Actions: Combines with phosphate to form phosphocreatine; converted in the gut to creatinine.

Standard dose: 0.1 g/kg daily; maximum 10 g/day.

Contraindications: Hypersensitivity, impaired kidney function, dehydration, and concurrent diuretic use.

Main drug interactions: Caffeine may adversely affect the efficacy of creatine supplementation. Concomitant use with agents that impair its excretion may increase serum levels.

Main side effects: GI upset, diarrhea, cramping, and dehydration.

Special points: Primary use is as an ergogenic agent.

CYCLOPHOSPHAMIDE

Actions: Cyclophosphamide is an alkylating agent with powerful and varied immunosuppressant properties. It is widely used as a chemotherapeutic agent to treat a variety of autoimmune and inflammatory diseases and cancers.

Standard dose: 600–1000 mg/m^2 intravenously, administered monthly with the minimum dose required to decrease white blood cell counts to less than 3000/mm^3 (measured at days 7, 14, and 28 post infusion). Dosages should be modified based on CBC nadir, hemoglobin, and serum creatinine. Prophylaxis for nausea and vomiting should be used. Oral dosing is 50–100 mg daily.

Contraindications: Hypersensitivity, severe bone marrow suppression. Cyclophosphamide is contraindicated in pregnant patients. Vaccinations should be updated prior to initiation when possible. The risks and benefits of cyclophosphamide should be discussed with all patients and their parents or legal guardians.

Main drug interactions: Enhances the adverse effects of other immunosuppressive agents and live vaccines. Allopurinol may enhance side effects.

Main side effects: Nausea, vomiting, anorexia, diarrhea, susceptibility to infection, stomatitis and mucositis, alopecia, leukopenia, anemia, thrombocytopenia, amenorrhea, and hemorrhagic cystitis. Long-term risk for bladder cancer may be mitigated by the use of mesna, vigorous hydration, and limiting the lifetime dose of cyclophosphamide to less than 100 g. Follow-up complete blood count (with differential) and urinalysis should be performed yearly, even after cessation of treatment, to monitor for hematologic or bladder malignancies.

Special points: Cyclophosphamide is a potent immunosuppressant with potentially serious adverse effects. Pregnancy screening in women of childbearing age should be done before initiation of cyclophosphamide.

DANTROLINE

Actions: Acts directly on muscle by inhibiting calcium release from sarcoplasmic reticulum causing the uncoupling of electrical excitation from contraction.

Standard dose: Start at 0.5 mg/kg once/day and increase gradually over 3–4 weeks to a target dose of 2 mg/kg 3 times/day.

Contraindications: Active hepatic disease.

Main drug interactions: Drugs with probable interaction include codeine, fentanyl, merperidine, morphine, and verapamil.

Main side effects: Liver failure, seizures, fatigue, weakness, and ataxia.

Special points: Liver function tests should be checked before starting and periodically while on treatment. Treatment may facilitate conversion of muscles to a type 2 fiber predominance, which can adversely affect weight-bearing. It may be prudent to use only in children who are expected to remain wheelchair-dependent.

FLUPHENAZINE

Actions: Dopamine D1 and D2 receptor antagonist.
Standard dose: Start at 0.5–1 mg at bedtime. Increase gradually up to 3–5 mg/day, divided 2 times daily.
Contraindication: Documented hypersensitivity (also see pimozide and haloperidol).
Main drug interactions: Caution with simultaneous use of compounds that prolonged the QT interval, cause sedation, or have an anticholinergic effect. Fluphenazine may increase serum concentrations of tricyclic antidepressants and the hypotensive action of antihypertensive agents. Concomitant lithium may cause an encephalopathy-like syndrome.
Main side effects: Extrapyramidal reactions, neuroleptic malignant syndrome, parkinsonism, tardive dyskinesia, drowsiness, restlessness, anxiety, agitation, euphoria, insomnia, confusion, weight gain, headache, seizures, tachycardia, galactorrhea, gynecomastia, hyperglycemia, hypoglycemia, sexual dysfunction, blurred vision, retinopathy, and visual disturbances.
Special points: Fluphenazine has been well tolerated and effective in treating tics. Use smallest dose and shortest duration possible; evaluate continued need periodically.

GABAPENTIN

Actions: Anticonvulsant structurally similar to gamma amino-butyric acid (GABA); has affinity for the alpha-2-(delta) sub-unit of the sodium channel.
Standard dose: Gabapentin: 50–300 mg QD-BID. Gabapentin enacarbil (extended release preparation of a gabapentin precursor with improved absorption through the GI tract): (600–1200 mg/day).
Contraindications: Hypersensitivity.
Main drug interactions: Antacids may decrease the serum concentration.
Main side effects: Sedation, dizziness, weight gain, vision changes, depression, suicidal behavior, and ideation. Potentially serious, sometimes fatal multiorgan hypersensitivity (also known as drug reaction with eosinophilia and systemic symptoms [DRESS]) has been reported with some antiepileptic drugs, including gabapentin.
Special points: Effective in restless legs syndrome and essential tremor.

GUANFACINE

Actions: Alpha-2a-adrenergic agonist in prefrontal cortex.
Standard dose: Guanfacine 1 mg should be administered at bedtime and should be increased by one-half to one tablet every 5–7 days, if necessary, to a dosage of one to three tablets given once or twice a day.

Contraindications: Hypersensitivity. Caution should be used in patients with cerebrovascular disease and cardiac, renal, or hepatic insufficiency.

Main drug interactions: May potentiate the CNS-depressive effects of alcohol, barbiturates, or other sedating drugs. Increases effect of other hypotensive agents.

Main side effects: Dizziness, drowsiness, confusion, fatigue, headache, hypotension, and mental depression. Constipation and dry mouth are common.

Special points: Less sedating and less hypotensive than clonidine. Abrupt withdrawal may cause rebound effects (increased blood pressure, headaches, and tics). Guanfacine is helpful in reducing tics and ADHD.

HALOPERIDOL

Actions: Dopamine receptor antagonist.

Standard dose: Start with 0.25–0.5 mg/day in the evening; if tolerated and symptoms warrant, can increase dose in 0.25–0.5 mg increments on weekly bases, administered once or twice a day. Total daily dose ranges from 0.75–5 mg.

Contraindications: Hypersensitive reaction to this class of medications, prolonged QT syndrome, narrow-angle glaucoma, Parkinsonism, severe cardiac or liver disease, severe CNS depression, or history of an acute extrapyramidal syndrome including acute dystonia and neuroleptic malignant syndrome.

Main drug interactions: Caution with the simultaneous use of compounds that prolonged the QT interval, cause sedation, or have an anticholinergic effect. Haloperidol may increase serum concentrations of tricyclic antidepressants and the hypotensive action of antihypertensive agents. Concomitant use of lithium may cause an encephalopathy-like syndrome. Fluoxetine may inhibit metabolism and increase the effect of haloperidol whereas rifampin or carbamazepine may reduce levels.

Main side effects: Extrapyramidal reactions, neuroleptic malignant syndrome, Parkinsonism, tardive dyskinesia, drowsiness, restlessness, anxiety, agitation, euphoria, insomnia, confusion, weight gain, headache, seizures, tachycardia, galactorrhea, gynecomastia, hyperglycemia, hypoglycemia, sexual dysfunction, lactation, gynecomastia, depression, urinary retention, blurred vision, retinopathy, and visual disturbances. Rarely causes photosensitivity reactions.

Special points: Although other typical neuroleptics tend to have a slightly better patient tolerance, haloperidol remains a useful medication for hyperkinetic movement disorders.

IVIG

Actions: Impede ability of pathological antibodies to bind to their epitope. Some effects are potentially mediated by the antigen-binding fragment (Fab) and others by the crystallizable fragment (Fc).

Standard dose: 2 g/kg administered intravenously over 1–5 days, redosing monthly as needed. Elimination half-life of IVIG is 14–24 days. Infusion should be initiated at a slow rate and increased as tolerated as per protocols. Especially on maintenance protocols 2 mg/kg may be infused in one day.

Contraindication: Hypersensitivity to IVIG, IgA deficiency with anti-IgA antibodies. Use with caution in patients with renal impairment or a history of thrombotic events.

Main drug interactions: IVIG may diminish the efficacy of live vaccines.

Main side effects: Common side effects are site pain/reaction, nausea, headache, and vasomotor symptoms. Serious complications include myocardial infarction, congestive heart failure, rash, thrombosis, aseptic meningitis, autoimmune hemolytic anemia, deep venous thrombosis, pulmonary emboli, acute respiratory distress syndrome, acute tubular necrosis, and anaphylaxis.

Special points: Risk of anaphylaxis is increased with immunoglobulin A (IgA) deficiency. Check IgA levels before initiation of therapy. Generally considered investigational for the treatment of movement disorders, although some evidence suggests IVIG may be as effective as oral prednisone in decreasing the severity of chorea in SC.

LEVETIRACETAM

Actions: Anticonvulsant; binds to SV2A, a synaptic vesicle protein.

Standard dose: Starting dose of 250–500 mg/day, divided into two daily doses, and increasing as tolerated by 250–500 mg/week. Anticonvulsant dosages in children range from 20 to 60 mg/kg/day.

Contraindications: Hypersensitivity to levetiracetam. Lower doses should be used in patients with impaired renal function.

Main drug interactions: No significant drug interactions have been identified.

Main side effects: Common side effects are somnolence, dizziness, headache, ataxia, fatigue, irritability, and emotional liability. Uncommon, but potentially serious side effects include depression and/or suicidality, psychosis, pancreatitis, and pancytopenia.

Special points: Helpful for action-induced and stimulus-induced cortical myoclonus, controversial benefit for tics.

METHYLPHENIDATE

Actions: DAT reuptake inhibitor and increases dopamine release.

Standard dose: For hypersomnia starting dose is 10 mg daily, given in two to three divided doses, 30–45 min before meals to aid absorption. Usual dose 10–60 mg/day in one to two divided doses. Relatively short duration of action (about 3–4 h). Extended-release formulation exists.

Contraindications: Avoid in patients on monoamine oxidase inhibitors due to risk of potentiating life-threatening hypertensive crisis. Structural heart defects, advanced heart disease, hyperthyroidism, or history of drug abuse.

Main drug interactions: Carbamazepine may reduce efficacy. Methylphenidate may increase serum levels of phenobarbital, primidone, phenytoin, warfarin, and SSRIs.

Main side effects: Tachycardia, hypertension, palpitations, sweating, irritability, anorexia, weight loss, tremors, seizures, and increased anxiety. At high dose may precipitate psychosis.

Special points: Schedule II restrictions. Abuse potential may be less than amphetamines. Approved for the treatment of hypersomnia because of narcolepsy.

MODAFINIL/ARMODAFINIL

Actions: CNS stimulant.

Standard dose: Armodafinil is a racemic enantiomer of modafinil with a longer half-life and once a day dosing. Armodafinil dosage is between 150 and 250 mg daily and for modafinil between 100 and 400 mg/day, the later given in two divided doses, daily. Medication is taken as early in the morning as possible, before eating.

Contraindications: Hypersensitivity.

Main drug interactions: Alters the efficacy of oral contraceptive agents.

Main side effects: Headache, nausea, rash, anxiety, depression, dry mouth, and insomnia. Should be used with caution in pregnant and breastfeeding women.

Special points: Schedule IV controlled substances. First line medication for excessive daytime sleepiness (EDS), but has limited efficacy on cataplexy and the symptoms of abnormal REM sleep.

OLANZAPINE

Actions: Atypical neuroleptic.

Standard dose: Start with 2.5 mg orally every evening, and then escalate gradually as necessary up to 5–10 mg/day in divided doses.

Contraindication: Hypersensitivity. Caution is recommended when there is concern regarding hyperglycemia and diabetes.

Main drug interactions: Use with caution in the presence of other CNS depressants because there may be an additive effect. The simultaneous use of olanzapine with dopamine agonists may decrease its therapeutic effects and olanzapine with antihypertensive medications may increase the risk of hypotension. Drugs that induce CYP1A2 or glucuronyl transferase enzymes (e.g., carbamazepine, omeprazole, and rifampin) may reduce olanzapine plasma levels. Drugs that inhibit CYP1A2 (e.g., estrogens, fluvoxamine) may elevate olanzapine plasma levels.

Main side effects: Hypotension, somnolence, weight gain, hyperglycemia, akathisia, Parkinsonism, or tardive syndromes, hyperprolactinemia, dizziness, fatigue, elevated liver enzymes, dysregulation of body temperature, neuroleptic malignant syndrome, and seizures.

Special points: Case reports and very small series have reported a beneficial effect in the treatment of tics and tardive dystonia. The risk of tardive syndromes with atypical antipsychotics is less than with traditional antipsychotics, but nevertheless exists.

PENICILLAMINE

Action: Chelator that increases the excretion of copper.

Standard dose: 20 mg/kg administered in 3 doses daily at least 1 h before or 2 h after meals. Slow dose increases to avoid neurological worsening.

Contraindications: Hypersensitivity to penicillamine; can usually be overcome by concomitant use of steroids, by lowering the dose, or by stopping the drug for a period of time.

Main drug interactions: Interacts with zinc, rendering both drugs less effective. Interferes with the action of vitamin B_6.

Main side effects: Penicillamine has a long list of side effects, including an initial hypersensitivity syndrome, subacute effects (e.g., bone marrow suppression, nephrotic syndrome, proteinuria), and chronic side effects (e.g., wrinkling, abnormal scar formation, elastosis perforans serpiginosa). Penicillamine also produces autoimmune disorders such as systemic lupus erythematosus and Goodpasture's syndrome. In animals, medication is associated with weakening of blood vessel collagen and elastin.

Special points: Associated with a high risk of developing neurological worsening in patients with Wilson's disease who present with neurological symptoms. Vitamin B_6 should be given as a 25-mg daily supplement. Penicillamine is associated with a significant list of acute, subacute, and chronic toxicities and teratogenicity.

PIMOZIDE

Actions: Dopamine receptor antagonist.

Standard dose: Start with 0.5–1 mg preferably in the evening; may be increased every 5–7 days. Usual range: 2–4 mg/day; in divided doses. Do not exceed 10 mg/day.

Contraindications: Documented hypersensitivity, history of cardiac arrhythmias, and prolonged QT syndrome. Prior history of neuroleptic malignant syndrome, tardive dyskinesia, CNS depression, or Parkinson's disease.

Main drug interactions: Use with caution in combination with QTc-prolonging agents and those with anticholinergic side effects. Increases the toxicity of monoamine oxidase inhibitors and CNS depressants. Concurrent use of macrolide antibiotics or azole antifungals increases the risk of cardiotoxicity and sudden cardiac death. Concurrent use of sertraline, paroxetine, and escitalopram, is contraindicated, since it may produce increased toxicity or attenuate therapeutic response.

Main side effects: Sedation, dysphoria, constipation, dry mouth, cognitive blunting, school refusal, acute anxiety with somatizations, personality change, weight gain, gynecomastia, or lactation, orthostatic hypotension, and blurred vision. Extrapyramidal reactions include akathisia, oculogyric crisis, drug-induced Parkinsonism, and a risk of tardive dyskinesia. Rare, but potentially serious adverse effects include cardiac arrhythmia (torsades de pointes), cardiac arrest, neutropenia, neuroleptic malignant syndrome, and seizures.

Special points: Typical dopamine receptor blocking agents have long been the mainstay of suppression of severe tics. An electrocardiogram should be done at baseline and periodically thereafter during the period of dosage adjustment. Any indication of prolongation of a corrected QT interval beyond 0.45 s (children) or 0.52 s (adults) should be considered a basis for stopping additional dosage increases and for considering a lower dosage. Monitor regularly for extrapyramidal side effects. Avoid the consumption of grapefruit juice with pimozide. Sudden unexplained deaths have occurred in patients taking high doses (>10 mg). To decrease the risk of tardive dyskinesia, use the smallest dose and shortest duration possible; periodically, evaluate continued need for medication.

PIRACETAM

Actions: Nootropic agent, mechanism of action in the treatment of myoclonus is not known.

Standard dose: Substantial variation in dosage requirements. Start with a dosage of 7.2 g/day (divided into two or three daily doses), and increase by 4.8 g/day every 3–4 days to the usual effective dose of 4.8–24 g/day.

Contraindications: Severe renal insufficiency or hepatic impairment. It is not recommended for use in children less than 16 years of age or in pregnant women. Avoid abrupt discontinuation, which may trigger withdrawal seizures.

Main drug interactions: Increases the serum levels of warfarin, thyroid hormone, and CNS stimulants.

Main side effects: Hyperkinesias, insomnia, weight gain, nervousness, diarrhea, and rash. May cause reversible thrombocytopenia and leukopenia. Do not discontinue abruptly, since may precipitate seizures.

Special points: Not currently approved by the United States Food and Drug Administration. Used for cortical myoclonus.

PRAMIPEXOLE

Actions: Non-ergot selective D2 and D3 dopamine agonist.

Standard dose: Titration is required to avoid side effects; start at 0.125 mg, titrate up by 0.125 mg every 3 days to efficacy. Most studies show improvement in symptoms in a dose range of 0.125–1.5 mg/day. Medication should be slowly tapered.

Contraindication: Hypersensitivity.

Main drug interactions: Antipsychotics may diminish the therapeutic effect. Decreased clearance of pramipexole may occur with cimetidine, ranitidine, verapamil, and quinine. If an atypical neuroleptic is required, consider quetiapine or clozapine because of lowered interaction.

Main side effects: Nausea, vomiting, abdominal pain, headache, fluid retention, dizziness, rhinitis, dyspnea, rash, daytime sleepiness, sleep attacks, insomnia, hallucinations, and orthostatic hypotension. Potential risk of heart failure.

Special points: Pramipexole has been shown to be effective in RLS symptoms and PLMS.

PREDNISONE AND METHYLPREDNISOLONE

Actions: Anti-inflammatory agents.

Standard dose: Prednisone: 1–2 mg/kg/day in children. Methylprednisolone: intravenous, 25–30 mg/kg/day (children; maximum daily dose of 1000 mg) for 3–5 days.

Contraindications: Hypersensitivity; systemic fungal infection.

Main drug interactions: Barbiturates and phenytoin may decrease the therapeutic effect of prednisolone. The concomitant use of corticosteroids and anticoagulants has been associated with both enhanced and diminished anticoagulant effects. Fluroroquinolones may increase the risk of tendon rupture.

Main side effects: The most common include changes in appetite and behavior, irritability, and difficulty sleeping. Potentially serious side effects are hypertension, impaired skin healing, fluid retention, hyperglycemia, hypernatremia, increased risk for infection, gastrointestinal ulceration, weight gain, nervousness, steroid psychosis, and depression. Other long-term issues include Cushing's syndrome, adrenocorticoid insufficiency, cataract, glaucoma, osteoporosis, avascular necrosis, and obesity. Patients should receive GI prophylaxis with an antacid and blood pressure and glucose should be monitored.

Special points: Trials in Sydenham's chorea have suggested steroid accelerated recovery, but no change in rate of remission or recurrence. Prednisone is generally reserved for patients with persistent, disabling chorea refractory to antichoreic agents.

PREGABALIN

Actions: Antiepileptic medication, isomer to gabapentin; has affinity for the alpha-2-(delta) subunit of the sodium channel.

Standard dose: 150–600 mg/day. Safety and efficacy in pediatric patients has not been established.

Contraindications: Hypersensitivity to pregabalin.

Main drug interactions: Reduced anticonvulsant effectiveness of ketorolac and orlistat.

Main side effects: Dizziness, weight gain, peripheral edema.

Special points: Helpful in essential tremor and restless legs syndrome.

PRIMIDONE

Actions: Anticonvulsant effects may be due to an alteration of transmembrane calcium and sodium ion fluxes. Primidone has little effect on gamma-aminobutyric acid (GABA) or glutamate receptors.

Standard dose: Start with 25–50 mg by mouth at night and gradually increase to 125–250 mg at night, if necessary.

Contraindications: Hypersensitivity to barbiturates, porphyria. Caution in patients with impaired hepatic, renal, and pulmonary function.

Main drug interactions: Anticoagulants, corticosteroids, doxycycline, phenytoin, carbamazepine, valproic acid, acetazolamide, central nervous system depressants, monoamine oxidase inhibitors, estrogen and progesterone, isoniazid, haloperidol, cyclosporine, theophylline, tricyclic antidepressants. Phenobarbital, a metabolite of primidone has been shown to decrease the anticoagulant effects of warfarin.

Main side effects: Drowsiness, fatigue, lethargy, somnolence, ataxia, dizziness, nausea, vomiting, cognitive dulling, confusion, hyperirritability, emotional disturbances, impotence, diplopia, nystagmus, weakness, granulocytopenia, red cell hypoplasia, and Stevens–Johnson syndrome.

Special points: Helpful for action-induced and stimulus-induced cortical myoclonus and tremor. Primidone metabolizes into two major compounds, phenylethylmalonamide and phenobarbital, however, serum concentrations of metabolites do not correlate with improvement.

PROPRANOLOL

Actions: Nonselective beta-adrenergic receptor antagonist.

Standard dose: Available as immediate release or long-acting preparation. Children, 1–2 mg/kg/day; adults, 80–320 mg by mouth per day, taken in three divided doses. Propranolol LA 60–320 mg by mouth per day.

Contraindications: Hypersensitivity to β-blockers, sinus bradycardia, second- or third-degree heart block, congestive heart failure, cardiac failure, bronchial asthma, severe chronic obstructive pulmonary disease, and insulin-dependent diabetes mellitus.

Main drug interactions: Blood levels and/or toxicity of propranolol may be increased by co-administration with substrates or inhibitors of CYP2D6, CYP1A2, and CYP2C19. Blood levels of propranolol may be decreased by co-administration with inducers such as rifampin, ethanol, phenytoin, and phenobarbital. Propranolol can inhibit the metabolism of diazepam, resulting in increased concentrations of diazepam and its metabolites.

Main side effects: Nonspecific weakness and fatigue. Other potential adverse reactions include weight gain, nausea, irritability, insomnia, vivid dreams, diarrhea, bradycardia, dizziness, headache, rash, impotence, depression, sexual dysfunction, and hypotension.

Special points: Received "effective" (Level A recommendation from the AAN practice guideline for treatment of essential tremor). β-2 blockade appears necessary for maximal tremor suppression. Propranolol is most effective against hand tremor. An extended-release formulation may provide satisfactory relief with once-daily dosing.

QUETIAPINE

Actions: Atypical antipsychotic, dopamine D2, D3 receptor antagonist, has mild anti-muscarinic, anti-serotoninergic, anti-adrenergic, and anti-histaminergic effects, and no effect on the D1 receptor.

Standard dose: 75–500 mg/day, average 360 mg/day in adults.

Contraindication: Avoid in combination with drugs that increase the QT interval. Use with caution in patients with congestive heart failure.

Main drug interactions: Worsen drowsiness associated with dopamine agonists, diphenhydramine hydrochloride, and sleep medications.

Main side effects: Sedation, dizziness, dry mouth, constipation, weight gain, worsening of Parkinson's disease, induction of diabetes, stroke, and heart attacks.

Special points: Better safety profile than other atypical neuroleptics. A high dose (up to 600 mg/day), but not a low dose (25 mg/day), improves levodopa-induced dyskinesia.

RESERPINE

Actions: Catecholamine-depleting drug.

Standard dose: Start at a low dosage 0.25 mg/day and increase by 0.25 mg/day every few days according to clinical response and tolerability. Reserpine can be given in dosages of 1–9 mg/day in divided doses.

Contraindications: Depression, Parkinson's disease, orthostatic hypotension, and pregnancy. Should not be used concurrently with monoamine oxidase inhibitors.

Main drug interactions: Caution with concomitant use of drugs that lower blood pressure or have an additive effect on somnolence and depression.

Main side effects: Sedation, orthostatic hypotension, depression, drug-induced Parkinsonism, insomnia, anxiety, akathisia, cardiac arrhythmia, and impotence.

Special points: Usually reserved for patients with severe tardive dystonia and hemiballismus that is unresponsive to other treatments.

RISPERIDONE

Actions: Atypical antipsychotic.

Standard dose: Begin with 0.25 or 0.5 mg in the evening and gradually titrate up to 2–4 mg/day divided twice daily.

Contraindication: Hypersensitivity. Known history of QT prolongation or concomitant use of other drugs known to prolong QT interval. Caution is recommended when there is concern regarding hyperglycemia and diabetes.

Main drug interactions: Beware of an additive effect with other CNS depressants or drugs that prolong the QT interval. Fluoxetine and paroxetine may increase the serum concentration of risperidone and decrease concentrations of 9-hydroxyrisperidone. Carbamazepine and similar enzyme inducers (e.g., phenytoin, rifampin, and phenobarbital) may decrease plasma concentrations. Dopamine agonists may decrease therapeutic effects.

Main side effects: Hypotension, somnolence, fatigue, weight gain, hyperglycemia, akathisia, Parkinsonism, or tardive syndromes, hyperprolactinemia, dysregulation of body temperature, neuroleptic malignant syndrome, tremor, drooling, headache, and seizures.

Special points: Use smallest dose and shortest duration possible and monitor regularly for extrapyramidal side effects. Risperidone is effective in reducing tics in children and adults.

RITUXIMAB

Actions: Rituximab is a monoclonal IgG targeting the CD20 surface antigen of B lymphocytes; eliminates B lymphocytes prior to differentiation to plasma cells.

Standard dose: Rituximab should be administered at a dose of 375–750 mg/m^2 once weekly for a period of 4 weeks. Alternatively, it can be administered at 1000 mg once, followed by a further 1000 mg dose 2 weeks later. Infusion should be started slowly and advanced according to protocol. Due to the allergic risk, patient should be pre-medicated with acetaminophen and diphenhydramine.

Contraindications: Patients who have had progressive multifocal leukoencephalopathy, hepatitis B, or are pregnant.

Main drug interactions: Rituximab may enhance the toxic/adverse effects of other immunosuppressants, and may reduce the efficacy of live vaccines.

Main side effects: Infusion reactions (hypotension, angioedema, bronchospasms, urticarial, anaphylaxis), edema, hypertension, fever, fatigue, chills, headache, insomnia, rash, pruritus, nausea, diarrhea, weight gain, cytopenias, neutropenic fever, increased liver enzymes, weakness, arthralgias, cough, rhinitis, epistaxis, reactivation of hepatitis B.

Special points: Originally developed as a treatment for B-cell lymphoma, it is effective in antibody mediated disorders. Patients who have high risk for hepatitis B infection should be screened before treatment. Screening for tuberculosis should also occur before treatment.

ROPINIROLE

Actions: Non-ergot selective D_2 and D_3 agonist.

Standard dose: Titration is required to avoid side effects; start at 0.25 mg taken 2 h before bed, titrate up by 0.25 mg every 3 days to efficacy. Effective dose range is 0.5–4.6 mg/day. An additional dose 1–2 h before symptom onset can be taken (i.e., at 4–6 pm).

Contraindication: Hypersensitivity.

Main drug interactions: Drugs that affect cytochrome P1A2 may interfere with the metabolism of ropinirole. Estrogen reduces the clearance of ropinirole. Antipsychotics may diminish the therapeutic effect. Decreased clearance of ropinirole may occur with cimetidine, ranitidine, verapamil, and quinine.

Main side effects: Nausea, vomiting, abdominal pain, headache, fluid retention, dizziness, somnolence, rhinitis, dyspnea, rash, daytime sleepiness, insomnia, hallucinations, depression, and orthostatic hypotension.

Special points: Used for the control of RLS symptoms and PLMS.

SODIUM OXYBATE

Actions: Sodium salt of gamma-hydroxybutyrate (GHB). Central actions may be mediated via GHB receptors, agonist effect on $GABA_B$ receptors, or through its metabolite GABA.

Standard dose: Dosing range is between 3 and 9 g every evening given in divided doses; first dose at bedtime and second dose 2–4 h later. The serum half-life of sodium oxybate is very short and twice-per-night dosing usually is required. Food should not be taken within 2 h of taking the drug.

Contraindications: Succinic semialdehyde dehydrogenase deficiency, and use of sedative/hypnotic agents, CNS depressants, and alcohol. Caution in patients with a history of psychiatric disorders or drug abuse. Central and obstructive sleep apnea syndromes should be identified and treated prior to initiating this medication. Avoid in alcoholics.

Main drug interactions: Additive effects on central nervous system depressants, e.g., all benzodiazepines, barbiturates, and sedative hypnotics.

Main side effects: Headache, nausea/vomiting, dizziness, somnolence, tremor, sleep walking, dissociative feelings, enuresis, constipation, and suicidal gesture. An unpleasant taste can be masked by mixing the solution with flavored water, but not juice which may reduce medication efficacy. Sodium overload is a concern with coexisting renal and cardiovascular diseases.

Special points: Sodium oxybate is a schedule III controlled substance beneficial for narcolepsy, excessive daytime sleepiness (EDS), sleep fragmentation, and cataplexy. First choice, if the patient is having both EDS and cataplexy. Because of its euphorigenic, amnestic, and behavioral disinhibitive properties, GHB has a high potential for misuse/abuse. One should avoid alcohol and have a regular sleep–wake cycle. Prescription requires registration and training and is only available through a centralized pharmacy.

TETRABENAZINE

Actions: Presynaptic monoamine-depleting drug that also acts as a postsynaptic dopamine receptor blocker and dopamine reuptake inhibitor.

Standard dose: Start with 12.5 mg daily, and increase by 12.5 mg/day every 3–5 days according to clinical response and as tolerated, divided into three daily doses. The usual effective dose is 50–150 mg/day and the maximum recommended dose is 200 mg/day.

Contraindications: Patients with a history of depression, suicidality, Parkinsonism, and hepatic function impairment. Discontinue promptly at the first signs of depression. Do not initiate treatment within 14 days of use of monoamine oxidase inhibitors (risk of hypertensive crisis).

Main drug interactions: Potentiates the systemic and neurologic effects of other amine depletors (reserpine and alpha-methylparatyrosine) and dopamine antagonists. Concomitant treatment with fluoxetine and paroxetine requires the reduction of tetrabenazine dose. Tricyclic antidepressants may accentuate adverse effects. Central excitation and hypertension have been reported when tetrabenazine was added to existing therapy with desipramine or MAO inhibitors.

Main side effects: Common side effects include Parkinsonism, drowsiness, fatigue, sedation, anxiety, depression, akathisia, tremor, nausea, vomiting, insomnia, and orthostatic hypotension. Less common but potentially serious side effects include suicidality and neuroleptic malignant syndrome.

Special points: US FDA approved for the treatment of chorea in patients with Huntington's disease. Reports suggest it may also be helpful in the treatment of tics, tardive dystonia, hemiballismus, and subcortical myoclonus.

TETRATHIOMOLYBDATE (TM)

Actions: Forms a tripartite complex with copper and protein; given with food, it prevents the absorption of copper and given between meals, is absorbed into the blood and complexes blood copper with albumin, rendering the copper nontoxic.

Standard dose: 20 mg 6 times daily, 3 times with meals and 3 times separated from meals.

Contraindications: None.

Main drug interactions: None.

Main side effects: Reversible anemia.

Special points: TM is experimental and not commercially available. TM is often combined with zinc for patients with Wilson's disease presenting with neurological symptoms. Combination of TM and zinc is used for approximately 8 weeks and then the patient is continued on zinc for maintenance therapy.

TIZANIDINE

Actions: A centrally acting alpha-2 adrenergic stimulant that reduces polysynaptic spinal stretch reflexes.

Standard dose: No established dosage in children, but 0.1–0.3 mg/kg/day is sometimes used.

Contraindications: Hypersensitivity or concurrent use of ciprofloxacin or fluvoxamine.

Main drug interactions: Avoid other anticholinergic or sedating medications.

Main side effects: Common side effects include somnolence, dry mouth, dizziness, increased liver transaminases, vomiting, and flu-like symptoms. More serious side effects include hepatotoxicity, bradycardia, hypotension, hypertension, and confusion. There is an increased risk of prolonged QT interval, especially when used in combination with other medications that are known to affect the QT interval.

Special points: Not extensively studied in children.

TOPIRAMATE

Actions: Anticonvulsant; multiple mechanisms of action including inhibiting voltage-gated sodium channels, augmenting the inhibitory chloride ion influx mediated by GABA, increasing endogenous GABA production, modestly inhibiting carbonic anhydrase activity, and antagonizing the AMPA/kainate subtype of the glutamate receptor.

Standard dose: Start with a dose of 25 mg/day, gradually increasing until benefit or side effects. The usual effective dose is 50–300 mg/day, given in divided doses. (Children, 5–9 mg/kg/day.) The maximum recommended dose is 400 mg/day. Titrate slowly.

Contraindications: Use lower doses in renal impairment. Monitor serum bicarbonate levels.

Main drug interactions: May decrease the efficacy of estrogen-based oral contraceptives. Concomitant use with phenytoin may increase the levels of phenytoin and decrease the levels of topiramate. Combined use with other carbonic anhydrase inhibitors (such as acetazolamide) may increase the risk of nephrolithiasis.

Main side effects: Confusion, cognitive impairment, paresthesias, altered taste, ataxia, diplopia, somnolence, dizziness, fatigue, depression, nervousness, ciliary edema, and weight loss. Uncommon but potentially serious side effects include nephrolithiasis, metabolic acidosis, oligohidrosis, hyperthermia, and acute angle closure glaucoma. May require monitoring of kidney function.

Special points: Second-line agent for the treatment of cortical myoclonus and essential tremor.

TRIENTINE

Actions: Chelator that increases the excretion of copper.

Standard dose: 250 mg 4 times a day at least 1 h before or 2 h after meals.

Contraindication: None.

Main drug interactions: Interacts with zinc, rendering both drugs less effective.

Main side effects: Gastritis, sideroblastic anemia, proteinuria and autoimmune disorders such as systemic lupus erythematosus and Goodpasture's syndrome.

Special points: Used in Wilson's disease to establish a more rapid negative copper balance and to reduce the body's copper burden relatively quickly. Trientine is often combined with zinc for patients presenting with hepatic disease and continued for approximately 4 months, followed by maintenance therapy with zinc alone. Trientine is moderately toxic and neurological deterioration has been reported, but may be safer than penicillamine. Has known teratogenicity.

TRIHEXYPHENIDYL

Actions: Centrally acting anticholinergic.

Standard dose: Start at a low dosage of 0.5–1 mg/day and increase gradually by 1 mg every 3–5 days, until benefit or adverse effects. Usually administered in three divided doses. The usual effective dosage is highly variable ranging from 6 to 60 mg/day, but some patients require higher dosages.

Contraindications: Narrow-angle glaucoma, severe constipation, gastroparesis, pyloric or duodenal obstruction, achalasia, urinary retention, myasthenia gravis, confusion, and dementia.

Main drug interactions: Use with caution in patients taking other drugs with anticholinergic activity, such as antihistamines, tricyclic antidepressants, or amantadine, since these may cause increased confusion or side effects. Reduces plasma levels of antipsychotic medications.

Main side effects: Dry mouth, dry eyes, sedation, pupil dilatation, blurred vision, nausea, constipation, urinary hesitancy or retention, fatigue, confusion, hallucinations, weakness, tachycardia, increased intraocular pressure, precipitation of narrow angle glaucoma, impaired concentration and memory, delirium, and anhidrosis with susceptibility to hyperthermia. Other side effects may include dizziness, nausea, vomiting, and anxiety. Patients may develop tolerance to these effects with continued low-dose treatment.

Special points: Trihexyphenidyl, may be more effective and better tolerated in children than adults. No evidence that trihexyphenidyl is superior to benztropine. Increase dosage very slowly to avoid side effects; relatively low doses may be helpful. Anticholinergics may exacerbate tardive dyskinesias and chorea, but have been helpful for tardive dystonia. Rapid taper can cause malignant hyperthermia, worsening dystonia, or cholinergic symptoms. Not highly recommended in Segawa's disease because levodopa therapy actually replaces the primary deficiency. Anticholinergic drugs should be discontinued gradually.

VALPROIC ACID

Actions: Anticonvulsant; mechanism includes modulation of sodium channels and potentiating GABAergic transmission.

Standard dose: Start with 125 mg twice daily and gradually titrate as tolerated. Antimyoclonic doses in children are typically in the range of 15–25 mg/kg/day, given in three divided doses.

Contraindications: Hepatic dysfunction, urea cycle disorders, and children younger than 2 years of age.

Main drug interactions: Increases levels of lamotrigine, carbamazepine, phenobarbital, primidone, amitriptyline, warfarin levels and decreases levels of rifampin. Valproate level decreases with hepatic enzyme-inducing AEDs (carbamazepine, phenytoin, phenobarbital). Cimetidine may increase the serum levels of valproic acid. A significant reduction in serum valproic acid concentration has been reported in patients receiving carbapenem antibiotics (e.g., ertapenem, imipenem, meropenem).

Main side effects: Common side effects include nausea, vomiting, diarrhea, weight gain, drowsiness, fatigue, peripheral edema, tremor (postural and action), ataxia, hyperammonemia, nystagmus, depression, alopecia, and livedo reticularis. Uncommon, but serious side effects include hepatic injury, pancreatitis, rashes (Stevens–Johnson syndrome), anaphylaxis, bone marrow suppression, and polycystic ovary disease. Reversible Parkinsonism has also been reported.

Special points: Liver function tests should be monitored closely. Valproate has been used in Sydenham's chorea and may be helpful for action and stimulus-induced cortical myoclonus. Avoid use of sodium valproate in women of childbearing age to prevent teratogenesis.

ZINC

Actions: Induces metallothionein, which in the intestinal cell blocks absorption of copper. Hepatic metallothionein will also sequester some potentially toxic copper in the liver and possibly protect it from further damage.

Standard dose: For children younger than 6 years of age dose is 25 mg twice daily and for children between the ages of 6 and 16, or with a body weight of 125 pounds or less, 25 mg 3 times daily. Administer more than 30 min before a meal.

Contraindication: None.

Main drug interactions: Interacts with either trientine or penicillamine during maintenance therapy; penicillamine is partially occupied by zinc, as is trientine.

Main side effects: Gastric irritation, mitigated by taking the first dose of the day in mid-morning or taking with a small amount of protein.

Special points: Zinc is often combined with trientine for patients with Wilson's disease presenting with hepatic disease and with tetrathiomolybdate for treatment of the patient presenting with neurological disease. However, beyond the initial treatment period, combination of more than one anti-copper drug is not recommended. Zinc does not have the propensity to cause the neurological worsening that can occur with penicillamine.

Anti-copper agents control only copper and its toxicity and have no immediate direct effect on symptoms.

ZIPRASIDONE

Actions: Atypical neuroleptic.

Standard dose: Start with 20 mg orally every evening, and then titrate as necessary. Effective dose is usually 20–40 mg daily but may increase as high as 100 mg.

Contraindications: Hypersensitivity. Known history of QT prolongation or concomitant use of other drugs known to cause torsades de pointes or prolong QT interval. Caution is recommended when there is concern regarding hyperglycemia, orthostatic hypotension, and diabetes.

Main drug interactions: Beware of an additive effect on prolongation of the QT interval with concomitant use of other anti-psychotic agents. Ziprasidone may enhance the effects of certain antihypertensive agents. CYP-450-3A4 inhibitors, such as erythromycin and ketoconazole, may increase serum levels; CYP-450-3A4 inducers, such as carbamazepine and rifampin, may decrease serum levels. Drugs that prolong QT/QTc intervals increase the risk of life-threatening arrhythmias.

Main side effects: Hypotension, somnolence, weight gain, dizziness, hyperglycemia, akathisia, Parkinsonism, tardive syndromes, hyperprolactinemia, insomnia, dysregulation of body temperature, neuroleptic malignant syndrome, anxiety, and seizures. Ziprasidone causes more prolongation of the QT interval than risperidone, olanzapine, or haloperidol.

Special points: A baseline electrocardiogram is recommended. Monitor patient regularly for extrapyramidal side effects. A placebo-controlled study has shown that ziprasidone may be beneficial in reducing tics.

ZONISAMIDE

Actions: Anticonvulsant; mechanism of action involves blockade of sodium and/or calcium channels.

Standard dose: Start with a dose of 25 mg by mouth twice a day, and gradually increase as tolerated to a usual effective dosage of 300–400 mg/day, given in divided doses.

Contraindications: Zonisamide is a sulfonamide and is contraindicated in the presence of an allergy to sulfa. Titrate slowly in renal disease.

Main drug interactions: The serum levels of zonisamide are decreased by hepatic enzyme-inducing drugs (phenobarbital, carbamazepine, oxcarbazepine, phenytoin, and rifampin) and increased by enzyme-inhibiting drugs (erythromycin, fluvoxamine, protease inhibitors).

Main side effects: Drowsiness, dizziness, ataxia, confusion, cognitive symptoms, depression, headache, anorexia, nausea, vomiting, abdominal pain, and weight loss. Uncommon but potentially serious side effects include Stevens–Johnson syndrome, hepatic necrosis, agranulocytosis, aplastic anemia, psychosis, suicidality, nephrolithiasis, oligohidrosis, and hyperthermia.

Special points: Second-line drug for myoclonus of subcortical or unknown origin. Conflicting results for the treatment of essential tremor.

Appendix B: Search Strategy for Genetic Movement Disorders

Making a precise genetic, molecular diagnosis provides substantial value to families, even if there is no disease-specific treatment. A specific diagnosis narrows the horizon of prognostic possibility, helps individuals and families to identify and network with other similarly affected persons, and, in some cases, provides a rationale for disease-specific therapies. In diseases with incomplete penetrance or anticipation, it can also clarify risks and provide useful information for relatives of the affected individual.

Because the molecular genetic causes of movement disorders and the complexity of genotype–phenotype relationships are ever-expanding, an efficient online search strategy is essential for neurologists. As discussed throughout this book, careful history of present illness, three-generation family history, and characterization of movement disorder phenomenology are vital. Not uncommonly, a finding outside of the nervous system, e.g., splenomegaly, may substantially narrow the differential diagnosis. A variety of online sites and search strategies may be used to arrive at a diagnosis more expeditiously. Two, OMIM and Simulconsult, will be discussed in this Appendix. Resources to use after the search will also be discussed.

USING OMIM TO AID IN DIAGNOSIS

The database Online Mendelian Inheritance in Man (OMIM), available at http://www.omim.org/, is an online catalog of human genes and phenotypes. This resource is provided without a user-fee and is intended for use primarily by physicians, other professionals, and researchers concerned with genetics. It is updated daily, and a table of entry statistics can be found at http://omim.org/statistics/entry. For example, in March 2015, there were 22,817 entries. These included 14,850 gene descriptions (autosomal 14,078, X-Linked 689, Y-Linked 48, and mitochondrial 35). There were 4368 entries with "phenotype description where the molecular basis is known" (4046 autosomal, 290 X-linked, 4 Y-linked, 28 mitochondrial). Each number serves as a link to that gene list, and lists can be downloaded into spreadsheets. There are also entries for "phenotype description or locus, molecular basis unknown" and for "phenotypes with suspected Mendelian basis."

OMIM can be used as a diagnostic search engine when faced with a difficult diagnosis. OMIM can be searched using any term or "phrase" in quotations, and multiple terms can be combined with *and*, *or*, or *not*. Helpful advice is provided on the main page including example searches and a link to a tutorial. Using a single movement disorder phenomenology as a search term generates hundreds of entries. Adding *and (another key feature)* narrows the number of possibilities.

To make this a practical clinical tool, it is worth taking a few actual patient diagnoses where the molecular basis is known and exploring the three types of available advanced OMIM searches in turn: OMIM, Clinical Synopses, and Gene Map. To do this, we will work through three examples of actual patients who presented with particular symptoms and signs. The point of the exercise is to use OMIM to generate a differential diagnosis in hopes of determining the molecular basis for the disease. There are many search options, but these searches will be fairly simple and straightforward.

EXAMPLE 1 ADVANCED SEARCH: OMIM

Case description: 11-year-old female with a 6-year history of progressive tremor, gait ataxia, and loss of cognitive skills. Family history is negative. Neurological examination is notable for psychomotor slowing, vertical gaze palsy, dysarthria, limb tremor and dysmetria, and gait ataxia. General examination is notable for questionable splenomegaly. Brain MRI shows diffuse cerebellar and, to a lesser extent, cerebral atrophy. One approach would be to order in stepwise fashion a microarray, an ataxia gene panel, and then if necessary whole exome sequencing. However, there is enough clinical data to support a more targeted, less expensive testing approach.

Steps for the Advanced Search OMIM

1. Search for OMIM in any web browser and select link to OMIM.org.
2. Select Advanced Search: OMIM.
3. Type at least two features in the search box. Because ataxia is a useful broad category and vertical gaze palsy is fairly specific, a useful choice would be to type *ataxia and "vertical gaze palsy."* Other findings, including *splenomegaly*, also work well to narrow differential diagnoses.
4. By clicking/selecting other boxes, restrict the search if desired (these are optional)
   a. Choose any special areas to search in, such as "Title" (can be helpful if *ataxia* alone is the search term, but not when searching with several symptoms or signs).
   b. Choose whether to restrict the search to certain types of records, e.g., only those with a clinical synopsis (helpful because the results will all have a phenotype description).
   c. Choose a MIM number prefix. For example select "# phenotype description, molecular basis known" (helpful because the results should be diseases that have links to genetic testing).
   d. Restrict the search to a chromosome or other pattern of inheritance (can be useful if pedigree suggests specific inheritance pattern, e.g., mitochondrial).
5. Click on the search box, which generates the results—*ataxia and "vertical gaze palsy"* restricted to "# phenotype description, molecular basis known" yields a list of three diagnoses (in 2015). In this case, the #1 diagnosis is #257220 Niemann–Pick Disease, Type C; #256000 Leigh Syndrome; #605899 Glycine Encephalopathy. These are listed with their cytogenetic location(s). Review the list.

TABLE B.1 OMIM Search for Example 1—Clinical Synopsis result for Niemann–Pick Disease, Type C1; NPC1

Clinical synopsis item	Information displayed as popup (partial list)
Inheritance	Autosomal recessive
Head and Neck	Vertical supranuclear gaze palsy
Abdomen	Hepatomegaly, Splenomegaly
Neurologic	Hypotonia, Developmental delay, Dysarthria, Dementia, Spasticity, Dystonia, Seizures, Cerebellar ataxia, Neuronal loss—particularly of Purkinje cells, Behavioral problems
Laboratory abnormalities	Normal or mildly reduced sphingomyelinase activity, foam cells in visceral organs and CNS
Miscellaneous	Genetic heterogeneity (see NPC2, 607625), Disease usually becomes apparent in early childhood, death usually in teenage years. Four major age groups: early infantile, late infantile, juvenile, adult), Incidence 1 in 150,000 live births in the general population. Estimated carrier frequency of 10–25% in Yarmouth County, Nova Scotia—variant type D is considered a genetic isolate,
Molecular basis	Caused by mutation in the NPC1 gene (NPC1, 607623.0001)

6. Click on the Clinical Synopsis box. The disease list now contains additional information by system, which the searcher can access two ways:
   a. Placing the cursor over each item creates a popup screen. This makes it easy to quickly focus in on key elements that may differentiate the diagnoses on the result list.
   b. Click on the disease name—this links to a table containing all of the clinical synopsis information organized by systems.

In the case of NPC1 for example the following information (excerpted) is available in the popups and table (Table B.1):

7. Use the clinical synopses information to narrow the differential diagnosis. There are often links within this section to help the clinician incorporate key features of the physical examination. For example, if a feature like "clinodactyly" may be present, there will be a link from that term directly to a picture and the clinical description of that term on the National Human Genome Research Institute morphology page http:// elementsofmorphology.nih.gov/

8. Each reasonable possibility may now be investigated further as discussed later. This patient's diagnosis was NPC1.

EXAMPLE 2 ADVANCED SEARCH: CLINICAL SYNOPSIS

Case description: 7-year-old female presents for a second opinion after extensive investigation elsewhere, with history of progressive "balance problems" and unusual eye movements.

Three generation family history is negative. Neurological examination reveals slow, impaired initiation of horizontal saccades and subtle nystagmus, intention tremor, chorea, dystonic posturing, gait ataxia. General examination reveals short stature. Brain MRI shows diffuse mild cerebellar atrophy. One approach would be to order in stepwise fashion a metabolic screening, microarray, an ataxia gene panel, and then if necessary whole exome sequencing. However, there is enough clinical data to support a more targeted testing approach.

Steps for the Advanced Search Clinical Synopsis

1. Search for OMIM in web browser and select link to OMIM.org.
2. Select Advanced Search: Clinical Synopsis. This will provide results that have a phenotype with clinical synopsis.
3. Type at least two features in the search box. Because ataxia is a useful broad category and the oculomotor problems are less so, a useful choice might be to type *ataxia and oculomotor*.
4. Restrict the search if desired to entries that have specific systems in the clinical synopsis (these are optional)
   a. Choose *Inheritance* to limit to entries where an inheritance pattern is specified.
   b. Choose *Growth* if the short stature in the example is considered a potentially important feature.
   c. Choose *Molecular basis* to limit results to those for which the molecular basis is known and for which genetic testing may be available.
5. Click on the search box, which generates the results—*ataxia and oculomotor* with boxes checked for *Inheritance*, *Growth*, and *Molecular basis* yields a list of six diagnosis (in 2015). These are listed with their clinical synopsis features. In this case, the #1 diagnosis is #208900 Ataxia-Telangiectasia; AT. Review the list.
6. Note that some diagnoses from a short list may be clearly incorrect or extremely unlikely. For example, this search generated #612716 Dystonia, dopa-responsive, due to sepiapterin reductase deficiency. For other possibilities, placing the cursor over the systems and comparing these findings to the patient's may narrow the differential diagnosis.
7. The Laboratory Abnormalities link may be especially helpful. For example, for the first diagnosis, AT, the first item in Laboratory Abnormalities is "elevated alpha fetoprotein." Reviewing the laboratory abnormalities across items in the differential diagnosis can aid in selection of further tests which are generally less expensive than genetic tests, to narrow the differential diagnosis.
8. Each reasonable possibility may now be investigated further as discussed later.

The next step in this patient's diagnostic evaluation was serum AFP, which was markedly elevated, consistent in this clinical setting with a diagnosis of AT.

Note—this search was somewhat contrived. The actual diagnosis was strongly suspected based on clinical experience and pattern recognition and made without an OMIM search. In fact, in this case, combining many pairs of symptoms through a large number of possible OMIM searches result in diagnosis lists that miss AT. So it is worth here pointing out several potential pitfalls of OMIM searches.

1. A single search term like *ataxia* has very high sensitivity but leads to too many results to investigate.
2. A search with two or more terms has higher specificity and reduces the number of results, but this short list may not contain the actual diagnosis if the wording differs from the wording used in OMIM. For example:
   a. The search *ataxia* and *chorea* yields a diagnosis list that includes Ataxia-Telangiectasia-Like Disorder (ATLD1) but not AT. The same result (not AT) occurs with *ataxia* and "oculomotor apraxia."
   b. The search *ataxia* and *choreoathetosis* yields a diagnosis list that includes AT, but not ATLD1.
3. The location of certain findings within the clinical synopsis may be unexpected. For example, as seen in the prior example, for the entry Niemann–Pick Disease Type 1 (NPC1), "vertical supranuclear gaze palsy" is listed under the synopsis system "Head & Neck." In this case, no oculomotor control problems are listed under the system "Neurologic."

EXAMPLE 3 ADVANCED SEARCH: GENE MAP ADVANCED SEARCH

Case description: 30-month-old female presents for evaluation of mild global developmental delay, poor walking and balance, and with microarray results showing a large chromosome 10q26 deletion. Three generation family history is negative. Neurological examination reveals normal oculomotor function, normal tone and reflexes, normal-range hand coordination with no limb dysmetria but very mild intention tremor. Vibratory and light touch sense seems normal (difficult). Gait is broad based and lurching, with irregular rate, high stepping, and frequent falls. Brain MRI shows subtle vermian atrophy/hypotrophy.

Steps for the Advanced Search Gene Map

1. Search for OMIM in web browser and select link to OMIM.org. Select Advanced Search: Gene Map. This goes to a search page with instructions on syntax. The page also provides some additional options to narrow the search and explains which Genome Reference Consortium source is used (e.g., GRCh37) from http://www.ncbi.nlm.nih.gov/projects/genome/assembly/grc/.
2. Following the recommended syntax, type the chromosome, colon, and lower boundary of the deletion (provided in the test result document) in the search box, i.e., from this case one would type: "10:128,000,000"
3. Restrict the search by selecting the box for "Phenotype exists."
4. Click on the search box, which generates the results—in this case (2015) one condition: %166760 Otitis Media, Susceptibility To.
5. As this is not helpful, there are several choices to move forward.
   a. Return to the main OMIM search page and type in *chromosome 10q26 deletion syndrome*. This yields over 3000 results but those with the closest cytogenetic location are listed first, including the entry "#609625 chromosome 10q26 deletion syndrome." Clinical

synopsis can be selected, as above, to aid in determining the similarity between the patient and the described findings in this contiguous gene deletion syndrome.

b. Repeat the Gene Map search with "10:128,000,000"but without selecting "Phenotype exists." This yields 25 entries, with the previously mentioned single established phenotype. This list can be downloaded and used for further investigation into the medical literature or for research purposes.

Note that this patient's syndrome fits broadly within the published 10q26 contiguous gene deletion syndrome. Reading through the individual genes deleted in an individual case is not definitive, but may provide some guidance with regard to affected body systems or guide individual treatment decisions. It may also help clarify whether the deletion is the likely source of the child's problem, or whether additional investigation is warranted.

Note that another webpage which can be used for this purpose is the University of California, Santa Cruz Genome Browser, found at http://genome.ucsc.edu/index.html.

NEXT STEPS AFTER THE OMIM SEARCH

A great strength of OMIM searches is easy links to more information. To read more about the diseases which seem most clinically relevant, there are several helpful options.

1. From the Clinical Synopsis search, arrow back to the cytogenetics section and click on the disease name. Alternatively, copy the disease name or number and paste it into the main OMIM search page box. This takes you to the OMIM disease entry which has a table of contents. A disease entry typically includes:
   a. A table of phenotype–gene relationships and text describing the disease, which may include its clinical features, inheritance, diagnosis, mapping, pathogenesis, molecular genetics, population genetics, nomenclature, history, and animal model.
   b. Narrative about the history of investigation into disease that can provide a lot of clinical descriptions of individuals and families with this disease. This can be helpful for discerning whether this disease merits further investigation.
   c. References, linked to PUBMED.
2. Select the "Links" to the right of the disease of interest. This provides direct links to useful clinical and scientific resources. Particularly useful links include:
   a. Gene Reviews. This contains expert disease reviews and invaluable descriptions of disease symptoms and signs, diagnostic testing strategies, differential diagnosis considerations, multiple aspects of disease management, therapies under investigation, genetic counseling strategies, patient and family groups.
   b. GTR. This stands for Genetic Testing Registry, a free resource maintained by the National Center for Biotechnology Information. This link yields a page with Clinical Tests and Research Tests, linked to laboratories where tests may be performed. This list may be long, but the list can then be restricted based on specific needs. For example:
      i. Test Purpose (Diagnosis, Pre-symptomatic testing, etc.)

    ii. Test Method (Cytogenetic, Sequence analysis of the entire coding region, deletion/duplication analysis, etc.)

    iii. Test services (Carrier, Prenatal)

    iv. Lab certification

    v. Lab location (by country, state)

c. Genetics Home Reference—a resource guide and central repository for information for patients, families, and doctors. This contains easy to understand information about symptoms, prevalence, inheritance, other general information, and clinical trials.

d. GARD. This stands for Genetics and Rare Disease Information Center, a free resource maintained by the NIH National Center for Advancing Translational Sciences. This also contains information about the disease, symptoms, tests, treatments, healthcare services, organizations, and research. The public can also send in questions for expert responses and these may be posted on the page.

e. POSSUM. This stands for Pictures of Standard Syndromes and Undiagnosed Malformations. This database contains pictures of syndromes and diagnoses but requires a paid subscription.

f. Other links for Protein information, Cellular Pathways, and Animal Models, etc.

USING SIMULCONSULT TO AID IN DIAGNOSIS

Simulconsult, available at http://www.simulconsult.com, is diagnostic decision support software for medical professionals. There is no user fee for the "phenome" version, but creating a unique account with a login is required. This software interfaces with a database containing over 5500 diagnoses with phenotypes in OMIM. Disease information is referenced and expert-reviewed.

The search strategy for Simulconsult is incredibly easy and versatile. It allows easy entry of both positive and pertinent negative findings from the examination as well as test results. The symptom entry allows for selecting age of symptom presentation, and the algorithm takes this into account in generating a differential diagnosis. This is particularly helpful for neurogenetic conditions with onset in childhood.

The site has helpful tutorials and worked out case examples. Another useful feature is that patient search entries can be saved for later use, so that as additional information becomes available this can be entered to update the differential diagnosis. This search engine helps efficiently reduce the diagnostic possibilities from many to few, thereby guiding a more rapid path to diagnosis for many patients. Because the tutorials are very clear, this next section will provide just one actual example.

EXAMPLE 1 SIMULCONSULT SEARCH

Case description: 2-year-old female with 18 months of failure to achieve developmental milestones. She babbles only. She crawls but walks only with support. Family history positive for older sister with similar presentation, but with clear regression of skills. On examination, she babbles but does not speak clearly. Walking is broad based with prominent asymmetric dystonic posturing noted standing and when moving legs while sitting. General examination is normal. Brain MRI shows diffuse cerebellar and brainstem atrophy (sibling has same findings).

Steps for the Simulconsult Search

1. Search for Simulconsult in web browser and select link to simulconsult.com
2. Signup/Login
3. Start new patient, enter sex—female; age—2 years; affected family members 1 of 1 sister.
4. Select neurology for list of symptoms. Select pertinent positives and negatives with age of onset, e.g., positive gait disturbance, ataxia, dystonia, hypotonia, regression, sleep disturbance, negatives hyperreflexia.
5. Select bundle MRI and select pertinent positives and negatives with age of onset, e.g., pan-cerebellar atrophy or hypoplasia, brainstem/pontine atrophy; negative white matter abnormality, brain cysts, corpus callosum hypogenesis; set unmarked absent.
6. Click differential diagnosis. Multiple diagnoses are listed. Top 4 are pontocerebellar hypoplasia, Aicardi-Goutieres syndrome, NBIA2A: INAD; CDG1A: PMM2-related.
7. Select the top choice, is pontocerebellar hypoplasia, EXOSC3 related.
   a. Click Assess Disease to review pertinent positive and negative findings.
   b. Click Profile Disease to see multiple findings which were not previously indicated. Add additional negative or positive findings from examination, e.g., the following signs—tongue fasciculations, muscular atrophy—are not present in this child, so check them as "absent now".
8. Select subsequent choices. Review findings. Lab tests are listed along with approximate costs. Thus the investigator may use this information in a cost-effective diagnostic approach. For example, testing for congenital disorders of glycosylation is inexpensive.
9. As with OMIM testing, use this differential diagnosis as a reading guide, then use Genetic Testing Registry (GTR) to identify laboratories for targeted genetic testing.

Final diagnosis for this patient and sibling was PLA2G6-Associated Neurodegeneration, the classic infantile neuroaxonal dystrophy (INAD) form. A likely reason this diagnosis was not first on the list was the absence of iron deposition in subcortical areas in the MRI scan.

SUMMARY

The number of diagnostic possibilities for heritable movement disorders in childhood has become increasingly daunting. Good clinical skills and medical knowledge remain invaluable for accurate diagnosis. Use of search engines and computer databases hold potential to make the diagnostic process more rapid. This reduces the emotional burden on families as well as the time necessary for physicians. See table B.2 for a list of useful websites for physicians and patients, including those discussed in this appendix.

TABLE B.2   Useful Websites for Clinicians and Patients

Site Name	Website	Description
FOR CLINICIANS		
Gendia	http://www.gendia.net/	Site for large network of genetic diagnostic laboratories, based in Belgium
GeneReviews	http://www.ncbi.nlm.nih.gov/books/NBK1116/	Expert authored, peer-reviewed disease descriptions
Genetests	http://www.genetests.org	Genetests lists genetic tests and laboratories
Genetic Testing Registry[a]	http://www.ncbi.nlm.nih.gov/gtr/	Searchable registry of genetic tests and laboratories
Genomic Research site	www.genome.gov	NIH National Human Genome Research Institute
Morphology	http://elementsofmorphology.nih.gov/	NIH National Human Genome Research Institute site for human malformation morphology
Neurological Diseases and anatomy	http://neuromuscular.wustl.edu/ataxia/aindex.html	Diagnostic information on ataxias
OMIM[a]	http://www.omim.org/	Online Mendelian Inheritance in Man - catalog of human genes and genetic disorders
POSSUMweb	http://www.possum.net.au/	Database of images of malformations and syndromes, for learning and diagnosis
SimulConsult[a]	http://simulconsult.com/	diagnostic decision support software
UCSC Genome Browser[a]	http://genome.ucsc.edu/index.html	University of California Santa Cruz Genomics Bioinformatics site containing reference data for genomes, with many tools and links
FOR PATIENTS AND FAMILIES		
GARD	https://rarediseases.info.nih.gov/gard	Site to help public find information about rare and genetic diseases
Genetic alliance United Kingdom	www.gig.org.uk	An alliance of patient organizations in the UK for persons with genetic diseases
Genetics Education Center	www.kumc.edu/gec/	University of Kansas Genetics Education Center
Genetics Home Reference	http://ghr.nlm.nih.gov/	A consumer-friendly reference guide for information about genetic conditions
National Organization for Rare Diseases	http://rarediseases.org/	Rare disease education, advocacy, and research support group
Undiagnosed Disease program	http://rarediseases.info.nih.gov/research/pages/27/undiagnosed-diseases-program	NIH program for undiagnosed diseases

[a]See discussion and examples in text.

Appendix C: Video Atlas

CHAPTER 6 TRANSIENT AND DEVELOPMENTAL MOVEMENT DISORDERS IN CHILDREN

- 6-1 This 12-year-old boy with genetically documented Friedreich's ataxia has congenital torticollis associated with fibrotic contracture of the clavicular portion of the right sternocleidomastoid muscle restricting his range of movement. This case was reported as part of a series of patients with congenital muscular torticollis. (Collins A, Jankovic J: Botulinum toxin injection for congenital muscular torticollis presenting in children and adults, *Neurology* 67:1083–1085, 2006.)
- 6-2 Home video of a young girl showing repetitive, stereotypic flexion of the right leg associated with some pelvic movements. This stereotype represents a self-stimulatory or masturbatory behavior, almost exclusively observed in girls before the age of 5 years.

CHAPTER 7 TICS AND TOURETTE SYNDROME

Eye and Facial Tics

- 7-1 This boy demonstrates frequent blinking, which is associated with alternating facial contractions, tongue protrusions, and mouth openings, typical of Tourette syndrome.
- 7-2 This girl demonstrates facial tics manifested by repetitive, sustained contractions of facial muscles resulting in grotesque grimacing, as well as neck muscle contractions, typical of dystonic tics.
- 7-3 This boy with Tourette syndrome demonstrates persistent blinking and more sustained contractions of the eyelids in a form of blepharospasm, an example of a dystonic facial tic. In addition, he demonstrates facial grimacing and oculogyric deviations.
- 7-4 This boy demonstrates oculogyric deviations, typical of ocular tics associated with Tourette syndrome.

Cervical Tics

- 7-5 This girl demonstrates dystonic tics of the neck resulting in repetitive neck flexion, which could be possibly wrongly diagnosed as anterocollis due to cervical dystonia.

Shoulder Tics

- 7-6 This young man demonstrates repetitive movements of either the left or right scapula, an example of a dystonic tic often preceded by a premonitory sensation in the region of the shoulder. This shoulder movement is very characteristic of and relatively specific for Tourette syndrome.

Trunk-Abdominal Tics

- 7-7 This girl with severe Tourette syndrome and obsessive-compulsive disorder demonstrates dystonic contractions of the rectus abdominus, resulting in a side-to-side movement of her abdomen, the so-called belly dancer dyskinesia.
- 7-8 This boy with Tourette syndrome demonstrates repetitive, complex movements produced by contractions of his shoulder and trunk muscles, preceded by an intense premonitory sensation of a chill.

Complex Motor Tics

- 7-9 This young boy with Tourette syndrome exhibits complex motor tics manifested by trunk bending and hopping.

Simple Phonic Tics

- 7-10 This boy with Tourette syndrome demonstrates a dystonic extension of his neck associated with repetitive expiratory grunting sounds. In addition, he demonstrates a holding or blocking tic during which time he stops breathing and is completely motionless.
- 7-11 This boy with Tourette syndrome demonstrates continuous grunting sounds associated with repetitive extensions of his neck, the so-called whiplash tics.
- 7-12 This 17-year-old girl with severe Tourette syndrome exhibits complex motor tics and loud screaming phonic tics.

Complex Phonic Tics

- 7-13 This boy with severe Tourette syndrome exhibits complex motor tics and loud phonic tics, including vocalizations.

CHAPTER 8 MOTOR STEREOTYPIES

- 8-1 Young boy with otherwise normal development and normal neurological examination demonstrates side-to-side head movement, believed to be normal, "physiological" stereotypy.
- 8-2 This young girl with Rett syndrome, an autistic disorder found predominantly in girls due to a mutation in the MECP2 gene on the X chromosome, demonstrates typical hand washing, hand clapping stereotypic movement along with toe walking.

- 8-3 This young girl with Rett syndrome demonstrates classic hand stereotypies and dystonic flexion of her toes, typically associated with this autistic disorder.
- 8-4 This boy with Norrie's syndrome manifests head stereotypy, which may represent a form of self-stimulatory behavior. He also exhibits self-injurious behavior.
- 8-5 This boy demonstrates an arm flapping stereotypy during excitement. The child flaps or waves hands and arms, includes larger-amplitude, rhythmic movements. Video from Mahone, E.M, et al. Repetitive arm and hand movements (complex motor stereotypies) in children. *Journal of Pediatrics* 2004;145:395–5; http://www.us.elsevierhealth.com/jpeds.
- 8-6 This child demonstrates a rapid, smaller-amplitude, back-and-forth movement of hands and arms or trunk characterized by overall smaller range of motion, includes tremulousness; while pacing. Video from Mahone, E.M, et al. Repetitive arm and hand movements (complex motor stereotypies) in children. *Journal of Pediatrics* 2004;145:395–5; http://www.us.elsevierhealth.com/jpeds.
- 8-7 This girl demonstrates a pattern of clenching-stiffening-posturing—repeated tensing of hands, arms, or head that mimics dystonia and includes prolonged facial grimacing or shoulder raising. Video from Mahone, E.M, et al. Repetitive arm and hand movements (complex motor stereotypies) in children. *Journal of Pediatrics* 2004;145:395–5; http://www.us.elsevierhealth.com/jpeds.
- 8-8 This boy has a ritualized sequence of purposeful behaviors usually involving a pattern of volitional movements (e.g., repetitive bending over or pacing). Video from Mahone, E.M, et al. Repetitive arm and hand movements (complex motor stereotypies) in children. *Journal of Pediatrics* 2004;145:395–5; http://www.us.elsevierhealth.com/jpeds.
- 8-9 This 4-year-old boy with normal cognitive function and social skills presents for episodes of repetitive, rhythmic, continual-type movements, sometimes accompanied by repetitive verbalizations. These physiological stereotypies occur more when he is engrossed in tasks and resolve with distraction. They are not bothersome, do not cause pain, and do not interrupt his activities. The video demonstrates repetitive, brief episodes of rhythmic, continual hand-rubbing lasting seconds, sometimes associated with pacing or marching. There is also a hand opening-closing stereotypy and rhythmic bilateral rubbing of the area below his nose.
- 8-10 This is a 13-year-old girl with a history of seizure disorder due to cortical dysplasia status post temporal lobectomy and autism and has a long history of repetitive, coordinated movement, typical of stereotypies. The video shows intermittent repetitive hand movements, including hand flapping movements consistent with stereotypies. She also had head shaking, head bending and facial contortion. These movements are distractible and are not persistent. Courtesy Amber Stocco, MD.

CHAPTER 9 PAROXYSMAL DYSKINESIAS

- 9-1 Young man with paroxysmal kinesigenic dystonia manifested by transient truncal dystonia triggered by sudden voluntary movement.
- 9-2 A girl with paroxysmal kinesigenic dystonia manifested by transient facial dystonia imitating a smile and right arm flexion precipitated by voluntary movement such as

jumping jacks. The patient also has a family history of infantile convulsions, a seizure disorder, and migraines.

- 9-3 This adolescent has many brief episodes per day of involuntary, asymmetric dystonic posturing. Here, after sitting for several minutes conversing, an episode is triggered when he stands and begins to walk. Consciousness is preserved throughout. Treatment with carbamazepine was successful.
- 9-4 This 12-year-old boy with paroxysmal kinesigenic dystonia manifested by bilateral, left more than right, dystonic stiffness in his legs and dystonic posturing of his left arm precipitated by sudden movement.

CHAPTER 10 CHOREA, ATHETOSIS, AND BALLISM

- 10-1 This 6-year-old girl with adoptive parents was developing well until age 3.5 years when she gradually stopped talking, became ataxic, and developed facial and generalized chorea. She was found to have juvenile Huntington disease with over 100 CAG repeats in the Huntington gene. Over the next year she developed myoclonic jerks, seizures, progressive ataxia; became bedridden in a fetal position; and died about one year after this video.
- 10-2 This teenage girl with documented lupus erythematosus has severe chorea of the face and the entire body, including some involuntary expiratory sounds and dysarthria. The chorea markedly improved with tetrabenazine.
- 10-3 Young girl with mitochondrial encephalomyopathy manifested chiefly by generalized chorea, dystonia, and ataxia.
- 10-4 This 10-year-old boy with chorea and some tics was found to have a de novo chromosome 15 paracentric inversion.
- 10-5 This girl has predominantly distal chorea following streptococcal infection with serologic evidence of Sydenham chorea.
- 10-6 This boy has Sydenham chorea manifested by left hemichorea involving chiefly his left hand.
- 10-7 This 8-year-old girl, a product of an alcoholic mother who was a heavy cocaine abuser, was born prematurely and now manifests generalized chorea and cognitive impairment.
- 10-8 This 7-year-old boy with FOXG 1 mutation has a history of global developmental delay, agenesis of the corpus callosum and seizures beginning at the age of 10 months gradually evolving into generalized chorea. The chorea interferes with his ability to reach and hold objects. Examination shows generalized chorea involving left more than right side of his body. His chorea failed to improve with tetrabenazine but markedly improved status-post bilateral GPi deep brain stimulation.
- 10-9 This 18-year-old girl with lupus chorea has a history of "meningitis" at age 10 and subsequent arthralgias, myalgias, and pericarditis. She presented with a 10-day history of involuntary movements and incoordination. Anti-DS DNA Abs titer was 160 (normal less than 10). She improved markedly with tetrabenazine.

CHAPTER 11 DYSTONIA

- 11-1 This boy with strong family history of DYT1 dystonia developed rapidly progressive generalized dystonia which evolved into a dystonic storm (or status dystonicus), associated with muscle breakdown, myoglobinuria, and despite three thalamatomies he eventually succumbed to the disease. He is a proband of a family first reported in 2002. (Opal P, Tintner R, Jankovic J, et al: Intrafamilial phenotypic variability of the DYT1 dystonia: from asymptomatic TOR1A gene carrier status to dystonic storm, *Mov Disord* 17:339–345, 2002.)

- 11-2 This girl with DYT1 dystonia manifested by oromandibular, truncal, and leg dystonia, as well as camptocormia, is the first reported case of marked improvement of generalized dystonia following bilateral pallidotomy. (Ondo WG, Desaloms M, Jankovic J, Grossman R: Surgical pallidotomy for the treatment of generalized dystonia, *Mov Disord* 13:693–698, 1998.) She later required bilateral pallidal deep brain stimulation to sustain the improvement. (Diamond A, Shahed J, Azher S, Dat-Vuong K, Jankovic J: Globus pallidus deep brain stimulation in dystonia, *Mov Disord* 21:692–695, 2006.)

- 11-3 This girl has autosomal dominant DYT1 dystonia, manifested by dystonic rapid movements and dystonic gait disorder, requiring assistance of her mother, who is also affected by DYT1 dystonia. She markedly benefited from bilateral pallidal deep brain stimulation.

- 11-4 This 17-year-old Latin American girl with childhood history of hyperactivity and aggressiveness, and progressive cognitive and language deficit, developed dystonia of her left foot at age 10, which later evolved into generalized dystonia. In addition, she manifests stereotypic touching of the ear and nose, and restless movements. Her T2-weighted MRI showed hypointensity of the globus pallidus consistent "eye-of-a-tiger" sign, and genetic studies confirmed a mutation in the PANK2 gene. Her brother had onset of symptoms at age 17 with difficulty with handwriting, tightness of fingers, and foot dystonia. He later developed gait difficulties, falls, dysarthria with unintelligible speech, difficulties with chewing, and oro-lingual dystonia. The proband's cousin has had progressive parkinsonism and dystonia. This family was reported in 2004. (Thomas M, Hayflick SJ, Jankovic J: Clinical heterogeneity of neurodegeneration with iron accumulation–1 (Hallervorden-Spatz syndrome) and pantothenate kinase–associated neurodegeneration (PKAN), *Mov Disord* 19:36–42, 2004.)

- 11-5 This 9-year-old boy with oromandibular, jaw opening, dystonia, which improved with injections of botulinum toxin into bilateral masseter muscles, has a rapidly progressive generalized dystonia and MRI of the brain consistent with PANK2 mutation.

CHAPTER 12 MYOCLONUS

- 12-1 This young woman has Baltic myoclonus, also known as Unverricht-Lundborg disease, due to a gene mutation, called EPM1 on chromosome 21, manifested by jerk-like, myoclonic movements involving the face and upper body.

- 12-2 This girl has dystonia-myoclonus syndrome due to epsilon-sarcoglycan mutation on chromosome 7, manifested by jerk-like, myoclonic movement predominantly affecting her left arm, associated with dystonic writer's cramp. Both her father and her brother are similarly affected by this jerk-like dystonic movement.

- 12-3 This 16-month-old girl presents with a 3 month history of progressive incoordination and jerk-like movement. She has myoclonus and opsoclonus, manifested by multi-directional but conjugate eye movements. Extensive evaluation for neuroblastoma was negative and she improved markedly with steroids. Courtesy Amber Stocco, MD.

CHAPTER 13 TREMOR

- 13-1 Home video of an infant girl with hereditary chin tremor.
- 13-2 Young boy with multiple sclerosis and severe cerebellar outflow tremor benefited markedly from contralateral thalamic deep brain stimulation.
- 13-3 This 18-year-old boy with a long-standing progressive gait difficulty and a 3-year history of head, hand, and leg tremor. In addition to the lateral head oscillation and hand tremor, he manifests stork-like gait and distal leg and foot deformity consistent with Charcot-Marie-Tooth disease.
- 13-4 This young man manifests symptoms of essential tremor, a bilateral, regular tremor of the hands present maintaining posture and on finger to nose testing approaching the target.
- 13-5 This boy has developmental delay, with fine motor skill clumsiness, low tone, and tremulousness. His hand tremor is brought out by posture, fatigue, finger to nose testing, and manipulating small objects.
- 13-6 This adolescent has learning disabilities, tall stature, and resting and postural tremor associated with 48, XXYY chromosomal aneuploidy.

CHAPTER 14 ATAXIA

- 14-1 This home video shows a 22 month old boy with Ataxia Telangiectasia. He was referred for evaluation of delayed gait and involuntary movements. Although he has a broad based, lurching gait, his predominant symptoms are intrusive choreic and dystonic movements.
- 14-2 This boy has an early onset, progressive, and severe phenotype of a spinocerebellar ataxia (SCA), affecting gait, fine motor control, finger to nose testing, postural maintenance of limbs, and eye movements. He has autosomal dominant SCA 5.

CHAPTER 15 PARKINSONISM

- 15-1 Young girl with documented Huntington disease, manifested by parkinsonism, myoclonus, chorea, and ataxia.
- 15-2 This 15-year-old boy, previously diagnosed with "intellectual disability" because of cognitive impairment since age 6 years, began to develop involuntary jerk-like

movements at age 9, followed by problems with his balance and generalized slowness, dysarthria, myoclonus, ataxia, and generalized seizures. The video demonstrates parkinsonian bradykinesia, blepharospasm, and stimulus-sensitive myoclonus. His father committed suicide at age 41. DNA test confirmed the diagnosis of juvenile Huntington disease with 89 CAG repeats in the Huntington gene.

- 15-3 This 15-year-old girl has juvenile Huntington disease with 67 CAG repeats in the Huntington gene. She manifests marked hypomimia and bradykinesia consistent with parkinsonism.
- 15-4 This 12-year-old boy with genetically confirmed Huntington's disease has had a seizure disorder, progressive cognitive deterioration, bradykinesia, spasticity, and increasing incoordination and gait difficulties. He has had two MRIs of the brain, which showed atrophy of the basal ganglia, particularly the caudate nucleus.

CHAPTER 17 INHERITED METABOLIC DISORDERS WITH ASSOCIATED MOVEMENT ABNORMALITIES

- 17-1 This 10-year-old girl with genetically confirmed neurodegeneration with brain iron accumulation (PLA2G6) has a history of mild global developmental delay presents and progressive leg spasticity. MRI showed bilateral gradient echo susceptibility changes in the substantia nigra and globus pallidus bilaterally. Courtesy Amber Stocco, MD.

CHAPTER 18 MOVEMENT DISORDERS IN AUTOIMMUNE DISEASES

- 18-1 This 3-year-old boy with subacute onset of myalgias, frontal headaches, malaise, and vomiting; followed by confusional state, insomnia, hallucinations, dysarthria and motor aphasia. Admitted with diagnosis of "viral encephalitis". During the hospitalization he developed generalized seizures and dysautonomia. On examination he had orofacial stereotypies, dystonic contractions of the left side of his face, blepharospasm, dystonic flexion of the right hand and generalized chorea. Further investigation found anti-NMDAR encephalitis. His condition resolved with immunotherapy and tetrabenazine. Courtesy Amber Stocco, MD.
- 18-2 This 12-year-old right-handed boy presented for an evaluation of muscle spasms involving his back, chest and abdominal muscles. His symptoms started with leg stiffness at the age of 5 years. The episodes of muscle spasm are usually triggered by a startle response. His GAD antibody titer was greater than 250 and he was diagnosed with stiff-person syndrome. He benefitted from IVIG treatments.

CHAPTER 20 CEREBRAL PALSY

- 20-1 This boy has generalized chorea and ataxia with preserved cognitive function, characteristic of "extrapyramidal" cerebral palsy.

CHAPTER 22 DRUG-INDUCED MOVEMENT DISORDERS

- 22-1 This 9-month-old girl developed orofacial stereotypy at age 2 months after 17-day treatment with metoclopramide for gastroesophageal reflux. This is the youngest reported case of tardive dyskinesia. (Mejia N, Jankovic J: Metoclopramide-induced tardive dyskinesia in an infant, *Mov Disord* 20: 86–89, 2005.)
- 22-2 This girl has severe generalized dyskinetic movements due to rapid withdrawal from haloperidol – a drug withdrawal dyskinesia.
- 22-3 This boy developed generalized dyskinesia after approximately 5 years of treatment with risperidone and fluphenazine. Symptoms resolved completely over 12–18 months.
- 22-4 This boy with Asperger's Disorder developed progressive, asymmetric dystonia with dystonic tremor after prolonged treatment with risperidone. Two years after discontinuing risperidone, symptoms resolved nearly completely.

CHAPTER 23 FUNCTIONAL MOVEMENT DISORDERS

- 23-1 This girl has a resting, postural, and kinetic tremor of the right arm. The psychogenic origin of the tremor is suggested by its distractibility and variable frequency and amplitude. Following a placebo challenge, there is immediate and complete resolution of the tremor.
- 23-2 This patient with psychogenic dystonia manifests violent limb and trunk posturing "when she lets go" and no longer tries to suppress the movements. Her affect is inappropriately cheerful, the so-called *la belle indifference.*
- 23-3 This 16-year-old girl suddenly developed generalized shaking of the body which occurred shortly after other girls in her school developed similar shaking, suggestive of "mass hysteria."
- 23-4 This girl has an asymmetric, predominantly unilateral tremor with variable amplitude and frequency, affected by posture in ways not characteristic of a neurologic postural tremor. The tremor resolves briefly during distraction. The tremor frequency can be entrained (modulated to match) by voluntary tasks with the same or contralateral hand.
- 23-5 This girl had a unilateral tremor which stopped and started suddenly and was not present during this neurology consultation. Home video shows a unilateral hand and arm tremor with variable direction and rate characteristic of psychogenic tremor.

Index

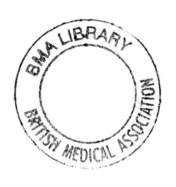